Principles and Practice of
Pharmaceutical Medicine

J

Principles and Practice of Pharmaceutical Medicine

Andrew J Fletcher
Temple University, Pennsylvania, USA

Lionel D Edwards
Novartis and Pharma Pro Plus Inc, New Jersey, USA

Anthony W Fox
EBD Group Inc, Carlsbad, California, USA

Peter Stonier
Consultant in Pharmaceutical Medicine, Surrey, UK

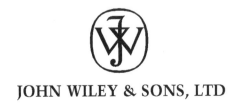

JOHN WILEY & SONS, LTD

National   01243 779777
International (+44) 1243 779777
e-mail (for orders and customer service enquiries): cs-books@wiley.co.uk
Visit our Home Page on: http://www.wiley.co.uk or http://www.wiley.com

Other Wiley Editorial Offices

John Wiley & Sons, Inc., 605 Third Avenue,
New York, NY 10158–0012, USA

WILEY-VCH Verlag GmbH, Pappelallee 3,
D-69469 Weinheim, Germany

John Wiley & Sons Australia, Ltd., 33 Park Road, Milton,
Queensland 4064, Australia

John Wiley & Sons (Asia) Pte, Ltd., 2 Clementi Loop #02–01,
Jin Xing Distripark, Singapore 129809

John Wiley & Sons (Canada), Ltd., 22 Worcester Road,
Rexdale, Ontario M9W 1L1, Canada

Library of Congress Cataloging-in-Publication Data

British Library Cataloguing in Publication Data

A catalogue record for this book is available from the British Library

ISBN 0-471-98655-0

Typeset in 10/11.5 pt Times from the author's disks by Kolam Information Services Pvt. Ltd., Pondicherry, India
Printed and bound in Great Britain by Antony Rowe Ltd, Chippenham
This book is printed on acid-free paper responsibly manufactured from sustainable forestry,
in which at least two trees are planted for each one used for paper production.

Contents

About the Editors

ANDREW J. FLETCHER, MB, BChir, (Cantab), MS (Columbia), FFPM, DipPharmMedRCP, is Senior Assistant Editor of The Merck Manuals, Merck & Co. Inc. and Adjunct Professor of Pharmaceutical Health Care at Temple University School of Pharmacy. He graduated from Cambridge University and St. Bartholomew's Hospital, London, briefly trained in Neurosurgery, joined CIBA-GEIGY in the UK as Medical Advisor, then European Medical Director, for Syntex, then joined Merck, first in the international division after graduating in business from Columbia University, New York City, he joined the Merck Manual as Assistant Editor. He teaches pharmaceutical medicine, bioethics, and medical and scientific writing at Temple University's School of Pharmacy. He is a founder member and ex-trustee of the American Academy of Pharmaceutical Physicians.

LIONEL D. EDWARDS, MB, BS, LRCP, MRCS, Dip RCOG and FFPM., is President of Pharma Pro Plus Inc., a drug development consulting company and Director Medical Affairs Novartis USA. Previously, he was Vice President of Clinical Research at Bio-Technology Pharmaceutical Corporation, a small Biotech firm making a profit with operations in the US and International marketplaces. Prior to this he worked at Noven, Inc., a small Skin Patch Technology firm with large internationally licensed partners—Ciba and Rhone Poulenc Rorer. He was Assistant Vice-President, International Clinical Research at Hoffman-La Roche, and Senior Director of Schering-Plough International Research, and Director of US Domestic Gastrointestinal, Hormonal and OTC Research Departments. Dr. Edwards has been involved in all aspects of clinical trials over the years on many different research drug devices in 10 therapeutic areas.

He served as Chairman of the PMA Special Population committee for 5 years, also he was on the Institute of Medicine Committee for Research in Women, sponsored by the NIH. He served on the efficacy subcommittee Topic 5 (Acceptability of Foreign Clinical Data) of the International Committee on Harmonization (ICH).

He is a Fellow of the Faculty of Pharmaceutical Medicine and an Adjunct Professor at Temple University Graduate School of Pharmacology. He has taught 'Drug Development' for PERI for over ten years and is on the teaching faculty of the National Association of Physicians. He is a founder member of the American Academy of Pharmaceutical Physicians.

ANTHONY ('Tony') W. FOX, BSc, MBBS, FFPM, MD (Lond), DipPharmMedRCP, CBiol, FIBiol, is President of EBD Group, San Diego. From The Royal London Hospital, after general clinical training he was Rotary International Fellow at Emory University (Atlanta), and CIBA-Geigy Fellow at Harvard. Industrial positions at Procter and Gamble and Glaxo came next. He was then Vice-President of a small pharmaceutical company. Among many societies, Tony is Charter Member, Trustee, and Education VP of the American Academy of Pharmaceutical Physicians. Publications span several areas of pharmaceutical medicine, e.g., regulation, pharmacology, clinical trials, pharmacovigilance, analgesics, migraine, genotoxicology, and metabolism. He has four patents, and five journals use his reviews.

PETER D. STONIER, BA, BSc, PhD, MBChB, MRCPsych, FRCP, FRCPE, FFPM has 24 years experience in pharmaceutical medicine. He was Medical and Board Director of the UK Hoechst Group of companies until he became a consultant in 2000. He is immediate past-President of the Faculty of Pharmaceutical Medicine of the Royal Colleges of Physicians UK. Formerly he was President of the International Federation of Associations of Pharmaceutical Physicians and Chairman of the British Association of Pharmaceutical Physicians. He is Visiting Professor in pharmaceutical medicine at Kings College, London and at the University of Surrey, which under his direction introduced the first MSc degree in Pharmaceutical Medicine in 1993. His publications include edited works in human psychopharmacology, clinical research, medical marketing and careers in the pharmaceutical industry. He is a graduate of Manchester Medical School, qualifying in 1974, following a BSc degree in physiology and a PhD in protein chemistry.

List of Contributors

Anbar, Dan *Millennium Biostatistics Inc., Bound Brook, NJ, USA*

Bohaychuk, Wendy *Good Clinical Research Practices Consultants, Lakehurst, Ontario, Canada*

Boyer, Gregory J. *Pharmacia Corporation, Stokie, Illinois, USA*

Castle, Win M. *Glaxo Smithkline, Philadelphia, PA, USA*

Chaponis, Robert J. *Global Medical Affairs, Pharmacia Corporation, Peapack, NJ, USA*

Choi, Han W.

Croft, Sara *Shook, Hardy and Bacon, MNP London, UK*

Cullen, Donna *Auditrial, Fairlawn, NJ, USA*

Curry, Stephen H. *President Stephen H. Curry, Consulting, Professor of Pharmacology and Physiology, University of Rochester, NY, USA*

DeCory, Heleen H. *Astra Arcus USA Inc., Rochester, USA*

Dreskin, Howard J. *Glaxo SmithKline Philadelphia, PA, USA*

Drucker, R. *Technomark Consulting Services, London, UK*

Dziewanowska, Zofia *La Jolla, CA, USA*

Edwards, Lionel D. *Novartis, East Hanover, USA*

Fox, Anthony W. *EBD Group Inc, 6120 Paseo del Norte, Suites 52–L2, Carlsbad CA 92009, USA*

Gabrielsson, Johan *Pharmacokinetics and Pharmacodynamics Section, AstraZeneca R+D Sodertalie, Sweden*

Graham, Ball *Good Clinical Research Practices Consultants, Lakehurst, Ontario, Canada*

Griffin, John P. *Quartermans, Welwyn, UK*

Hanson Divers, Christine *US Scientific Initiatives and Customer Support, Health Economics and Outcomes Research, AstraZeneca, Apex, NC, USA*

Hammad, G. *Watford, UK*

Hughes, Graham R. *Technomark Consulting Services, London, UK*

Husson, J.M. *Paris, France*

Johnson-Pratt, Lisa R. *Merck & Co. Inc., North Wales, PA, USA*

Kennedy, William *Consultant Delaware, USA former V.P. Regulation Affairs*

Labbe, Etienné *Sanofi-Synthelabo, Paris, France*

Lee, T.Y. *ACER/EXCEL Inc., USA*

Lilley, Roy *Independent Health Analyst, former NHS Trust Chairman, Camberley, Surrey, UK*

Linda, Packaid *La Jolla, CA, USA*

Lopez, Gabriel *Basking Ridge, NJ, USA*

Marler, Matthew *Astra Arcus USA Inc., Rochester, USA*

McCarthy, Dennis J. *Drug Metabolism and Pharmacokinetics, AstraZeneca Pharmaceuticals LP, Wilmington, Delaware, USA*

Métry, Jean-Michel *AARDEX Ltd, Zug, Switzerland*

Miller, Jay D. *Amgen Inc., Thousand Oaks, California, USA*

Minor, Michael *ACER/EXCEL Inc., USA*

Molony, Leslie J. *Biotechnology Business Strategies, Pleasant Hill, CA, USA*

Naito, C. *Teikyo University, Japan*

Ostechaus, Jane T. *Wasateh Health Outcomes, Park City, Utah, USA*

Papaluca, Amati M. *EMEA, London, UK*

Pratt, Timothy *Shook, Hardy and Bacon LLP, Kansas City, USA*

Price, Gill *VP MedImmune Inc., USA*

Reno, Frederick *Merritt Island, FL, USA*

Spilker, Bert *Pharmaceutical Research and Manufacturers of America, 1100 fifteenth street NW, Washington DC 20005, USA*

Starkey, Paul *Former Vice President Smithkline Beecham Consumer Healthcare, Morris Plains, NJ, USA*

Shapiro, David *Scripps Clinic, La Jolla, CA, USA*

Tilson, Hugh H. *University of North Carolina School of Public Health, Chapel Hill, NC, USA*

Toland, Susan *Wardell Associates International, LLC Princeton, NJ, USA*

Townsend, Raymond J. *Wasatch Health Outcomes, Park city, Utah, USA*

Turner, Nadia *AstraZeneca, Macclesfield, Cheshire, UK*

Vogel, John R. *John R. Vogel Associates, Kihei, HI, USA*

Walker, S. *Centre of Medicine Research, Carshalton, UK*

Wardell, William *Wardell Associates International LLC, Princeton, NJ, USA*

Wells, Frank *Medicolegal Investigations Ltd, Ipswich, UK*

Wells, Marilyn J. *Department of Health, Physical Education, and Recreation, Hampton University, Virginia, USA*

Williams, R. *US Pharmacopia, Rockville, USA*

Yasurhara, H. *Teikyo University, Japan*

Yeon, Howard B.

Young, Michael D. *Strategic Healthcare Development, Wayne, PA, USA*

Preface

Pharmaceutical medicine is a relatively new, but rapidly growing, academic discipline in the USA. The American Academy of Pharmaceutical Physicians (AAPP) was founded in 1993 and hosted, in 1999, a meeting of the International Federation of Associations of Pharmaceutical Physicians (IFAPP). The birth of AAPP coincided with many ongoing changes in the pharmaceutical industry in the USA, as health care delivery began to move more towards managed care, and large corporations began to amalgamate and downsize. As these trends continue into the 21st century, pharmaceutical physicians are increasingly regarding consultancy work and contract research organization (CRO) affiliation as good career opportunities, and now recognize the need for continuing education and training in this broad spectrum discipline.

This textbook, which represents a collaborative effort of international experts, is dedicated to the more than 3,500 pharmaceutical physicians and all the other professionals working in the US pharmaceutical industry and allied fields. It is also intended to be useful for those outside the USA because the basic tenets of the specialty have, for a long time, become global.

As editors, we would like to thank our contributors for their expertise, their dedication, and their vision. We would like to thank and acknowledge the work and counsel of our colleague Robert Bell, MD, MRPharmS, who helped us greatly during the early part of this project. We would also like to thank and acknowledge the enormous help, encouragement, and patience of the team at John Wiley & Sons, Inc., UK, with whom we have worked closely over these past few years, among whom we have particularly stressed (!) Michael Davis, Deborah Reece, Hannah Bradley, Lewis Derrick, and Hilary Rowe.

Lastly, we would like to thank our families, and friends, who have withstood the frequent telephone calls, e-mails, and meetings, often late into the night. Indeed, to all who made this project possible, both authors and non-authors, we thank you. We are certain that this specialty, and our patients, even though we may help them vicariously, will benefit because of your contributions.

Andrew Fletcher
Lionel Edwards
Tony Fox
Peter Stonier

Section I

Overview of Pharmaceutical Medicine

Pharmaceutical Medicine as a Medical Specialty

Michael D. Young

Celltech Chiroscience PLC, Slough, UK

Medicine is an art that has been practiced since time immemorial. The use of herbs and natural medicaments to relieve pain or to aid the sick in coping with their afflictions has been a part of all societies. In the Western world, medicine has developed at least since the time of the Greeks and Romans—the Hippocratic oath reminds us of this nearly 2500 year history. However, the progress of medicine has been very different from that of many other arts within society. It has come of age after an incredibly long maturation period. As a function capable of offering a successful treatment for an human ailment, medicine is very much a development of the last 100–150 years. Indeed, the major advances have come in the last 50–75 years.

The role of physicians in society has changed over the centuries. It may have reached its nadir during the early renaissance, when the general attitude was, as Shakespeare said, 'Trust not the physician; his antidotes are poison'. From the nineteenth century onward, as their diagnostic understanding has grown and as their therapeutic agents have become increasingly effective, physicians have come to be increasingly valued. Today, much of the practice of medicine in all of its subspecialties is based on a physician's diagnosis and treatment with drugs, devices, or surgery. This radical change to an era of focused treatments, after aeons of using homespun remedies and then watching hopefully for the crisis or the fever to pass, has accompanied the recent revolutions in the understanding of biological processes and in technical and biotechnical capabilities. These developments have allowed us to produce pure therapeutic agents and to establish how to use them safely and effectively.

The exponential growth in scientific knowledge, particularly over the last 100 years, has brought about a paradigm shift in our approach to pharmaceuticals. Until the twentieth century, the sale and use of medicines and medical devices was almost entirely unregulated by governments. It was a case of *caveat emptor*, with only the drug-taker's common sense to protect against the dangers of the so-called patent medicines and 'snake oils'. The obvious abuses in these situations led eventually to government intervention, to professional regulation, and to requirements that drugs be pure and unadulterated. With advances in science and in the ability to define and establish drug efficacy came a requirement to demonstrate that drugs were also safe. Finally, as late as the second half of the twentieth century came the legel requirement to establish that pharmaceuticals were effective before they were marketed. These legal requirements reflected changes in social attitudes and expectations grounded in the questions that the development of biological and basic sciences had made it possible to ask and to answer. The response to these changes has led to the development of the specialty of pharmaceutical medicine.

Pharmaceutical medicine can be defined as: 'the discipline of medicine that is devoted to the discovery, research, development, and support of ethical promotion and safe use of pharmaceuticals, vaccines, medical devices, and diagnostics'. (By-laws of the American Academy of Pharmaceutical Physicians). Pharmaceutical medicine covers all medically active agents from neutraceuticals, through cosmeceuticals and over-the-counter (OTC) pharmaceuticals, to prescription drugs. Furthermore, the specialty is not confined to those

Principles and Practice of Pharmaceutical Medicine. Edited by A. J. Fletcher, Lionel D. Edwards, Anthony W. Fox and Peter Stonier © 2002 John Wiley & Sons Ltd.

physicians working within what is classically considered the pharmaceutical industry, but includes those involved in the clinical management or regulation of all healthcare products. It is the basic specialty for physicians within the cosmetics and nutrition industry for those in the device industry and for those in 'not-for-profit' companies, such as those responsible for the national blood supplies and/or for specialized blood products. Furthermore, it is the fundamental discipline for physicians who are in government health ministries, insurance companies, National Health Trusts or HMO management, drug regulatory agencies or any other oversight or regulatory function for healthcare.

In the early part of this quarter-century, for a medicine to be adopted and for it to sell, it was sufficient that science could conceive of a new treatment, that technology could deliver that treatment, and that clinical research could prove it effective and safe for the physician to use. This is no longer the case.

Over the past three decades we have seen the emergence of two major influences in decisions about new advances in healthcare. These are the payer–providers and the patient–consumers. Their role in the decision-making process has increased rapidly in the last 25 years, as can be seen in Figure 1.1

With an increasing proportion of society's healthcare budget going on pharmaceuticals, even a growth in the percentage of the gross national product that governments are willing to allocate to healthcare has been unable to meet the demands of unbridled development. This has made the payer/provider a major determiner of the use of pharmaceuticals. All possible treatments cannot be freely available to all and a cost-to-benefit consideration has had to be introduced. This in turn has ensured that pharmaceutical medicine involves pharmacoeconomics training and even media training to deal

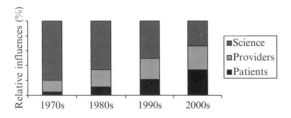

Figure 1.1 The influencers of healthcare provision

with what, for some, may be seen as the rationing and/or the means-testing of access to the totality of healthcare options. These are significant ethical and social issues and physicians within the pharmaceutical industry or the health regulatory agencies will inevitably be required to provide a perspective, both internally and to those outside.

The second new decision maker in the provision of healthcare has arrived even more recently as a crucial component. These are the end-user or patient groups. The rising status of the physician since the nineteenth century encouraged a paternalistic doctor–patient relationship, with the physician clearly in the lead. In recent times the nature of this relationship has come under question. The advent of holistic medical concepts focused on the whole patient, and taking into account the entirety of an individual patient's life has forced changes in the focusing of any therapeutic interaction. The general increase in educational standards within the developed world and the massive increase in available information culminating today with the electronic media and the Internet has inevitably produced a more informed patient. This has empowered the patient and led to the formation of all kinds of public interest and patient groups. Furthermore, the ability in this century to think in terms of the maintenance of good health and even of the abolition of disease (e.g. smallpox and polio) has changed the patient's and society's attitude to what they can and should expect of physicians. Today we are very much moving towards a balance in the therapeutic interaction, if not to a patient–doctor relationship. This change is a seminal one for the delivery of healthcare and for the development of new therapeutic agents.

For prescription drugs, the major factor bringing about the involvement of patient groups was probably the revolution in the new drug evaluation process caused by the AIDS epidemic. This terrible affliction occurred at a time when groups within society were forming to fight for their recognition and/or rights quite independent of the occurrence of a life-threatening disease. Nonetheless, within the Western world, it is clear that these groups rapidly came to form a vanguard for patients rights with respect to AIDS. They challenged the paternalism within medicine and insisted on access and full disclosure of what was going on in pharmaceutical medicine and within academic medical politics.

Without this openness such patients had lost confidence in pharmaceutical companies, in academia, and in the medical and regulatory establishment. Having forced a re-evaluation and a greater respect for patients' needs, AIDS Coalition to Unleash Power (ACTUP) and others have brought patient representatives into the drug development process. Such educated and involved patients have, in their turn, come to understand the scientific methodology and the requirement for the adequate testing of new drugs. Indeed, the requirements have consequently become much more acceptable to patients in general. Nevertheless, there is no doubt that these proactive patient representative groups have changed forever the role of the patient in the development of therapeutics and of healthcare within society.

Pharmaceutical medicine is the discipline that specializes within medicine in overseeing the process of developing new therapeutics to improve the standard of health and the quality of life within society. Inevitably, then, it was one of the first medical specialties to feel this change in patients' view of the quality of their care. An integral part of all progress in healthcare is evaluating the needs of patients and society and the gaps in the present provisions for those needs. In order to oversee this progress, pharmaceutical medicine involves the combination of first, the medical sciences to evaluate disease; second, the economic sciences to evaluate the value with respect to costs; and third, the ethical and social sciences to evaluate the utility of any new drug to patients and to society as a whole.

As with all products, truly successful therapeutic agents are those that meet all the customers' needs. In today's and tomorrow's world the concept that all that is needed is for medicines to meet the scientific requirements of being effective and safe is essentially an anachronism. It is not just the scientific factors and customers that must be satisfied. Table 1.1 shows that the two other critical factors or influences outlined in Figure 1.1 produce many more customers to be served.

As members of the public become generally more and more informed, it is inevitable that they will want to take more of a role in deciding on their own health and how any disease they may have is to be treated. It is important to realize that this is likely to change the demand for healthcare. Some of the focus will move to areas not classically considered

Table 1.1 Controlling factors in the adoption of new therapeutic agents

Influences	Controllers/'GateKeepers'
Medical science	Regulatory agencies Physicians Health professionals
Healthcare providers	Politicians National health services/HMOs Insurance companies
Consumers	Patient groups Pharmacists Media

diseases or to health areas considered today an inevitability of life or a condition for which the patient should 'just take charge'. Typical examples will be, on the one hand, an increased focus on quality of life or on the effects of aging (such as cognitive dysfunction, the menopause, osteoporosis, and waning immunological function, with consequent increasing vulnerability to disease) and, on the other hand, disorders such as obesity, attention deficit, hyperactivity, and even anorexia/bulimia. As the patients or their representatives respond and 'take charge', we should not be surprised to see a change in what are considered therapeutic modalities and how they are made available. We might expect a demand for products that do not need prescriptions (e.g. minerals, neutraceuticals, and cosmeceuticals) or for patients to be able to self-diagnose and use prescription drugs moved to a 'pharmacy only' or to a full OTC status. Some of these moves may well fit within one or more governments' desire to reduce the national pharmaceutical bill and hence may be something that has both patient and provider endorsement.

Those seeking to develop therapeutic products will need to understand these dynamic interactions and the consequent potential changes in one or more society's approach to its healthcare. Indeed, this is another opportunity for pharmaceutical medicine to broaden. The speciality should cover all pharmacologically active treatments, all disease preventions and all health maintenance modalities. The objective is to maximize patient benefits and extend product lifecycles, as well as company sales. Clearly, pharmaceutical medicine requires an ability to read the direction society is taking and an understanding that, on a global basis, various

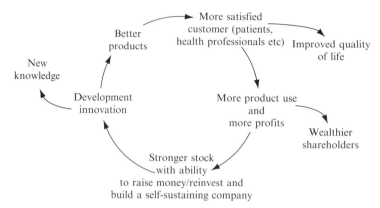

Figure 1.2   The cycle that drives the pharmaceutical industry

societies can take different attitudes to how they will regulate and/or classify a therapeutic agent. However they are classified or regulated, new therapeutic agents will continue to be needed, health benefits to deliver *now*, and to be potentially significant revenue generators for a business, allowing investment in future therapeutics. This is the basic cycle (Figure 1.2) that drives the pharmaceutical industry.

The R&D process is moving forward as biomedical science progresses and disease processes are better understood. The process of developing a therapeutic agent is much more than the better understanding of a disease leading to a new approach to its management. The process includes: first, state-of-the-art technical manufacturing sciences to ensure a drug substance is pure; second, appropriate and innovative pre-clinical science to ensure that a new chemical entity is as safe as possible before being used by humans; third, the most sophisticated clinical evaluation methodology. This methodology must establish the efficacy and safety of a new treatment in humans and include a multidisciplinary approach to the medical, social, and economic issues of quality of life and cost–benefit. Finally, the process includes the business management of the social and political issues inherent in establishing, communicating and assuring the value of the new drug within a global economy.

The amount spent on R&D by the pharmaceutical industry has grown logarithmically over the last few decades and now the industry outspends the National Institutes of Health in the USA (Figures 1.3, 1.4).

Similar growth in R&D investment has been seen outside America, e.g. in the UK. With such a massive R&D effort, the process has inevitably become subdivided into several functional sections, the most obvious being:

- *Basic chemical or structural research*—exploring the genetic basic of a disease or the microstructure of a receptor or enzyme active site, and from that, developing tailored molecules to provide specific interactions and potential therapeutic outcomes.
- *Preclinical research and development*—using biological systems, up to and including animal models, to explore the causes of diseases and the potential safety and efficacy of new therapeutic agents.
- *Clinical development*—using humans, both the healthy and those with a disease, to evaluate the safety and efficacy of a new drug. This section is itself, by convention, subdivided into three phases.
- *Regulatory and societal development*—ensuring that the entire development of each new therapeutic is seen in the context of its need to meet governmental requirements and that the appropriate value-added components (e.g. quality of life, cost–benefit, evidence-based medicine, relative competitive positioning) over and above the basic demonstration of safety and efficacy are integrated into the product's database.

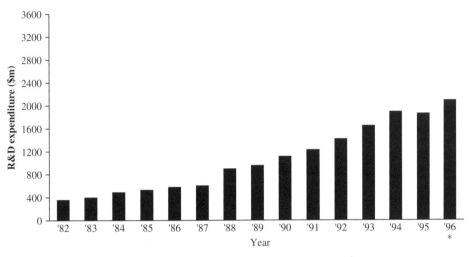

Figure 1.3 Total UK pharmaceutical R&D expenditure (including capital), 1982–1996 (*estimated for 1996). (From Centre for Medicines Research Report, 1996)

- *Post-market approval medical affairs*—this involves the promotion of each product bymarketing and sales functions and the oversight of this process by pharmaceutical physicians. Two other critical postmarketing components are first, continued learning about the safety and efficacy of the product in normal medical practice, as opposed to clinical trials; and second, the development of new or improved uses of the product as more is learned about it and as medical science moves on. The former of these two functions is termed 'pharmacovigilance' and the latter 'product evergreening'.

So the whole process of developing a new drug is extremely expensive and time-consuming. It is a also very difficult and risky process. Indeed, the majority of initial new product leads never reach the level of being tested in humans, and over 80% of products that are tested in man never become licensed drugs. Of course, all the many failed research and development efforts must be paid for, as well as the relatively few successful projects. As Figure 1.3 shows, this can only be done from the earnings on the new treatments that are developed. This, and the need to return to shareholders a profit on their long-term investment in the R&D process, are the basic factors in the cost of new drug. A major role of pharmaceutical medicine is to ensure that the value of new therapies is clearly demonstrated so that society can see the cost–benefit of new medicines.

Overall, the process of moving from a research concept through development to a marketed drug and then further refining the drug's value throughout what marketing would call the product's life

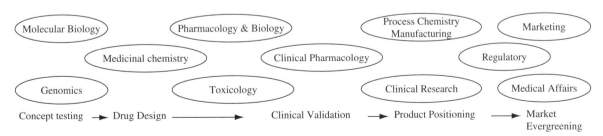

Figure 1.4 Integrated drug discovery and development. (Adapted from Taylor, 1993)

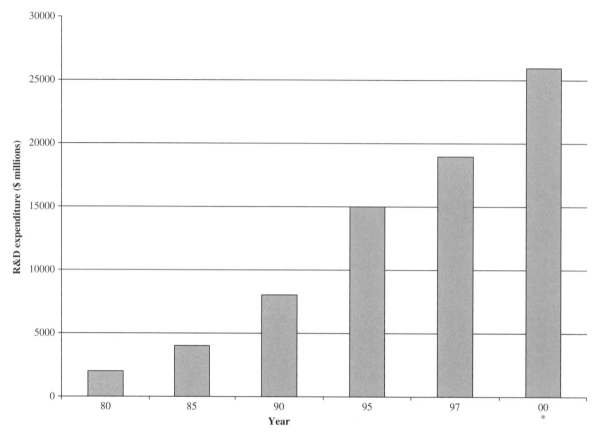

Figure 1.5   R&D expenditures, ethical pharmaceuticals, research-based pharmaceutical companies, 1980–2000. (From PhRMA Annual Survey 1997; 2000 expenditure from Ernst and Young, 2001)

cycle involves many disciplines. It can be seen in the terms shown in Figure 1.5. The basic responsibility for establishing and maintaining the safety and efficacy of a drug involves knowing where all of these differing functions can impact on the risks and benefits of medicines for patients.

In the 1950s and 1960s random screening and serendipity was the basis of the approach to new drug discovery. The structure–activity relationships were rudimentary and used simplistic pharmacophores and animal 'models of diseases'. This approach had essentially thousands of chemicals chasing a few models to hopefully find a new drug. The 1970s and 1980s have seen the impact of receptor science. They have seen the development of protein chemistry and elucidation of many enzymes and cell surface structures. Finally, the 1990s have seen the impact of enabling biomolecular technolo-

gies, such as combinatorial chemistry, genomics and high-throughput screening, and computer-assisted drug design, and so in the 1990s we have basic pharmaceutical discovery being carried out at the molecular and disease mechanism level. As such, we now have many models to evaluate and have probably reversed the development paradigm to one that Dr Stanley Crooke, the Chief Executive Officer of Isis, has described as 'target-rich [but] chemical-poor'.

Inevitably, in today's world, where science seems to be producing amazing advances almost weekly, the focus is on R&D and on further improvements in healthcare in the future. This should not cause us to take our eye off the needs of today and the ability of today's medicines to be used most effectively. The value of a new therapeutic agent is not maximal at the time of its first approval. Much can be done after market approval to ensure that a new drug's utility is both fully understood and is actually realized. The physicians within pharmaceutical medicine need to oversee and lead this process. This requires that they are trained in economics and business as well as medicine. Indeed, some may well go on to specialized courses in those areas leading to diplomas and even university degrees.

The rapid advances in the biosciences and our gains in the understanding of diseases offer the opportunity of new benefits or uses for drugs to be developed after they have been marketed. Consequently, there is a real and ongoing role for those in pharmaceutical medicine to follow the advances of medical sciences and to improve the value of the drugs of today within the medical and healthcare practices of tomorrow. This 'evergreening' process is analogous to physicians in their practice learning about a therapy and, as they come to know more about the use of the treatment, and as their practice dynamics change, modifying the use of that therapy to the maximal benefit of patients.

The management of a drug on the market is a professional challenge for which no medical school trains its physicians. The overall process and skill is an important part of the training within the speciality of pharmaceutical medicine. This effort may include the issues of quality-of-life evaluations, together with the appropriate development of evidence-based medicine, of outcomes research and of cost–utility sciences. All of these are techniques needed within pharmaceutical medicine. Used appropriately, they can help not only to establish the curative value of a new medicine but also to ensure that the therapy gets delivered optimally.

Just as is one's personal practice of medicine, there is no more rewarding experience than the optimal use of a treatment modality in a complex clinical case with a successful outcome and a happy patient; there is an equivalent reward in pharmaceutical medicine for a physician who: positions a product to deliver the best benefit for all patients; convinces all those delivering the care to use the product; and sees a consequent real improvement in society's level of healthcare. In the past, many good therapeutic agents have not been used as or when they should be. This was not because patients in trials have not been benefited; rather, it was because the value message had not been positioned

adequately for the care providers and/or for those who have to manage the healthcare resources of our societies. Even when well-developed and appropriately used for their approved indication, many drugs take on a new lease of life as the medical sciences change and new therapeutic uses become possible; e.g. lidocaine was a very well known local anesthetic and was decades old when it found a new role as an antiarrhythmic within the new context of cardiac resuscitation and coronary care units.

By the same token, as medicine moves forward, the acceptability and safety of a drug can change. It is a basic axiom of pharmaceutical medicine that no drug can ever be considered completely safe. This is true no matter how much human use data is available. For example, Phiso-Hex (hexachlorophene) gained broad usage as a skin wash and scrub to combat the spread of infection. It was used in pediatric and neonatal units in hospitals, by nurses and surgeons as a scrub and was even sold over the counter as a teenage acne remedy. Notwithstanding all this, it became a safety issue. This was because, as medical science advanced, more and more premature babies were able to survive. The skin of those babies was more permeable than that of full-term babies, children or adults. There was therefore a new potentially 'at-risk' group. Hexachlorophene toxicity in humans was considered to have resulted and this led to the product being modified or removed in many markets worldwide.

The scale of the response to this issue provides a case history that highlights another skill and training required within pharmaceutical medicine, namely crisis management. This is a very important technique which is critical in addressing substantive health issues. In the relatively recent history of healthcare, there have been several such issues, e.g. Zomax, Oraflex, Tylenol tampering, toxic shock syndrome, Reye's syndrome, the Dalcon shield, contaminated blood supply, silicon implants and the so-called 'generic drug scandal', to mention but a few.

Today, as much as being a leader in R&D, it is part of the role of the pharmaceutical physician to recognize new opportunities and to be alert for any emerging evidence of potential added benefits and/or new safety issues, as products and those of competitors are used more broadly outside the confines of clinical trials.

Many of the areas of expertise needed in pharmaceutical medicine overlap with the expertise of other medical disciplines. The most obvious overlap has perhaps seemed to be with clinical pharmacology. Indeed, clinical pharmacologists have a real interest in the R&D of the pharmaceutical industry and their training is a good one for entry into the industry. However, clinical pharmacology is by no means the entirety of pharmaceutical medicine. Indeed, some pharmaceutical physicians will work in even more basic and theoretical science settings, whilst others will be in more commercial settings. Of course, many within the specialty can and do focus on the development of disease models and the evaluation of new chemical entities in these diseases. The most modern methods in such areas are vital to the successful development of new drugs, and the continued and continuous interaction between the industry and academia is absolutely necessary. Indeed, the distinction between academia and pharmaceutical medicine is becoming blurred. The pharmaceutical industry R&D effort is now leading to Nobel prizes being awarded to those in the industry for pioneering work on subjects as diverse as prostaglandins, anti-infectives, and pharmacological receptors such as the histamine and the β-adrenergic receptor. The direct interaction within a company between those involved in basic research on receptors, active sites or genetic code reading sites; those synthesizing new molecules; and those testing them in the clinic, leads to the potential for a very fruitful research effort. Naturally, the industry as a prime inventor has the opportunity to carry out seminal work with entirely unique concepts, even if many of them do not become therapies for humans. The human is a unique animal which can, and does, exhibit unique responses to a new chemical entity. No pre-clinical work can be entirely predictive of a successful response in the clinic, and there can, in the end, be no substitute for human testing. Some products fail because of safety problems specific to man, and some because the early promise of efficacy in model systems is not realized in man.

Those who join this new specialty may come from many medical backgrounds and can well spend much of their time doing things other than pharmacology. In a very real way, those in pharmaceutical medicine are practicing medicine. They are responsible for the products of the pharmaceutical industry that are in use today. As such, they are influencing the health of far more people globally than they ever could in the context of their own individual clinical practice.

Any discussion of the discipline of pharmaceutical medicine today would be incomplete without a comment on the impact of biotechnology and the burgeoning biotechnology revolution. This is a revolution that is driven in a very different way than that in which the pharmaceutical industry has classically been run. The prime drivers are a multitude of small venture capital companies which are espousing the very cutting edges of research in biologics, genetics, and technology. They are largely managed by a combination of bioscientists and financiers. In this context the role of pharmaceutical medicine takes on its most extreme variants. At one end are physician/scientists, who are the research brain of the venture, and at the other end are physicians/businessmen, who are the money-raising voice of the venture. In either of these settings, pharmaceutical medicine is needed and the specialist will apply all of the training components that, as I have already indicated, compose this new discipline. The biotechnology industry is carrying forward some of the best and brightest projects of the world's leading academic institutions. It is moving pure research concepts through applied research into development and finally to the production of remarkable new therapeutic products. This industry has already created two or three new companies of substance, with sales of over $1 billion/year and a capitalization measured in billions. More than these obvious and huge successes, the industry has spawned literally thousands of venture capital efforts and new companies developing drugs, devices, diagnostics and all manner of medical technologies. Amazingly, this is an industry which has come into being in the last decade or two. Like the PC and software industry, it is revolutionizing society's approach to new product development and even to what a new therapeutic agent actually is. Already, companies are finding that the major transition points in the therapeutic product development process, from molecular to biochemical system, to cellular system, to organ model, to intact organism, to mammalian model, to humans, are all real watersheds. Pharmaceutical medicine provides the required understanding of each of these processes and particularly of the transition points. In a very real sense, the success of these emerging companies will be determined by the quality of their pharmaceutical medicine efforts.

The new discipline of pharmaceutical medicine is a specialty which has only very recently become recognized in its own right as a specialty within medicine. Indeed, the Faculty of Pharmaceutical Medicine of the Royal College of Physicians was only founded in 1990 in the UK and the Academy in the USA even more recently in 1994. Like many new ventures, this new medical speciality is not seen by all today as one of the premiere medical roles. However, there is a growing involvement of academics within the pharmaceutical industry and Nobel prize-winning work is being done within the industry. Furthermore, there is a growing understanding within academia that in the past someone else was capitalizing on their intellectual endeavours, so we are seeing more medical and bioscience academics patenting their discoveries and going into business. As this progress continues, the two disciplines of research and business are coming to realize that neither can do the other's work. Pharmaceutical medicine is the natural common pathway and the integrating specialty which will fill this need and will deliver the healthcare advances of the future. If this is so, then pharmaceutical medicine will become a leadership medical function in the twenty-first century. The speciality lies at the conjunction of changing societal needs for healthcare, the burgeoning biosciences and the understandings of how to provide improved quality of life and cost–utility for patients today. The expertise it contains and provides includes basic sciences such as chemistry and mathematics, applied sciences such as engineering, economics and business, biological sciences such as pharmacology and toxicology, and the medical sciences from paediatrics to geriatrics and from family medicine to the individual subspecialties. As such, pharmaceutical medicine is one of the most challenging, exciting and rewarding areas of medicine. It is a career for those who wish to be in the vanguard of research on multiple fronts.

REFERENCES

Centre for Medicines Research (1996). *UK Pharmaceutical R & D expenditure 1982–1986*. Monograph, London.

Taylor JB (1993) In: D'Arcy RF et al (Eds) *Textbook of Pharmaceutical Medicine*. Queen's University: Belfast.

Erast & Young (2001). *Biotechnology Annual Report*. http://www.ey.com

Pharmaceutical Research Manufacturers Association (1997) *PhRMA Annual Report 1999–2000*. Monograph. Washington DC. http://www.phrma.org

What Pharmaceutical Medicine Is, and Who Does It

William Wardell[1], Susan Toland[1], and Anthony W. Fox[2]

[1]Wardell Associates International, Princeton, NJ, USA, and[2] EBD Group Inc, Carlsbad, CA, USA

Pharmaceutical medicine deals with the discovery, development, evaluation, and monitoring of drugs and devices, as well as with medical aspects of their commercial promotion. Although the main focus of this chapter is on the activities of pharmaceutical physicians in pharmaceutical companies, it should be remembered that other arenas occupied by this discipline include regulatory authorities, universities, and clinical investigators in their clinical practices. Overlapping disciplines include clinical pharmacology, pharmacoeconomics, and biostatistics. In the USA, it could be further argued that those who operate managed care organizations also require many of the same skills as pharmaceutical physicians. In most countries, public health physicians and pharmaceutical physicians share at least some concerns and methodologies. If there is any specialty that has been practicing evidence-based medicine for decades, then it is pharmaceutical medicine (it is nice to watch the rest of the profession catching up with us!). However, it is typically within pharmaceutical companies where one finds the full spectrum of pharmaceutical medicine being practiced.

Pharmaceutical medicine is a medical specialty in which both physicians and non-physicians take part. This is not unusual. For example, various medical specialties require specialist nurses, nuclear medicine requires physicists, pathology requires histologists, and venereology requires contact tracers. In our case, pharmaceutical medicine requires pharmacists, clinical research associates, statisticians, administrators, and financiers. Interaction with a diverse set of other types of professional can be one of the most rewarding (and educational) aspects of a career in pharmaceutical medicine.

Pharmaceutical medicine is a young specialty, in its organized form. It is true that physicians have worked with pharmaceutical companies for many decades, but during the first two-thirds of the twentieth century they were often viewed as either a necessary evil or a window dressing for respectability. In the early 1970s, the British Association of Pharmaceutical Physicians (BrAPP) was formed. In 1975, BrAPP introduced a 2 year program of part-time study, and this may be viewed as the beginning of organized pharmaceutical medicine. The Royal Colleges of Physicians (RCP; London, Edinburgh, and Glasgow) then promptly supported this initiative by providing examinations for a diploma in pharmaceutical medicine, based upon the BrAPP syllabus.

Elsewhere, many countries are now following where the UK has led. In 1999, Belgium introduced a diploma modeled closely on that of the RCP. At the time of writing, Switzerland will probably next to introduce its diploma. Elsewhere, the American Academy of Pharmaceutical Physicians (chartered in 1994) has become the largest single group of doctors organized in this specialty, and its Board has approved an educational syllabus that is also compatible with the RCP model; learning resources for this American syllabus are currently being marshaled.

The large number of national associations of pharmaceutical physicians worldwide are coordinated by the International Federation of Associations of Pharmaceutical Physicians (IFAPP). This Federation concerns itself with various global aspects of the specialty, e.g. the International Conference on Harmonization. A conference on pharmaceutical medicine is held every 2 years,

Principles and Practice of Pharmaceutical Medicine. Edited by A. J. Fletcher, Lionel D. Edwards, Anthony W. Fox and Peter Stonier © 2002 John Wiley & Sons Ltd.

being co-sponsored by IFAPP and the national association where the conference takes place.

Given the global, and cross-professional, aspects of pharmaceutical medicine, what, then, can a medically-trained person specifically contribute? A degree in medicine, and some years as a junior doctor, require training that is of unusual breadth among academic pursuits. This breadth of training, perhaps fairly termed a 'jack-of-all-trades but master of none', leads to the capability to contribute thought to the overall scope of development programs. An important part of interacting with the diversity of other professionals is to be able to see, and explain when necessary, how one aspect can impact on others. Furthermore, in drug development and postmarketing surveillance, it is the physician who is most likely to be able to estimate the clinical hazards and anticipate the clinical condition of the patients (or normal subjects) who are exposed to the drugs. Most important of all, it is the physician who is the guardian of the patient from an ethical standpoint.

SUBSPECIALIZATION

There are any number of rôles that pharmaceutical physicians can play (see Table 2.1). Later chapters in this book consider drug discovery, clinical trials, regulatory affairs, marketing, etc. Suffice it to say that pharmaceutical physicians are found in all these subspecialties. They are also found at the next higher level of complexity, the coordination and leadership of all these individual activities, using integrated development plans. Physicians usually find it easy to move between such subspecialties and, indeed, between different companies: this is further evidence of the value of the breadth of training in medicine.

The number of subspecializations has increased in recent years. Examples include the recent tremendous advances in pharmacoeconomics and information science. At least one pharmaceutical physician is now both a part-time regulator and a part-time private barrister in the UK. The increasing interaction between pharmaceutical companies and health maintenance organizations in the USA has led some pharmaceutical physicians into the worlds of finance, contract, and epidemiology.

Table 2.1 Some sub-specializations in pharmaceutical medicine.

Administration
Advertising
Biostatistics
Clinical pharmacology
Clinical trialist
Consulting
Finance
Futurism
Genomics
Industrial intelligence
Informatics
Information technology
Journalism
Legal affairs
Licensing
Lobbying and Politics
Marketing
Medical monitor
Medical writing
Patent law
Pharmacology
Pharmacoeconomics
Pharmacoepidemiology
Pharmacovigilance
Regulation (governmental)
Regulatory affairs
Toxicology

WHY DO CLINICIANS JOIN INDUSTRY?

Industry, or government employment, are not for everyone. Doctors, pharmacists, nurses and others who enjoy diversity should be especially attracted to this specialty. Versatility and adaptability, *vice versa*, are required for a successful career in this discipline.

Another personality trait that must be considered is the capability to cooperate and listen. The typical clinician is usually in sole charge of the patient, and needs brook little disagreement in decision-making from his/her staff. The bombastic surgeon is an international phenomenon; the pharmaceutical physician has to be the exact opposite in his/her approach. The really successful doctor in industry will be someone who actually enjoys receiving opinion from people who are not medically qualified.

For pharmaceutical physicians involved in drug development (a large subset of the specialty), there are also product-related satisfactions. These can be relatively vicarious (e.g. a reduction in spontaneous adverse event report frequency after a labeling change). More directly, occasionally, we have friends or relatives who benefit from the drugs that we develop. One of the authors of this chapter has been hugged to the point of assault by a complete stranger in Georgia (USA), a patient who judged him responsible for 'curing' her migraine. Neither protests that the reality is teamwork, nor perfume-induced sneezing, deterred this extra-verted Southern lady!

Some join the industry for only a short period, and then decide that they would prefer to return to their original clinical callings. This, too, can be of professional benefit. One's clinical skills do not decline much in the first 2 or 3 years away from patients, and they can, in any case, be maintained with part-time or *locum tenens* clinical employment while one holds a position in a pharmaceutical company. Upon leaving industry, it is likely that the physician will take back to the clinic some new skills, e.g. better management techniques and how to approach clinical data with scientific scepticism; this experience is not usually available in the ordinary clinical situation. Such a physician will also have inside knowledge of how to increase the probability of industrial sponsorship of his/her clinical research project! One author of this chapter, when approached by a doctor with trepidation or vacillating on whether to accept an industry position, has a standard response: 'Now is not make-your-mind-up time. That will be in 2 or 3 years because then you must probably decide whether to *stay* in the industry'.

In 2000, the American Academy of Pharmaceutical Physicians surveyed its members. One of the questions asked about personal fulfillment, and more than 90% of respondents indicated high degrees of satisfaction with pharmaceutical medi-cine as a career. Lest one suspect that this was seeking the opinions of the already converted, it should be pointed out that other specialist colleges have conducted similar surveys. No other medical specialty in the USA contains such a large propor-tion of doctors with such positive views.

FURTHER READING

Berde B (1985) Physicians as employees of the pharmaceutical industry. *Eur J Clin Pharmacol* 28: 363–5.

Bootman JL, Townsend RJ, McGhan WF (eds) (1996) *Principles of Pharmacoeconomics*, 2nd edn. Harvey Whitney Books: Cincinatti, OH.

Dollery C (1994) Medicine and the pharmacological revolution (the Harveian oration of 1993). *J R Coll Physicians (Lond)* 28: 59–69.

Dziewanowska ZE (1990) Globalization of the pharmaceutical industry; opportunities for physicians in clinical research. *J Clin Pharmacol* 30: 890–92.

Fox AW (2001) What is pharmaceutical medicine? *Clin Res* 1: 28–30.

Gabbay FJ (1987) Consolidating the discipline of pharmaceut-ical medicine in the United Kingdom. In Burley D, Haasard C, Mullinger B (eds), *The Focus for Pharmaceutical Know-ledge: The Proceedings of the Sixth International Meeting of Pharmaceutical Physicians*. Macmillan: London; 286–92.

Jefferis JJ (1985) The pharmaceutical industry and academic medicine: opportunities for physician collaboration. *Circula-tion* 72 (suppl 1): 21–4.

Sampson MC (1984) Career Opportunities in Industrial Clinical Research. In Matosen GM (ed.), *The Clinical Research Pro-cess in the Pharmaceutical Industry*. Marcel Dekker: New York; 479–505.

Shaw L (1991) A misunderstood specialty: a survey of physicians in the pharmaceutical industry. *J Clin Pharmacol* 31: 419–22.

Spilker B (1989) Career opportunities for physicians in the pharmaceutical industry. *J Clin Pharmacol* 29: 1069–76.

Young MD (1990) Globalization of the pharmaceutical indus-try: the physician's role in optimizing drug use. *J Clin Phar-macol* 30: 990–93.

Competency-based Training System for Clinical Research Staff

Jay D. Miller

Amgen Inc., Thousand Oaks, California

The pharmaceutical industry is a highly regulated industry in which many of the activities and tasks performed by staff are defined by regulations and guidelines issued by various regulatory authorities around the world. The training requirements for sponsor companies can therefore be fairly well defined. In addition, international initiatives by regulatory authorities and trade organizations have further defined the role of staff involved in clinical research.

The International Conference on Harmonization (ICH) guideline for Good Clinical Practice (GCP; 1997), for example, describes a minimum standard for the ethical and scientific standards for designing, conducting, and reporting clinical research. The ICH GCP guideline is the unified standard for the European Union (EU), Japan and the USA to facilitate mutual acceptance of clinical data. The ICH GCP guideline, together with other ICH guidelines, provides an operational definition of the core competencies needed by clinical staff to conduct world-class clinical research.

One of the principles of ICH GCP is that 'each individual involved in conducting a trial should be qualified by education, training, and experience to perform his or her respective task(s)'. Specifically regarding the selection and qualifications of monitors, the ICH GCP guideline states that 'monitors should be appropriately trained and should have the scientific and/or clinical knowledge needed to monitor the trial adequately'. Most major pharmaceutical firms have always had varying degrees of in-house education and training for staff, supplemented (as appropriate) by external workshops, courses and training meetings. The ICH GCP guideline formalizes the requirements for credible education programs to comply with current GCP requirements.

WHAT IS A COMPETENCY-BASED TRAINING PROGRAM?

Few people come to the pharmaceutical industry from academia with the requisite knowledge and skills necessary to plan, conduct, and report clinical research to regulatory authority standards. This knowledge and skill usually needs to be provided to the new staff by the way of in-house training.

One approach to education and training in the industry is what is called 'competency-based training'. A competency is a skill, knowledge or behavior required to undertake effectively the tasks and responsibilities for which an individual is responsible.

A competency-based education and training system (CBETS) details the essential knowledge and skills needed by sponsor's staff to complete the requirements of GCP. The concept of a CBETS is different from traditional educational and training approaches. Traditional approaches tend to address the training needs of individuals based on their job descriptions, e.g. within a sponsor company, a monitor will receive training on how to monitor a clinical trial, and a physician will receive training in protocol development. In this traditional education and training model, the required tasks are functionally defined. The monitor may not learn much about preparing protocols and the physician may not learn much about monitoring. However, each may be intimately involved in both tasks.

Principles and Practice of Pharmaceutical Medicine. Edited by A. J. Fletcher, Lionel D. Edwards, Anthony W. Fox and Peter Stonier © 2002 John Wiley & Sons Ltd.

The CBETS asks *what* tasks the sponsor needs to have done to meet its drug development goals and objectives. The primary tasks of clinical research and good clinical practice can be described rather precisely. Once one knows what the major tasks are and what activities are needed to accomplish these tasks, one can define the knowledge and skills needed by staff to complete the tasks and, finally, what education and training should be provided to understand the knowledge and skills.

When the tasks and activities are fully defined, a CBETS will ask who is going to do these tasks and how competent (e.g. expert, fundamental skills) they need to be to complete the tasks. In the example provided above, it is useful for the physician to have a fundamental knowledge of the monitoring process, even though he she will not be performing the tasks. The physician may, however, be supervising the monitors. It is appropriate for the monitor to receive advanced training in the requirements of monitoring, since this is one of his/her major functions. In terms of protocol development, the physician and monitor each need expert competency to develop the protocol, since the sponsor may be investing hundreds or millions of dollars in the program. The monitor only needs fundamental skills in protocols, since his/her responsibility may be limited to implementing the protocol at the clinical site.

The CBETS can apply to behavioral and management training as well as technical training. Education and training programs in the pharmaceutical industry can be designed to provide the competencies necessary to prevent or remove obstacles to staff performance. These obstacles can be well defined in advance in a CBETS.

COMPETENCY-BASED TRAINING PROGRAM FOR CLINICAL STAFF

The following is a description of the typical essential competencies needed to plan, conduct, and report a clinical research program in a regulated environment. Each competency is described, as well as the knowledge and skills a sponsor's representative would need to be successful in completing the task. Judgment can then be applied to the most

urgent needs in providing education and training around the knowledge and skills.

While many readers will be thoroughly familiar with the tasks described below and described in more detail throughout the chapters of this book, a brief explanation of the task is provided, together with the success factor in completing the task.

General Clinical Competencies

Understanding of the drug development process

All new clinical staff need to understand the overall drug development process. Before new investigational products can be introduced into man, extensive preclinical and toxicological studies are performed. Staff who will be responsible for the clinical portion of drug development need to have an appreciation of the work that has been undertaken to progress the compound through to the clinical phases.

This includes understanding the vision, mission and objectives of the sponsor's clinical development strategy. Most sponsors have a unique investigational product development system. Being familiar with this system is important in understanding the sponsor's decision-making approach, its internal milestones, and its methods for budgeting and resourcing clinical programs. Individuals new to industry should identify and understand the function of the major departments comprising the clinical research and development process, as well as understanding the operation of sponsor management bodies.

To gain this knowledge, new staff members should attend the sponsor's orientation program on drug development and the appropriate Pharmaceutical Education and Research Institute Inc. (PERI) or Drug Information Association (DIA) overview courses on investigational drug development. There is considerable literature available that discusses the drug development process, such as the *Guide to Clinical Trials* by Dr Bert Spilker. Regulatory authorities provide important guidelines on registration expectations. In addition, many sponsors have internal documentation explaining the company's systems and processes. Senior-level staff can also attend the advanced course on international investigational product development and regulatory issues sponsored by Tufts University.

Understanding the US FDA regulations

The Food and Drug Administration (FDA) in the USA remains the dominant regulatory authority in the world. An understanding of the FDA regulatory structure, operations and functions is very important to individuals new to the pharmaceutical industry or new to the industry within the USA. The different approaches of the Drug and Biologics Divisions should be understood. Staff need to identify and understand FDA investigational drug IND and biologic regulations and FDA guidelines and regulations.

Knowledge and skills are required for the specific regulations governing drug development in the USA. These include Title 21, Code of Federal Regulations Parts 50,56,312 and 314.

Senior-level staff need to understand how the communication process works with the FDA, for example, End-of-Phase II Meetings, IND Annual Report, FDA Advisory Committee meetings, Pre-New Drug or Biologic Licence Applications (NDA/BLA) Meetings, clinical holds, IND termination, and FDA audits.

Understanding Good Clinical Practices (GCP)

Understanding the responsibilities and obligations of sponsors in terms of GCP is fundamental knowledge, essential to conduct clinical research. Currently, most pharmaceutical firms reference the ICH GCP guideline as the minimum standard for conducting clinical trials.

The responsibilities and obligations include knowledge of the elements of informed consent, the role and responsibilities of institutional review boards/independent ethics committees (IRB/IEC) and the importance of clinical study quality assurance.

All sponsor staff have a specific and direct responsibility for the safety and welfare of subjects participating in clinical trials. A full and complete understanding of GCP is requisite for all sponsor staff. Most sponsors provide internal training on these issues. There are excellent PERI or DIA overview courses covering GCP.

Competencies Associated with Planning Clinical Research

Conceptualization and Development of Clinical Research and Development Plans (CRDPs)

Developing an international CRDP to answer questions defined by the investigational product target profile is a key activity of senior-level industry personnel. This competency requires an understanding of toxicology and clinical pharmacology to identify clinical target profile criteria. The CRDP defines the critical path for the clinical program and the clinical budget. The CRDP also defines investigational drug development assessment and decision points, and the project resource (personnel and budget) estimates.

CRDPs will cover:

- Preparing the clinical section of IND/CTX submission.
- Preparing clinical reports needed to support IND/CTX submissions.
- Clinical research and scientific methodology.
- Phase I studies.
- Phase II studies.
- Phase III studies.
- Phase IV studies and safety surveillance studies.
- Pilot efficacy studies.
- Pharmacokinetic and bioavailability studies.
- Dose-ranging studies.
- Dose-titration studies.
- Registration studies.
- Marketing and safety surveillance studies.

The goal of these plans is to provide an efficient NDA/BLA with the minimum studies needed for registration and approval in the world markets. The medical, scientific, regulatory and marketing opinions must be weighed and balanced in the plans.

Understand and Conceptualize Clinical Study Design

To successfully create a CRDP, the individual must know the basic concepts of research design and statistics, the concepts of clinical research and investigational drug development; possess an in-depth understanding of the concepts of clinical pharmacology, pharmacokinetics, pharmacodynamics, toxicology, state-of-the-art therapeutic medicine and methodology, and FDA/EU/ICH therapeutic research guidelines and regulatory issues; and understand basic concepts of project planning and scheduling.

Preparation of the Investigator's Brochure (IB)

The IB is a summary of clinical and preclinical data on the investigational product which is relevant to the study of the investigational product in human subjects and the investigator's assessment of risk in participating in the study. The sponsor compiles clinical information for the preparation of the IB.

The preparation of an IB may be performed by clinical staff or a medical writing group. The activities included in preparing the IB include: coordination of the compilation of clinical and preclinical data from contributing departments (e.g. clinical pharmacology, toxicology); describing the physical, chemical and pharmaceutical properties and formulation; preparing a clear, concise summary of the information relating to the safety and effectiveness of the investigational product; providing a detailed description of possible risks and benefits of the investigational product; and a clear rationale for the dosage and dosing interval.

To prepare an IB, the sponsor's representative must understand: the fundamental purpose and uses of the IB; the basic format and content of sponsor IBs; the clinical pharmacology and toxicology findings; the investigational product–disease relationships; the international regulatory requirements governing IBs; and the indications and safety profile of the investigational product.

Design and Preparation of Clinical Protocols

The clinical protocol describes the objectives, design, methodology, statistical considerations, and organization of the trial. The sponsor is usually responsible for developing the protocol in industry-sponsored clinical trials. However, internal and external content experts are frequently consulted. Protocols must be written ensuring medical soundness and clinical practicality.

Often the sponsor uses a template to complete the sections of the protocol. The tasks of developing a protocol include: defining clear protocol objectives, identifying primary efficacy and safety parameters and appropriate subject selection criteria, and identifying correct dosages and route.

To prepare appropriate protocols, staff must understand: research design and statistical inferences for clinical research; state-of-the-art research designs and trials; therapeutic area guidelines; GCP; regulatory requirements, guidelines and country-specific issues; national and international medical practices; sponsor protocol review and approval procedures; and possess in-depth investigational product-disease knowledge.

Clinical protocols are the building blocks of the clinical research plan and the NDA/BLA. Protocols specify the conditions that permit and lead to meaningful and credible results in clinical programs. Operationally, protocols provide a written agreement between the sponsor and the investigator on how the trial is going to be conducted. This agreement allows the sponsor to ensure that the study will be done to the highest ethical and medical standards and that the quality of the data can relied upon as credible and accurate.

All clinical protocols and supporting documents are reviewed and approved internally by a group of senior clinical research managers. This group assesses the overall study design and ability of the study to meet its objectives, as well as the quantity and quality of the data. In addition, the group reviews the procedures for the safety and welfare of the subjects, to ensure compliance to GCP and ethical principles. The quality of a clinical protocol can be assessed by how well the elements of the protocol are prepared. The elements of clinical protocols are described in Table 3.1.

Table 3.1 Elements of clinical protocols

Background and rationale
Study objectives
Experimental design and methods
Schedule of assessments
Subjection selection criteria
Screening procedures for entry
Study parameters
Trial medication
Premature withdrawal
Subject replacement policy
Criteria for excluding data
Statistical analysis plans
Signatures

The extent of a background section will vary with the drug's stage of development. New clinical data not already included in the IB should be emphasized. The rationale provides a concise statement of the reasons for conducting the study and the basis for the dosage selection and duration that will be used in the trial. Quality protocols should target relevant information in the background and convincing rationale for the study.

Every protocol must state a primary, quantifiable, study objective. Secondary objectives should be limited in scope and related to the primary question. Objectives must be specific and capable of answering a key clinical question required by the clinical research plan.

The study design is an important element in assessment of quality protocols. The overall purpose of the study design is to reduce the variability or bias inherent in all research. Good study design will always address control methods that reduce experimental bias. These control methods will often include treatment blinding, randomization and between- or within-patient study designs. The schedule of assessments describes a schedule of time and events and provides a complete profile of the overall trial design. Good quality schedule of assessments sections also include acceptable time windows around the variables being collected.

The inclusion and exclusion criteria are described in the subject selection part of the protocol. To a large extent, the success or failure of a particular clinical trial can often be traced back to how well the criteria were developed. Protocol authors strive to include the most appropriate patient population to satisfy the study objective and still include those kinds of patients that will ultimately receive the drug. Therefore, selection criteria can be unreasonable and unnecessary in some cases and vague and non-specific in other cases. The management of concomitant medications is particularly problematic. The protocol must attempt to define those medications that are permitted for intercurrent illnesses and those that are prohibited, since they will interfere with the interpretation of the test medication. While there are no easy answers, quality protocols are able to justify with some precision the rationale for each inclusion and criteria. How these criteria are applied is handled in the screening for study entry section.

The efficacy and safety parameters describe how and when the variables are going to be recorded, usually in relation to drug administration and follow-up periods. How adverse events are managed and recorded are particularly important to the sponsor and regulatory authorities. Protocol authors should ensure that the study defines the criteria for success or failure of treatment. End-points should be clear and defined. Since many clinical phenomena are open to interpretation, protocols should provide definitions of variables and time windows for their collection. If the assessments are purely subjective, then methods to prevent observer bias (so-called "observer truing") must be employed. Addressing these issues will improve the quality and meaningfulness of the results of the study.

The description of the management of trial medication is often a source of confusion. Protocols must include clear directions for dosing intervals and adjustments. Since patients will never follow a protocol precisely in all cases, provisions for missing doses or "what-if?" situations should be anticipated. Good protocols always include, in addition, adequate compliance checks of drug consumption by the subjects of the study.

Protocols should predetermine how subjects will be replaced following dropping out of the study. This is important, because the means by which subjects are replaced can adversely affect the statistical analysis. Similarly, a decision concerning the conditions under which a subject would not be evaluable must be stated explicitly before the study starts. This is intended to minimize intentional or unintentional data manipulation.

Design of the Format and Content of Case Report Forms (CRFs)

The CRF is the document used to record all of the protocol-specified data used to describe individual subject results. Many sponsors use standard modules to prepare the CRF.

To prepare successful CRFs, the sponsor's staff must know: typical clinical practices; therapeutic conventions; investigator and staff needs; data management and analysis plans; project-specific definitions and procedures; CRF completion problem areas; remote-data entry and review; and approval procedures for CRFs. Ideally, CRFs should be pre-tested with internal and external experts.

The quality of a clinical trial can be influenced by how well the CRF is designed. If the investigator's staff cannot enter the protocol data as required, the sponsor will have a considerable challenge in trying to interpret the results.

There are a number of design principles that facilitate the use of CRFs in clinical trials. These principles include the concepts of standardization and minimization. The sponsor standardizes the design of CRFs in one consistent international format. This permits uniform databases, consistency in collection and more rapid data entry. In addition, standardization facilitates the monitoring process and therefore increases accuracy of the data. While efficiency is an important variable in the design process, the systems must also be sufficiently flexible to account for the variances between projects. Finally, an important principle of both protocol and CRF design is to collect only the data needed to satisfy the objectives of the protocol. The inherent temptation to collect more data must be resisted.

There are several CRF design characteristics which define quality CRFs. Some of these include:

- Limiting the amount of space for free text.
- Providing instructions on the CRF for its completion.
- Consistent layout of information within the CRF.
- Simple, unambiguous language.
- Collecting only raw data, letting the computer do transformation calculations.
- Intensive monitor training in the use of the CRFs.
- Use of the project-specific procedure manual to document conventions and CRF decisions.

High-quality CRF design is probably the cheapest investment in big returns on a clinical trial.

Packaging and Labeling of Investigational Products

The investigational product is the active ingredient or placebo being tested in a clinical trial. Forecasting investigational drug supplies is important, in that it must be done well in advance of the start date of the clinical trial. To make this forecast, it is necessary to estimate, from the CRDP, the bulk investigational product supply needs.

To handle drug supplies successfully, the sponsor's representative must know: the procedures for ordering bulk investigational product supplies; models for bulk investigational product quantity estimation; investigational product packaging time frames; protocol-specific and country-specific requirements for packaging and shipping investigational product supplies; procedures for packaging international investigational product supplies; investigational product supply tracking systems; investigational product ordering and packaging processes; general investigational product formulation and packaging processes and configurations; protocol design; randomization procedures; and investigational product dispensing and accountability.

Identification and Selection of Clinical Investigators for Study Placement and Conducting Prestudy Evaluation Visits

Selecting investigators. The proper selection of clinical investigators is one of the key success factors for any clinical program. The principal investigator has the primary responsibility for the success of the trial. His/her leadership and direction of co-investigators and study staff is critical in performing the requirements of today's trials. Time spent in learning who are the best investigators is well spent and pays significant dividends in the end.

To successfully identify and select clinical investigators, the sponsor's representatives need to: identify internal and external sources for potential investigators; define investigator selection criteria, protocol requirements, expected cost of the study, and investigator and facility qualifications; interview potential investigators; and, finally, schedule and conduct prestudy site evaluation visits.

The clinical team has an important role in determining the quality selection of clinical investigators. Selection criteria will be based upon the needs of the clinical research and development plan (CRDP) and the individual protocols. Quality investigators can be identified by:

- Previous clinical research experience.
- Previous performance on sponsor and other company trials.

Table 3.2 Sources of quality investigators

Clinical leaders/therapeutic area heads
Country company heads
Consultants
Colleague recommendations
Investigator recommendations
Scientific and medical literature
Physician directories
Speakers at professional meetings

Table 3.3 Prestudy visit questions

How will the protocol specifically operate at the prospective center?
How will informed consent be obtained? By whom?
How will source documents be managed?
How will adverse events be handled and followed up (serious and non-serious events)?
How many studies is the investigator conducting currently?

- Their reputation among peers and the quality of their publications.
- The experience and training of their support staff.
- The quality and reputation of their research facilities.

Potential sources of quality investigators are shown in Table 3.2.

Many physicians may need to be considered before the best investigators can be identified. Preliminary contact should be done by telephone. Only those investigators who satisfy the primary selection criteria need to be visited.

Prestudy visits. The purpose of the prestudy visit is to evaluate the investigator's interest and ability to conduct the study to the required sponsor standards. Special attention is paid to the quality of the investigator's staff and facilities, as well as to the availability of the required patient population. In conducting the prestudy site evaluation visit, the sponsor's representative determines whether or not the investigator is qualified by training and experience to conduct the trial.

The prestudy visit is a professional exchange of information. The investigator is informed of the preclinical and clinical background of the drug. Of primary importance to the investigator is the rationale for use of the drug and the expected safety profile. Much can be inferred from the investigator's preparation and questions about the investigational drug. The protocol should be explained, including the requirements for the patient population, the study design, and a description of the safety and efficacy variables.

Other aspects of the study are also discussed with the investigator, such as the completion of the CRF, access to source documents, and management of

drug supplies. The nature and form of informed consent is reviewed. In these discussions, the monitor is attempting to identify aspects of the study which present difficulties or problems for the investigator. Quality investigators usually have clear understanding and strategy for the above activities. Examples of the questions that require answering during prestudy visits are shown in Table 3.3.

Some objective measure of the availability of the correct patient population is important during a prestudy visit. This can often be best accomplished through a chart or hospital census review by the monitor. The time spent doing this aspect of a clinical trial will invariability result in better and more timely results in clinical programs.

Assuming that the outcome of the prestudy visit(s) is successful, the sponsor's representative will need to develop and negotiate study contracts and secure essential documents.

Competencies Associated with Conducting Clinical Research

Conducting Study Initiation

The study initiation visit is sometimes confused with the prestudy visit. The purpose of the study initiation meeting is to orientate the study staff to the requirements of the protocol. At the point of the study initiation visit, the study site should be fully ready to begin all aspects of the trial. The monitor must ensure that the study medication and materials are available at the site. In addition, all essential documentation must be completed and available. Key study documentation is shown in Table 3.4.

All study staff who will have direct involvement in the trial should participate in the study initiation visit. This usually includes: the investigator and

Table 3.4 Key Study Documentation

Approved protocol and CRF
Informed Consent Form and Subject Information Sheet
Investigator's *Curriculum Vitae*
Written IRB/IEC approval
Local regulatory approval
Signed study contract
Laboratory ranges and accreditation

subinvestigator(s), the study coordinator or research nurse, pharmacist, and laboratory personnel or specialists as needed.

During the meeting, all major points and requirements of the protocol are reviewed and discussed. Procedures for subject enrollment are particularly important, since this is the area which may cause the most problems for the site. During the presentation, participants may raise important medical or logistical issues that have or have not been anticipated by the protocol authors. It is important to note these concerns and communicate them to the protocol authors, as appropriate.

The sponsor's representative should be competent in the basic medical and scientific issues of the investigational product and protocol, know the target disease or symptoms, be able to train the investigative staff on the conduct of the study, confirm facility capabilities, conduct the site initiation meeting, describe adverse event reporting requirements, and be able to resolve protocol issues during and after meeting.

Conducting Clinical Trial Monitoring

Clinical trial monitoring includes those activities that ensure that the study is being conducted according to the protocol. Monitoring permits an in-process assessment of the quality of the data being collected. The first alert to safety issues is often revealed during the process of monitoring the clinical trial.

Monitoring clinical studies involves the act of overseeing the progress of a clinical trial. Monitors ensure that the study is conducted, recorded and reported in accordance with the protocol. This is accomplished by the review of CRFs on-site for possible errors, inconsistencies, and omissions. The monitor identifies errors and discrepancies

that require discussion with the investigator or staff and any safety questions or issues. The monitor compares CRFs with source documents, confirming that source data are consistent with CRF entries, identifies all serious adverse events, resolves previous and current CRF queries, and confirms completeness of investigator records and files.

To be a successful monitor, the sponsor representative should know: how to interpret hospital/clinic records/charts, laboratory tests, and interpretations; has to query resolution procedures; protocol and CRF data requirements; medical nomenclature; Serious adverse event (SAE) procedures; and health authority requirements. In addition, a monitor needs to have excellent interpersonal communication and problem-solving skills.

Clinical monitoring requires clinical, interpretive, and administrative skills. The monitor needs to confirm subject selection and patient enrollment compliance. Quality monitoring will always include and confirm the following activities:

- Properly obtained informed consent.
- Adherence to the protocol procedures and inclusion/exclusion criteria.
- Transcription of data from source documents to the CRF that is both consistent and logical.
- Identification of any safety issues, including serious adverse events.
- Proper accountability and reconciliation of drug supplies.
- Continued adequacy of facilities and staffing.

The frequency of clinical monitoring depends on the actual accrual rate of the patients. Complex studies may need to be visited more frequently, depending on the accrual rate of subjects, the amount of data, and the number of visits. Generally, most investigators should be monitored every 4–6 weeks. Sufficient time for good monitoring practices should be anticipated by the monitors. Following a monitoring visit, the monitor will prepare a monitoring report for sponsor records and follow-up correspondence to the trial site. The monitor may need to plan intervention and possible replacement of non-performing or non-compliant trial centers.

Managing Drug Accountability

The sponsor is responsible for providing the investigator with investigational drug(s). Both the sponsor and the investigator have a role in drug accountability. The sponsor's representative inspects storage of investigational product supplies; checks study site investigational product dispensing records; checks randomization and blinding; and maintains records of investigational product shipments. The monitor reconciles investigational product shipped, dispensed and returned; arranges for shipment of investigational product to core country or investigative sites; checks investigational product supplies at site against enrollment and withdrawals; maintains investigational product accountability records; resolves investigational product inventory problems; implements tracking system for investigational product management on a study and project level; arranges for the return and/or destruction of unused investigational product supplies; and ensures final reconciliation of investigational product supplies.

GCPs require sponsors to be able to account for the drug supplies prepared and shipped to the investigator, the investigator's use of those supplies, and the return and destruction of remaining drug supplies. Planning drug supplies is a detailed and complex activity. Bulk and formulated drug requests must typically be made at least 6 months in advance of the need for those supplies. This is to account for the ordering of intermediates or finished drug, purchasing of comparator agents, and for quality control testing.

Drug packaging should follow as consistent a format as possible within a project and must be identical within multicenter trials. Regulatory documents required for investigational drug use in the core countries must be anticipated and made available when needed, e.g. methods of analysis, stability data, customs declarations. The typical requirements for drug labels is described in Table 3.5.

Once the study is under way, the use of the investigational drug must be accounted for by the investigator's staff. Subjects should return unused medication and empty containers to the investigator. The amount of drug dispensed and the amount used by the patients are compared for discrepancies. This provides a measure of compliance by the study subjects. Monitors must also check that drug

Table 3.5 Typical labeling requirements for investigational drug

Local language	Route of administration
Name of investigator	Dosage
Study number	Dosage form
Bottle number	Quantity or volume
Lot number	Storage precautions
Drug name or code	Directions for use
Manufacturer name	Note: 'For Clinical Trial'
Manufacturer address	Caution statement
Local affiliate name	Expiry date

supplies are being kept under the required storage conditions.

Study drug must be dispensed according to the randomization schedule. Failure to do so can result in some of the data having to be discarded during statistical analysis. This issue can prove to be problematic when a single site is studying patients at different locations. Finally, the double-blind code must not be broken, except when essential for the management of adverse events. The breaking of treatment codes can make that patient's data unusable for efficacy analyses.

Handling Adverse Drug Experiences (ADEs)

Safety concerns are present throughout the drug development process. From the filing of INDs, through the conduct of clinical trials, to the approval process of the NDA/BLA and the marketing of the drug, safety is the primary concern of any clinical program.

Management of safety is a principal responsibility of the sponsor monitor. The monitor has responsibility for informing the investigator about the safety requirements of the study. This will include a discussion of expected and unexpected adverse events, how to report adverse events should they occur, and how to characterize the adverse events in terms of project-specific definitions.

Monitors are expected to review CRF and source documents with particular attention to potential safety problems. On the CRF, the adverse events section and laboratory results section are reviewed for important findings. Often, relevant notes are made by the investigator in the comment section of the CRF. In source documents, safety issues may be uncovered in the progress notes of hospital charts or the interpretative reports of various diagnostic tests, e.g. chest X-rays, ECGs. Safety problems can manifest themselves in many ways. Monitors must be alert to exaggerated changes from baseline with expected pharmacological effects, acute and chronic effects and multiple drug treatment reactions.

Monitors are often the first company representatives to learn about an adverse event. The timeliness of reporting the event to management is important in satisfying regulatory reporting requirements. In general, the expectation is that the sponsor will learn of the event within 24 h of its occurrence. The sponsor monitor will transmit the information about the event to headquarters within 24 h and headquarters will get the information to the drug safety department within 24 h. The monitor should immediately notify appropriate senior managers of serious ADEs that are unexpectedly discovered. These strict timelines are designed to keep us in compliance with the regulatory authorities. Failure to adhere to the reporting timelines required for regulatory authorities is evidence of negligence on the part of the sponsor. The sponsor monitor is responsible for assuring adherence to reporting systems for managing serious adverse events.

The sponsor monitor is responsible for the timely follow-up of all serious adverse events. The cases must be followed to completion. The monitor needs to collect all required follow-up information on ADEs.

To be successful, monitors need to be competent in:

- Basic medicine and therapeutics.
- Recognizing clinical signs and symptoms.
- Interpretation of laboratory findings.
- Medical practice, nomenclature, and terminology.
- Relevant regulatory requirements.
- Protocol requirements.

The sponsor needs to provide on-going review of safety data for investigational products.

Closing Down the Center

Closing down a study is important, because it may represent the sponsor's last and best chance to obtain the data required in the trial. The study close-down visit usually occurs after the last subject has completed the trial, including any post-treatment follow-up visits. Drug supplies should be reconciled and the integrity of the double-blind treatment codes should be confirmed. Any outstanding queries should be resolved and documented.

Arrangements for retaining source data should be confirmed with the investigator. In addition, the investigator should notify the IRB/IEC of the completion of the study. When the final draft of the clinical study report is available, it should be given to the investigator for signature. In multicenter trials, a single lead investigator may sign a pooled study report.

Reviewing, Editing and Verifying In-house Case Report Data and Databases

While the goal of monitoring is to provide complete and accurate ("clean") CRFs, it is necessary to review CRFs for consistency and unrecognized errors once they are received in-house. The use of computer edit and logic checks supports this effort, where computer output is verified against CRF data. Discrepancies are identified and CRF queries are generated for resolution.

The goal of managing CRFs is to get the data from the CRFs to a clean database in the fastest time possible, while maintaining the highest level of quality. To accomplish this task, CRFs must be ready for data entry at the site. CRFs must be cleaned on an ongoing basis during the study. To do this, efficient systems must be incorporated to simplify the query process. The approach used by some sponsors permits electronic exchange of CRF data between the investigator, monitor, and data entry personnel. Computerized checking programs and edit checks make the process more value-added for the monitors.

Clinical teams should design database before the trial begins, reduce the amount of data collected, use standardized CRFs, and complete the review process on an on-going basis. The philosophy is, 'Do it right, first time' at the source.

To be successful, staff must know how to prepare CRFs for data entry, be able to verify database consistency with original records and CRFs, and assure that queries are handled effectively.

Competencies Associated with Reporting Clinical Research

Preparing Clinical Study Reports

The requirements for reporting clinical trials to international regulatory authorities are similar in intent but differ in detail. Sponsors approach preparation of NDA/BLA documentation in a modular format. Each module satisfies a specific documentation need. The modules are generally organized as follows:

- *Module I.* Includes a basic summary of the study, not unlike a publication. It includes: study rationale, objectives, methods, results, and conclusions. Module I also has a large appendix, which includes: list of investigators; drug lot numbers; concomitant diseases and medications; intent-to-treat analysis; patient listings of adverse events and relevant laboratory abnormalities; and publications on the study.
- *Module II.* Includes the protocol and any modifications, case report form, detailed methodology, and the glossary of original terminology and preferred terms.
- *Module III.* Presents the detailed efficacy findings, including the intent-to-treat analysis population and the efficacy data listings.
- *Module IV.* Presents the detailed safety findings, including the intent-to-treat analysis population and the safety data listings.
- *Module V.* Includes individual center summary reports, quality assurance measures, statistical methods and analyses, and randomization lists.

The skills necessary to prepare a clinical study report include:

- Advanced research design, methodology, and statistics.
- Preparation and review of study tabulations.
- Ability to confirm that study tabulations conform to protocol design.
- Ability to verify study tabulations against computer data listings.

- Clarification of outstanding issues regarding data analysis and presentation.
- Drafting of assigned study report sections according to the clinical study report prototype.
- Interpretation of adverse events.
- Interpretation of laboratory findings.
- Interpretation of efficacy findings.
- Ensuring that data support the conclusions.
- Ensuring that reports satisfy regulatory requirements.
- Developing clear, simple graphs, tables, and figures to illustrate and support findings.
- Ability to write a clear, concise report that accurately summarizes and interprets the results.

Preparing Annual Safety Reports

Sponsors in the USA are required to submit annually to the FDA a summary of safety findings of investigational products. This involves verification of AE tabulations against computer data listings and the preparation of safety tables. The current findings are reviewed and compared with AE data from the past reporting period.

The sponsor's representatives must be able to clarify any outstanding issues regarding safety interpretation and presentation of the data. Since this information is of critical importance to the FDA, the annual report must be written in a clear, concise manner that accurately summarizes and interprets the safety results. The annual report should provide clear, simple graphs, tables, and figures to illustrate and support safety findings. Following the submission of the annual report, safety findings are usually integrated into an updated version of the IB.

To be able to prepare annual reports, the sponsor's representative should know how the reports satisfy FDA requirements and those of other regulatory authorities. The clinical representative should be able to interpret clinical safety and laboratory findings. The ability to understand computer-generated clinical output and the organization and structure of the NDA/BLA safety database is important.

The annual report and NDA/BLA safety update review and approval procedures must be understood as well as the procedures for the preparation of the IB.

Preparing Clinical Sections of NDA/BLA

The knowledge and skill needed to prepare an NDA/BLA/PLA includes the ability to:

- Verify individual study tabulations against overall summary computer listings.
- Prepare brief descriptions of the studies.
- Interpret critical clinical safety and efficacy results.
- Interpret laboratory findings.
- Develop clear tables and figures to illustrate and support clinical findings.
- Summarize, interpret, and integrate the overall safety and efficacy results.
- Prepare NDA/BLA clinical study summaries, benefit–risk summary, expert reports, and package insert.

In addition, an understanding of electronic NDA/BLAs (CANDA/BLAs) and EU/FDA data presentation requirements are useful.

The expert report usually generates considerable discussion within a project. The document is most often prepared by sponsor under the guidance of an external expert. Whilst internal experts are acceptable, it should be remembered that the regulatory authorities are looking for an individual who knows the drug thoroughly and can express an unbiased opinion of its medical importance. The expert report is not just a summary but a critical assessment of the clinical evaluation of the drug.

The expert report provides an independent assessment of the risk–benefit of the drug and its use. The text is limited to 25 pages, but may include an 'unlimited' number of attachments. Many companies have been creative in font size and two-sided preparation of the document.

Certain trends and directions can be recognized in the preparation of NDA/BLAs. The ICH has the long-term goal of harmonizing the content of European, US and Japanese NDA/BLAs. EU registration dossiers are becoming more detailed in the process and are expected to include integrated summaries in the future. The US FDA will accept more non-US data for drug approval as common high standards for clinical trials become well established in the world. Finally, electronic NDA/BLAs will be the norm and are already required in the USA.

REFERENCES

International Conference on Harmonization (1997) Good clinical practice: consolidated guideline. *Fed Reg* 62 (90).

International Conference on Harmonization (1997) Draft guideline on general considerations for clinical trials. *Fed Reg* 62 (104).

International Conference on Harmonization (1996) Guideline on the structure and content of clinical study reports. *Fed Reg* 61 (138).

CFR 21 (50, 56, 312, 314).

Spilker B (1991) *Guide to Clinical Trials*. Raven: New York.

Section II

Drug Discovery and Development

Introduction to Section II

Lionel D. Edwards[1] and Anthony W. Fox[2]

[1]Basking Ridge, NJ, and [2]EBD Group Inc, Carlsbad, CA, USA

This section of the book is concerned about the events that must take place in the conversion of a drug into a medicine that can be approved by regulatory authorities. It is important to know what does and does not comprise these events.

First, the chapters here may be regarded loosely as the premarketing phases of a successful drug's life cycle. This not congruent with the whole of drug development. What is needed to get a drug approved is not the same as what is needed to make that drug into a commercial success.

Second, the overall emphasis here is clinical development, how this is done, and what preclinical information is needed in order to carry it out. Necessarily, we have here had to be general, and these chapters are mostly written to describe, and assist with, typical development issues. However, for some disciplines, this is impossible; for example, there is little preclinical pharmacology in this section, since this discipline is really product-specific. In contrast, the general principles of toxicology (for example), and what the pharmaceutical physician needs to know about toxicology before starting any clinical trial, may be usefully stated in the general case.

Third, while some clinical developers erroneously view regulatory affairs as the implementation of their clinical development plans (and probably vice versa), the proper constraints imposed by regulatory authorities are so fundamental that they deserve a section to themselves (see Section III). However, we would emphasize that this division is artificial in comparison to how real drugs get developed, which requires intimate coordination of clinical development with regulatory compliance. Similarly, the financial and legal underpinnings of the drug development process are described in later sections of this book, but are constraints that constantly govern the thinking of the good pharmaceutical physician during clinical development.

Fourth, the chapters on Phase I clinical trials and pharmacoeconomic research have been written by experts in these fields. These are very rapidly-developing disciplines. The typical pharmaceutical physician has usually paid little attention to these aspects of clinical development, but it is our belief that these will dictate his/her clinical development plans to an ever-increasing degree in the future. Phase I studies can shorten overall clinical development time, and the pharmacoeconomic leveraging of (especially) Phase III and Phase IV studies (with preparatory Phase II work) are now essential in the modern competitive environment.

The integration of the activities described in these chapters is essential to good clinical development. Some cross-referencing and overlap between these chapters is deliberately included to emphasize such integration. Pharmaceutical physicians, specialized though they may be in one discipline or another, are well-advised to keep an observant eye on the interactions between their own and other company departments. Experience is probably the best teacher of integration. But we hope these chapters convey some idea.

4

Drug Discovery: Design and Serendipity

J. Leslie Molony

ProPharma Partners, Inc., Hayward CA USA

How is it that medicines are discovered? In ancient times, and even today, tribal peoples knew the healing or hallucinogenic properties of indigenous plants and animals. The knowledge was accumulated through generations, recorded by chant and living memory, and was derived largely from human experience. Although many of the drugs in use today were discovered by chance, most drug discovery scientists engage in directed research, based on a series of steps, each requiring substantial scientific input. While available facilities, resources, technology focus, or even corporate culture can define the procedures followed by researchers at particular institutions, there are some obvious, generally applicable milestones in this process leading to the discovery of therapeutics.

DESIGNING A DRUG DISCOVERY PROJECT

An outline of the thought processes involved in designing and implementing a Drug Discovery program is diagrammed in Figure 4.1. This chapter will discuss the process, and give practical examples from contemporary drug discovery scenarios.

All drug discovery projects depend on luck to be successful, but research and careful planning can improve chances of success and lower the cost. Project teams can streamline the discovery process by mapping the most direct methods that will yield a discovery. Using the tools available from modern biology, chemistry, robotics, and computer simulations, years can be eliminated from the search for new drugs. The costs of getting a new therapeutic into the marketplace in 1997 were estimated at $300–400 million and the average discovery and development time is still 7 years.

UNMET CLINICAL NEED

Usually, scientists are directed to research new targets in specific therapeutic areas based on unmet clinical needs. Once a need is identified and a particular therapeutic area chosen, the biological research begins. It is during this first stage of drug discovery that anecdotal clinical observations, empirical outcomes, and 'data' collected from folk medicine are often employed—if only as direction-finding tools.

Once a direction is chosen, it must be validated scientifically, within a defined biological system. Because human disease or pathology is usually multifactorial, the first task of the researcher is to narrow down the search to better defined mechanisms, preferably a small number of pathophysiologically observable processes, e.g. pinpointing one or two types of cells which can be considered causes of the pathology. From the cellular stage, the researcher next defines specific molecular targets, such as receptors or cellular enzymes that comprise the destructive phenotype.

Researchers will target systems which are affected by, or may be directly involved with, a particular disease. The treatments arising from these types of approaches can be palliative, or may find a market or need as disease-modifying drugs. Prime examples of palliative therapies are drugs designed to alleviate side effects of treatment with toxic chemotherapeutic drugs, such as nausea and wasting. In these cases, drug discovery scientists search for drugs which alleviate each symptom as if it were an isolated pathology.

Disease-modifying drugs are those which directly affect the primary disease. Examples of DMDs are the chemotherapeutic agents themselves, which destroy tumors by preventing their growth.

Principles and Practice of Pharmaceutical Medicine. Edited by A. J. Fletcher, Lionel D. Edwards, Anthony W. Fox and Peter Stonier © 2002 John Wiley & Sons Ltd.

CELLULAR MECHANISMS OF DISEASE

Drug discovery biologists and pharmacologists research and evaluate the physiological mechanisms of the disease to be addressed by a therapeutic substance. Initially, research takes the form of literature searches and intense reading. The first step of the biologists is to identify potential physiological, genetic or cellular mechanisms which could explain the pathological outcomes. In many cases, preliminary research has been published on several aspects of the pathology. It is then the task of the biologists to design and implement experiments which further define or eliminate potential drug targets.

This process can begin with the identification of a particular type of cell that can be used for cell biological, molecular and biochemical investigations. Is there an anomaly in a cell derived from a tumor, to use a cancer example, which renders that tumor cell unique from normal cells derived from the same tissue? If the difference is significant and can be reproducibly observed in the laboratory, it can be exploited for drug discovery. In other diseases, the cell which is identified can be normal, but activated to a destructive state by stimulation with disease pathogens. In rheumatoid arthritis, for example, the normal T lymphocyte is stimulated to react to antigens present in the joint, thus developing a destructive phenotype.

Once a target cell is identified and the pathological mechanism described, molecular targets can be evaluated. Modern drug discovery usually requires identification of a particular molecule whose function can be modified by a chemical substance. The choice of the molecular target is an important milestone in the drug discovery process.

MOLECULAR TARGET IDENTIFICATION

Combining Basic and Applied Research

Molecular target identification is critical to the discovery process. Often, the molecular targets are not obvious, although cellular and histological disease pathologies have been described in the literature. At this point, the researcher returns to the laboratory bench to design critical experiments.

Common types of target identification experiments involve raising monoclonal antibodies to proteins (receptors) on the surface of cells derived from diseased tissue, then screening the hybridoma supernatants for activity in preventing a cellular manifestation of the disease. Referring back to the cancer example, tumor cells often contain overexpressed, mutated, or absent 'oncogenes'. Oncogenes are proteins which regulate the signaling from a particular receptor in normal cells, but are mutated, and thus are constitutively active or constitutively inactive, in different tumor cells. They are known as 'oncogenes' because their modification is often the cause of the abnormal behavior of tumor cells. Examples of oncogenes are *RAS* and *SRC*. The normal *RAS* is known to regulate cellular division and link the nuclear changes to alterations in the cellular architecture required for mitosis (cytoskeleton and cell motility). *SRC* is known as a key signaling molecule which can affect cell growth by modulating the responses of the epidermal growth factor (EGF) receptor to its ligand. Many recent cancer drug discovery efforts in the cancer area have targeted *SRC, RAS* or the EGF receptor. The molecular targets chosen for these discovery efforts ranged from the EGF receptor itself, the EGF receptor enzymatic signaling activity, the SRC molecule itself or its enzymatic activity, or any of the enzymes which regulate key interactions in this signaling cascade. RAS inhibitor discovery projects have focused on the biological requirement that RAS be translocated from the cytosol to the membrane before its enzymatic activity is functional. Prevention of the enzymatic event which allows translocation of RAS to the plasma membrane in cancer cells will prevent activation of events mediated by RAS.

Other examples of molecular target identification can be derived from following some thought processes that a discovery scientist would follow to design a novel approach to treating inflammatory diseases. A cell or molecular biologist beginning a program in arthritis in 1997 would have access to literature from clinical trials of anti-TNF antibodies, and data describing transgenic mice which, when genetically engineered to cause monocytes to express constant levels of the cytokine (TNF), will develop arthritis. Also available would be large volumes of data on the cellular infiltrates in the inflamed joint: monocytes and T lymphocytes are the most prevalent, and data regarding the elevation in levels of other cytokines, such as IL-1β, and other mediators of inflammation, such as leukotrienes and phospholipases. After an exhaustive review of the recent literature, a drug discovery scientist might conclude that inhibitors of TNF receptors might provide a significant benefit to those with arthritis, and to those in the developmental stages of the disease. At that point, the scientists then decide which target to approach: the TNF receptor itself, the ligand TNF, the signal transduction enzymes regulating the function of the receptor or, perhaps, expression of TNF itself via regulating the TNF gene.

Hypothetically, because we also know that steroids, a currently used therapeutic, works by inhibition of gene expression of many of these mediators, it will probably be successful to target the gene transcription pathways leading to expression of TNF in the joint. However, other considerations exist. Are the transcription mechanisms known, and if so, are there any other required enzymes or proteins which are regulated by those same mechanisms? As it turns out, the mechanisms which regulate TNF transcription are common to pathways of inflammation, but are not common to proteins and enzymes required for cellular functions.

Because anti-TNF treatments and TNF-overexpressing transgenic mice have already been developed, it is known that TNF itself can cause destructive arthritis. Preventing TNF-receptor activation by using antibodies to TNF will prevent arthritis, and even reverse the destruction.

The investigators may seek the counsel of marketing experts and physicians regarding the use of the antibodies, and any clinical trial data available through the literature on the anti-TNF antibodies. These antibodies will be competing against any product which comes out of a TNF antagonist drug discovery program. Antibodies may present significant delivery problems because they are not orally bioavailable, i.e. they cannot be taken in pill form, but must be injected. Other problems associated with non-human antibodies result from elicitation of immune responses to antibodies themselves after several doses, thus limiting the number of times the antibody can be administered. The goal of the discovery group would be to discover a therapeutic with better properties than the existing antibodies, such as one that could be formulated into a pharmaceutical product, i.e., an orally bioavailable TNF antagonist.

The next question to be answered is what individual regulatory enzyme will be the most effective and most specific target. To answer this question, biochemists studying the transcription regulation of inflammatory mediators may be consulted. Literature on the subject is available. However, part of the goal of drug discovery researchers is to take a unique, less obvious angle. This involves exhaustive literature searches, attendance at meetings, and working with competitive intelligence teams to determine what approaches are being taken by the competition. Unless a company can work faster or better than the competition by taking a direct approach, it is, perhaps, a better strategy to approach the target identification issue less directly.

Each individual laboratory working on TNF as a therapeutic target is approaching the problem from a different direction. For example, one group may seek to inhibit transcription factor activation by phosphorylation or proteolysis, while another group seeks to inhibit the binding of the transcription regulatory complex to the DNA. Key decision points will be made when targets are cloned, and assays are set up for screening. Those assays which can be related directly to cellular events, which allow screening of the required number and type of chemical compounds, and which are predictive of *in vivo* responses, will be chosen for follow-up by the screening team. Other assays that are developed during this exploratory stage may be used as secondary screens, or will be used for validation of targets. Figure 4.2 generally outlines the process that has been developed in the scenario in this section. Target Identification requires further elaboration, and will be discussed next.

METHODS OF NEW TARGET IDENTIFICATION

The ideal molecular drug target is one which has been discovered in-house and is proprietary. Alternatively, a receptor or enzyme discovered by a researcher at a university, the cDNA of which is available for licensing by the drug company, could also provide an effective and proprietary target. These targets are often discovered serendipitously, or could be the result of extensive 'fishing expeditions' using protein biochemistry, immunology (antibody targeting), pharmacology, or molecular biology methods.

Cell and molecular biologists can identify a gene or genes responsible for the cellular variations seen in certain techniques employing subtractive cloning. Total mRNA from normal cells are compared with total mRNA from diseased or modified cells (called normalization). Usually, numerous genes are found to be modified or alternatively expressed, and the mRNA will be detected in the hybridization reactions. The real work comes in sequencing and identifying these genes, and ascertaining which are the unknown, novel sequences. Regarding the newly discovered genes, e.g. potential causes of cell transformation into cancerous tissue, many biochemical and cell biological experiments will be required to determine the function of the protein coded for by the new gene.

Another method of target identification is to raise monoclonal antibodies to cell-surface receptors derived from a cell suspected to be involved in the pathology targeted. Antibodies then identified by FACS (fluorescence activated cell sorting, or labeling techniques) as binding to the target cell are then used in functional assays to prevent a response thought to be critical for disease development. If an antibody can inhibit this response, the antibody is then used by protein biochemists to isolate the culpable receptor.

Genomics and New Target Identification

Drug companies have recently become involved in the use of genomics to identify new genes which might have some role in disease pathology. Molecular biologists can seek mutations or alterations in genetic signatures which are predictive of the targeted disease in a large population. If this mutation is always associated with the disease, they can then map this gene to the disease. This is known as 'linkage analysis'. When linkage analysis can predict that a disease-regulatory gene falls within a certain region of a chromosome bounded by other known genes, scientists can determine the genetic sequence of the causative gene. This process is known as 'positional cloning' because the cloning begins and ends at certain chromosomal locations. Positional cloning, coupled with global epidemi-

ological studies and linkage analysis, will provide molecular targets for the few diseases which are derived from hereditary alterations in the human genome, often the result of inbreeding in isolated populations. An example of new target identification using these methods was the identification of ApoE as an important causative factor in Alzheimer's disease (Pericak-Vance et al 1991).

The pharmaceutical industry can further exploit this genomic technology by choosing specific diseases, performing epidemiological research to find families with patterns of hereditary disease, and mapping the transmission of the disease to find the specific genes that cause the pathology. Genes are then identified using positional cloning.

However, other researchers are not closing in on suspected mutations, but identifying all the genes expressed by human cells, and then sequencing short segments of each one. These 'expressed sequence tags' (ESTs) can then used as starting points to derive full-length cDNA for a newly identified gene.

Genomics may, with the completion of the Human Genome Project, become a mainstay of new target identification for drug discovery. The Human Genome Project is a consortium of government and industry-funded laboratories, which sequenced the entire human genome using both EST and positional cloning methods. This project identified and sequenced all of the estimated 60,000 to 30 000–100 000 human genes (3 billion nucleotides) by the year 2001.

At the time of writing complete genomic sequences are available for atleast 141 viruses, 51 organelles, two eubacteria, one eukaryote and most mammalian mitochondria. Several organisms for which complete genome data are available include *Haemophilus influenzae, Mycoplasma genetalium*, and *Saccharomyces cervisiae*. The volume of this information may be illustrated by almost the simplest case: the yeast, *S. cerevisiae* contains approximately 6000 genes (Schuler et al 1999), the sequences of which are available to scientists at FTP sites on the internet. It is expected that by maps for the common bacteria *E. coli* and *B. subtilis*, and the *C. elegans* will also be complete and soon publicly available.

The sequencing of unknown genes will not directly identify new molecular targets for disease. However, the availability of sequences will permit rapid identification of genes once a target protein is identified, without having to sequence more than a few peptides of the protein. The access to gene sequence information should shave months off of the discovery process, allowing rapid cloning of new targets for assay development.

Genomics and epidemiology will identify genes that are altered or mutated in certain diseases. However, this molecular biological breakthrough will not permit the mapping of a function to the genes. That task is assigned to the cell biologists, who will have to study basic cellular mechanisms with normal and diseased genes, or study transgenic animals expressing the disease-specific gene in certain tissues, before a function can be attributed to the newly identified gene.

Yet another group of biotechnology companies is exploiting this niche, to provide 'functional genomics' services which allow identification of biological functions associated with their clients' newly-identified disease genes. Functional genomics takes advantage of cell or developmental biology, and measures the effects of modified vs. normal gene sequences in functional assays. These functional assays are not, themselves, drug screens. They are methods of validating new targets, which must then be developed further for the discovery of drugs.

Physiological Systems

Drug discovery scientists must bear in mind what the broader effects of inhibiting, modifying, or eliminating this new target would be on the organism. The perfect target is organ-, tissue- or cell-specific, thereby limiting effects to the system involved in the disease. The choice of a target for a disease will be critical to the outcome and performance of the drug, and will determine what organs or tissues will be susceptible to side effects.

CRITICAL IMPORTANCE OF *IN SITU* AND *IN VIVO* STUDIES

Pharmacologists are often able to develop tissue and whole animal models of human disease. In some instances, studies on isolated tissues, such as blood vessels, heart muscle or brain slices, will allow a tissue or organ-specific understanding of the effects of potential new drugs. Cardiovascular pharmacologists often study isolated arteries, which are maintained in a physiological salt solution. Electric stimulation can induce contraction of the vascular smooth muscle, and the effects of hypertensive drugs on vascular contraction can then be measured. Historically, these systems were often used as primary drug screening tools. Because these methods are much less direct than molecular screening, they are now relegated to secondary or tertiary roles as validation of the targets or drugs discovered.

Transgenic Technology

Recently, the pharmaceutical industry has adopted transgenic technology, allowing researchers to engineer rats and mice whose physiology mimics a disease on a molecular and tissue-specific level. Transgenic animals are used in the pharmaceutical industry for two major purposes: target validation and protein expression. The expression of recombinant proteins in large quantities by genetically engineered animals is a common method of obtaining recombinant proteins or enzymes to be used as therapeutics or nutritional supplements. Sheep, goats, and cattle have been engineered to produce recombinant proteins in their milk, for example. These types of transgenic animals will not be discussed here.

In the pharmaceutical industry, as in basic research, the cause of a disease can be identified by introducing a suspect gene into the genome of a rodent. This technology utilizes the plasticity of the embryonic stem cells derived from fertilized ova. Embryos are removed at the 4–8 cell-stage, micro-injected or transfected with a plasmid containing the gene to be expressed, probably engineered to be dependent upon a promoter which limits expression to specific organs or tissues, and engineered to confer upon those ES cells carrying the plasmid resistance to the selectable marker. After selection of the population, genetically altered embryonic stem cells are grown to the 6–8 cell stage and placed *in utero*. The resultant rodents will express the introduced gene if the plasmid was incorporated into the host DNA. Using this method, researchers can then determine if an overabundance or restriction of a specific factor will result in a disease, or will prevent one.

In contrast, the 'knockout mouse' was engineered to determine the functions of unknown genes. The test gene is targeted for deletion in the mouse embryo, and its DNA is replaced with plasmid containing a disrupted gene which cannot be expressed, and a marker gene which confers resistance. After positive selection, embryos are then reintroduced into mothers and carried to term. However, in most cases, homozygous knockout mice (mice which lack the gene in both sets of chromosomes) develop abnormalities that are incompatible with life beyond an early embryonic stage. In some cases, however, the knockout mouse which lacks specific genes, thus does not express the resultant receptor or enzyme, and will give unique insight into the function of the previously unknown gene.

Spontaneously Arising Phenotypic Models

Mutations which cause disease can arise spontaneously. Genetic mapping methods utilizing positional cloning can help identify disease-causative genes and their proteins in animals which have spontaneously developed diseases similar to those of humans. An example of this type of technology is the *ob/ob* genetic mouse, which is obese, and has mutations in a gene for a peptide hormone known as leptin. This mouse, and its counterpart the *db/db* mouse, which has mutations in the leptin receptor, can be used as animal models for obesity. A similar mouse, the Agouti strain, is also obese and has defects in melanocortin receptors, which regulate hair color as well as appetite, and the expression or release of leptin by adipose tissue. The Agouti mouse develops type II diabetes, and therefore can be used as an animal model of that disease in humans. Of course, human disease is rarely as simple as a single genetic misread, so these models must be used with some caution when testing drugs or when identifying the causative genes.

In Vivo Models of Disease

Human pathology is inevitably more complex than those of rats and mice. Thus, it is often necessary to induce a pathological state by introduction of a pathogen or stimulant directly into a healthy animal.

Whether the disease is induced endogenously (genetically) or exogenously by manipulation or administration of a disease-producing agent, the development of new animal models is a time-consuming process. Pharmaceutical researchers are supervised by veterinary medical doctors, and by committees which review the protocols to be used. These veterinary professionals and committees oversee the issues related to humane use, as well as updating researchers on more efficient methods which might allow reduction in the number of animals used.

Why are *in vivo* (whole animal) studies still important to drug discovery? While new technologies are becoming available to develop computer-generated models of whole organisms, this has not eliminated the need for animal use. Until reliable computer models accurately predict the effect of each chemical compound on the cell, the tissue and the organism as a whole, physiological studies will remain critical. New chemical or biological therapeutics are often broad-acting, affecting perhaps unrelated physiological systems. The effects of new compounds on one system may negate or enhance its therapeutic effect, thereby eliminating or identifying a drug discovery lead candidate. In addition, results from testing novel drugs in historical animal models of disease are often required by regulatory agencies prior to allowing testing in humans.

TARGET VALIDATION

The next logical step, once a molecular target has been identified, is the validation of the molecular target and the evaluation of this target for possible effects in other systems. This stage of the project may involve developing antibodies which inhibit actions of the target molecule, and testing these antibodies in animal models of disease. In experimental systems where a receptor is expressed in the mouse or rat, and its elimination will not be fatal, the genetic knockout technology can be employed.

There may be fortunate scenarios where drugs, often developed for other uses, have broad-acting effects which include preventing a newly identified molecular interaction causing a known pathology. This drug, while not an ideal candidate to treat the pathological state, may be used as a positive control for *in vitro* and *in vivo* assay validation. Alternatively, antibodies which inhibit the function of a targeted receptor or ligand may be used *in vivo* to evaluate the pharmacological and physiological effects of inhibiting that particular interaction.

If the outcome of target validation experiments is promising, drug screens will be established to identify new chemical entities which will serve as specific therapeutics in place of antibodies or the broader-acting drugs. Usually, these target validation models will be used to validate the drug screening assays as they are developed, and can be used as decision-making points for any new drugs identified using the *in vitro* assays.

IN VITRO ASSAY DEVELOPMENT

An assay, or screen, is the primary tool used to integrate a biological system with chemical compounds that will become drugs. Assays are experimental systems which allow rapid and reproducible measurements of the effects of chemicals on the molecular target. These can take many forms, from whole cell-based assays to one-enzyme colorometric-readout assays. Critical components of any assay system are the availability of positive and negative controls, and quality control parameters obtained from experimenting with multiple possible parameters. Assays or screens are, in themselves, experimental systems, therefore good scientific method must be applied. Data generated by screens must meet criteria of statistical significance. A drug screening decision tree is diagrammed in Figure 4.3. The importance of those decision points is described further in this section.

Technological Considerations

Assay development for drug screening requires the creative flexibility to integrate the assay or assays into existing technology. Prior to the technological breakthroughs resulting in robotic high throughput screening and combinatorial chemistry, most drug screening was performed manually. These assays were competitive, because drug companies had limited numbers of proprietary substances in their libraries, and medicinal chemists were limited in the number of new chemical entities they could design and synthesize manually.

For example, a biotechnology division has established a novel high-throughput robotics system which is integrated with data analysis and data storage computers. There are usually limits to the types of assays that can be run using this integrated technology. If, for example, a novel assay has been developed using measurements of fluorescently labeled cells flowing through a detector (FACS), the equipment must be redesigned or the assay must be modified to use existing technology—a fluorescent plate reader using a 96-well format, for example. In smaller, more technology-driven companies, assay developers will construct their assays specifically to make use of certain proprietary platforms, e.g. some companies use proprietary cell lines and cell-based screening, while others use robotics and high throughput screening, but restrict their targets to certain classes of molecules, such as 7 transmembrane domain G-protein linked receptors.

Primary vs. Secondary Screens

The keys to a successful drug discovery program are the assays used to evaluate chemical or biological compounds. Assays will be prioritized based on several scientific considerations. If the chosen target is a receptor whose ligand is known, and we are seeking a drug which will inhibit the receptor from binding to its ligand, a simple receptor/ligand screen may be established. If the target is a signal transduction enzyme which modifies another intracellular protein, an enzyme-substrate screen can be established using a simple colorimetric readout. These are often designed to be primary, or first round, screens.

Before any novel chemical entities are screened in the primary assay, known compounds and controls from many classes of drugs, known as pharmacophores, are often tested in the assay. This will provide a set of controls, both negative and positive, for developing new compounds based on chemical structures. Pharmacophores are often

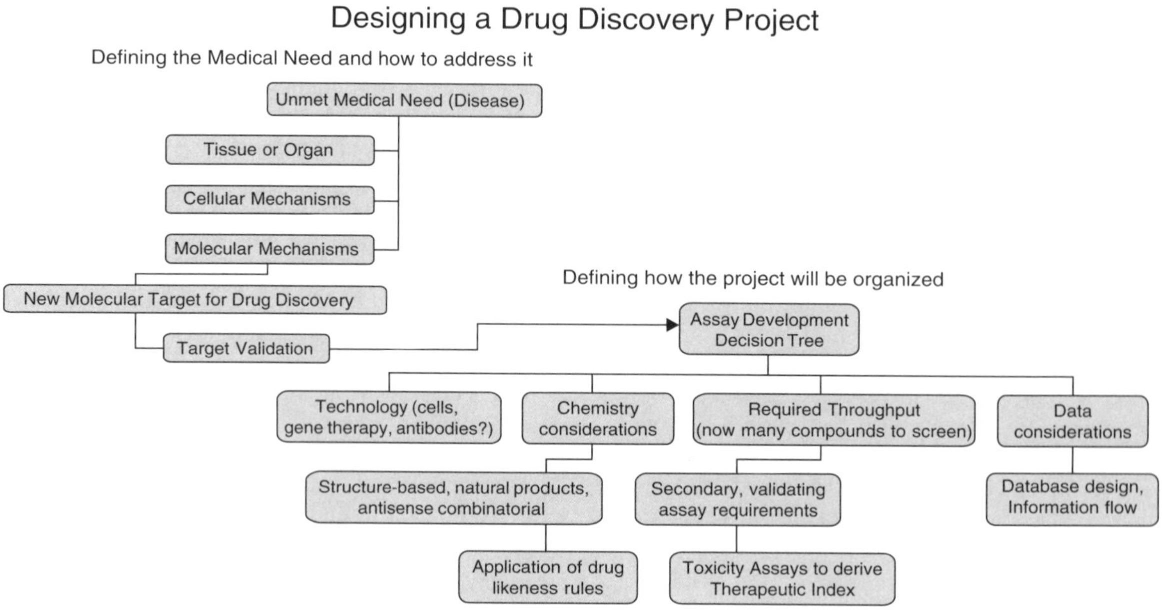

Designing a Drug Discovery Project
Defining the Medical Need and how to address it
Unmet Medical Need (Disease)
Tissue or Organ
Cellular Mechanisms
Molecular Mechanisms
New Molecular Target for Drug Discovery
Target Validation
Defining how the project will be organized
Assay Development Decision Tree
Technology (cells, gene therapy, antibodies?)
Chemistry considerations
Required Throughput (now many compounds to screen)
Data considerations
Structure-based, natural products, antisense combinatorial
Secondary, validating assay requirements
Database design, Information flow
Application of drug likeness rules
Toxicity Assays to derive Therapeutic Index

Figure 4.1 The drug discovery process

Clinical need = therapeutic target
Physiological target, system or organ
Cellular target
Molecular target
Drug discovery

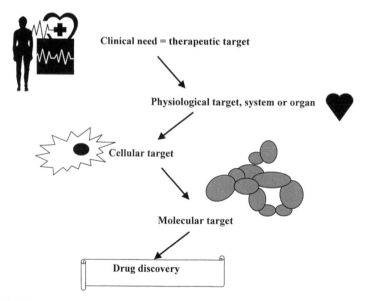

Figure 4.2 Target identification

used to find chemical backbones with some activity. These backbones can then be optimized using rational design or methodical medicinal chemistry. Often, antibodies are used as controls because no existing chemical inhibits the interaction.

Most primary assays are used in high-throughput screening systems, and can be adapted for use with robotics. The assay should then be highly reproducible, and contain both negative and positive controls. Because the reagents used for assays

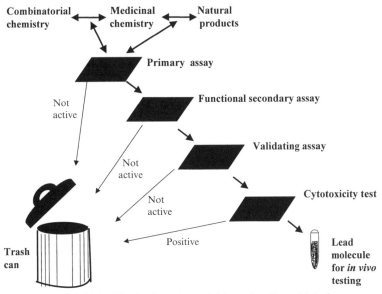

Figure 4.3 Drug screening flowchart

may present some variability, quality control parameters are often used to validate reagents before employing them in screens.

Primary assays are used for the first round of testing drugs which may or may not have activity. It is important that secondary, or validation, assays be established. These secondary screens will allow a second criterion (or more) for accepting a compound as active. These assays are often related to the primary assay, but contain more of the entire cellular system. Often, secondary assays utilize live cells in which the enzyme and/or receptor are crucial for a specific cellular response.

Secondary assays can also be used to evaluate a molecular interaction which the researcher does, or does not, want to inhibit with a drug. This can select for compounds that are more specific. Examples where 'elimination' type of assays are used are receptor systems which have very similar structures but have unique functions. G-protein-coupled receptors, such as the β-adrenergic or serotonin receptors, have similar structures but quite different functions. In these and many other examples, specificity can be engineered into the discovery process by the addition of secondary screens. Compounds that are active against any

receptors other than the target would be eliminated. In most cases, the drugs will have broad activity at very high doses, but will be quite specific at pharmacological doses.

In addition to evaluating and validating *in vitro* activity of a new compound, the drug discovery program must validate that newly discovered chemicals are not toxic. Cytotoxicity assays are usually included in a drug discovery flow chart. Drugs which have good activity in the *in vitro* assays, but are cytotoxic, may prove difficult to develop further. Often, medicinal chemists can modify them to eliminate the toxic side effects. Once the toxic effects are "engineered away," the active compounds can then be tested in animals.

Considerations Regarding Specific Types of Compounds

The four major sources of starting material for drug screens are chemical libraries, natural products, specifically designed medicinal chemistry-derived drugs—often modified and synthesized using directed combinatorial chemistry—and computationally designed drugs.

Large pharmaceutical companies often have their own libraries of compounds, collected after decades of manual synthetic chemistry, which are used as starting points for random screening. In addition to these proprietary compounds, test compounds can be obtained commercially and are derived from the Fine Chemical Database. Usually, these chemicals are organic—only partially soluble in water. The amount of organic solvent required to solubilize the chemical will often determine whether or not it can be evaluated in an aqueous-based assay. Random screening of broad compound collections or mixtures of natural products is a common method of seeking new chemical leads.

For companies which do not use large compound collections or sources of natural products, combinatorial chemistry and molecular modeling are both used to discover leads. Medicinal chemists use "drug-likeness" rules, or physical properties of the starting components, to define what types of chemicals are tested and progressed through development. These rules, developed by C.A. Lipinski at Pfizer, provide guidelines to assist with selection of compounds that possess physical properties re similar to existing drugs.

Considerations Regarding Throughput and Assay Cycles

There are four basic types of classical assays: receptor/ligand assays, enzyme/substrate assays, antibody/antigen assays, and cell-based assays, which use live cells and measure a cellular response. Assays which measure the association of two molecules are the simplest types of assays to develop, because the binding reaction can be followed by radioactivity or colorimetric or fluorescent readouts. There are several technical developments which reduce or eliminate the need for radioactivity.

Classical receptor/ligand assays measure the binding of a radio-labeled ligand to its receptor. The type of radioactivity will depend on factors such as the structure of the ligand, the affinity of the binding reaction, and environmental factors such as disposal of radioactive waste. ^{125}I, ^{3}H, ^{35}S, ^{32}P and, infrequently, ^{14}C, have been used for receptor/ligand screening. Briefly, the assay measures the binding of a known amount of radio-

active ligand to a known amount of receptor. Receptors can be presented as components of a membrane preparation, or can be purified from natural or recombinant sources. Ligands can be either purified natural or recombinant ones, or can be prepared from synthetic ligands, such as peptide sequences or drugs known to bind to the receptor. There are numerous formats available for assay set-up, such as filters, multiwell plates, or beads, to which the receptor is bound. Radiolabelled ligand is incubated with the receptor in the presence of test compounds. Unbound material is removed by washing plates or filtering wash solutions through filters, then radioactivity is quantified, either in solution, using scintillation counters, or using the filter format and scintillation counters made to detect radioactivity in that format.

An assay technology which combines radioactivity with bead technology is known as the scintillation proximity assay (SPA) system, which works by binding a receptor to a bead which contains a scintillant. Membrane preparations or purified receptors are linked to beads, often using wheat-germ agglutinin lectin. The receptor–bead complex is then incubated in a solution containing radioactively labeled ligand. When ligand binds, radioactivity is in proximity to the scintillant, and thus stimulates a response. If the ligand is inhibited from binding, no response is observed. This technology is also effective for enzymatic assays, in which the radioactively labeled substrate is bound to the bead and is then cleaved, removing the radiation and the signal if the enzyme is active. In this case, however, a positive signal indicates inhibition of the enzyme. For SPA assays, the readout is quantified using a scintillation counter that can measure filters or multiwell plates. The SPA screening format is often used for high-throughput screening, since it is easily scaled up.

ELISAs (enzyme-linked immunoabsorbent assays) are another common framework used for drug screening. An enzyme-linked-antibody takes the place of a ligand, whose receptor is bound to a plate or filter. The mixture of drug and enzyme-linked antibody is incubated in the well with the receptor. After a series of washes to remove unbound material, the substrate for the enzyme is added to the well. A common enzyme/substrate pair is alkaline phosphatase and pNPP (*p*-nitrophenyl phosphate), which results in a yellow color. Another enzyme commonly used is horseradish peroxidase (HRP). Substrates for HRP include 2,2′-azino-bis(3-ethylbenzthiazoline-6-sulfonic acid (ABTS: green), tetramethylbenzidine (blue), and o-dianisidine (yellow-orange).

Signal transduction enzymes such as tyrosine kinases can be assayed in high-throughput screens. These screens often measure the binding of a substrate, either the ATP at that binding site, or a more specific site where the enzyme recognizes its substrate and transfers the phosphate. In these assays, a synthetic peptide substrate is often synthesized. To detect whether or not the substrate has bound, one can use either ^{32}PATP or enzyme-linked antibodies recognizing the phosphorylated amino acid. Some assays are designed for fluorescence or luminescence readouts using probes with those properties.

Recombinant vs. Natural Proteins

Molecular target enzymes or receptors must be highly purified, and must be obtained in sufficient quantities and with consistent activities. Proteins used in assays may be derived from recombinant expression systems or from natural sources. The choice will be made according to the amount of material needed and the ease of extraction from the source. Usually, recombinant proteins are over-expressed in bacterial, yeast insect or mammalian systems, resulting in much greater yields of pure protein per gram of starting material than can be obtained from natural tissues. Care must be taken to normalize the activity or binding affinities for each preparation, requiring biochemical quality control monitoring That will permit comparison between assays run, and thus relative activities of compounds tested, using different batches of target protein.

Cell-based Assays

A more direct method of screening compounds for cellular activity, while simultaneously determining that the compound can access the receptor or enzyme in its cellular environment, is by assaying the effects of drugs on whole cells. This type of assay will eliminate at least one step in the process of drug screening, since all drugs will eventually have to be tested with whole cells. However, because there are multiple cellular systems that could be affected, it becomes more difficult to define a mechanism of action for a compound discovered using a cell-based assay.

The Drug Screening Process

Once assays are developed and characterized and sources of new compounds chosen, the screening process begins. This is the most routine and least creative task of drug discovery. At the same time, the more efficient the screening process, the more likely it will be to discover new chemical entities that have therapeutic value. Screening can be performed manually or can be totally automated; most screening groups are somewhere in the middle of that spectrum. Often, drugs are weighed out by hand and put into solution, then loaded into liquid sample handlers for dilution and delivery. Robots can also be used to set up 96-well plates to which receptors are bound, or cells attached. Depending upon the format of the assay, the screening and data collection process may also be performed automatically.

Spectrophotometric devices, called microplate readers, collect raw data resulting from colorimetric or fluorescent screens. Similarly, scintillation devices measure the amount of radioactivity in samples from drug screens. The computer format of the data will then allow it to be exported into a spreadsheet or statistical analysis computer program for analysis.

First-round screens based on random compounds or natural products are usually performed by testing one concentration of a new compound or natural product mixture. In some cases, the test is done in duplicate or triplicate, depending on factors such as space and time. Active compounds are then titrated for dose–response analysis. If a dose–response is observed, the active compounds are tested in the secondary assays, and tested for toxicity. Once a compound has proven active, not cytotoxic (if required), and dose–responsive, it can be analoged using combinatorial chemistry or medicinal chemistry methods. Small modifications in the side chains of active molecules will be produced, and these modified compounds tested in the assays.

Chemical structure modifications which enhance activity and refine specificity will be followed up using medicinal chemistry methods, relating structures of compounds to activity in certain assays. These exercises will result in the definition of a quantitative structure–activity relationship (SAR) for the series of compounds active in the assays.

The development of quantitative structure–activity relationships (QSARs) is made more efficient by the use of computer databases into which are integrated chemical structures. Compounds synthesized for other discovery programs can be related to activities from new assays to help researchers build specificity and activity profiles for novel drugs.

The screening process itself can take between 2 weeks and over a year, depending upon the throughput available. The most rapid technology screened 10 000 compounds or more each week. At that rate, new assays can be cycled through screening rapidly for lead identification. New technology is being developed which will increase that screening potential to 100 000 compounds/month. Therefore, screening of one molecular target with a large collection of compounds will take on the order of a few weeks. Optimization and QSAR analyses for 'hits' can be performed using the manual screening methods, or robotic screens with lower throughput ranges.

Sources of New Chemical Entities

Existing Drugs

Chemical diversity is a critical variable in drug discovery. To obtain diversity, chemists have turned to natural products, have used random screening of broad chemical collections such as the Fine Chemical Directory and their corporations' own chemical directories, and have developed methods of combinatorial chemistry to deliver more compounds. Random screening is performed when there are no starting points—no peptide or natural product leads, and no drugs known to bind to the receptor or enzyme target.

Medicinal chemists often begin by finding a chemical structure, either from a previous patent or literature report, that is an antagonist or agonist of a receptor target. They can design compounds with similar charge distributions, but with unique structural features, that can be considered new chemical entities (NCEs). This traditional medicinal chemistry represents the scientific basis of many pharmaceutical breakthroughs in the last several decades. Novel methods for discovery or identification of NCEs from computer-generated models were not developed until the 1980s.

Because random screens will generate leads with quite varied structures, chemists then turn to computer analyses to help them narrow down the most critical chemical components of a potential new drug. Many statistical and analytical programs are available.

Once a significant number of structures is obtained, chemists can employ QSARs to map chemical structures with the most desirable activities. These algorithms can also be used to eliminate undesirable activities, such as cytotoxicity or lack of specificity. QSAR analysis is a very powerful tool in drug discovery. These methods have significantly reduced the number of compounds a chemist must synthesize, by directing and focusing chemical efforts.

Designing Novel Drugs

Computer-assisted design (CAD) of drugs is a similar method of making use of the structural attributes of the receptor or enzyme target. Using data obtained from X-ray diffraction of crystalline arrays of the receptor (usually bound to a ligand or antibody), the computational chemist can construct a three-dimensional model of the target, complete with charge distributions and conformational variations. This model can then be used to predict which chemical structures will have the desired properties to fit into the active sites on the molecule. One biotechnology company that has been successful using this CAD method is Agouron Pharmaceuticals, Inc. in San Diego (Now a division of Pfizer, Inc.) California. Interested readers should refer to work performed by Agouron, and to reviews of CAD provided in the reference list.

Pharmacognosy is not yet a redundant source of molecules. The Pacific Yew has recently yielded the lead for successful therapies for ovarian cancer. One large pharmaceutical company has recently concluded an agreement with a Central American country to preserve its entire flora and give that company exclusive rights to any pharmacophores within it.

Combinatorial Chemistry. The breakthroughs in technology that have allowed sequencing of genes 'on a chip' and high throughput screening of compounds in microtiter plate format have also caused a revolution in chemical synthesis, known as combinatorial chemistry.

Biological Therapeutics. The chapter on biotechnology drugs enlarges on this subject in more detail, but suffice it to say here that vaccines, antibodies, proteins, peptides, and gene therapies all now exist. These biological drugs bring with them specific, regulatory, clinical trials and manufacturing difficulties. Gene therapy, in particular, carries human safety risks that do not apply to other classes of therapy, e.g. the infective nature of some types of vector that are employed, and the potential for incorporation of the test genetic material into the genome in males, leading to expression of gene products in offspring.

New Uses for Old Drugs. Lastly, opportunities still exist for astute clinicians to find new uses for old drugs, and for these newly-discovered uses to lead to new and unexpected drugs. The recent approval of bupropion as a smoking cessation agent is a good example of a chance observation while the drug was being used for its initial indication, which was as an antidepressant. This has led to realization of the influence of nicotine on depression, and investigational drugs of a new class, based on this alkaloid molecule, are now being designed.

SUMMARY

This chapter began with a survey of the modern methods of drug discovery. Figure 4.4 describes the relationship between screening of compounds, chemical modifications, drug formulations (pharmaceutics), preclinical testing, and clinical trials. Pharmaceutical physicians should be aware of some of the techniques employed and the rapid rate at which genetic information is becoming available. It should be noted that this modern revolution has not quite completely swept away

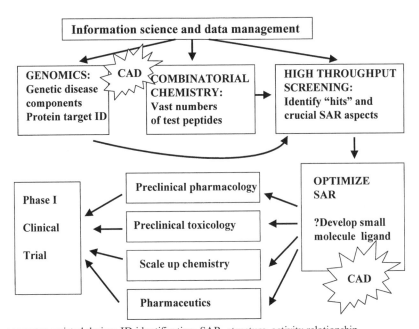

Figure 4.4   CAD, computer-assisted design; ID identification; SAR, structure–activity relationship

the occasional new drug found by serendipidity or astute clinical observation.

As the human genomic map has been deciphered, and target discovery streamlined, the decision-making process now involves additional hurdles. There is a wealth of newly identified molecules available from the genome project, and few novel methods to effectively sort them into "druggable" targets. And, the discovery methods for identifying new, novel chemical backbones with drug-like properties are still being developed.

One thing to note is that the field has moved on since the genome has been sequenced. Chemistry is still the rate-limiting step. In other words, new chemical structures that have unique activities are still hard to come by.

REFERENCES

Amersham Life Science (1993) Brochure on scintillation *Drug Discovery* proximity assays. Publication No. S 593/657/4/93/09. Amersham International:

Beeley LJ, Duckworth DM (1996) The impact of genomics on drug design. *Drug Discovery Today* 1(11): 474–80.

Chapman D (1996) The measurement of molecular diversity: a three dimensional approach. *J Computer-Aided Mol Design* 10: 501–12.

Goffeau A et al (1996) Life with 6000 Genes. *Science* 274: 546–67.

Kozlowski MR (1996) Problem solving in laboratory automation. *Drug Discovery Today* 1(11): 481–8.

Lipinski CA et al (1997) Experimental and Computational approaches to estimate solubility and permeability in drug discovery and development settings. Advanced Drug Deliv. Rev. 23: 3–29.

Lipper RA (1999) How can we optimize selection of drug development candidates from many compounds at the discovery stage? Modern Drug Discovery 2(1): 55–60.

Pericak-Vance MA, Bebout JL, Gaskell PC et al (1991) Linkage studies in familial Alzheimer disease: evidence for chromosome 19 linkage. *Am J Hum Genet* 48: 1034–1050.

Schuler GD et al (1996) A gene map of the human genome. *Science* 274: 540–46.

Van Drie JH (1997) Strategies for the determination of pharmacophoric 3D database queries. *J Computer-Aided Mol Design* 11: 39–52.

Wainer IW (1993) Stereoisomers in clinical oncology: why it is important to know what the right and left hands are doing. Ann Oncol 4 (Supp 2): 7–13.

5

Pharmaceutics

Anthony W. Fox

EBD Group Inc., Carlsbad, CA, USA

It is a triumph of modern pharmaceutics that most physicians think, both when conducting clinical research and in ordinary clinical practice, that 'a drug is a drug is a drug'. The typical pharmaceutical physician never makes a pharmaceutical (or galenical) drug formulation. Nevertheless, understanding at least some elements of this science is important because:

- A suitable formulation permits the conduct of clinical trials.
- Formulations constrain clinical trial design, e.g. whether a well-matched placebo is likely to be available, or whether special procedures to mask an infused, colored solution might be needed.
- Packaged white powders are probably not marketable, and overcoming galenical problems is a *sine qua non* for product feasibility.
- Formulation can strongly influence patient acceptability and thus probability of commercial success.
- Product storage and stability (or lack thereof) can bias clinical trials results.

For all these reasons and more, marketing and clinical input on suitable formulations should be included in the earliest considerations of project feasibility, and it behooves the pharmaceutical physician to be able to provide such input in an informed manner. Equally, the pharmaceutical physician should understand the constraints and difficulties that his colleagues work under, even though the physician is not him/herself qualified for a position in the company's pharmaceutics department. At the end of the day, product licences are awarded and new drug applications (NDAs) are typically approved after the resolution of at least as many questions about 'chemistry and manufacturing' (for which read 'pharmaceutics') as about clinical efficacy and safety.

THE CONSTITUENTS OF A MEDICINE

'A drug is not a drug is not a drug' because, when administered to a human being, in the general case, it contains:

- Active compound at a dose within a limited range, sometimes as a racemic mixture.
- Manufacturing impurities.
- One or more excipients.
- Degradants of the active compound.
- Degradants of the impurities.
- Degradants of the excipients.

An *impurity* is defined as a compound which is the by-product of the manufacturing process used for the active compound, and which is not removed prior to formulation. Impurities can have their own toxic potential, and control of impurity content is therefore a highly important feature in any New Drug Application (NDA). An *excipient* is defined as a material that is incorporated into the formulation to aid some physicochemical process, e.g. tablet integrity, dissolution, or taste; excipients are typically chosen from among many compounds without pharmacological properties (e.g. lactose), although there are examples where pharmacokinetics change with the excipient used. There are specialized examples of excipients; e.g. *propellants* are excipients that assist in the delivery of inhaled drugs to the respiratory tract. A *degradant* is defined as a compound that accumulates during the storage of bulk drug or finished formulation.

Principles and Practice of Pharmaceutical Medicine. Edited by A. J. Fletcher, Lionel D. Edwards, Anthony W. Fox and Peter Stonier © 2002 John Wiley & Sons Ltd.

Not even this list, however, comprehensively describes a formulation. Many tablets carry printed identification markings or are color-coated; dyestuffs are outside the definition of an excipient, and allergies to them have been documented. Differential efficacy exists among differently colored placebos, and this should therefore also be expected for active formulations. Furthermore, formulations have more subtle but nonetheless differential characteristics, such as whether the tablet was compressed at a higher or lower pressure.

THE FORMULATION CHOICE

Clearly, the formulation chosen for particular drugs is not random. Furthermore, the degree to which it is critical varies from drug to drug. For example, hydrocortisone is available for at least seven routes of administration, as tablets, several creams and ointments, intraocular solutions, suppositories, intra-rectal foams, injections, and eardrops. Even newer drugs, with fewer indications than hydrocortisone, seek greater market acceptability by providing a variety of alternative formulations (e.g. sumatriptan is available as an injection, intranasal spray, suppository, and tablets).

One commonly-used principle is to target drug delivery to the organ where beneficial effects are likely to occur. This can achieve:

- Relatively fast onset of effect.
- Locally high drug concentrations.
- Relatively low systemic drug concentration, avoiding toxicity.

Probably the most common applications of this principle are the administration of β-adrenergic agonists bronchodilators by inhalation, and the use of topical hydrocortisone creams.

Impurities and degradants may possess their own toxicological properties. Early in development, the structures of these impurities and degradants may be poorly characterized. Typically, both bulk drug and finished product become more refined as clinical development proceeds. Thus, in order to preclude any new toxicology problems developing later during clinical development, it is common practice to use the least pure bulk drug for toxicology studies. This is commonly accomplished by using drug removed from the production process before the last step, for example, before the last recrystallization. This usually guarantees that a lower purity, i.e. mixture with greater molecular diversity than the drug of interest, will be tested toxicologically than that to which patients will actually be exposed.

The evasion of formulation and toxicological testing by 'herbal medicine' manufacturers is completely illogical in this context. For example, *Petasites hybridus* (the butterbur or bog rhubarb) contains well-characterized carcinogens. Butterbur extract tables are sold as chronic oral therapies for bladder dysfunction and migraine prevention, and claimed to be innocuous on chemical purity grounds. Similarly, oral melatonin has an absolute bioavailability of about 15% maximum, and has been withdrawn in the UK and Japan due to concerns about safety (DeMuro et al 2000).

Various physicochemical properties of bulk drug can be measured. Some will be reasonably familiar from medical school biochemistry, e.g. the *pH* of drug solutions, and the pK of particular molecules in aqueous solutions. *Log P* is a measure of lipophilicity, usually being measured as the octanol/water distribution coefficient when the aqueous phase is buffered at pH 7.4. *Powder density* is the ratio of weight to volume occupied by a powder; some powder particles pack together more efficiently, and a comparison between table salt and talcum powder is an illustration. *Particle size and distribution* is measured typically using an infra-red device. *Solubilities* in various solvents are also helpful to those whose task is to make drugs into prescribable pharmaceutical formulations. *Hygroscopicity* is a measure of the capability of a drug to absorb water from the atmosphere; such drugs gain weight with time, and are often less stable than drugs which do not have this capability. Standard manuals such as the *Merck Index* provide many of these data.

SPECIFIC FORMULATIONS

Tablets, Syrups, Wafers and Oral Suspensions

The excipients of oral formulations vary according to the physical state of the desired finished product, as well as how it must be manufactured. *Binders* are used to hold the various components together, and include starches and polyvinylpyrrolidine (to which many dogs exhibit a species-specific allergy). *Bulking agents* (sometimes called dilutants, or, confusingly for a solid formulation, diluents) include lactose and cellulose, and increase tablet weight, which may improve production uniformity. *Coatings* are often sugar- or cellulose-based and may be employed when a drug tastes foul, or to create a particular color scheme. Silica and starch may also be used to improve the flow of powder in mass production, when it is known as a *pro-glidant*, and stearic acid salts are used to enable tablets to escape the press when finished, this being an unusual use of the term *lubricant*.

The large majority of generic drugs are tablets designed for systemic delivery of drug. The regulation does not require that innovative and generic drugs have identical excipients. Exemption from demonstration of efficacy may be obtained, provided that bioequivalence can be demonstrated with another drug that is the subject of an ordinary NDA. The regulation Title 21, Code of Federal Regulations (21 CFR) 320.1 – 320.63 defines bioequivalence as: '...demonstrated if the product's rate and extent of absorption, as determined by comparison of measured parameters, e.g. concentration of active drug ingredient in the blood, urinary excretion rates, or pharmacological effects, do not indicate a significant difference from the reference material's rate and extent of absorption'. Although, theoretically, it may be possible to demonstrate bioequivalence using a well-validated *in vitro* or animal method, per 21CFR320.24 (ii)–(iii), the data that has traditionally been most persuasive has been a pharmacokinetic comparison of the generic and reference drugs in man. The commonest study design is to compare two oral formulations with the following optimal design features (21CFR320.26):

- Normal volunteers in the fasting state.
- Single-dose, randomized, cross-over, with well-defined reference material.
- Collection of blood samples for at least three half-times of elimination, and at a frequency that captures distribution phase, C_{max} and T_{max}, and at identical times for the two formulations.

- When there are major metabolites, then collections should accommodate at least three half-times of their elimination.

In this case, the T_{max}, C_{max}, AUC, and half-time of elimination for parent drug and principal metabolites become the end-points of the study. For combination therapies, these end-points have to be measured and fulfilled for all active components, and they should not be administered separately.

The regulation does not define what a significant difference might be, although a commonly applied standard seems to be a formulation whose mean T_{max}, C_{max}, and AUC is within 20% of the reference material, and is also within the 95% confidence interval. However, these limits are tightened when:

- The therapeutic ratio of the drug is low.
- The drug has solubility < 5 mg/ml.
- Tablet dissolution *in vitro* is slower than 50% in 30 min.
- The absolute bioavailability is < 50%.
- There is extensive first-pass metabolism that makes rate of absorption, as well as extent, a factor governing exposure.
- There are special physicochemical constraints, such as chelation, complex formation, or crystallization to consider (see 21CFR320.33).

It should be noted that there are other ways to demonstrate bioequivalence, and in the United States of the Food and Drug Administration (FDA) will advise, in advance, on adaptations to 'standard' measures of bioequivalence, in the interests of promoting the right clinical trial design. For example, two oral formulations can be compared with an intravenous dose. If the drug is concentrated in the urine, but has negligible concentration in the blood (e.g. nitrofurantoin antibiotics), then urine sampling with a frequency that matches the blood samples above can be employed. Multiple dose bioequivalence study designs are also available. Rarely, the testing of bioequivalence at steady-state is required, because patients cannot be withdrawn from therapy, and normal volunteers would face an undue hazard. The regulation also permits bioequivalence to be demonstrated using chronopharmacological effect, i.e. pharmacodynamic data, and specifies the frequency and timing of endpoints in much the same way as for blood samples (see above). This can be useful for drugs that are not intended to be absorbed systemically, e.g. the rate of onset and offset of topical anesthesia to a standardized experimental injury.

Bioequivalence studies do not always require the filing of an Investigational New Drug application (IND). An IND is needed always if the generic drug is without an approved innovator in the USA, is radioactive, or is a cytotoxic. However, when single- or multiple-dose studies do not exceed the approved clinical dose sizes, and when there will be retention samples available for inspection, then an IND need not be filed. An IND is needed for a multiple dose bioequivalence study, when a single-dose study has not preceded it. The usual protections for human subjects are required, and, of course, these include an Institutional Review Board approval.

By definition, sustained release formulations differ pharmaceutically and pharmacokinetically from the innovator drug. Delayed or sustained re-lease oral formulations are used for chronic ther-apy, and may have two principal advantages: (a) reduction in dose frequency (and thus, hopefully, improved compliance; see Chapter 21); and (b) re-duction of C_{max} for a standard AUC, which can improve tolerability when adverse events are plasma concentration-related. The demonstration of bioequivalence usually hinges on the following factors: (a) equivalence of AUC to an innovator drug at steady state; (b) the absence of any chance of 'dose dumping'; (c) consistency of performance from dose to dose [see 21CFR320.25(f)].

Various tactics can be employed in the pursuit of the sustained-release strategy, including mixtures of granules with different thicknesses of polymer coating, all contained within a single capsule; os-motically driven tablets, which slowly release drug through a small aperture during the entire traverse of the small bowel; layered tablets with deliberately delayed dissolution; and tablets designed to release their contents only in relatively alkaline environ-ments (i.e. beyond the ampulla of Vater). It is illogical to seek sustained-release formulations for drugs with relatively long half-times of elimination.

Gases

Gases are usually administered in the context of general anesthesia, either alone or in combination with a variety of infusional agents. In most situ-ations, the gas is made by vaporizing a liquid (usu-ally a halogenated hydrocarbon or ether). Validated vaporizers, usually designated for use with a single liquid, are required. In addition, many patients are paralyzed during surgery and mechanical ventilators (including a hand-squeezed bag) must consider drug economy, occupational exposure of the staff, carbon dioxide scrubbing, and other pharmacokinetic features that are rarely encountered elsewhere. This is quite apart from the usual considerations of tidal and minute volumes, oxygen supply, blood pressure management, etc. Gas flow can be measured with various devices, and exhaled gas concentrations (including for carbon dioxide) can now be measured real-time. Malignant hyperthermia is an adverse event that is almost always associated with the inhalation of a halogenated hydrocarbon, and which can be treated with dantrolene (Strazis and Fox, 1993).

The theory relating physicochemical properties of gases and the partial pressure at which they can achieve anesthesia is beyond the scope of this chap-ter. Indeed, this question hinges on how the state of anesthesia can itself be measured, one of the more difficult pharmacodynamic endpoints in pharma-ceutical medicine. One wit, also a famous cardi-othoracic anesthesiologist, has commented: 'If you can tell me what consciousness is, then I will tell you what anesthesia is!'.

There are some uses for gaseous drugs outside of surgery. Nitrous oxide and oxygen mixtures are sometimes used as analgesics during labour, or when transferring patients in pain by road or heli-copter. In very cold weather, nitrous oxide can liquify, reducing the delivered dose; shaking the container helps.

Helium/oxygen mixtures are used to improve oxygenation in patients with subtotal airways ob-struction, exploiting the superior flow characteris-tics of the lighter gas. The use of this mixture as prophylaxis against nitrogen narcosis in the deep sea, while minimizing fire hazard, is also well-de-scribed. Fire hazard from oxygen (arguably a gas-eous drug under some circumstances) is important; the disastrous fire inside the command capsule of Apollo 3, during a lift-off rehearsal on the pad at Cape Kennedy, took place within a pure oxygen atmosphere. Reduction in total atmospheric pres-sure, to reduce fire hazard, has since been employed in all pressurized American space vehicles, but they still contain supra-atmospheric partial pressures of oxygen.

Metered Dose Inhalers and Nebulized Drugs

In general, and with a few rare exceptions (see below), the inhaled route of administration is the most difficult that is commonly encountered. Metered dose inhalers and nebulizers are considered together here because they have many features in common. These formulations, in both cases, are administered as aerosols of drug solution.

It is customary, in textbooks for a general audience, to insert at this point a graph that relates aerosol particle size to the various levels of the airway where drugs can impact. Particles $> 10\,\mu m$ are stated to be commonly impacted in the pharynx; $< 5\,\mu m$ particles are assumed to be ideal for alveolar delivery, and $< 0.05\,\mu m$ particles are said not to impact at all, being liable to be exhaled. This is an oversimplification. Particle deposition is dependent on a large number of other factors, attested to by a vast literature that has accumulated over at least the last 25 years, straddling the border with the disciplines of pulmonology and industrial hygiene. Other factors governing particle deposition (and example studies) include:

- Coughing (Camner et al 1979)
- Mucociliary action (Lippmann et al 1980)
- Exercise and minute ventilation (Bennett et al 1985)
- Mucous production and ability to expectorate (Agnew et al 1985)
- Apnoeic pause at the end of inhalation (Legath et al 1988)
- Whether a patient is actually having an asthma attack (Patel et al 1990)
- Breathing pattern, airway calibre, spacers and reservoirs (Bennett 1991)
- The physicochemical properties of the drug(s) (Zanen et al 1996)
- Lung morphometry (Hofmann 1996)
- Sampling techniques, on which exposure calculations are based (Cherrie and Aitken 1999).

The truth is that it is practically impossible to measure the lung deposition of inhaled drugs in man. Furthermore, *in vitro* studies use apparati that do not model the anatomy of the human respiratory tree, let alone the diseased respiratory tree. The British Association for Lung Research have recognized this complexity and issued a consensus statement (Snell and Ganderton 1999) which recommends, at a minimum, a five-stage collection apparatus, examination of a range of particle sizes ($0.05 - 5\,\mu m$), a range of flow rates and patterns to mimic the various physiological states, the development of an apparatus modeled on the shape of the human pharynx, the concomitant use of swallowed activated charcoal in clinical studies to minimize absorption by swallowing drug impacting on the oropharynx, regional lung assessments in three dimensions, and further development of useful statistics to describe such findings.

The metered dose inhaler has been in use for about 50 years and doubtless forms the mainstay for the treatment of asthma, as well as for patients with chronic bronchitis with a reversible component. Great technical challenge has been experienced in the last few years, due to the need to change their propellants into non-fluorohydrocarbon materials, as part of the global effort to protect the atmospheric ozone layer. The contribution of metered dose inhalers to this problem, in comparison to vapour escaping from refrigerators and car air conditioners, must have been negligible. Nonetheless, indirectly, these huge costs are now being borne by healthcare systems worldwide. The clinical studies had to rely on efficacy parameters because of the inability to quantitate lung deposition and the general aim of avoiding systemic drug absorption.

A wide variety of nebulizers are now available. They all have their own physicochemical properties. In the absence of the ability to quantitate lung deposition, the Food and Drug Agency (FDA) has now said that it will approve only combinations of new drugs with specified nebulizers; labeling for α-dornase is the first to exhibit this change in policy. This requires that the clinical development plan be implemented, as early as possible, with the nebulizer that is intended to be marketed.

Inhalational toxicology is generally required to support inhalational clinical trials and product approvals. This highly specialized field requires the validation of the nebulizing system for each drug and species separately. The scaling from animals to man in the selection of initial doses is something of an imponderable, given the complexities in measuring lung deposition described above.

Oral Transmucosal

The best drugs for oral transmucosal administration are those that do not taste bad, and which have high potency. For example, among opioids, the two drugs that have been successfully developed using this type of formulation are buprenorphine and fentanyl. Formulations vary, but include sublingual pellets, chewable gums, and solid formulations that are held on a stick, somewhat like a lollipop. Most wafer formulations dissolve in the mouth and are actually converted into a solution for swallowing and gastrointestinal absorption (e.g. rizatriptan wafer). Benzocaine lozenges are intended for the same purpose but to dissolve more slowly, thus bathing the oesophagus as a symptomatic treatment (e.g. for radiation oesophagitis); a similar approach is used with anti-fungal drugs.

Intranasal

The absorptive capacity of the nasal mucosa has been known for centuries. Even if unexploited by pharmaceutical scientists, the abuse of cocaine (including by primitive peoples), and nicotine (snuff) has routinely used this route of administration for systemic delivery. Vast annual tonnages of anti-allergy and decongestant drugs are now administered to the noses of the developed world. These are intended to treat local symptoms, and avoidance of systemic absorption is a favourable feature. α-Adrenergic agonists, antihistamines, and steroids probably lead the list for this topical route of administration.

Therapeutically, interest in the nasal mucosa for systemic absorption of drugs initially centered on its capability to absorb small to moderately sized polypeptides. For example, vasopressin-like drugs (nonapeptides) may be used to treat diabetes insipidus in patients with panhypopituitarism. This avoids repeated parenteral injections, and avoids the digestive capacity of the gut.

In the USA, the FDA has issued a draft guideline on establishing the bioequivalence of nasal sprays and aerosols for local absorption. This intent of this guideline is to facilitate the development of generic products for use by this route of administration. This guideline has been challenged on several scientific and technical grounds (e.g. Harrison 2000). While this situation is not yet resolved, many guidelines in the USA remain in draft status for long periods of time, and are treated as definitive.

Transdermal vs. Topical

The principal distinction between transdermal and topical drugs is that only the former are intended for systemic delivery. Both formulations are, however, subject to the same skin irritancy testing prior to human exposures.

The skin is biologically intended to be a barrier. Evading this barrier is not easy, because drugs must traverse dead epithelium and live dermis; the former is hydrophobic, while lipophilic drugs tends to form a reservoir in the latter. As in oral transmucosal administration, potent drugs, with modest requirements for mass absorbed and reasonable lipophilicity, are the best candidates for transdermal delivery. Fentanyl, nicotine, and scopolamine are good examples.

Rectal

The use of suppositories is probably one of the clearest examples of cross-cultural differences in the approach to pharmaceuticals. A surgeon on a famous ocean liner has commented that: 'Part of the problem of stocking one's pharmacy is that one needs three times as many drugs as when working on land: tablets for the Brits, shots (injectables) for the Yanks, and suppositories for the French!' However, the route of administration is eminently logical, e.g. for the acute treatment of migraine, where drugs are often vomited.

In the UK and USA, peri-operative antibiotics (especially metronidazole), theophylline for pediatric nocturnal asthma, and topical treatments for proctitis and inflammatory bowel disease are the most commonly used rectally-administered drugs.

Paraldehyde remains an effective way to abort seizure in pediatric patients in the emergency room, without the need to find a vein. Use a glass syringe. In the USA, diazepam can be administered by the same route, for the same purpose.

Vaginal

An intravaginal suppository is more accurately termed a *pessary*. Most are designed for topical or local use, including for *Candida albicans* and *Trichomonas* infections, as well as for preparation of the cervix prior to induction of labour. Contraceptive devices are outside of the scope of a chapter on pharmaceutics, although the nonoxyl-containing sponge pessary is a unique formulation.

Injectates (s.c., i.m, i.v.)

The solubility of a drug, and the compatibility of a particular solvent with the site of injection, are inter-related factors governing the suitability of this route of administration, and the pharmaceutical formulation that is employed.

Water-soluble drugs are usually also hygroscopic, and need to be stored in an anhydrous environment to maintain their stability. These are most easily supplied as lyophilized powders, which can be reconstituted with water or saline immediately prior to injection. This applies to early development as well, when the filtration of drug solution through micropore nylon filters prior to lyophilization can be a convenient way to ensure sterility. Lyophilizates in stoppered vials can also be subjected to γ-irradiation to ensure sterility. Stability studies should include not only the range of temperatures and humidities (see below), but also with the vials inverted.

Intravenous formulations are probably the least demanding of all injectates. Solutions of thiopental sodium are routinely administered at the induction of anesthesia, but are extremely alkaline and would be very damaging if administered subcutaneously or intramuscularly. Unfortunately, this occurs occasionally as an iatrogenic adverse event when the injection (pH 9) extravasates; serious injury can easily occur to the structures in the cubital fossa (including the median nerve).

The route of administration may also be governed by tolerability aspects associated with the formulation. If a drug cannot be dissolved in a concentrated manner in a suitable vehicle, then often dose size must increase. Intravenous injections of penicillin-type antibiotics are much more comfortable than when the same dose is administered intramuscularly.

Organic solvents are often used to enhance the rate of absorption from the subcutaneous or intramuscular site of administration. For example, benzyl alcohol and sodium benzoate are used to dissolve diazepam, and extravasation of this formulation is not as serious a problem as for thiopental.

Rarely, adverse events are reported when an apparently innocuous formulation is administered by the wrong route. Usually these problems arise because of excipients that the typical physician takes little interest in. Intravenous remifentanil is formulated with glycine, and hence it is not well-suited for epidural administration.

The development of an injectate is often one tactic used for obtaining a patent. Even though a composition of matter patent (i.e. the structure of the drug molecule itself) may be old, the development of a non-obvious injectate, and its method of use for a new indication, may be sufficient to obtain a further patent and thus extend effective proprietary coverage. Such patents are usually stronger in North American than in European jurisdictions.

Packaging

The selection of an inert package is an essential part of the pharmaceutical development of a drug. There are many standard stoppers, plastic and glass bottles, etc., with which regulatory authorities are very familiar. Stability studies must be conducted, of course, in the same sorts of packaging.

Packaging nonetheless varies, and over a period of months or years an apparently impervious material may, permit the ingress of water. Foil wraps are generally available for all tablets, although they are inconvenient to arthritic hands; these are usually the most impervious of all materials. PVC blister packs are at the other end of the spectrum; Padfield (1985) has provided one example where a 0.8% increase in tablet weight within a PVC package occurred within 12 weeks.

Drugs, both investigational and prescription, are today transported over great distances. Airlines often advertise their cargo holds as pressurized and temperature-controlled, but even so require special arrangements for the conveyance of livestock. The potential for condensation in the air, after degradation when the pallet sat for several hours on the unshaded tarmac in Dakkar, is great.

STABILITY TESTING

Stability testing of drugs is an entire subspecialty within the pharmaceutical professions and cannot be covered in depth here. However, suffice it to say that it is the pharmacist's duty to ensure that drugs are being used when they have been tested with various challenges, which may be considered as factorial combinations of:

- Low and high temperatures.
- Low and high humidity.
- Exceeding the labeled drug shelf-life.
- In contact with all feasible components of the packaging (e.g. both the glass and the stopper of a vial, the latter by inverted storage).
- Exposure to bright and subdued light (in some case clear and amber glass bottles).

It is these data that justifies approval and continued marketing of a drug that complies with the 'quality' criterion of the oft-quoted triad, 'safety, efficacy, quality'. This is usually not a trivial exercise.

INNOVATION IN PHARMACEUTICS

Innovation has always been a very visible activity in pharmaceutics. As noted above, we very rarely administer powders out of paper cones today. The dry-powder inhaler used for sodium cromoglycate was developed because that drug is almost insoluble, but is also now being revived in the post-hydrofluorocarbon era. The intravenous emulsion of propofol is also unique, again being invented out of necessity. Pharmaceutical physicians should not underestimate the scale of these technological achievements, even if the drugs involved are very familiar.

What are we likely to see in the future? Novel pharmaceutical formulations seem to fall into two groups, those being used for gene therapy and those being used elsewhere.

Investigational gene therapies are now commonplace, and are comprised of two components: the DNA itself (the 'construct') and usually a method of delivery ('the vector'). Naked DNA can be injected but its expression is inefficient. Vectors may include viruses. However, such viruses have to be human, and their attenuation sometimes is lost after administration, leading to very serious adverse events. Non-viral vectors can include targeted liposomes, microspheres, and emulsions.

There are several other examples of truly unique formulations or routes of administration that we may expect to be further exploited in the future. AIDS-associated infective retinitis is treated with a drug administered by intraocular injection, and the current parlous state of retinal detachment treatments suggests that this route of administration may find wider use. It turns out that cell membranes become leaky when exposed to high voltages: otherwise insoluble or excluded drugs can enter the cell under these conditions, and this uses a multi-tined stimulator, known as an electroporator. Needleless injectors have been available for decades, yet still seem to be under-used (the needleless injector used by Dr 'Bones' McCoy of the 'USS Enterprise' is clockwork, develops several thousand pounds pressure per square inch, and feels like a mild middle-finger percussion when used over the deltoid).

SUMMARY

The objective of this chapter has been to provide the pharmaceutical physician with some appreciation of the complexity of pharmaceutical development. Understanding the vocabulary will help participation in team meetings, where pharmaceutical and clinical development must be coordinated. A chapter on this scale will never equip a pharmaceutical physician to conduct pharmaceutical development. At the very least, it should now be clear that a drug is not a drug is not a drug.

REFERENCES

Agnew JE, Pavia D, Clarke SW (1985) Factors affecting the 'alveolar deposition' of 5 microns inhaled particles in healthy subjects. *Clin Phys Physiol Meas* 6: 27–36.

Bennett WD (1991) Aerosolized drug delivery: fractional deposition of inhaled particles. *J Aerosol Med* 4: 223–7.

Bennett WD, Messina MS, Smaldone GC (1985) Effect of exercise on deposition and subsequent retention of inhaled particles. *J Appl Physiol* 59: 1046–54.

Camner P, Mossberg B, Philipson K, Strandberg K (1979) Elimination of test particles from the human tracheobronchial tract by voluntary coughing. *Scand J Resp Dis* 60: 56–62.

Cherrie JW, Aitken RJ (1999) Measurement of human exposure to biologically relevant fractions of inhaled aerosols. *Occup Environ Med* 56: 747–52.

DeMuro RL, Nafziger AN, Blask DE et al (2000) The absolute bioavailability of oral melatonin. *J Clin Pharmacol* 40: 781–4.

Harrison LI (2000) Commentary on the FDA draft guidance for bioequivalence studies for nasal aerosols and nasal sprays for local action: an industry view. *J Clin Pharmacol* 40: 701–7.

Hoffmann W (1996) Modeling techniques for inhaled particle deposition: the state of the art. *J Aerosol Med* 9: 369–88.

Legath L, Naus A, Halik J (1988) Determining the basic characteristics of aerosols suitable for studies of deposition in the respiratory tract. *J Hyg Epidemiol Microbiol Immunol* 32: 287–97.

Lippmann M, Yeates DB, Albert RE (1980) Deposition, retention, and clearance of inhaled particles. *Br J Indust Med* 37: 337–62.

Padfield JM (1985) Making drugs into medicines. In Burley DM, Binns TB (eds), *Pharmaceutical Medicine*. Arnold: London and New York; 51.

Patel P, Mukai D, Wilson AF (1990) Dose–response effects of two sizes of monodispersed isoproterenol in mild asthma. *Am Rev Resp Dis* 141: 357–60.

Snell NJ, Ganderton D (1999) Assessing lung deposition of inhaled medications. Consensus statement from a workshop of the British Association for Lung Research, held at the Institute of Biology, London, UK, April 17 1998. *Resp Med* 93: 123–33.

Strazis KP, Fox AW (1993) Malignant hyperthermia: A review of published cases. *Anesth Analg* 77: 297–304.

Zanen P, Go LT, Lammers JW (1996) Optimal particle size for -2 agonist and anticholinergic aerosols in patients with severe airflow obstruction. *Thorax* 51: 977–80.

6

Non-clinical Toxicology

Frederick Reno

Merritt Island, FL, USA

The evaluation of the safety of new pharmaceutical agents through non-clinical studies is a critical aspect of any development program. Usually in the discovery stage, or what can be considered the 'research' phase of research and development, either *in vivo* or *in vitro* studies have established the pharmacological profile of the new drug and a rationale for its potential clinical efficacy. At this stage, the potential agent can be considered a new chemical entity (NCE) or perhaps an analog or metabolite of an existing one. Preliminary studies are also made with respect to drug absorption, metabolism, and excretion. In many companies, drug metabolism is a separate entity from the toxicology function but, for the sake of completeness of this chapter, a discussion of this important research area will be included. At some point, a decision is made to move the agent into the 'development' phase, and the initiation of non-clinical toxicology studies necessary to establish safety for initial clinical trials is begun.

Over the past two decades, separate regulatory authorities in the USA, Europe, and Japan have established their own guidelines for the types and extent of preclinical studies that are necessary. Although often quite detailed, these jurisdictions were rarely similar, and designing a non-clinical toxicology program that would be universally accepted was difficult, if not impossible. The International Conference on Harmonization (ICH), a tripartite group that consists of regulators and pharmaceutical company representatives from the three geographical areas, has been meeting for several years to address the harmonization of many aspects of the drug development process. These meetings have resulted in the issue of many guidelines (in either draft or final form) for non-clinical studies and applicable in all three jurisdictions. These guidelines will be identified throughout this chapter. In addition, all non-clinical toxicology studies that are intended to support clinical trials or marketing applications must be conducted in compliance with good laboratory practices (GLP; Federal Register December 1978). The volume edited by Williams and Hottenderf (1997) provides more information on the subjects that are discussed below.

CONSIDERATIONS RELATED TO THE CLINICAL DEVELOPMENT PLAN

The nature, timing, and extent of the initial non-clinical toxicology program depend on the clinical development plan that it must support. The ICH guidelines further specify the extent and duration of non-clinical studies that are required to initiate or continue clinical studies (*Federal Register* November 1997, and see below). Therefore, it is important that the clinical development plan, at least the initial stages, be clearly delineated.

Initial Clinical Studies

Usually, the initial clinical goals are to study tolerability and to provide initial pharmacokinetic assessments. These studies may only involve single doses of the drug administered to normal volunteers. Such a clinical study would require a restricted set of toxicity studies to support the safe use of the drug in this situation. On the other hand, some companies achieve economies by having the initial toxicology program be sufficient to support not only initial clinical studies but also Phase II. The toxicology studies may then involve repeated doses over a period of weeks. Thus, the initial clinical studies must be determined before the non-clinical program can be designed.

Principles and Practice of Pharmaceutical Medicine. Edited by A. J. Fletcher, Lionel D. Edwards, Anthony W. Fox and Peter Stonier © 2002 John Wiley & Sons Ltd.

Initial Proof of Principle

In most cases, a proof of principle (i.e. initial indication of clinical efficacy) during early Phase II clinical studies will require clinical treatment for some period of time, ranging from days (diagnostic agents, etc.) to weeks or months (for other types of drug). Since exposure of patients in clinical trials (in most cases) cannot last beyond the duration of the animal studies, careful consideration of the development schedule must be made, so that no delays are caused through lack of toxicological coverage. This requires that the appropriate preclinical reports are available prior to the planned initiation of the clinical trial.

Enrollment of Women

Most regulatory agencies now request that women be enrolled into the clinical studies as early in Phase II as possible. Since thalidomide, reproduction, and teratology studies have been required prior to enrollment of large numbers of women in clinical studies. In some cases, depending upon the proposed indication for the drug, postmenopausal or otherwise reproductively incapable women can be used. However, the timing of the enrollment of women needs to be understood well in advance so that the lack of appropriate non-clinical reports does not hinder clinical development.

CONSIDERATION OF REGULATORY STRATEGY

It is common, particularly for American companies, to carry out initial Phase I studies abroad. This is because these studies can often be initiated outside the USA with little regulatory involvement, and with safety considerations being reviewed by an Institutional Review Board or Ethics Committee. Consequently, the company accepts the entire responsibility for any hazards or risks to the study subjects. This has the effect of allowing Phase I studies to be initiated more rapidly and thus obtaining information on preliminary safety and pharmacokinetic data earlier. Awareness of such a strategy dictates a different scenario to the preclinical manager than would a strategy requiring

the filing of an investigational new drug application (IND) for the first study in man.

INITIAL NON-CLINICAL CONSIDERATIONS

Of equal importance to the successful initiation of a non-clinical program are several factors that can have a great impact on the rapidity with which a program can be implemented. Experience has shown that overlooking the importance of these factors can result in unanticipated delays, costing time and money.

Formulation Aspects

It is desirable for the pivotal non-clinical studies to be carried out using the proposed clinical route of administration and with a formulation that best approximates that anticipated for initial clinical usage, although, of course, this is unlikely to be the formulation that is eventually marketed when the program is successful. Factors such as method of synthesis, excipients and appropriate vehicles usually evolve from bench-scale drug supplies and simple vehicles, to more sophisticated galenicals as the program proceeds. Scale-up of manufacturing processes can result in bulk drug with different impurities, and adverse effects may be due to parent drug, metabolites or impurities. Furthermore, tablets or capsules cannot be given to most animal species, and the non-clinical studies are therefore carried out using dosing solutions or suspensions. The type of formulation can affect the pharmacokinetics of the drug, thus altering the toxicological profile, making comparison of animal and human pharmacokinetics, in the context of the formulations used, into a critical element in the evaluation of human safety.

Impurities/Stability

Early-stage small-scale synthesis methods will often create a different profile of impurities or degradants than drug supplies produced by scaled-up processes. Every batch of drug used in non-clinical studies must have a certificate of analysis that clearly specifies the purity levels and the quantities of impurities (which may include residual solvents, unreacted starting materials or degradants). The impurities must be reviewed in terms of the potential contribution that they can make to toxic effects that may be manifested in the non-clinical studies. There are ICH guidelines that pertain to impurities, and the extent to which additional toxicity studies need to be performed in impurities (*Federal Register* January 4 1996, March 19 1996).

Of equal importance is the stability of the drug in the non-clinical formulation. This can determine whether the non-clinical formulations must be prepared daily or can be prepared weekly. If drugs are to be given orally, it is obvious that they must be resistant to degradation of gastric acids and must be stable in the formulation itself (water, carboxymethylcellulose suspensions, etc.). As will be discussed in more detail later, this requires the availability of an analytical method at the earliest stages of development.

Drug Requirements

The amount of bulk drug that is typically required to carry out the non-clinical studies may be a big surprise, in comparison to that needed for initial clinical studies. While many biologically derived drugs may require relatively small quantities, due to the potency of the material or the limited number of non-clinical studies that are possible (see below), a typical program need for 'first time in man' drugs that are relatively non-toxic may require 2–3 kg of active drug. For many companies, this can be difficult from either a manufacturing standpoint (small quantities synthesized prior to scale-up) or cost.

Analytical Methods for Dose and Plasma Determinations

GLP regulations require confirmation of the potency of all formulations used in non-clinical studies. Furthermore, current ICH guidelines also require toxicokinetic data (i.e. animal pharmacokinetics determined at one or more time points during a non-clinical toxicology study). Both the potency and toxicokinetic assays require an analytical

method for the determination of parent drug (and possible major metabolites) in solvents and plasma, usually validated for multiple non-clinical species.

Appropriate Species

In the early stages of the development of any drug, there is little, if any, information on which to make a scientific judgment relative to the most appropriate animal species for non-clinical studies that will best predict responses in the human. In these cases, since regulatory agencies require the use of both a rodent and a non-rodent species, the typical approach would be to use the rat and the dog for the toxicity studies, and mice or rabbits for other more specialized studies. Primates may be needed when there is availability of considerable background data in these species in terms of the parameters of interest (hematology, blood chemistry, histopathology, etc.). When candidate drugs are proteins (e.g. animal-derived monoclonal antibodies), then antibody formation may be major issue and may dictate the choice of species. For example, it may be known that only the chimpanzee does not develop neutralizing antibodies to the drug, which would lead one to select that species as the non-clinical model. Topical formulations are another special case, and the rabbit is commonly employed. The selection of the animal species for the non-clinical program is often not straightforward.

TOXICOLOGICAL SUPPORT PRE-IND AND FOR PHASE I CLINICAL STUDIES

The preliminary evaluation of the safety assessment of any new drug requires multiple studies, some of which evaluate general and multiple endpoints (such as toxicity studies). Other studies evaluate more specific and defined endpoints (such as mutagenicity studies and safety pharmacology studies). Drugs that are derived from a biological origin, such as proteins, monoclonal antibodies, or drugs produced by biological vectors (or what are generally referred to as 'biotechnology products'), present additional problems that require a significantly modified approach. The ICH guidelines recognize that unique approaches may be needed, has addressed this in a further guideline (ICH 1997), and poses additional problems for the toxicologist (Terrell and Green 1994). This section will elaborate on those studies needed to support the safety of a typical xenobiotic agent, although the same general principles follow for biotechnology products, often being necessary but not sufficient. There are two types of guidelines that must be considered in initiating the non-clinical program. The first relates to the types of studies required; the second relates to protocol requirements for the studies themselves.

The types of studies needed are dictated by national regulatory requirement, although the ICH has promulgated a international guideline (*Federal Register* November 25 1997) that is progressing through the final review stage at the present time. These studies, outlined in Tables 6.1 and 6.2, vary somewhat by the phase of the clinical trial, and may still vary among countries where the trial is being conducted. The US Food and Drug Administration (FDA) has also published guidelines that outline the requirements necessary to initiate initial clinical studies (FDA 1995). This latter document focuses more on the extent of study documentation required than the study types, and allows for data to be submitted that is not in final report form.

The following sections briefly describe the studies that would typically be performed to support

Table 6.1 Duration of repeated-dose toxicity studies to support Phase I and Phase II clinical trials in the EU, and Phase I, II, and III clinical trials in the USA and Japan[a]

Duration of clinical trial	Minimum duration of repeated-dose toxicity studies	
	Rodents	Non-rodents
Single dose	2–4 weeks[b]	2 weeks
≤ 2 weeks	2–4 weeks[b]	2 weeks
≤ 1 month	1 month	1 month
≤ 3 months	3 months	3 months
≤ 6 months	6 months	6 months[c]
> 6 months	6 months	Chronic[c]

[a] In Japan, if there are no Phase II clinical trials of equivalent duration to the proposed Phase III trials, then non-clinical toxicology studies of the durations shown in Table 6.2 should be considered.
[b] In the EU and USA, 2 week studies are the minimum duration. In Japan, 2 week non-rodent and 4 week rodent studies are needed. In the USA, with FDA concurrence, single-dose toxicity studies with extended examinations can support single-dose human exposures.
[c] Data from 6 months of administration in non-rodents should be available before clinical exposures of more than 3 months. Alternatively, if applicable, data from a 9 month non-rodent study should be available before clinical treatment duration exceeds that supported by other toxicology studies.

Table 6.2 Duration of repeated-dose toxicity studies to support Phase III clinical trials in the EU, and product marketing in all jurisdictions[a]

Duration of clinical trial	Minimum duration of repeated-dose toxicity studies	
	Rodents	Non-rodents
≤ 2 weeks	1 month	1 month
≤ 1 month	3 months	3 months
≤ 3 months	6 months	3 months
> 3 months	6 months	Chronic

[a] The above table reflects the marketing recommendations in all three ICH regions, except that a chronic non-rodent study is recommended for clinical use > 1 month in Japan.

initial studies in man. Additional specialized studies might be needed in order to study the potential for an effect that might be characteristic of drugs in the particular class in question (e.g. antibody determinations for some biological products; neurotoxicity studies for drugs acting on the central nervous system, etc).

Acute Toxicity Studies

Single-dose studies in animals are an important first step in establishing a safety profile. Note, however, that the calculation of an LD_{50} is no longer required or scientifically necessary. The aim of single-dose studies is to explore a range of doses. Identification of doses without drug-related effects, a dose that produces some level of exaggerated effect (not necessarily death) that helps identify potential side effects, and other doses in between helps all further toxicological (and clinical) tolerability assessments. These studies can be designed using 'up-and-down' or other tactics to reduce the time and number of animals required. These studies may then guide dose selection for the first repeated-dose studies. Various guidelines for the performance of these studies are available, and the ICH has also published its own guideline (*Federal Register* August 26 1996).

Repeated-dose Toxicity Studies

Repeated-dose studies are designed to identify safe levels of the drug following treatment regimens that are designed to provide continuous exposure of the animals to the test drug. Ideally, the route of administration should mimic that planned in man, and the animal studies should involve longer durations of exposure and higher doses than those planned clinically. The type and duration of specific studies, and which ones are needed relative to different stages of clinical development, were mentioned previously (*Federal Register* November 25 1997). Protocols must specify the number of animals per group, numbers of groups and experimental procedures to be carried out, and standard versions of these have been available for some time. In general, for initial repeated-dose studies, protocols require the use of three dose groups plus a control, and a minimum of 10 rodents and three non-rodents per sex per group. Doses must be selected that will allow for the identification of toxic effects at the highest dose as well as a no-effect level at the middle or lowest dose.

Usual experimental procedures include the determination of body weights and food consumption on at least a weekly basis, evaluation of hematology and blood chemistry parameters during the treatment period, ophthalmoscopic examinations, the recording of macroscopic examinations at necropsy, and the determination of organ weights. A complete histopathological examination of tissues from animals is required. In rodent studies, this can take the form of examination of all high-dose and control animals and the examination of target organs at the two lower doses. In non-rodent studies, it is typical to examine tissues from all animals in the study.

It is crucial that plasma concentrations of drug are measured in these studies to allow for determination of effects on the basis of exposure. Frequently this is a more appropriate measure of comparing effects in animals and man, since rates of absorption, distribution, and excretion can vary extensively between these species. This aspect, now commonly referred to as 'toxicokinetics', has been outlined in an ICH guideline (*Federal Register* March 1 1995). This guideline specifies minimum requirements in terms of number of time points examined, number of animals per time point, and the requirements for calculation of various pharmacokinetic parameters such as C_{max}, AUC, etc. These will become important for comparison with human data as it becomes available later.

Mutagenicity Studies

Mutagenicity studies are highly specialized. There are multiple hereditary components in both somatic and germinal cells that may be affected by drugs. During the 1970s, it was thought (somewhat naïvely) that these studies may be replacements for the long and costly carcinogenicity studies that are required for many drugs. Although this goal was never realized, mutagenicity studies nonetheless provide useful indications of the ability of a drug to alter genetic material, which may later be manifested in studies of carcinogenic or teratogenic effects (Kowalski, 2001). Genotoxicity studies are relatively inexpensive and may also serve, early in the drug development process, to assure drug developers and regulators that no obvious risk of such adverse effects exists, albeit knowing that more definitive studies to evaluate teratogenic and carcinogenic effects will not come until later.

An exhaustive review of the various components of a mutagenicity evaluation will not be attempted here. Multiple guidelines are available. Those issued by the ICH include general guidelines (*Federal Register* April 24 1996) and specifics related to the core battery of studies required (*Federal Register* April 3 1997). Tennant et al (1986) have summarized the correlation between the results of a battery of mutagenicity assays and the probability of the material producing a positive carcinogenic response in long-term rodent studies. Obviously, mutagenicity studies cannot address issues of non-genetic carcinogenicity or teratogenicity.

Positive results in one or more mutagenicity assays do not necessarily translate into human risks. Mechanistic studies may show that such responses would not occur in the human cell population, or the concentrations at which positive responses occurred may far exceed any concentration of drug that may occur in the clinical setting. Many drugs are on the market today that have produced some type of positive response in these studies and yet it has been concluded that no human risk is present or the potential risk is not known (e.g. aspirin causes chromosomal breaks). A Fairly standard worked example is provided by Fox et al, 1996.

Pharmacokinetic Studies

In the early stages of drug development, it is important to identify important parameters that relate to the absorption and excretion pathways for the drug. In the later stages of development, studies on the extent of tissue distribution and the identification of metabolites become important. Another reason why this is important is that it assists the investigator in knowing that the appropriate species has been selected for the non-clinical toxicology program. It is important to human safety evaluation that the non-clinical models chosen are representative of the metabolism of the drug in man. Therefore, it is necessary to have pharmacokinetic information early in the program, so that it can be compared to the data generated in the early clinical studies.

Drug metabolism is a highly specialized field, and is increasing in sophistication all the time. A relatively new technique that is available to the preclinical investigator is the use of *in vitro* methods to establish and confirm similar mechanisms in drug metabolism between animals and man (see Chapter 10). These procedures involve the use of liver slices and/or liver hepatocyte homogenates and can be done in human and animal cultures at the earliest stages of drug development.

Toxicokinetic data is generally obtained from repeated-dose toxicity studies, and generally determines whether: (a) the plasma concentrations of the drug increase in a linear fashion over the range of the increasing doses used in the studies; and (b) plasma concentrations increase over time, suggesting an accumulation of the drug in plasma or tissues; (c) there is a relationship between the plasma concentrations of the drug (or metabolites) and the toxicity associated with higher levels of the drug; and (d) the effects are more closely related to peak concentrations or to overall exposure (measured by the area under the concentration time curve, AUC).

Toxicokinetic data are generally collected on the first day of dosing in a repeated-dose study, and near the last day of dosing, i.e. during the last week, of a 90 day toxicity study. In rodent studies, satellite groups of animals are required due to the blood volumes needed for assay. For larger non-rodents the main study animals can usually provide the samples. Guidelines have been made available covering most aspects of the collection and analysis of these data (*Federal Register* March 1 1995)

Lastly, pharmacokinetic assessment requires tissue distribution studies in non-clinical models to determine the extent of localization of the drug in tissues. In some situations, where single-dose tissue distribution studies suggest drug localization, a tissue distribution study following repeated dosing may be indicated. The conditions under which such studies may be necessary have been delineated in an ICH guideline (*Federal Register* March 1 1997)

Safety Pharmacology

Studies related to safety pharmacology (sometimes confusingly termed 'general pharmacology' studies) tend now also to be performed earlier in the drug development process than was previously the case. While in some respects considered an aspect of the discipline of pharmacology, the purpose of safety pharmacology is to evaluate the potential pharmacological properties that may be unrelated to the intended indication for the drug. An example of this would be significant effects of a drug on the cardiovascular system that may actually be under development for the treatment of gastric ulcers.

Most major developed countries have stated guidelines indicating that safety pharmacology studies are required. Table 6.3 lists the guidelines from major countries. As can be seen from these guidelines, it is not always clear when such studies are required. All of the major organ systems need to be evaluated, and therefore studies need to be performed that would identify potential effects on the central nervous, cardiovascular, and gastrointestinal systems, as well as an evaluation of renal function and possibly immunogenicity.

Like many other disciplines, there are a multitude of protocols and procedures that can be followed for each pharmacology study. A decoiled review of each available procedure is outside the purview of this discussion.

Table 6.3 International regulatory guidelines for safety pharmacology studies. Excerpts from international regulatory documents

USA—'Studies that otherwise define the pharmacological properties of the drug or are pertinent to possible adverse effects'
(21CFR314.50, para 2)
EU—'A general pharmacological characterization of the substance, with special reference to collateral effects' (EC Directive 91/507/
EEC)
UK—'A general pharmacological profile of the substance is required, with special reference to collateral effects ... the aim should be to
establish a pattern of pharmacological activity within major physiological systems using a variety of experimental models' (MAL2,
p. A3F-1)
Canada—'Secondary actions—studies related to secondary pharmacological actions of the new drug which may be relevant to
expected use or to adverse effects of the new drug' (Canada RA5, exhibit 2, p. 21).
Australia—'Studies should reveal potentially useful and harmful properties of the drug in a quantitative manner, which will permit an
assessment of the therapeutic risk ... Investigations of the general pharmacological profile should be carried out' (Guidelines under
the Clinical Trial Exemption Scheme, pp. 12, 15)
Nordic countries—'New drugs should be studied in a biological screening program so as to define any action over and above that which
is desirable for the therapeutic use of the product'
Japan—'The objective of general pharmacological studies is to examine extensively the kind and potency of actions other than the
primary pharmacological actions, predict potential adverse effects likely to manifest in clinical practice ...' (Japanese Guidelines, 29
January 1991).

Non-clinical Summary Documents

Prior to the initiation of initial studies in man, it is important that all of the non-clinical information available is made into an integrated summary. This information must be included in the clinical investigators' brochure and so that the clinical protocol can be modified to include relevant biochemical or other markers to minimize human risk. The regulatory authority and ethics committees are further target audiences, and the company may wish to use this for formal, internal proceedings to justify the decision to proceed with initial human exposure.

TOXICOLOGICAL SUPPORT FOR PHASE II–III STUDIES

Non-clinical toxicology studies required to support Phase II and Phase III stages of the program depend upon a variety of factors. First, as shown in Tables 6.1 and 6.2, the ultimate clinical regimen, i.e. duration of therapy or treatment, determines the ultimate duration of the animal studies. For example, a diagnostic agent or a drug with a 3–4 day regimen [as might be the cases for disease or trauma situation that are handled in the intensive care unit may require little in the way of additional repeated-dose toxicity studies. In comparison, a new antihypertensive agent may require all of the longer-term studies.

Second, the drug development strategy established by the company may call for the availability of proof of absorption and perhaps even preliminary proof of efficacy (sometimes called 'proof of principle') before expending resources for the longer and more expensive studies. On the other hand, the company may have determined that the drug in question is on a 'fast track', and is willing to expend resources early in the hopes of getting an earlier approval, and thus to the market faster. The following sections will summarize the areas that need to be addressed.

Chronic Toxicity Studies

As discussed above, the extent of additional repeated-dose studies are generally outlined in Tables 6.2 and 6.3. The maximum duration of chronic studies is generally 6 months. The ICH guidelines describe situations where studies of 9–12 months duration in a non-rodent species may be necessary, particularly for the US FDA. The ICH has issued a guideline relative to the duration of chronic toxicity studies.

Protocols for these studies are similar to those for studies of shorter duration, except that a minimum of 10–15 rodents/group and four non-rodents/sex/group are required. Toxicokinetic measurements are still required. The usual in-life and post-mortem observations are performed.

Reproduction and Teratology Studies

The Thalidomide tragedy demonstrated the need to evaluate new drugs in reproductive toxicology studies. Some of the earliest guidelines were issued by the US FDA (the 'Goldenthal guidelines'). An ICH guideline now covers the performance of these studies (*Federal Register* September 22 1994), as amended in 1995 to address possible effects on male reproduction.

In general, there are three phases of the reproductive process that are evaluated. The first phase (historically referred to as Segment I study, and now under ICH as Stage A) evaluates the effect of the new drug on fertility and the early implantation stages of embryogenesis. In these studies, breeding animals of one species (usually rats or rabbits) of both sexes will be treated for 2 or more weeks prior to mating, and then the females will be further dosed until day 6 of gestation. The second stage (historically Segment II, now ICH Stage B) is the teratology study (sometimes termed 'the developmental toxicity study') and is done in both of the same two species. The third stage (Segment III or ICH Stage C) evaluates treatment during late gestation, parturition, and lactation. Behavioral and neurodevelopmental assessments in the offspring are often made in Segment III studies. In some cases, two of the studies can be combined and still satisfy the ICH guideline.

The period in the drug development process at which results of these studies are required varies somewhat from country to country, and is discussed in the ICH guideline. Hoyer (2001) reviews the current situation, and provides additional perspective.

Carcinogenicity Studies

Carcinogenicity studies involve the treatment of rodents for long periods of time (18 months to 2 years) in order to determine whether the material possesses the capability to initiate or promote the development of tumors. The relevance of these models to the human situation has been debated for many years. Carcinogenicity studies have been required for all drugs where clinical therapy may extend for 6 months or longer. While the scientific debate about relevance of these studies continues, they remain required by regulation.

Several different ICH guidelines have been issued that address the various aspects of the carcinogenicity testing of drugs, including when studies are needed (duration of clinical therapy; *Federal Register* March 1 1996). Other features of the new drug may mandate carcinogenicity testing, such as structure–activity similarities to known carcinogens, evidence of preneoplastic lesions in repeated-dose non-clinical studies, or long-term tissue sequestration of the drug. Another guideline (*Federal Register* March 1 1995) addresses the complex issue of the selection of doses for these studies; this responds to much criticism of the prior recommendation to use the maximum tolerated dose (which had been suggested by the National Toxicology Program; Haseman and Lockhart 1994). The current ICH guideline recommends a high dose causing up to a 25-fold greater plasma AUC in rodents compared to the AUC in man at steady state. A subsequent amendment to this guideline (*Federal Register* December 4 1997) adds a further proviso that the highest dose in a carcinogenicity study need not exceed 1500 mg/kg/day when (a) there is no evidence of genotoxicity and (b) the maximum recommended human dose is no bigger than 500 mg/day. The basis for species selection, circumstances needing mechanistic studies, and exploitation of pharmacokinetic information in carcinogenicity testing is described in yet another guideline (*Federal Register* August 21 1996).

Modern protocols for carcinogenicity studies have changed little since first established in the early 1970s. In recent years, the use of mice (historically the second of the two required species in addition to rats) has come under scrutiny because they may be inappropriate models, with unusual sensitivity to certain classes of chlorinated hydrocarbons. The most recent ICH guideline (*Federal Register* August 21 1996) allows for the option of using transgenic mice and study designs of somewhat shorter duration.

Of growing importance is the interaction of factors that are critical to a successful toxicology programme. For example, if a transgenic mouse model is selected, then the choice of strain is important and may depend upon whether the drug is non-genotoxic (TG.AC model) or genotoxic (p53 model). Metabolic and pharmacokinetic data are important to ensure that the selected models handle and metabolize the drug in a fashion at least reasonably similar to man, and may vary for the same drug according to the toxic effect of interest. Perhaps the most important factor is the relevance of the doses selected to those in man. While this has been a subject of controversy for years, a recent ICH guideline allows for the use of toxicokinetic measurements, and states that doses that produce an AUC in the carcinogenicity model that are 25 times that seen in man at steady state may no longer have to be used under some circumstances. A recent review of the status of carcinogenicity testing (Reno 1997) addresses the many factors that should be considered in a carcinogenicity program.

Special Studies

It is not uncommon in drug development programs for specific toxicities to be uncovered. In most cases, additional studies are then carried out that will attempt to elucidate additional information with regard to the mechanism of the effect. For example, the identification of a non-specific behavioral effect (e.g. tremors and/or convulsions) may trigger the performance of a neurotoxicity study, which includes an exhaustive evaluation of the potential effects on central and peripheral nervous tissues. The identification of an effect on reproduction may warrant the performance of detailed studies to identify the specific mechanism or phase of the reproductive cycle that is affected. In-depth metabolic studies may prove that the effect is related to a metabolite in animals that has no relevance to man, and prevent the abandonment of an otherwise promising drug. It is rare that a drug development program does not involve some type of special study.

NDA REQUIREMENTS

Format and Content of the Application

The FDA, in what was referred to as the 'New Drug Application (NDA) Rewrite', issued guidelines for how a non-clinical section of an NDA should be organized (the guideline contains not only requirements on what is required but also a basic table of contents for this document). Of par-

ticular importance is the integrated summary. This document contains an overview of all studies that were conducted, how the pharmacology, pharmacokinetic, and toxicology study information is interrelated (Peck et al, 1992), and what significance the data has to human safety. A well-written integrated summary can be beneficial not only to the agency reviewer, but also to the NDA Sponsor. Some of the information in this summary is also needed for the product's package insert. Crucially, it should include comparisons between effects seen in animals and the likelihood that such findings would be expected in clinical usage. These comparisons are often quantitative, and must be made both on a mg/kg and a surface area (mg/m^2) basis (Voisin et al 1990).

CANDA Requirements

The Computer Assisted NDA (CANDA) refers to the submission of data to the FDA in machine-readable form. At the present time, it is required that, at a minimum, the data from the carcinogenicity studies be submitted to the agency in a specified format that is available from the FDA. This allows the agency to apply its own criteria and statistics to the data and independently confirm the sponsor's conclusions. This agency review is then submitted to the FDA's Carcinogenicity Assessment Committee for final review and conclusions.

Expert Reports

The European Community, and other countries, require several expert reports in each dossier, one of which examines the non-clinical toxicology of the new drug. These documents are typically about 20–30 pages long and summarize all the toxicology data, as well as the clinical implications.

Much from the integrated summaries described above may be reused in this report, with the exception of the expert, who must personally sign the report. Expert reports contain the expert's curriculum vitae, and part of the regulatory review process is to evaluate whether the expert is actually qualified for this role. The choice of expert is important, and his/her independence is crucial because the role is that of a reviewer, not of a sponsor. Experts may nonetheless be drawn from within the sponsoring company with appropriate protections, although those from outside may carry more credibility in some jurisdictions.

REFERENCES

Hoyer PB. Reproductive toxicology: current and future directions. *Biochem Pharmacol* 2001. 62: 1557–1564.

Fox Aw, Yang X, Murli H, Lawlor TE, Cifone MA, Reno FE, Absence of mutagenic effects of sodium dichloroacetate. *Fund Appl Tox* 1996; 32: 87–95.

Kowalski LA. In vitro carcinogenicity testing: present and future perspectives in pharmaceutical development. *Cure Opin Drug Discov Devel* 2001; 4: 29–35.

Tennat RW, Stasiewicz S, Spalding JW. Comparison of Multiple parameters of rodent carcinogenicity and in vitro genetic toxicity *Environ Mutagen* 1986; 8: 205–227.

Peck CC, Barr WH, Benet LZ et al. Opportunities for integration of pharmacokinetics, Pharmacodynamics, and toxicokinetics in rational drug development. *Clin Pharmacol Ther* 1992; 51: 465–473.

Reno FE (1997) Carcinogenicity Studies. In *Comprehensive Toxicology*, vol 2, *Toxicological Testing and Evaluation*, Williams PD, Hottendorf GH (eds), Elsevier: London; 121–31.

Terrell TG, Green JD (1994) Issues with biotechnology products in toxicologic pathology. *Toxicol Pathol* 22: 187–93.

Voisin EM, Ruthsatz M, Collins JM, Hoyle PC (1990) Extrapolation of animal toxicity to humans: interspecies comparisons in drug development. *Regulat Toxicol Pharmacol* 12: 107–16.

Williams PD, Hottendof GH, (Eds.) *Comprehensive Toxicology Vol.2: Toxicological testing & Evaluation.* Elsevier: London, 1997.

Informed Consent

Anthony W. Fox

EBD Group Inc., Carlsbad, CA, USA

There is a tendency to assume that the principles of informed consent are self-evident. In fact, evidence that this is not the case comes from many sources, such as ethics committees, who are frequently dissatisfied with proposed informed consent documents, and sophisticated Western governments that, from time to time, have conducted clinical trials without it (e.g. the Tuskeegee travesty).

Informed consent was first formulated under international law through the Declaration of Helsinki, and in response to the atrocities of the Second World War. The principles of informed consent are under continuous review and discussion (e.g. Marsh, 1990). This is to be expected when reasonable standards of informed consent are dependent not only upon the design of a particular study, but also on environmental factors, the current state of medicine, and particular local characteristics of clinical trials populations, all of which are themselves continuously changing.

ETHICAL BASIS

Although enlarged upon elsewhere in this book, two ethical principles guiding informed consent are those of *autonomy* and *equipoise*. *Autonomy* is the concept that the patient is an individual who is under no duress, whether subtle or obvious, actual or inferred, and is competent to make a choice according to his/her free will. Clinical trials conducted on persons in custody, or on subordinate soldiers, may both violate the patient's autonomy. *Equipoise* is the concept that the investigator, and those sponsoring the trial, are truly uncertain as to the outcome of the study; in practical terms, this is a guarantee to the patient that an unreasonable hazard cannot result from unfavourable randomization because the treatment options are not known to be unequally hazardous.

WRITTEN INFORMED CONSENT

The large majority of clinical trials use a written informed consent document. In the absence of any special circumstances, the essential elements of such a document are:

1. A clear statement that the study is a research procedure.
2. A clear statement that participation is voluntary and that there will be no repercussions, either in the patient's relationship with the investigator, or with the patient's other caregivers, should the patient decide not to take part in the study.
3. A description of the scope and aims of the research, and whether or not there may be benefits to patients exposed to the test medications. The foreseeable risks and discomforts should also be disclosed. The possibility of placebo treatment, and the probability of being treated with each test therapy, should be stated.
4. Clear descriptions of alternative therapies or standard therapies or procedures (if any), in order that the patient can judge whether to enter the study.
5. The methods for compensation that may be available in the case of injury (these often have marked international variations).
6. Names and telephone numbers of persons who the patient may contact in case of any difficulty during the study. Also, the identity of person(s) of whom the patient may ask questions during the day-to-day conduct of the study, and an

Principles and Practice of Pharmaceutical Medicine. Edited by A. J. Fletcher, Lionel D. Edwards, Anthony W. Fox and Peter Stonier © 2002 John Wiley & Sons Ltd.

expression of willingness on the part of the investigator to provide answers to any questions that the patient may have.

7. A confidentiality statement. This should include the degree to which the patient's identity could be revealed to an inspecting regulatory authority, and whether information from the clinical study will automatically be communicated to the patient's primary care or referring physician. In any case, there should be an assurance that no patient identity information will be made public.

8. A statement of the circumstances under which the patient will be withdrawn from the study (e.g. non-compliance with test procedures).

9. A clear statement that the patient may withdraw from the study at any time and for any reason, again without repercussions to his/her relationship with any clinical caregiver.

10. A statement that the patient will be required to give a full and accurate clinical and treatment history on study entry and periodically thereafter (according to the study design).

11. Assurance that any new information that arises (e.g. in other studies) and which may alter the assessment of hazard of study participation will be communicated to the patient without delay.

12. A statement about the number of patients taking part in the study, and a brief summary of how many patients in the past have been exposed to the test medication.

Written informed consent documents should be signed by both the patient and the investigator, and ideally the patient should sign before an impartial witness. Informed consent documents should be written in a language that is understandable to the patient, and ideally at a level of complexity that could be understood by a young adolescent of average intelligence from the same community as the patient. There should be adequate time for the patient to review the document. All written informed consent documents should be approved by an ethics committee or an institutional review board.

UNWRITTEN INFORMED CONSENT

Informed consent, in law, must be informed, but need not be written. Ethics committees and institutional review boards may sanction specific methods for the documentation of oral informed consent. This is a very rare clinical situation.

SURROGATE INFORMED CONSENT

Some patients are incapable of providing informed consent, whether written or not. These patients are often in demographic subgroups which are medically underserved. Consequently, these are patients for whom there is encouragement to the pharmaceutical industry by governments, activists, and others to increase research into experimental therapies. Children, those with various types of neurological disease (e.g. Alzheimer's disease), and emergency patients (e.g. unconscious head injury, stroke, multiple trauma, etc.) are good examples. Many of these patients have a very poor prognosis, and epitomize the concept of unmet medical need. For these patients, clinical research would be impossible if written informed consent was an essential prerequisite.

For children, most ethics committees agree that provision of written informed consent by a parent or guardian is acceptable. If the child is of sufficient age, then his/her concurrence may also be sought; while this is not sufficient evidence of informed consent, the refusal to provide concurrence by a child who is likely to be competent to understand the clinical trial conditions should be sufficient to exclude the child from a study.

In the case of studies in legally incompetent adults, again most ethical committees will accept a legal guardian or custodian *in lieu* of the patient him/herself, provided that there is sufficient evidence that the custodian has a *bona fide* and independent interest in the patient's welfare. Again, forms of concurrence can be employed when possible. The ordering of a patient's participation in a clinical trial by a Court Order would usually be a form of duress and thus violate the concept of autonomy described above.

WHEN INFORMED CONSENT IS IMPOSSIBLE

Emergency patients have as much right to taking part in clinical research as any other type of patient. For example, patients with acute head injury and a low Glasgow Coma Score have a dismal prognosis, and therapeutic interventions (if ever likely to be successful) must be instituted quickly. Under these conditions there is often not even the time to find relatives to provide surrogate informed consent. Even if relatives can be found quickly enough, then their emotional state may not be suited to becoming truly informed before giving consent.

Experiments are now under way to investigate whether some substitute for informed consent may be used. One set of guidelines suggests that such clinical trials can be conducted when:

1. There is clinical and public agreement that the disease merits clinical investigation with the investigational therapy.
2. There has been advertising and publicity in the likely catchment area of suitable patients that such a study is being undertaken.
3. The ethics committee or institutional review board has approved, in detail, the methods used in pursuit of local publicity.
4. An independent, clinically experienced individual will confirm that the patient is a member of the well-defined population that is the subject of the clinical research, and that it is not unreasonable to include the patient in the study for any other reason.
5. No relative (if any is available in a timely fashion) objects.

It is likely that these guidelines will be refined, possibly on an international basis, in the near future.

RESPONSIBILITY OF PARTIES TO INFORMED CONSENT

It is the responsibility of all parties to the informed consent that all parties remain within its ethical and practical constraints. The Informed Consent document is essentially an agreement between Ethics Committee, investigator and patient. However, for example, an investigator is also responsible for the patient's role in the informed consent; if the investigator suspects that the patient is not truly informed, even in the absence of any deficiency on the part of the investigator, then the investigator should nonetheless police the patient's part of the agreement. This is entirely different from the notion of a contract, where each party to the contract is responsible only for fulfilling its own commitments.

Audit and policing of some of the elements listed above may also form part of the duty of a regulatory authority. For example, in the USA, the Food and Drug Administration (FDA) will audit institutional review boards (IRBs) and issue citations if the IRB is not ensuring that written informed consent documents are complete and appropriate. FDA will also audit study sites, and discipline investigators (including prosecution) who do not ensure that appropriate informed consent procedures are being followed.

Although under law it is not the primary responsibility of the typical pharmaceutical company, it nonetheless behoves pharmaceutical physicians to ensure that appropriate informed consent is being obtained in all company-sponsored studies. Many companies recognize this within their own Standard Operating Procedures, and create patient files that require a copy of the signed informed consent. Investigators will often be grateful if the company will draft an informed consent document that complies with the guidelines, which the investigator can submit to the ethics committee or IRB.

REFERENCES

Marsh BT (1990) Informed consent. *J R Soc Med* 83: 603–6.

8

Good Clinical Practices

Wendy Bohaychuk and Graham Ball

Good Clinical Research Practices Consultants, Lakehurst, Ontario, Canada, and Oxford UK

The aim of this chapter is to describe the general framework for conducting good clinical practices (GCP)-compliant clinical research, particularly pharmaceutical industry clinical research. Since it is difficult to cover this broad topic in such a short chapter, the authors will focus on those areas that are most discussed, most problematic, and most critical to achieving a GCP-compliant clinical study. Thus, there is particular emphasis on ethical issues, source data verification and data integrity, monitoring and safety review, and study medication/device management.

THE CURRENT RULES FOR CONDUCTING CLINICAL RESEARCH

Conducting GCP-compliant clinical research is a serious undertaking, and this has been recognized by numerous authorities internationally. It is difficult to achieve a fully GCP-compliant a clinical study, but the expectation today is that the greatest effort will be made nevertheless and the documentation to provide evidence of this effort must be available.

The Basic Tenets of GCP

The primary reason for the presence of a GCP code of practice is to safeguard human rights, as the welfare of current study subjects and future patients is at stake. Therefore, systems must be in place (such as ethics committee review and informed consent) to protect study subjects. Collecting honest and accurate data is also a major objective of GCP to ensure that data have integrity and that valid conclusions may be drawn from those data. Fur-

ther, data should be reproducible, i.e., if the study were to be conducted in a similar population using the same procedures, the results should be the same. To assure the integrity and reproducibility of research results, the whole process should be transparent, i.e., everything must be documented so that an external reviewer may verify that the research was actually conducted as reported by the researchers.

The General Regulatory Framework for GCP

The regulatory framework for compliance with research procedures has essentially developed on an international basis only in the last two decades, except for the US where rules were first established in the 1930s. Today, most countries in the European Union, other countries in Europe (e.g. Hungary, Poland and Switzerland) and Japan have regulations on GCP. Other countries have regulations controlling clinical studies, with guidelines on GCP, such as Australia and Canada. In the 1990s, an attempt was made to harmonise GCP requirements in the form of the ICH GCP document which has since been adapted in regulation by many countries. Some countries have no guidelines or regulations, but guidance for researchers has been provided by oragnisations such as the Council for the International Oragnizations of Medical Sciences (CIOMS) and the World Health Organization (WHO). (A brief list of existing regulations and guidelines is presented at the end of this chapter.) Regulatory authority review and/or approval is usually necesary in all countries before, during, and after clinical studies.

In the last few years, there has been increasing interest in regulatory inspection of GCP compliance

Principles and Practice of Pharmaceutical Medicine. Edited by A. J. Fletcher, Lionel D. Edwards, Anthony W. Fox and Peter Stonier © 2002 John Wiley & Sons Ltd.

to ensure validity of the data and protection of study subjects, and to compare the practices and procedures of the investigator and the sponsor/CRO with the commitment made in the application for marketing. Although inspection has been a regulatory requirement in the USA for many years, inspectorates have only just started in countries such as Austria, Denmark, France, Finland, Germany, Japan, The Netherlands, Norway and Sweden. There are problems in finding good inspectors, in deciding on the final standards for inspections, and in imposing sanctions for non-compliance. An interesting recent development has been the initiation of inspections in Europe by the central regulatory authority, the European Medicines Evaluation Agency (EMEA). Regulation of compliance with requirements by ethics committees is also developing in some parts of the world (e.g. France and Denmark). To date, the US Food and Drug Administration (FDA) is the only authority that is actively checking on the activities of institutional review boards (IRBs) by inspection and licensing.

For non-compliance with regulations, only the USA has imposed serious sanctions to date. The 'blacklist' (list of all investigators who have been found to be non-compliant and were barred from clinical research for FDA submissions) is publicly available through freedom of information rules.

The USA has vast experience (thousands of inspections) compared to the handful of inspections in other countries.

Within a research organization, other independent review, auditing, is undertaken internally to check on compliance with standards and basically to pre-empt the inspectors. Auditing may be conducted at any time during a clinical study to ensure continued compliance with GCP. Almost all aspects of GCP could be audited. Auditing, by definition, must be undertaken by personnel who are independent of the research being audited.

SETTING UP CLINICAL STUDIES

To ensure that the standards for clinical research are established before studies begin and to check on compliance with those standards, many fundamental systems and processes must be defined by pharmaceutical companies and contract research organizations (CROs). These are outlined in Table 8.1.

The sponsor/CRO has a duty to place a study safely. That is, the sponsor (or the delegated CRO) must assess and choose a site where study subjects will not be harmed. Some companies report that, in practice, they have little choice in this process, as the marketing department has already selected the

Table 8.1 General systems and procedures for implementation of GCP

The following systems and procedures must be established by clinical researchers to ensure compliance with GCP requirements:

Quality assurance: systems for assuring quality and for checking quality must be established and followed at all stages
Planning: studies must be conducted for valid (ethical and scientific) reasons
Standard operating procedures (SOPs): research procedures must be declared in writing so that reviewers can determine the standards which are being applied and so that users have a reference point
Well-designed study: all studies must have a valid study design, documented in a protocol, so that it can be fully reviewed by all interested parties. The data collection plans, as described in the CRF, are part of the protocol
Qualified personnel: all personnel (sponsor/CRO and study site) must be experienced and qualified to undertake assigned tasks. Documentation of qualifications and training must be evident
Ethics committee review and approval: all studies must be independently reviewed by ethics committees/IRBs, to assess the risk for study subjects, before clinical studies begin. Review must continue throughout the study
Informed consent: all study subjects must be given the opportunity to personally assess the risk of study participation by being provided with certain information. Their assent to participate must be documented
Monitoring: a primary means of quality control of clinical studies involves frequent and thorough monitoring by sponsor/CRO personnel
Data processing for integrity of data: data must be honest. Data must be reviewed by site personnel, monitors and data processing personnel
Control of study medications/devices: the product being studied must be managed so that study subjects ultimately receive a safe product and full accountability can be documented
Archives: documentation of research activities must be securely retained to provide evidence of activities

investigators (often those most likely to influence use of the medications/devices). Another rationale for apparent lack of choice is that there are too few patients or investigators in a particular therapeutic area. None of these reasons is as important as compliance with the basic GCP principle, which requires the sponsor/CRO to assess, select and choose safe settings for research.

Setting up clinical studies is a lengthy process, as there are many documents to prepare [e.g. protocols and case report forms (CRFs)], study facilities to be assessed (e.g. study sites, CROs, clinical laboratories, Phase I units), regulatory review to be considered, and negotiations and agreements with study sites (e.g. contracts, finances, confidentiality, indemnity, insurance) to be undertaken. In addition, as will be dealt with in subsequent sections, ethical aspects of the study must be considered (e.g., ethics committee and IRB review and informed consent requirements) and study medications/devices must be organized.

Protocols and Case Report Forms (CRFs)

The protocol, with the accompanying CRF, is the key document governing a clinical study. It formally describes how a clinical study will be conducted and how the data will be evaluated, and it must include all the information that an investigator should know in order to properly select subjects, collect safety and efficacy data, and prescribe the correct study medication/device. Protocols must be prepared in accordance with a specified and standardized format that is described in guidelines and regulations (the reader is particularly advised to refer to the ICH GCP document). Protocols are usually prepared, at least initially, by the sponsor or the delegated CRO, although investigator input is obviously necessary.

Any document used to collect research data on clinical study subjects may be generically classed as a data collection form. These completed forms provide evidence of the research conducted. The most common type of data collection form is the CRF. Other types of data collection forms include diary cards, dispensing records, quality of life forms, etc. The CRF must allow for proper analysis of the data and proper reporting of the data in the final clinical study report and it must reflect the protocol exactly: no more and no less data must be collected. Thus, a CRF must be created for each clinical study and must be prepared in parallel with the protocol. CRFs are usually also prepared by sponsors/CROs in pharmaceutical industry research because of the demanding requirements for their design and contents.

Selection of Investigators and Study Sites

The sponsor/CRO must go through a formal assessment procedure before placement of a study. Some of the most important areas requiring assessment are described in Table 8.2. All studies involving research of investigational medications and devices require qualified investigators, and the internationally accepted standard for 'qualified' usually encompasses three main criteria: medically qualified, i.e. legally licensed to practice medicine as a physician; experienced in the relevant therapeutic speciality; and experienced in clinical research.

Many contracts or agreements must be prepared, understood and authorized before clinical studies begin. The most common contracts include: the protocol and CRF; agreements for finances, confidentiality, insurance, and indemnity; and contracts between the sponsor and the CRO. A separate investigator agreement, specifying all responsibilities,

Table 8.2 Selection of study sites

The following items should be assessed at study sites by sponsor/CRO monitors before studies begin:

Study site personnel, e.g. qualification, experience, training, availability; specific allocation of responsibilities

Facilities, e.g. offices, wards, archives, pharmacy, clinical laboratory; study medication/device storage areas; clinical laboratories; access to source documents; ethics committee/IRB requirements

Suitable study subject population, e.g. access to suitable subjects in sufficient numbers; method of subject recruitment; source, e.g. from investigator's subject population, or be referred by other physicians and, if referred, means by which investigator will obtain adequate evidence of medical history; use of advertisements; potential subject enrolment (recruitment) rate

Table 8.3 Investigator GCP responsibilities

The following investigator responsibilities must be declared in agreements or contracts:

Adhere to the protocol exactly. No changes to the protocol may be undertaken without following a formal protocol amendment procedure and without agreement by the sponsor/CRO

Be thoroughly familiar with the properties of the clinical study medications/devices as described in the investigator brochure

Have sufficient time to personally conduct and complete the study. If more than one investigator is involved at a specific study site, the specific responsibilities must be described for each investigator. The investigator must ensure that no other studies divert study subjects, facilities or personnel from the study under consideration

Maintain the confidentiality of all information received with regard to the study and the investigational study medication/device

Submit the protocol, information sheet and consent form, and other required documentation, to an ethics committee/IRB for review and approval before the study begins. During the study, the investigator is also responsible for submitting any new information, e.g. protocol amendments, safety information, which might be important for continuing risk assessment by the ethics committee/IRB

Obtain informed consent from each study subject prior to enrolment into the study

Inform the subjects primary care physician, e.g. general practitioner or family physician, of proposed study participation before enrolment into the study

Maintain study subject clinical notes, i.e. source documents, separately from the CRFs. The source documents must support the data entered into CRFs and must clearly indicate participation in a clinical study. If the study subject is referred by another physician, the investigator must ensure that sufficient evidence is available in the clinical notes to support the eligibility of the study subject

Maintain a confidential list identifying the number/code and names of all subjects entered into the study

Allow authorized representatives of the sponsor/CRO and regulatory authorities direct access to study subject clinical notes (source documents) in order to verify the data recorded on CRFs

Ensure CRFs are complete and accurate

Allow monitoring visits by the sponsor/CRO at a predetermined frequency. During these monitoring visits, the monitor must be allowed to communicate with all site personnel involved in the conduct of the clinical study

Report all AEs and SAEs to the sponsor/CRO and follow the special reporting requirements for SAEs

Maintain the security and accountability of clinical study supplies, ensure that medications/devices are labeled properly, maintain records of clinical study medication/device dispensing, including dates, quantity and use by study subjects; and return or disposition (as instructed by the sponsor/CRO) after completion or termination of the study

Archive all CRFs and documents associated with the study for a minimum of 15 years. Notify the sponsor/CRO of any problems with archiving in potential unusual circumstances, e.g. investigator retires, relocates, dies; study subject dies, relocates, etc.

Provide reports of the study's progress whenever required

Review the final clinical report, and sign and date the signature page after review

Allow an independent audit and/or inspection of all study documents and facilities

Agree to the publication policy

Agree to the sponsor's/CRO's ownership of the data

Agree to the stated time frames for the study, e.g. start and completion of recruitment, submission of completed CRFs

Work to GCP as defined by the ICH, FDA and local regulations

is usually necessary in addition to the protocol, to emphasize certain aspects of the protocol. Table 8.3 highlights some of the main investigator GCP responsibilities which might be included in contracts.

ETHICAL CONSIDERATIONS

Part of the selection process for a study site involves confirming that ethics committee/IRB review will be safe and that all study subjects will be properly informed prior to consent to study participation. If the sponsor/CRO cannot obtain documented evidence of compliance with these two fundamental requirements, it is not safe to work with that site.

Ethics Committee/IRB Review

All clinical studies require review by an independent ethics committee/IRB before, during and after the study. Before any study subjects are treated, review by the committee must be documented in compliance with international guidelines and the local regulations of the country in which the research is conducted. Clinical studies begin (for the study subjects) whenever any procedure is undertaken by study subjects that they would not normally undergo: ethics committee/IRB review must be sought before these events. Thus, if a study requires screening procedures, washout from normal treatment, and even completion of a questionnaire that poses personal questions, the study begins when those procedures are undertaken. It is a common misconception that studies begin only when study subjects are randomized to treatment.

Prior to selection of a clinical study site, the sponsor/CRO must confirm and document, in the prestudy assessment visit report, that the investigator has access to a local ethics committee/IRB. Local committees cannot be bypassed: the only official exception to this requirement is in France, where, by regulation, a central committee may rule for all sites in a multicentre study. However, in the USA, it appears to be common practice for a central IRB to rule for the widely geographically separated areas in the country, and researchers may not inform the local IRB.

Normally, the sponsor/CRO will prepare all necessary documentation for submission by the investigator to the ethics committee/IRB (it is not usual procedure for the sponsor/CRO to directly submit items to the committee, unless requested to do so by the committee). Whatever the local variations, the sponsor/CRO is usually responsible for ensuring the submission of the items in Table 8.4. Some committees require other additional items.

The membership of an ethics committee/IRB will vary nationally and regionally. However, the sponsor/CRO is only permitted to conduct studies that are approved by ethics committees/IRBs that have a sufficient number of qualified members to enable a medical and scientific review of the proposed study and to enable a review of all other ethical aspects of the study. Generally, ethics committees also have to be diverse in composition. Details of the membership of the ethics committee/IRB should be obtained and reviewed by the sponsor/CRO, prior to initiating the study, to ascertain the above and to determine that there is no serious conflict of interest (e.g. investigator voting on her/his study).

The sponsor/CRO should also request a written copy of the working procedures of the ethics committees/IRBs. These procedures should provide sufficient information to assure sponsors/CROs, investigators, auditors and inspectors of the integrity and independence of the ethics committee/IRB. Unfortunately, today, it is still difficult to obtain working procedures from many committees.

Ethics committees/IRBs also have responsibility for review during and after clinical studies (Table 8.5). In other words, committee review is an ongoing responsibility that extends beyond the initial submission and review of documents to proceed with the study.

Informed Consent

Potential study subjects may enter a clinical study conducted by the sponsor/CRO only after being properly informed and consenting to participate. The researchers must consider who does what, when, what sort of information must be provided, and how this will all be documented. The general principles for the conduct of informed consent are noted in Table 8.6. (See also Chapter 7). All information sheets and consent forms should include the items listed in Table 8.7 and they must be provided before study participation. Obtaining informed consent is a complex issue and it is not easy to comply with these requirements.

MONITORING AND SAFETY ASSESSMENT

The conduct of clinical studies is a cooperative undertaking between the sponsor/CRO and the investigator; each is responsible for ensuring that the study is in conformity with the protocol and in accordance with all applicable laws and regulations, and, of course, that study subjects are protected at all times. This responsibility involves regular and conscientious review of the progress of the study by the sponsor/CRO and by the investigator and study site personnel.

Monitoring

One of the most important means of quality control of a clinical study is managed by frequent and thorough monitoring. A monitor's aim is first to protect the agenda of the sponsor/CRO who employs him/her. Monitors (often referred to as CRAs or Clinical Research Associates or Assistants in the pharmaceutical industry) must ensure maintenance of proper standards, compliance with the

Table 8.4   Review by ethics committees/IRBs before clinical studies begin

The following items should be reviewed by ethics committees/IRBs before clinical studies begin:

Protocol (including annexes, such as the CRF)

Consent procedures (described in the protocol and the appended information sheet and consent form), which specify who will provide information and who will obtain consent, how consent will be documented, and whether or not a witness will be present

Consent form/information sheet. Most committees will be particularly interested in these documents to ensure that all necessary information is provided to study subjects

Suitability of investigator and facilities, including support personnel. Some committees may request a copy of investigator and other site personnel CVs. The committee will be particularly interested in allocation of resources, whether the investigator has enough time and study subjects to conduct the study, and whether use of resources for clinical studies will detract from normal medical care requirements

Delegation of responsibility by investigators

Source of study subjects and means of recruitment. The committee will wish to know if study subjects are known to investigators and, if not (i.e. referred patients), how investigators will confirm eligibility and whether primary care practitioners will be informed. The committee will wish to determine that advertisements are not unduly coercive or misleading or too 'inviting'

Appropriateness (eligibility) of study subjects (described in the protocol)

Primary care physician to be informed of study participation

Number of subjects to be studied and justification for sample size (this information should be in the protocol). The committee will be interested in how many subjects will be exposed to the risk of treatment. In a multicenter study, the local ethics committee/IRB should be informed of the number of subjects to be enrolled at each site and the total number of subjects to be enrolled in the study

Investigator brochure or other authorized summary of information (e.g. preclinical and clinical summaries) about the investigational products, including comparator products and placebo. If the study medication/device is a marketed product, the ethics committee/IRB must review the most current data sheet, product monograph, etc. The brochure is particularly important for confirming the formal declared safety profile of the study treatment and therefore is of great assistance to committees in assessing the relevance of AEs. Also, the committee can verify, by reviewing the brochure or product labeling, that the information sheet for obtaining consent provides sufficient information with regard to safety

Evidence of regulatory submission and review/approval (if applicable). Committees particularly wish to know whether the drug/device is on the market in their country or in other countries, and the details of the stage of the submission

Adequacy of confidentiality safeguards, with regard to protection of identification of the study subject (described in the protocol and the appended information sheet and consent form)

Insurance provisions, if any, for injury to study subjects (described in the protocol or provided as a separate document). Committees must confirm that there is insurance for protection of the study subjects

Indemnity/insurance provisions for the sponsor/CRO, investigator, institution, etc. (as relevant to the study and if required by local regulations)

Payments or rewards to be made to study subjects, if any. Committees must determine that the amount, and schedule of payments, is not unduly coercive

Benefits, if any, to study subjects

Payments or rewards to be made to investigators. Many committees are beginning to realize that the financial interests of the investigator might have a strong influence on some aspects of the study, particularly recruitment patterns

Assurance of quality/stability of medication/device to be administered

Review decision of other ethics committees/IRBs in multicentre studies

Duration of study

Plans to review data collected to ensure safety

protocol, accurate and complete data capture, and standardization across sites in a multicentre study. Basically, monitors will undertake the review noted in Table 8.8.

In general, study sites should be visited by a monitor at least every 4–6 weeks. The frequency of monitoring visits will be defined for each individual study and will depend on details such as the study phase, treatment interval and overall duration, enrolment rate, complexity of the study methodology, occurrence of adverse events (AEs) or other significant events, and the nature of the study medication/device. At the beginning of a study, monitoring may be even more frequent. The most time-consuming task at the study site is the review of source documents to confirm entries in CRFs and compliance with the protocol.

The monitor will be ever-vigilant for protocol violations which can occur during a study and which can have a serious impact on eligibility and evaluability. Many researchers confuse the terms

Table 8.5 Review by ethics committees/IRBs during and after clinical studies

The following items should be reviewed by ethics committees/IRBs during and after clinical studies:

Serious and/or unexpected AEs, if any occur during the study, including the follow-up period
Protocol amendments, if any, and reasons for amendments
Protocol violations which impact on subject safety, if any
Discontinuation of study, if applicable, and any reasons for premature discontinuation
Any new significant information, e.g. information arising from other studies, results of interim analyses, marketing approvals, changes in local procedures, updated investigator brochure, supply problems, during study, if any
Amendments to consent forms/information sheets, if any
Annual reports of the study. More frequent review may be necessary, depending on the working procedures of each individual ethics committee
Final clinical report/summary of study. Some ethics committees/IRBs also review publications, if any

Table 8.6 Principles for the conduct of informed consent

The following principles for conducting informed consent should be implemented for all clinical studies:

Informed consent must be obtained from each study subject. The person receiving the information and giving consent must sign the consent form. This is usually the study subject, but may be the study subject's legally acceptable representative (depending on national regulations) in the event that the study subject is incapable of providing informed consent, e.g. the subject is unable to write or understand the consent documents, or the study subject is in a 'vulnerable' population, e.g. children, elderly. Informed consent must be obtained before the start of the study
The person providing the information and obtaining consent must sign the consent form. This person should be an investigator who must be qualified to adequately inform the study subject, and her/his signature also indicates personal involvement in the consent process. If other personnel, e.g. study nurses assist in providing information or obtaining consent, they should also sign the consent form, clearly describing their role in the consent procedure
A witness or patient advocate should be present during the consent procedure at the times of providing information and giving consent, and should sign the consent form. The witness will ensure that there was no coercion in the obtaining of informed consent and that the study subject was given adequate time to consider participation in the study. The witness must be able to confirm that the consent procedure was adequate and must have no vested interest in the clinical study, i.e. the witness should be impartial, independent, or neutral, as far as this can be achieved. The relationship of the witness to the study subject and to the investigator and the study should be documented
All participants should personally date their signatures and all dates should precede the start of the study (for each subject)

Table 8.7 Information to be provided to study subjects before obtaining consent to participate in clinical studies

The information sheets and consent forms should contain the following items:

1. *Information about the consent procedure*:
   Consent to be given by the study subject's free will
   Adequate time (which should be defined in advance in the protocol) must be allowed for the study subject to decide on participation in study
   Adequate time must be allowed to ask questions
   Statement that participation is entirely voluntary
   Statement that refusal to participate will involve no penalties or loss of usual benefits
   Description of circumstances under which participation would be terminated
   Right to withdraw at any time without prejudice or consequences
   Study subject is allowed to keep the written explanation (information sheet and consent form) for future reference

2. *Information about the study and medications/devices*:
   Instructions on use and storage of study medication/device, if relevant
   Name of sponsor/CRO
   Explanation that the study is a research procedure
   Description of study type and research aims
   Description of study medications/devices
   Description of procedures to be followed

Table 8.7   *(contd.)*

Description of experimental procedures to be followed, if any. Experimental procedures might include those which are not normally used for the presentation under consideration or procedures which are new or have never been used before

Comparator treatments (including placebo) described. It is important to explain 'placebo' in simple terms

Randomization procedures. Randomization is not easily understood by many subjects and should also be explained in simple terms

Expected duration of participation

Required number of visits

Reason for selection of suitable subjects

Approximate number of other study subjects participating in the study

3. *Information about the risks/benefits*:

Foreseeable risks, discomforts, side effects and inconveniences

Known therapeutic benefits, if any. The benefits must not be 'oversold'

Availability of alternative therapies. If there are other treatments, this must be explained so that the subject does not feel the new treatment is the only option

Any new findings, which might affect the safety of the study subject, and that become available during participation in the study, will be disclosed to the study subject

Assurance of compensation for treatment-induced injury with specific reference to local guidelines (it must not be expected that the study subject is familiar with the guidelines, and therefore the guidelines must be explained and/or attached)

Terms of compensation

Measures to be taken in the event of an AE or therapeutic failure

Financial remuneration, if any. Patients, whether receiving therapeutic benefit or not, are not usually paid for participation in clinical research, except for incidentals such as travel costs. Healthy volunteers are usually paid a fee for participation, but this payment should never be offered to induce the prospective subjects to take risks they would not normally consider

Explanation of additional costs that may result from participation, if any (this normally only occurs in the USA)

4. *Other items*:

Ethics committee/IRB approval obtained (some debate about this)

Name of ethics committee/IRB (if applicable by local and/or national requirements) and details of contact person on the ethics committee/IRB (if applicable by local and/or national requirements)

Explanation that participation is confidential, but records (which divulge study subject names) may be reviewed by authorized sponsor/CRO representatives and may be disclosed to a regulatory authority

Name, address and telephone number (24 h availability) of contact person at study site for information or in the event of an emergency (this information may be provided on a separate card)

Requirement to disclose details of medical history, any medicines (or alcohol) currently being taken, changes in any other medication/device use, and details of participation in other clinical studies

Medical records will clearly identify study participation

Conditions as they apply to women of child-bearing potential

Primary care physician (or general practitioner or family doctor) and/or referring physician will be informed of study participation and any significant problems arising during the study. Some subjects may not be comfortable with this requirement, e.g. in a study of sexually transmitted diseases, they may not wish the doctor, perhaps a family friend, to be aware of their situation. If this is the case, the subject is not eligible for the study as it is vital to confirm history with the primary care physician.

The information sheet must be written in language which is understandable, e.g. technically simple and in the appropriate national language, to the study subject.

'protocol violations' and 'protocol amendments'. It is important to appreciate the differences between these terms and understand how to avoid protocol violations and how to manage protocol amendments. Perhaps the easiest way to explain the difference is to stress that violations are not planned changes (hopefully) to the protocol, whereas protocol amendments are planned changes and are enacted through a formal approval process (if violations are deliberate or planned, a case of fraud should be considered!).

Reporting and Recording Safety Events

An issue over which site personnel and monitors will be particularly watchful is the observation and recording of safety information. In many studies, safety information is under-reported because of the tendency to make judgments that are often based on subjective and biased clinical opinion. It seems difficult to teach clinical researchers to operate as 'scientists': that is, to observe and record all observations before making judgments. The monitor

Table 8.8 Objectives of monitoring visits

The following tasks should be undertaken by the sponsor/CRO monitor at each study site visit:

Verify accuracy and completeness of recorded data in CRFs, including diary cards, quality of life forms, registration forms, consent forms, etc., by comparing with the original source documents (clinic or hospital records). Where discrepancies are found, arrangements must be made for corrections and resolution. Resolve any outstanding queries, ensuring completion of any issued data queries, since the last monitoring visit

Verify compliance with entry criteria and procedures, for all study subjects, as specified in the protocol. If subjects are found to be ineligible or unevaluable, these events must be immediately brought to the attention of the investigator. There may also be implications for payment to the study site and requirements for reporting to ethics committees/IRBs. Finally, and most seriously, there could be implications for subject safety

Review all AEs, including clinically significant laboratory abnormalities, that have occurred since the previous visit. If a serious or unexpected AE has occurred, which was not correctly reported by the investigator, the monitor must ensure that the correct reporting procedure is followed immediately

Evaluate the subject recruitment and withdrawal/dropout rate. If recruitment is less than optimal, suggest ways in which it can be increased. In particular, query the reasons for withdrawals/dropouts, or unscheduled visits, in case these are related to AEs

Confirm that all source documents will be retained in a secure location. Source documents must be legible and properly indexed for ease of retrieval. Check the study site file to ensure that all appropriate documents are suitably archived. Check that the investigator files are secure and stored in a separate area which is not accessible to individuals not involved in the study

Conduct an inventory and account for study medications/devices and arrange for extra supplies, including other items, such as CRFs, blank forms, etc., if necessary. Resolve discrepancies between inventory and accountability records, and medication/device use, as recorded in the CRFs. If a pharmacy is involved in the study, the pharmacy and pharmacist must be visited. Check that the medication/device is being dispensed in accordance with the protocol. Check that the medication/device is being stored under appropriate environmental conditions and that the expiry dates are still valid. Check that the medication/device is securely stored in a separate area that is not accessible to individuals not involved in the study. Check that any supplies shipped to the site since the last visit were received in good condition and are properly stored. If applicable, ensure that randomization procedures are being followed, blind is being maintained, randomization codebreak envelopes are intact (sealed and stored properly) and a chronological sequence of allocation to treatment is being followed

Verify correct biological sample collection (especially number, type, and timing), correct procedures for assays (if applicable), and labeling, storage and transportation of specimens or samples. All clinical laboratory reports should be checked for identification details, validity and continued applicability of reference ranges, accuracy of transcription to CRFs (if any), comments on all out-of-range data, and investigator signatures and dates. The dates of sample collection, receipt, analysis and reporting should be checked to ensure that samples are analysed promptly, and that investigators are informed of results and review them promptly

Ensure continued acceptability of facilities, staff and equipment. Ensure that the reference range, documentation of certification and proficiency testing, licensing, and accreditation, for the clinical laboratory are still current. Document any changes in clinical site personnel and, if changes have occurred, collect evidence of suitability of new personnel. Ensure that new staff are fully briefed on the requirements of the protocol and study procedures and arrange any training of new personnel, if necessary. Document any changes in overall facilities and equipment and if changes have occurred, collect new evidence of suitability, maintenance, calibration and reason for change of new equipment

Advise the investigator and other site personnel of any new developments, e.g. protocol amendments, AEs, which may affect the conduct of the study

---

and all clinical research personnel must ensure that all safety information is documented. This means that all adverse events (AEs) occurring in clinical studies must be recorded in CRFs, their significance must be assessed, and other information must be provided, for reporting AEs externally (e.g. to regulatory authorities and ethics committees/IRBs). This applies to any study treatment (including comparator agents, placebo and non-medical therapy) and any stage of the study (e.g. run-in, washout, active treatment, follow-up).

All research personnel must search for clues about safety events from many sources, such as:

information in clinical records at the study sites; information in data collection forms (e.g. CRFs, diary cards, quality of life forms, psychiatric rating scales, etc.), occurrence of missed and/or unscheduled visits, dropouts and withdrawals; use of any concomitant medications/devices; and abnormal laboratory data. AEs may also occur simply as a result of study procedures and study participation. Information about definitions of AEs and requirements for reporting AEs must be clearly stated in the protocol and explained to the site staff, who must also be educated in the correct procedure and immediate requirement for reporting any adverse event suspected to be serious or unexpected per the regulatory definitions.

All investigators and other study site personnel, ethics committees/IRBs, and possibly study subjects, must be informed of all new significant safety information, including all events occurring with any treatment (e.g. washout, investigational product, comparator, placebo, etc.) in the study, even if these occurred in another study with the same treatment, or in another country. Significant safety information includes all SAEs and any other events (e.g. significant trends in laboratory data or new preclinical data) that might have an impact on the risk assessment of the study. Safety events may necessitate an update to the investigator brochure, the protocol and CRF, and the information sheet and consent form.

COLLECTING DATA WITH INTEGRITY

Collecting data that are accurate, honest, reliable and credible is one of the most important objectives of conducting clinical research. It is difficult to achieve. However, in general, data in CRFs are not credible to the regulators unless they can be supported by the 'real' documents (i.e. the source documents maintained at the study site for the clinical care of the study subject).

Source Data Verification

Source data verification is the process of verifying CRF entries against data in the source documents. Source data verification is only carried out at the study site, usually by the sponsor/CRO monitor (auditors will also conduct source data verification on a sample of CRFs; inspectors may conduct source data verification on a sample or all CRFs).

Source documents (and the data contained therein) comprise the following types of documents: patient files (medical notes where summaries of physical examination findings, details of medical history, concurrent medications/devices, and diseases are noted), recordings from automated instruments, traces (eg ECGs, EEGs), X-ray films, laboratory notes, and computer databases (e.g. psychological tests requiring direct entry by patient

onto computers or direct entry of patient information onto computers by physicians).

The primary purpose of source documents is for the care of the study subject from a clinical perspective: the primary purpose of CRFs is to collect research data. CRFs (and other data collection forms) generally cannot substitute as source documents. Data entered in CRFs should generally be supported by source data in source documents, except as specifically defined at the beginning of the study. Nevertheless, some data entered in CRFs may be source data (e.g. multiple blood pressure readings, psychiatric rating scales, etc.) and would not be found elsewhere. This may be acceptable, if these data would not normally be entered in medical records, and if knowledge of such data is not required by the investigator or other clinicians who concurrently or subsequently treat the study subject (the protocol should specify which data will be source data in the CRF).

How much information is expected to be documented in source documents? This is a difficult issue, but one that must be discussed and resolved before the CRFs are completed. Some guidelines are provided in Table 8.9.

Direct access to source documents is required for all studies—direct access means monitors, auditors, other authorized representatives of the sponsor/CRO, and inspectors are permitted to view all relevant source documents needed to verify the CRF data entries. Other restricted methods of access to source documents (e.g. 'across-the-table', 'back-to-back', 'interview method') are not acceptable, as they do not allow proper verification of the data in CRFs. To ensure direct access, the study subject consent form must clearly indicate that permission for access has been granted by the study subject.

Other Review to Assure Data Integrity

After retrieval from the study site, there are further means of assessing CRFs. First, there is the initial review at the sponsor/CRO premises: this process is sometimes referred to as 'secondary monitoring'. Thereafter, review by the data management department is another extremely important means of quality control. It is a lengthy and complex process and there are few guidelines and regulations for

Table 8.9 Source data verification

For all study subjects, source data verification requires a review of the following items:

Existence of medical records/files at the study site. There must be a medical file, separate from the CRF, which forms a normal part of the clinical record for the study subjects. The medical file should clearly indicate the full name, birth date, and hospital/clinic/health service number of the study subject

Eligibility of study subjects. The medical file must show compliance with the inclusion and exclusion criteria. At a minimum, demographic characteristics, e.g. sex, weight and height, diagnoses, e.g. major condition for which subject was being treated, and other 'hard' data, e.g. laboratory results within a specified range or normal chest X-ray, should be clearly indicated. All required baseline assessments must be evident. If the medical file has little or no information concerning medical history, it would not support selection of the subject

Indication of participation in the study. The medical file should clearly show that the subject was in a clinical study in case the information is necessary for future clinical care

Consent procedures. The original signed consent form should be maintained with the subject's medical files or in the investigator files and an indication that consent was obtained (with the date specified) should be noted in the medical files. Signatures and dates must be checked carefully to ensure that the correct individuals were involved in the consent procedure and that consent was obtained prior to any study intervention

Record of exposure to study medication/device. The medical file should clearly indicate when treatment began, when treatment finished, and all intervening treatment dates

Record of concomitant medications/devices. All notations of previous and concomitant medication/device use must be examined. All entries in the CRF should be verifiable in the medical file by name, date(s) of administration, dose and reason (or indication). All entries in the medical file during the time period specified by the protocol must be noted in the CRF. Concomitant medication/device use must be explicable by an appropriate indication and must be consistent from visit to visit. The reasons (indications) for use of concomitant medications/devices, newly prescribed during the study period, must be noted as AEs. The medical history should be reviewed to determine whether medical conditions arising during the study already existed at baseline. The dispensing records, which are normally separate from the medical file, must also be examined to determine consistency.

Visit dates. All visit dates should be recorded in the medical file. Interim visit dates recorded in the medical file, but not in the CRF, should be noted by the monitor in case they signify occurrence of AEs or protocol violations. The final visit date should be so indicated, e.g. 'study finished' or 'withdrew from study'

AEs. All AEs noted in the medical file during the time period specified by the protocol must be recorded in the CRF. The monitor must also carefully check other documents (e.g. diary cards, quality of life forms) for sources of information about AEs. Occurrence of out-of-range laboratory values, which are considered to be clinically significant by the investigator, must be reported and assessed as AEs

Major safety and efficacy variables (to be decided and documented in advance). It is not necessary for all measured variables to be recorded in the medical file. Present and future clinical care of the study subject is the most important factor in determining whether or not measured variables should be recorded in the medical file. The investigator should record what he/she would normally record to care for the study subject, but also take into account any recording needed because of the special circumstances of a clinical study. The entire medical file should be reviewed to ensure that no additional information exists in the medical file that should have been recorded in the CRF

reference. These processes will inevitably result in queries about the data. It is critical that all data review procedures be prompt. As time goes by, it becomes more and more difficult to correct data. Slow processing usually means that data lose credibility.

To ensure that the integrity of clinical research data is maintained and that there is total agreement between the data recorded on CRFs, the data entered on the computer, the data recorded in data listings and cross-tabulations, the data entered into statistical and clinical study reports, and finally the data in the sponsor/CRO and investigator archives, it is essential that the data must only be changed by following a formal procedure. Thus,

requests for data clarification and all resolution of queries must be documented. All data changes must be authorized by the investigator ultimately. Obviously, the sponsor/CRO cannot arbitrarily make changes of data.

Archiving

Systems must be in place to ensure that documents will be securely retained for a long period of time. The purpose of archiving is to safeguard all documentation that provides evidence that a clinical study has been conducted in accordance with the principles of GCP. Archives at both the sponsor/

CRO and investigator sites must be reasonably secure with regard to indexing, controlled access, fire-resistance, flood-resistance, etc.

The investigator must be held responsible for ensuring that all source documents, especially records acquired in the normal practice of care and treatment of a study subject, are safely archived and available for inspection by authorized company personnel or regulatory authorities. Further, the investigator must archive all necessary documents for a minimum of 15 years—the usual industry standard. All appropriate clinical study documents should be archived by the sponsor/CRO, essentially for the lifetime of the product. The specific documents to be retained are described in the ICH GCP document.

MANAGING STUDY MEDICATIONS/DEVICES

Management of clinical study medications and devices is a complicated activity, and many clinical researchers report that they are not particularly interested in this aspect of clinical studies: they assume that it is all handled by other personnel in the manufacturing facility. Meanwhile, personnel in the manufacturing facility usuall report that once the supplies are released, they assume no further responsibility!

Preparation of Study Medications/Devices

The preparation of study medications or devices for clinical studies is a time-consuming process and often rate-limiting in initiating the study, particularly with double-blind designs. Requisition, labeling and packaging are some of the important considerations.

Requisition of study medication/device (including placebo and comparator products, if relevant) must be initiated at an early stage to allow sufficient time to procure the study medications/devices and to prepare the final labeling and packaging, taking into account any special circumstances for blind studies and for import requirements.

The principles of safe labeling and packaging require compliance with the following principles: the contents of a container can be identified; a contact name, address and telephone number is available for emergencies and enquiries; and the study subject (or the person administering the medication/device) is knowledgeable about storing and administering the study medication/device, and that the packing process can be audited against a standard Operating Procedure.

Shipment of Study Medications/Devices

Clinical study medications/devices should not be dispatched to study sites until all prestudy activities have been completed and regulatory requirements satisfied. The receipt of each shipment of study medication/device should be confirmed in writing by the investigator or pharmacist (or other authorized personnel), who will be instructed to return a completed 'acknowledgement of receipt form' immediately. The recipient at the study site will be instructed to contact the sponsor/CRO immediately if there are any problems (e.g. missing or broken items, defects in labeling, evidence of excursion from temperature ranges) with the shipment. The recipient must be particularly instructed to record the exact date of receipt of the clinical supplies at the study site. This information is necessary so that the monitor can determine that the supplies were secure and correctly stored environmentally during the entire period of shipment.

After the clinical study supplies have been sent to the study site, the monitor must verify as soon as possible that the supplies have arrived satisfactorily. Supplies may not be dispensed to study subjects until the monitor has checked their condition. The monitor will verify that the amount shipped matches the amount acknowledged as received. If there is a lack of reconciliation, or if the shipment is not intact, recruitment may be delayed until the situation is resolved.

Control of Study Medications/Devices at Study Sites

Evidence of careful control at the study site is imperative and naturally it is difficult to standardize the situation across many study sites and many countries. Security, correct storage, and accurate documentation of dispensing and inventory are necessary. Systems to ensure and assess compliance with the required use of the product being studied must be established. Monitors must be trained to check on these features and ensure that all site personnel are fully briefed.

The expectations with regard to maintenance of study medications/devices at study sites focus on security and appropriate environmental conditions. Concerns for security require that supplies be maintained under locked conditions. All agreements between the sponsor/CRO and the study site must specify that supplies are only for clinical study subjects—this information must also be clearly stated on the labeling. The main concern for appropriate environmental conditions is usually temperature requirements, but other factors (e.g. light, humidity) might also be important. Terms such as 'room temperature' and 'ambient temperature', which have different meanings in different countries, should always be avoided and specific temperatures must be stated. At each monitoring visit, the monitor will ensure that the correct procedures are being followed.

Compliance with medication/device use (by the study subject) should be assessed in all studies. If supplies are dispensed to subjects for self-administration, methods to assure compliance (e.g., diary cards, instructions on labeling, supervised administration) and methods to check compliance (e.g. tablet counts, plasma/urine assays, diary card review) must be in place. At each study visit, the study subjects should be asked to return all unused supplies and empty containers to the investigator, who will check the supplies for assessment of compliance and store them for return to the sponsor/CRO. The monitor will review all relevant documents (e.g. source documents, CRFs, medication/device inventory, dispensing forms) to ensure that the data in the CRFs reflect the subjects' compliance with the study medications/devices.

Overall Accountability of Study Medications/Devices

Overall accountability must documented and reviewed. A reconciliation of the initial inventory and the final returns must be undertaken and all discrepancies must be explained. Final disposition and destruction must be carefully documented to also allow assessment of possible detrimental environmental impact. All unused and returned medications/devices, empty containers, devices, equipment, etc., which are returned to the investigator by the study subjects, must be stored securely and under correct environmental conditions at the study site until retrieval by the monitor. The monitor will check the supplies returned and verify that they reconcile with the written specifications. All discrepancies and the reasons for any non-returns must be documented and explained.

Generally, destruction of returned study medications/devices by the sponsor/CRO may not take place until the final report has been prepared and until there is no further reason to question the accountability of the study medication/device. The actual destruction process must be documented in a manner which clearly details the final disposition of the unused medications/devices and the method of destruction. The information is particularly necessary in case of any query regarding environmental impact. In exceptional circumstances, unused study medications (e.g. cytotoxics, radio-labeled products) may be destroyed at the study site, with appropriate documentation.

Randomization and Blinding

Randomization procedures are employed to ensure that study subjects entered into a comparative study are treated in an unbiased way. Blinding (or masking) procedures (e.g. single-blind or double-blind) further minimize bias by ensuring that outcome judgments are not based on knowledge of the treatment. If the study design is double-blind, it is essential that all personnel who may influence the subject or the conduct of the study are blinded to the identity of the study medication/device assigned to the subject, and therefore do not have access to randomization schedules.

SUMMARY

The code of Good Clinical Practice was established to ensure subject safety and arose because of biases inherent in clinical research (e.g. pressures to recruit subjects for payment, publication, etc.), which needed some counterbalance. It is hoped the reader will appreciate that GCP is not 'bureaucratic nonsense' (as argued by some researchers), but is a logical, ethical, and scientific approach to standardizing a complex discipline.

SOURCES OF INTERNATIONAL GUIDELINES/REGULATIONS FOR GCP

Australia
National Statement on Ethical Conduct in Research Involving Humans, National Health and Medical Research Council Act, 1992. **http://www.health.gov.au/nhmrc/publications/synopses/e35syn.htm**
Note for Guidance on Good Clinical Practice (CPMP/ICH/135/95). *Annotated with TGA comments*. Therapeutic Goods Administration [TGA] (Australia), Commonwealth Department of Health and Aged Care. The TGA has adopted CPMP/ICH/135/95 in principle but has recognised that some elements are, by necessity, overridden by the National Statement (and therefore not adopted) and that others require explanation in terms of 'local regulatory requirements', July 2000. **http://www.health.gov.au/tga/docs/html/ich13595.htm**
Note for Guidance on Clinical Safety Data Management (CPMP/ICH/377/95). *Annotated with TGA comments*. Therapeutic Goods Administration (Australia), Commonwealth Department of Health and Aged Care. The TGA has adopted the Note for Guidance on Clinical Safety Data Management: Definitions and Standards for Expedited Reporting in principle, particularly its definitions and reporting time frames. However, there are some elements of CPMP/ICH/377/95 which have not been adopted by the TGA and other elements which require explanation in terms of 'local regulatory requirements', 2000. **http://www.health.gov.au/tga/docs/html/ich37795.htm**

Canada
Code of Ethical Conduct for Research Involving Humans, Medical Research Council of Canada, Natural Sciences and Engineering Research Council of Canada, Social Sciences and Humanities Research Council of Canada, 1998. **http://www.nserc.ca/programs/ethics/english/policy.htm**
Clinical Trial Review and Approval, Drugs Directorate, Policy Issues, Health and Welfare Canada, 1995. TPP (Therapeutic Products Program, Canada) **http://www.hc-sc.gc.ca/hpb-dgps/therapeut/htmleng/whatsnew.html**
Clinical Trial Framework, Schedule 1024, Food and Drug Regulations. Therapeutic Products Directorate, Health Products and Food Branch, Health Canada, 2001. **http://www.hc-sc.gc.ca/hpb-dgps/therapeut/zfiles/english/schedule/gazette.ii/sch-1024_e.pdf**

European Union
Good Clinical Practice for Trials on Medicinal Products in the European Community, Committee for Proprietary Medicinal Products [CPMP] EEC 111/3976/88-EN, Brussels, 1990.

Commission Directive 91/507/EEC modifying the Annex to Council Directive 75/318/EEC on the approximation of the laws of Member States relating to the analytical, pharmacotoxicological and clinical standards and protocols in respect of the testing of medicinal products, Official Journal of the European Communities, 1991.
Commission Directive 2001/20/EC of the European Parliament and of the Council of 4 April 2001 on the approximation of the laws, regulations and administrative provisions of the Member States relating to the implementation of good clinical practice in the conduct of clinical trials on medicinal products for human use. **http://europa.eu.int/eur-lex/en/lif/dat/2001/en_301L0020.html**
Manufacture of Investigational Medicinal Products, Annex to the EC Guide to Good Manufacturing Practice, EEC 111/3004/91-EN, Brussels, 1992.
Biostatistical Methodology in Clinical Trials in Applications for Marketing Authorizations for Medicinal Products, Committee for Proprietary Medicinal Products [CPMP] EEC 111/3630/92-EN, 1994.

UK
Clinical Trial Compensation Guidelines, Association of the British Pharmaceutical Industry (ABPI), 1994.
Conduct of Investigator Site Audits, ABPI, 1993.
Good Clinical (Research) Practice, ABPI, 1996.
Good Clinical Trial Practice, ABPI, 1995.
Introduction to the Work of Ethics Committees, ABPI, 1997.
Patient Information and Consent for Clinical Trials, ABPI, 1997.
Phase IV Clinical Trials, ABPI, 1993.
Set of Clinical Guidelines, ABPI, 2000.
Structure of a Formal Agreement to Conduct Sponsored Clinical Research, ABPI, 1996. **http://www.abpi.org.uk/**
Fraud and Misconduct in Clinical Research, Royal College of Physicians of London, 1991.
Guidelines for Clinicians Entering Research, Royal College of Physicians of London, 1997.
Guidelines on the Practice of Ethics Committees in Medical Research Involving Human Subjects, Royal College of Physicians of London, 1997.
Research Involving Patients, Royal College of Physicians of London, 1990.
Research on Healthy Volunteers, Royal College of Physicians of London, 1986. **http://www.rcplondon.ac.uk/pubs/pub_print_by-title.htm**
Governance Arrangements for NHS Research Ethics Committees: (Section A – General Standards and Principles, Department of Health [DOH], Central Office for Research Ethics Committees [OREC], 2001 **http://doh.gov.uk/research/rec**
Guidelines for Good Pharmacy Practice in Support of Clinical Trials in Hospitals, Royal Pharmaceutical Society, 1994.
Guidance on Good Clinical Practice and Clinical Trials in the NHS, *National Health Service, 1999*. **http://www.doh.gov.uk/research/documents/gcpguide.pdf**
Research Ethics Guidance for Nurses Involved in Research or Any Investigative Project Involving Human Subjects, Royal College of Nursing Research Society,1998 **http://www.doh. gov.uk/research/rd3/nhsrandd/researchgovernance/govhome.htm**

USA
Regulations:
Code of Federal Regulations [CFR], 21 CFR Ch 1, Food and Drug Administration [FDA], Department of Health and Human Services [DHHS]:
Part 11 – Electronic Records; Electronic Signatures **http://www.access.gpo.gov/nara/cfr/waisidx_01/21cfr11_01.html**
Part 50 – Protection of Human Subjects **http://www.access.gpo.gov/nara/cfr/waisidx_01/21cfr50_01.html**
Part 54 – Financial Disclosure by Clinical Investigators **http://www.access.gpo.gov/nara/cfr/waisidx_01/21cfr54_01.html**
Part 56 – Institutional Review Boards **http://www.access.gpo.gov/nara/cfr/waisidx_01/21cfr56_01.html**
Part 312 – Investigational New Drug Application; **http://www.access.gpo.gov/nara/cfr/waisidx_01/21cfr312_01.html**
Part 314 – Applications for FDA Approval to Market a New Drug; **http://www.access.gpo.gov/nara/cfr/waisidx_01/21cfr 314_01.html**

Compliance Program Guidance Manuals for FDA Staff:
Compliance Program 7151.02. FDA Access to Results of Quality Assurance Program Audits and Inspections, 1996. [Same as Compliance Policy guide 130.300] **http://www.fda.gov/ora/compliance_ref/cpg/cpggenl/cpg130-300.html**
Compliance Program 7348.001 – Bioresearch Monitoring—In Vivo Bioequivalence, 1999. **http://www.fda.gov/ora/compliance_ref/bimo/7348_001/Default.htm http://www.fda.gov/ora/compliance_ref/bimo/7348_001/foi48001.pdf**
Compliance Program 7348.809 – Institutional Review Boards, 1994. **http://www.fda.gov/ora/compliance_ref/bimo/7348_809/irb-cp7348-809.pdf**
Compliance Program 7348.810 – Bioresearch Monitoring – Sponsors, Contract Research Organizations and Monitors, 2001. **http://www.fda.gov/ora/compliance_ref/bimo/7348_810/default.htm http://www.fda.gov/ora/compliance_ref/bimo/7348_810/48-810.pdf**
Compliance Program 7348.811 – Bioresearch Monitoring – Clinical Investigators, FDA, 1997. **http://www.fda.gov/ora/compliance_ref/bimo/7348_811/default.htm http://www.fda.gov/ora/ftparea/compliance/48_811.pdf**

Information Sheets:
Computerised Systems Used in Clinical Trials. FDA, 1999 **http://www.fda.gov/ora/compliance_ref/bimo/ffinalcct.htm**
Enforcement Policy: Electronic Records; Electronic Signatures— Compliance Policy Guide; Guidance for FDA Personnel, FDA, 1999 **http://www.fda.gov/ora/compliance_ref/part11/FRs/updates/cpg-esig-enf-noa.htm**
Guidance. Financial Disclosure by Clinical Investigators. FDA, 2001. **http://www.fda.gov/oc/guidance/financialdis.html**
Guidance for Institutional Review Boards and Clinical Investigators, FDA, 1998. **http://www.fda.gov/oc/ohrt/irbs/default .htm**
Guidance for Institutional Review Boards, Clinical Investigators, and Sponsors: Exceptions from Informed Consent Requirements for Emergency Research, FDA, 2000. **http://www.fda.gov/ora/compliance_ref/bimo/err_guide.htm**
Guideline for the Monitoring of Clinical Investigations, FDA, 1988. **http://www.fda.gov/cder/guidance/old006fn.pdf**
Guideline on the Preparation of Investigational New Drug Prod-

ucts (Human and Animal), Department of Health & Human Services, FDA, April 1991. **http://www.fda.gov/cder/guidance/old042fn.pdf**

Inspection and Warning Letters:
Clinical Investigator Inspection List **http://www.fda.gov/cder/regulatory/investigators/default.htm**
Debarment List **http://www.fda.gov/ora/compliance_ref/debar/default.htm**
Disqualified/Restricted/Assurances List for Clinical Investigators **http://www.fda.gov/ora/compliance_ref/bimo/dis_res_assur.htm**
Notice of Initiation of Disqualification Proceedings and Opportunity to Explain (NIDPOE) Letters **http://www.fda.gov/foi/nidpoe/default.html**
Public Health Service (PHS) Administrative Actions Listings **http://silk.nih.gov/public/cbz1bje.@www.orilist.html**
Warning Letters **http://www.fda.gov/foi/warning.htm**

Forms:
Form FDA 1571 – Investigational New Drug Application (IND) **http://forms.psc.gov/forms/FDA/FDA-1571.pdf**
Form FDA 1572 – Statement of Investigator **http://forms.psc.gov/forms/FDA/FDA-1572.pdf**
Form FDA 3454 – Certification: Financial Interests and Arrangements of Clinical Investigators **http://forms.psc.gov/forms/fda3454.pdf**
Form FDA 3455 – Disclosure: Financial Interests and Arrangements of Clinical Investigators **http://forms.psc.gov/forms/FDA/FDA-3455.pdf**

International
ICH:
Clinical Safety Data Management: Definitions and Standards for Expedited Reporting, International Conference on Harmonisation [ICH] of Technical Requirements for the Registration of Pharmaceuticals for Human Use, 1994. **http://www.ifpma.org/pdfifpma/e2a.pdf**
Clinical Safety Data Management: Periodic Safety Update Reports for Marketed Drugs, International Conference on Harmonisation [ICH] of Technical Requirements for the Registration of Pharmaceuticals for Human Use, 1996. **http://www.ifpma.org/pdfifpma/e2c.pdf**
Note for Guidance on Structure and Content of Clinical Study Reports, International Conference on Harmonisation [ICH] of Technical Requirements for the Registration of Pharmaceuticals for Human Use, 1995. **http://www.ifpma.org/pdfifpma/e3.pdf**
Guideline for Good Clinical Practice. International Conference on Harmonisation [ICH] of Technical Requirements for the Registration of Pharmaceuticals for Human Use, 1996. **http://www.ifpma.org/pdfifpma/e6.pdf**
General Considerations for Clinical Trials. International Conference on Harmonisation [ICH] of Technical Requirements for the Registration of Pharmaceuticals for Human Use, 1997 **http://www.ifpma.org/pdfifpma/e8.pdf**
Statistical Principles for Clinical Trials. International Conference on Harmonisation [ICH] of Technical Requirements for

the Registration of Pharmaceuticals for Human Use, 1998. **http://www.ifpma.org/pdfifpma/e9.pdf**

WHO:

Good manufacturing practices for pharmaceutical products supplementary guidelines for the manufacture of investigational pharmaceutical products for studies in humans, *1994.* **http://saturn.who.ch/uhtbin/cgisirsi/Thu+Sep++7+13:17:28+MET+DST+2000/0/49**

International Ethical Guidelines for Biomedical Research Involving Human Subjects, Council for

International Organizations of Medical Sciences [CIOMS] in collaboration with the World Health Organization [WHO], 1993. **http://saturn.who.ch/uhtbin/cgisirsi/Thu+Sep++7+13:17:28+MET+DST+2000/0/49**

Guidelines for Good Clinical Practice (GCP) for Trials on Pharmaceutical Products, Division of Drug Management & Policies, World Health Organization, 1994. **http://saturn.who.ch/uhtbin/cgisirsi/Thu+Sep++7+13:17:28+MET+DST+2000/0/49**

Operational Guidelines for Ethics Committees that Review Biomedical Research, World Health Organization, 2000. **http://saturn.who.ch/uhtbin/cgisirsi/Thu+Sep++7+13:17:28+MET +DST+2000/0/49**

World Medical Association:

Declaration of Helsinki. Recommendations Guiding Physicians in Biomedical Research Involving Human Subjects, Adopted by the 18th World Medical Assembly, Helsinki, Finland, June 1964, amended by the 29th World Medical Assembly, Tokyo, Japan, October 1975, the 35th World Medical Assembly, Venice, Italy, October 1983, and the 41st World Medical Assembly, Hong Kong, September 1989, the 48th General Assembly, Somerset West, Republic of South Africa, October 1996, and the 52nd General Assembly, Edinburgh, Scotland, October, 2000. **http://www.wma.net/e/policy/17-c_e.html**

Other Related Publications by the Authors:

Bohaychuk W, Ball G (1994) *Good Clinical Research Practices. An Indexed Reference to International Guidelines and Regulations, with Practical Interpretation* (available from authors).

Bohaychuk W, Ball G (1996) *GCP. A Report on Compliance.* (available from authors)

Bohaychuk W, and Ball G (1998), *GCP Audit Findings – Case Study 1*, Quality Assurance Journal, Volume 3, Issue 2.

Bohaychuk W, and Ball (1998), *101 GCP SOPs for Sponsors and CROs* (available from authors, paper and diskette).

Bohaychuk W, and Ball (1998), *GCP Audit Findings – Case Study 2*, Quality Assurance Journal, Volume 3, Issue 3.

Bohaychuk W, Ball G, Lawrence G, Sotirov K (1998) *A Quantitative View of International GCP Compliance. Appl Clin Trials* February: 24–29 (first in a series of articles published approximately every 2 months).

Bohaychuk W, Ball G (1999) GCP compliance assessed by independent auditing: international similarities and differences. In Hamrell M (ed.), *The Clinical Audit in Pharmaceutical Development* Marcel Dekker: New York.

Bohaychuk W, Ball G (1999) GCP compliance: national similarities and differences. In *Eur Pharmaceut Contract* September.

Bohaychuk W, Ball G (1999) Conducting GCP-compliant Clinical Research (available from John Wiley & Sons Ltd, Baffins Lane, Chichester, West Sussex PO19 1UD, UK, **www:interscience.wiley.com**).

Bohaychuk W, and Ball G (2000), GCP Compliance Assessed by Independent Auditing. International Similarities and Differences, In *The Clinical Audit in Pharmaceutical Development*, edited by M Hamrell. (Marcel Dekker publishers)

9

Quality Assurance, Quality Control and Audit

Donna Cullen

Auditrial, Fairlawn, NJ, USA

The Food and Drug Administration (FDA) and regulatory agencies throughout the world require assurance, from those who seek to market drugs, biologics, medical diagnostics or medical devices in their countries, that these products are safe and effective for their intended indications. Companies engaged in the research, development, licensing, and marketing of pharmaceuticals must comply with regulations governing the manufacturing and testing of their products. They must ensure that risks to test animals and human subjects are minimized throughout the research and development process and that the data generated in support of their objectives are true and accurate. Monitoring and inspection by companies and regulatory agencies are required to assess and control the integrity of research and development.

BACKGROUND

In 1963 a Brooklyn hospital undertook an investigation to determine whether pre-existing cancer or other debilitations in cancer patients compromised their ability to defend against cancer cells. Twenty-two control patients, without cancer, were given an injection of live cancer cells without their written consent, without being informed about the injections, and without the approval of the hospital's research committee. Both the investigator and the medical director were found guilty of fraud, deceit, and unprofessional conduct. In 1974 eight prisoners in a Maryland correctional facility were coerced into testing vaccines for typhoid and malaria. In 1977 a physician investigator claimed that all source records for patients enrolled in a clinical study at his location were lost in a rowboat accident. In 1978 three separate investigators were cited for either falsifying or inadequately documenting clinical study data. As recently as 1997, a physician investigator in California pled guilty to fraud after substituting his own blood for some clinical study tests. Another investigator in Georgia was convicted of fraudulently diverting approximately $10 million in grants for clinical studies, and was cited for failing to participate in the care of study subjects enrolled at his location and inadequately supervising his research staff. These are but a few of the historical cases that demonstrate the need for quality assurance in pharmaceutical research and development, despite years of regulation and control.

The FDA was established as a law enforcement agency in 1930. At that time, the Federal Food and Drugs Act of 1906, which prohibited false and misleading statements about a drug or its ingredients, and the Shirley Amendment (1911), which subsequently prohibited false therapeutic claims in drug labeling, were the only two substantive regulations governing the research and development of pharmaceuticals. In 1938 Congress passed the Federal Food, Drug and Cosmetic (FD&C) Act, both in response to recommendations from the FDA to revise the obsolete 1906 Federal Food and Drugs Act, and as a result of an elixir of sulfanilamide, which caused 107 deaths, mostly in children, because of its adulteration with glycol. The FD&C Act required that drug safety be established before marketing and extended regulations to cosmetics and therapeutic devices. It did not address the issue of drug efficacy, however. Factory inspections and standards for food quality and containers were also authorized.

Between 1941 and 1945, Congress amended the 1938 FD&C Act to reflect the development of insulin, penicillin, and other new antibiotics.

Principles and Practice of Pharmaceutical Medicine. Edited by A. J. Fletcher, Lionel D. Edwards, Anthony W. Fox and Peter Stonier © 2002 John Wiley & Sons Ltd.

The FDA was given authority to approve these products as both safe and effective and to require certification that each batch or lot conforms to the established standards of purity and potency. The regulation of biological products (serum, vaccines and blood products) began in 1944 with the Public Health Service Act and was supplemented in 1986 by the Childhood Vaccine Act, which required patient information on vaccines, and gave the FDA authority to recall biologics and authorized penalties for violations.

The Nuremberg Code, adopted in 1949, required voluntary consent for all research subjects, guaranteed their right to leave a research study at any time, protected them from remote possibilities of injury, disability, or death, and stipulated that the results of research studies must be intended for the good of society.

The Durham Humphrey Amendment (1951) defined the kinds of drugs that required medical supervision for safe use and restricted them to sale by prescription. Two years later, in 1953, the US Public Health Service issued a policy document entitled *Group Consideration of Clinical Research Procedures Deviating from Accepted Medical Practice or Involving Unusual Hazard*. This policy stated that the potential risks of clinical studies must be carefully assessed and that informed consent was essential. Ethical review of research proposals was also suggested. In this same year, the Factory Inspection Amendment was passed, requiring the FDA to give written inspection reports to manufacturers.

The Color Additives Amendments (1960) required manufacturers to establish the safety of these substances in foods, drugs and cosmetics. Following reports of birth defects associated with the use of thalidomide in Australia and Western Europe, public support for tougher drug regulation prompted the passage, in 1962, of the Kefauver–Harris Drug Amendment. Many US patients who had received thalidomide in clinical studies during this period were not informed that its status was investigational. This legislation required drug manufacturers, for the first time, to prove that their products were effective prior to marketing, and required the affirmative act of approval by the FDA. In the same year, President John F. Kennedy proposed the Consumer Bill of Rights, which include the rights to safety, information, choice, and the right to be heard.

The Declaration of Helsinki, published in 1964, established free and informed consent, preferably written, for research subjects, or consent by a legal representative if a subject is legally incompetent. It also required research to be supervised by competent medical persons.

Drug abuse and control amendments were enacted in 1965 in response to abuse of depressants, stimulants and hallucinogens. In 1966 the FDA, in cooperation with the National Academy of Sciences and the National Research Council, began an evaluation of the effectiveness of approximately 4000 drugs that had been approved between 1938 and 1962 on the basis of safety alone. The Fair Packaging and Labeling Act was passed in the same year and required true and informative labeling for all consumer products involved in interstate commerce. A review of the safety and effectiveness of over-the-counter drugs sold without prescription began in 1972, and was followed 10 years later by FDA-mandated tamper-resistant packaging regulations, in reaction to reports of deaths from Tylenol capsules laced with cyanide.

In 1971, in a move to affirm the Declaration of Helsinki, and further guarantee the protection of research subjects, the US Department of Health, Education and Welfare (DHEW) issued *The Guide to DHEW Policy on Protection of Human Subjects*. This publication required every institution receiving DHEW funds for research to establish a committee to monitor the ethical integrity of that institution's human research, and made both the institution and the investigator responsible for violations.

Congress passed the National Research Act in 1974 and created the National Commission for the Protection of Human Subjects of Biomedical and Behavioral Research. The commission was given the task of developing ethical guidelines for conducting research in human subjects, particularly children, prisoners, and the mentally impaired. The commission recommended to DHEW and Congress the enactment of federal regulations governing ethical review of all human research by institutional review boards, including accreditation and education. The commission also recommended that these boards be required to review informed consent procedures for research subjects, and that DHEW establish an office to monitor compliance. In response to these recommendations, the FDA and DHEW drafted regulations and guidelines for clinical investigators and institutional review boards.

QUALITY ASSURANCE

It is the responsibility of each company to identify and meet the regulatory standards and to follow the regulations and guidelines applicable to its products. Failure to do so will delay licensing and marketing approval. The company must give its promise or guarantee (assurance) of the character of its product with respect to the grade of excellence (quality). Compliance at each phase of the development and manufacturing process must be carefully documented. The FDA and most foreign regulatory agencies assess the degree of compliance with current accepted standards, and guidelines for manufacturing, preclinical/animal testing, and the conduct of clinical studies in human subjects. In the USA these standards are published as regulations under Title 21 of the Code of Federal Regulations 21 CFR for Good Manufacturing Practice (GMP) and Good Laboratory Practice (GLP), and Guidelines for Good Clinical Practice (GCP).

Elsewhere in the world, individual countries have established their own standards and guidelines or have formed alliances with other countries, such as the Commission of the European Community (CEC), to unify and facilitate approvals. The EU, Australia, Canada Japan, the Nordic countries, the USA and the World Health Organization (WHO) have already drafted an international ethical and scientific standard for designing, conducting, recording and reporting clinical trials with human subjects. The International Conference on Harmonization (ICH) Guideline of Good Clinical Practice, published in May 1997, has its roots in the Declaration of Helsinki and assures the rights, safety and well-being of human subjects participating in research.

GMP regulations encompass every phase of product development (manufacturing, testing, acceptance, etc.), from the purity of the raw materials to the quality of the finished product. Established procedures include staffing and training, quality control, facilities and maintenance, selection, calibration and maintenance of equipment, procurement, testing and storage of raw materials, containers and closures, production and process controls, laboratory and stability testing, packaging and labeling, holding and distribution, returned and salvaged drug products, and records and reporting. In addition, there are guidelines and regulations issued by the Occupational Safety and Health Administration (OSHA), the Environmental Protection Agency (EPA), the International Standards Organization (ISO) and the *United States Pharmacopoeia* (USP) that are also applicable to most phases of the manufacturing process.

The FDA has established regulations and requirements for extensive animal testing of a product before human investigations are permitted. GLP regulations govern every aspect of preclinical development, including the humane and proper care of the animals used in research and the qualifications of testing facilities.

Good clinical practice (GCP) guidelines ensure that risks to human subjects participating in research studies are minimized, that they are properly informed about these risks and that their participation is entirely voluntary. Procedures are established for preparing investigational new drug applications (IND), the responsibilities of sponsors and investigators, the composition and responsibilities of institutional review boards, and obtaining and documenting written informed consent. Special consideration is also given to prisoners used in research, drugs intended to treat life-threatening or debilitating illnesses, foreign studies, and administrative actions for non-compliance.

Compliance to applicable GMP and GLP regulations and GCP guidelines can be assured by establishing policies and standard operating procedures (SOPs) that address them, and by documenting that these procedures are followed. SOPs should be reviewed routinely and updated when required. Deviations from SOPs must be carefully explained and documented and should be addressed with a view towards correction and preventing recurrence. If a quality assurance unit or department exists within a company, it should be empowered to assure compliance to regulations, guidelines and SOPs. It should also be organized in a way that will permit the inspection and reporting of processes and procedures without the possibility of coercion or pressure from the personnel and departments that it monitors. For example, it should not be under the control of manufacturing or clinical research. Frequently, the organizational structure places it within regulatory affairs, but free-standing QA/QC departments are also common.

To assure that a final product meets recognized standards for safety and efficacy, the quality of the ingredients, the quality of the manufacturing processes, and the quality of the research and testing used to develop the product must be verifiable. The basic elements required to accomplish this include written quality standards, systems to inspect, control, validate, and maintain quality, systems to manage changes in quality, and records to document that these systems are in place and operating properly. The burden of proof rests with the holder of the IND and the supporting documentation.

QUALITY CONTROL

The proactive arm of quality assurance is quality control. Compliance to regulations throughout each phase of the research and development process can only be assessed by routine monitoring with repeated sampling and testing using validated methods, by comparing the results to the desired or accepted standards, and by making corrections when deviations from the standards are identified. To maintain quality, variability must be controlled. To improve quality, variability must be reduced.

Planning, good scientific methods, and validation are the first steps in a quality program, and quality control (testing and inspection) is the continuing verification that validated systems remain in control. Planned change and revalidation assure continuing quality improvement within the regulated environment.

Another important factor to consider in any quality control program is personnel. Procedures should be established to verify qualifications, provide and evaluate continuous training, and assess and document job performance. Education and training are essential to maintaining competency. Those individuals who perform the processes within research and development and those responsible for monitoring and control should be qualified, properly trained, and understand the accepted standards and guidelines. There must be a commitment on the part of employees to abide by them as well.

Quality control in manufacturing involves: physical and chemical testing of raw materials, intermediates, and the final product; potency testing; microbiological testing; product stability testing; environmental monitoring and analysis; process reliability; process validation; equipment qualification and validation; product disposition; complaint handling; auditing of suppliers; and periodic product review. Statistically valid sampling plans are needed to support the testing and inspection of raw materials, components and final product, as well as systems to identify each of these during the production process. The stability and reliability testing of these items before and after distribution must also be monitored. Regular communication with executive management is essential. There should be a system to identify trends and handle customer complaints, and there should be provisions for special situations that require updates on the quality of the system and to manage changes, both planned and unplanned. Unplanned changes within a system (ingredients, processes, equipment, documentation or personnel) require investigation and appropriate corrective action, and must be carefully documented.

The basic characteristics of a new product are determined in the preclinical development phase. This includes the development of new product formulation, identification of its physical, chemical, pharmacologic, and toxicologic properties, as well as pharmacokinetics, and metabolism and teratology studies in animals. This information must be gathered and reported to regulatory agencies before the first dose of the product can be administered for research in human subjects. Thus, it is imperative that quality control procedures are functioning at the beginning of the development process, to ensure that regulatory requirements are met and that the product safety information is accurate before proceeding to the next series of tests. Animals must be adequately fed and housed to ensure that they are free of diseases that might alter or invalidate the test results. The new product and controls must be administered according to established protocols, variables must be controlled during testing, data must be carefully recorded, and specimens must be collected and properly analyzed and stored. Data recorded in bound notebooks or recorded on electronic media must be archived.

In the clinical development phase, many of the development processes move 'off-site' and away from the immediate control of the sponsor company. The number of variables increases at a time when the responsibility for the quality of the operation must be shared with others at remote locations. Clinical investigators must be carefully selected after an indication for a product has been identified and a study plan or protocol has been prepared. A visit should be made to each investigator's location to evaluate the capabilities of the staff and inspect the facilities. The investigator and any subinvestigators or clinical study support staff who will assist with the evaluation and treatment of the research subjects should be qualified by training and experience to undertake the research. The investigator must be willing and able to personally oversee all of the staff who will administer treatments, conduct study-related tests, dispense the investigational product, and record the data. There should be secure, locked storage space available, away from patient traffic areas, for the investigational product. A laboratory with current certification and licensing is needed to perform the clinical tests required by the study protocol. The investigator must also have access to a qualified institutional review board (IRB) to review and approve the clinical trial, ensure that the rights of human subjects are protected and that they are exposed to no more than minimal risk.

In the early clinical development phases, human subjects, who will usually be healthy, will be confined for varying periods of time while single or multiple doses of the product are administered and safety data are recorded. These subjects receive little in the way of benefit, except monetary compensation. When a reasonably safe and reasonably effective dose or dose range has been identified, the safety and efficacy of the product will be determined by studying patients with the indicated symptoms, condition or disease. Some of these patients will, of necessity, receive no treatment or treatment with inactive substances (placebo).

The sponsor of a clinical study is responsible for ensuring that it is properly monitored. Monitors should be appropriately trained, and should have the scientific and clinical knowledge needed to monitor a study adequately. They should be familiar with the investigational product, the protocol, written informed consent, applicable SOPs and current GCP guidelines and regulatory requirements. They should also be capable of suggesting and directing corrective action when necessary.

Orientation of the investigator and clinical staff to the study design and test procedures and the investigational product characteristics is imperative, to ensure that everyone has a thorough understanding of the research goals. A meeting should be scheduled with the investigator and clinical staff prior to the enrollment of patients, to review and discuss the clinical study in detail. When more than one investigator is participating in the same study, as in a multicenter study, a formal investigator's meeting can be organized at a convenient time and location. In advance of the meeting the investigator should be provided an opportunity to review a copy of the study protocol and current investigator's brochure. The meeting agenda should include a thorough review of the protocol, case report forms for data collection, investigational product packaging and dispensing, the timing of clinical laboratory tests and other tests required by the study protocol (e.g. physical examination, electrocardiogram, etc.). The procedures for reporting adverse experiences, particularly those that are deemed serious or unexpected, should be thoroughly discussed. It is also helpful to provide an overview of the investigational product's development history, especially toxicology and prior clinical experience, as well as a review of the investigator's responsibilities, as outlined in the GCP guidelines.

The monitor should arrange a visit to initiate the clinical study after all of the necessary regulatory documents have been filed and the study materials have been delivered to the site. This visit will make it possible to verify their receipt and perform a complete inventory. If some time has elapsed since the prestudy or investigator's meeting, time should be set aside to review the protocol and any changes that have occurred since the meeting. An inspection of the investigator's regulatory documents should be made and deficiencies documented and corrected.

Regulations currently stipulate that an active clinical study should be monitored at a minimum of once each year, but in practical terms the rate of subject enrollment and the volume of data collected usually dictate a much higher frequency of monitoring visits. Each interim or periodic monitoring visit should include an inspection of the investigator's regulatory documents, a review of informed consent for subjects enrolled since the previous monitoring visit, and an inventory of the investigational product. The case report forms used for data collection should be compared to the information in the subject's chart, to ensure their accuracy and completeness. Adequate source documentation is imperative, so that clinical data can be independently verified, and should include evidence that a subject is enrolled in the clinical study, that the investigational product is being administered according to protocol, and that protocol deviations or violations and adverse experiences are properly documented. Source documents are defined as original documents, data, and records (e.g. hospital records, clinical and office charts, laboratory notes, memoranda, subjects' diaries or evaluation checklists, pharmacy dispensing records, recorded data from automated instruments, copies or transcriptions certified after verification as being accurate copies, microfiches, photographic negatives, microfilm or magnetic media, X-rays, subject files and records kept at the pharmacy, at the laboratories and at medico-technical departments involved in the clinical study). After reviewing all of these items, the monitor should be able to confirm that the protocol is being followed, that the data are true and accurate, that there is adequate supervision by the investigator and the institutional review board, and that regulatory obligations are being met. Deficiencies should be addressed at the time of the visit and the findings must be documented in a written report.

The monitor should arrange to close a study site after all subjects have completed the trial, all data have been verified on site, and all investigational products have been inventoried and reconciled. The investigator's regulatory document files must be current and complete and archived along with copies of the case report forms for data collection.

Provision should be made to communicate any changes to a study plan or protocol, and all serious adverse experiences, to all investigators involved in the trial in a timely fashion. These changes must also be reported to their respective institutional review boards. Additions, changes, or corrections to clinical data should be made only by the investigator, or individuals authorized by the investigator, and must be carefully documented.

An IRB is responsible for the protection of the rights and welfare of human subjects. It is authorized to conduct the initial review of research studies and approve, require modification of, or disapprove any activities covered under existing GCP guidelines. A research study includes the study plan or protocol, the content of the subject informed consent, and any advertising or other information that will be used to direct subjects to the clinical study. An IRB is obligated to continue to review and approve each research study at least annually, and significant changes to a study plan or protocol (i.e. changes that may affect or impact the rights and safety of the research subjects) before the investigator implements them. Investigators must provide periodic progress reports to the IRB as required, and submit a final report at the conclusion of the study. Serious adverse experiences must be reported promptly.

Guidelines for IRBs are defined in 21 CFR, Part 56. They are required to have and to follow written procedures. They must consist of at least five members of diverse backgrounds. These individuals should be sufficiently qualified through training and experience to consider the research in light of the community and institution that they represent, and be knowledgeable of applicable laws, regulations and standards for professional conduct and practice.

The investigator must ensure that the subjects selected for the study meet the inclusion criteria, and none of the exclusion criteria, and that they are treated according to the study plan. The IRB must ensure that the rights and welfare of the subject are protected. The monitor must ensure that the study plan is followed, that all data are true and accurate, and that all regulatory requirements are met. Maintaining the quality of clinical research depends upon their joint efforts.

AUDITS

To assure compliance with regulations, government and regulatory agencies throughout the world must perform official inspections of clinical facilities. The FDA employs approximately 1100 investigators and inspectors in 157 cities to inspect almost 95 000 FDA-regulated businesses within the USA. Audits are performed during clinical development to assure the quality of the research data, and routinely after product approval to assure adherence to GMP regulations.

Inspections of clinical study sites can be 'routine' or 'for cause'. The former is usually directed towards pivotal trials of a product that is awaiting approval, and investigators who enroll large number of subjects in a study. The latter is usually reserved for cases where there is reason to suspect the validity of data generated at a clinical site. Further, if significant deviations from regulations are discovered during an audit, a routine inspection may become a 'for cause' inspection and be intensified or expanded to include other studies. When violations are discovered, the FDA can request voluntary corrective action or recall a product from the market if it has already been approved. Failure to voluntarily correct a problem can lead to legal sanctions, seizure and destruction of a product, and criminal penalties. Audits by other regulatory agencies outside the USA follow similar procedures. Given the continuous evolution of oversight activities employed by these nations, their review may be either more or less stringent than that of the FDA.

During its continuing review of product development prior to marketing approval, FDA can request a hold on a clinical development program if it determines that:

- Human subjects would be exposed to an 'unreasonable and significant risk of illness or injury'.
- One or more investigators are not qualified by reasons of scientific training and experience.
- The investigator's brochure is determined to be erroneous, incomplete or misleading.
- The information submitted under the IND is insufficient, or the design of a study or clinical program is deemed to be deficient or lacking in scientific merit.
- The manufacturing, control, and labeling of the investigational product are substandard with respect to identity, quality, or purity, or insufficient quantities exist to adequately conduct a clinical trial.
- A satisfactory alternative therapy becomes available or evidence strongly suggests that the investigational product is unsafe or ineffective.

During a clinical hold, new subjects may not be enrolled in clinical studies or treated with the investigational product. However, in some instances, subjects already receiving the investigational product may be permitted to continue. If significant deviations from the study program occur or serious safety issues are encountered, FDA can request termination of a clinical program or withdrawal of an IND.

A routine investigator site audit will focus on two major areas. First, an auditor will examine the facts surrounding the conduct of the study to determine who did what, the degree of delegation of authority, where specific aspects of the study were performed, how and where data were recorded, how investigational product accountability was maintained, and how the monitor communicated with the investigator and evaluated the progress of the study. Second, the study case report forms for data collection will be compared to all available subject records and source documents that might support the study data. Subjects' records before and after the study can also be audited to evaluate medical histories that pre-date enrollment, and to determine what degree of follow-up occurred after treatment with the investigational product. Informed consent for all subjects enrolled at a site are routinely examined, and an auditor will also want to determine whether all adverse experiences have been properly reported. Nearly 10 000 inspections at more than 4000 investigative sites have been completed since 1964. The most frequently encountered deficiencies continue to be inadequate subject informed consent, failure to adhere to the protocol, inadequate and inaccurate records, and inadequate drug accountability. The most frequently encountered deficiencies in informed consent are failure to identify a contact person for questions about research subjects' rights, incomplete descriptions of study procedures and compensation/treatment for injury, inadequate confidentiality statements, and an incomplete description of available alternative procedures.

FDA can audit the records of the study sponsor, as well as contract research organizations (CROs), to review standard operating procedures and all of the documents related to a particular clinical study, including electronic databases. Since 1981, nearly 200 such inspections have occurred. Departures from regulations requiring voluntary corrective action were reported for 10% of the sponsors and CROs inspected. Two of the inspections resulted in official action. The most frequently reported deficiencies were records that were unavailable, inadequate or inaccurate, inadequate or improper informed consent, inadequate investigational product accountability, deviations from the protocol and, inappropriate payments to volunteer research subjects.

Since 1986, FDA has performed nearly 2100 audits of more than 1400 public (e.g. affiliated with a university, hospital or other institution) and private institutional review boards. Fewer than 20 of these were 'for cause'. Complete compliance was observed for only about 13% of these inspections and 1% uncovered violations that were serious enough to warrant regulatory or administrative sanctions, which included suspension of clinical studies. The most frequently encountered deficiencies have been inadequate meeting minutes, lack of a quorum at meetings; inadequate written procedures, and inadequate continuing review.

At the conclusion of a FDA audit, the inspector will conduct an exit interview to discuss deficiencies observed and, if appropriate, will issue an Establishment Inspection Report (Form 483). For many sites, voluntary action to correct deficiencies will then be requested, some in writing. Failure to voluntarily correct deficiencies, or the occurrence of serious deficiencies at some sites, may result in a delay in the approval of a new drug application (NDA), or disapproval of the application, disqualification of an investigator, restrictions on an investigator, or criminal charges, fines and imprisonment. There are currently about 80 physicians who are ineligible to receive investigational products and more than two dozen others who have agreed to some restriction of their use.

The quality assurance department within a company will frequently conduct audits of investigator sites, either during a clinical study or after it has been completed. Companies that do not have a quality assurance department or unit may contract this service from a consultant or a third party specializing in regulatory audits. The intent and scope of these audits are the same as the FDA, but they afford a company an opportunity to verify compliance and to correct deficiencies that might otherwise delay product approval. These audits

also provide a means to assess both the quality of the investigator site and the quality of the monitoring throughout the study. Audits performed outside the USA, in conjunction with multinational studies, can be problematic due to language and cultural differences, as well as a diversity of government regulations.

When the product development program has been completed and the NDA has been submitted for review, the FDA will likely perform routine inspections of the manufacturing facilities to verify GMP compliance and a sample of the clinical study sites to verify GCP compliance.

An audit of manufacturing and control processes will include a thorough review of all of the documentation required to demonstrate that a product meets the requirements for its intended use, including requirements for marketing and consumer use, technical design and performance, regulatory and quality assurance, and product safety. Equipment systems will also be inspected.

FUTURE TRENDS

Computer and electronic media, originally employed for databases and statistical analysis, have now expanded to include remote data entry at investigator sites and transfer of documentation of NDA submissions. This has prompted the development of regulatory guidelines to ensure that software systems are properly designed, tested, validated, and upgraded, that they include adequate security measures and provisions for documenting changes to data (an audit trail), and that the individuals who use the systems receive adequate training. Auditors will require training to keep pace with the development of these systems and to effectively audit them in the future.

The globalization of pharmaceutical research and development is expected to shorten the time required for product approval and registration, by increasing the number of subjects available for research studies and broadening an investigational product's exposure to ethnic intrinsic factors (genetic and physiological) and extrinsic factors (cultural and environmental).

The pharmaceutical industry is already establishing a presence in Central and Eastern Europe and is aggressively moving towards South America and

China. Japan remains focused on possible genetic differences, and continues to insist upon studies conducted in its own population as a condition for registration and approval. Regional variations, such as diet, alcohol and tobacco consumption, climate, exposure to pollution and other environmental factors, socioeconomic status, and differences in technology and health care standards, require creative planning for multinational trials.

As nations adopt more open trading policies throughout the world and form economic alliances, the trend toward multinational studies will require increased cooperation between governments and a greater degree of harmonization to level the playing field in drug development. In addition to the ICH Guideline for good clinical practice (GCP) already published, unified GMP and GLP guidelines have been drafted and some portions are already approved. Efforts such as these will hopefully pave the way for mutual acceptance of all research and development data by the regulatory authorities of these and other nations.

SUMMARY

Over the years, the pharmaceutical industry has endeavored to work in partnership with the regulatory agencies to perfect the laws and regulations that govern research and development. These laws and regulations will continue to evolve as technology and health care capabilities change to meet the growing needs of our world. Accompanying this growth will be the need for the continued assurance of human safety and well-being. This must remain the foremost consideration in pharmaceutical research and development.

BIBLIOGRAPHY

Barton BL (1990) FDA's inspections of US and non-US clinical studies. *Drug Inf Assoc J* 24: 463–8.

Buc NL, Hutt PB (1988) *Recent Changes in the FDA Drug Approval Process for Drugs and Biologics: Where We Have Been and Where We are Going*. Prentice Hall Law and Business: New York.

Code of Federal Regulations, Title 21, Ch. 1 (4-1-97 edn), Part 58, Good Laboratory Practice for Nonclinical Laboratory Studies.

Code of Federal Regulations, Title 21, Ch. 1 (4-1-97 edn), Part 211, Current Good Manufacturing Practice for Finished Pharmaceuticals.

CPG (1991) Compliance Policy Guide: Fraud, Untrue Statements of Material Facts, Bribery and Illegal Gratuities. CPG: 7150.09, September.

DeSain C (1993) *Documentation Basics That Support Good Manufacturing Practices*. Aster: Eugene, OR.

DeSain C, Sutton CV (1996) *Documentation Practices. A Complete Guide to Document Development and Management for GMP and ISO 9000 Compliant Industries*. Advanstar Communications: Duluth, MN.

Department of Health and Human Services, Public Health Service, Center for Drug Evaluation and Research, Office of Training and Communication (1998) *Freedom of Information Office Staff*. HFD-205, January.

Dumitriu H (1998) Impact of the ICH Guideline of Ethnic Differences. *Drug Inf J* 32: 141–4.

FDA (1991) Bioresearch monitoring—human drugs; clinical investigators. In *Compliance Program Guidance Manual*, Program 7348.811. September, Chapter 48.

FDA (1991) Bioresearch monitoring—human drugs, biologics, medical devices and radiological health products and veterinary drug products; sponsor, contract research organizations, and monitors. In *Compliance Program Guidance Manual*, Program 7348.810, October, Chapter 48.

FDA (1992) Bioresearch monitoring—institutional review boards. In *Compliance Program Guidance Manual*, Program 7348.809, January, Chapter 48.

FDA (1997) *The Food and Drug Administration: An Overview*. Publication No. BG95–13, July 15.

Guertler-Doyle V (1998) Taking clinical trials into China. *Appl Clin Res Trials* 7(6): 54–60. June.

ICH (1997) *International Conference on Harmonization: Guideline for Good Clinical Practice*, May 9.

Kingham R (1988) History of FDA Regulation of Clinical Research. *Drug Inf Assoc J* 22: 151–5.

Natoroff BL (1998) Clinical Trials in Central/Eastern Europe: Industry Viewpoint. *Drug Inf J* 32: 129–33.

Schoichet S, Creasy G, Kasay S (1998) A systems infrastructure for sponsor/CRO collaboration on international clinical trials. *Drug Inf J* 32: 155–61.

FDA (1997) *US Department of Health and Human Services, Food and Drug Administration, Center for Drug Evaluation and Research Fact Book*, May.

Warnock-Smith A (1998) Proposed EC harmonization directive would increase regulatory burden. *Appl Clin Res Trials* 7(1): 28–31.

10

Phase I: The First Opportunity for Extrapolation from Animal Data to Human Exposure

Stephen Curry[1], Dennis McCarthy[1], Heleen H. DeCory[1], Matthew Marler[1] and Johan Gabrielsson[2]

[1] *Astra Arcus USA Inc, Rochester, NY, USA, and* [2] *Astra Arcus AB, Sodertalje, Sweden*

There is a need to make reliable and rapid predictions of human responses from animal data. Although drug discovery is primarily designed to find compounds with desired efficacy, most research-orientated pharmaceutical companies also use data on absorption, metabolism and pharmacokinetics in the decision-making process (Welling and Tse 1995). Usually, the strategy is to use all available data to choose one or two candidates from a whole pharmacological class of new drugs for Phase I testing (Welling and Tse 1995). Thus, compounds are chosen on the basis of animal data, partly because of suitable bioavailability, half-life, and tissue penetration characteristics. The possibility of multiphasic plasma level decay patterns following intravenous doses is an important element in this selection process.

Data for chosen compounds will commonly also have been subjected to simultaneous modeling of pharmacokinetic and pharmacodynamic data from animals, again in an effort to optimize the chances that the drugs chosen will have the properties in humans specified in a pre-discovery product profile. The pharmacodynamic information available typically includes data from receptor-binding studies, *in vitro* functional assays, and *in vivo* pharmacological screening experiments. Pharmacokinetics, related when possible to observed drug effects, is a powerful and critical component of the pivotal step from animal research to human research in the drug development process. For many drug researchers, Phase I is an end-point

in itself, as both the end of the research and discovery process and the beginning of the clinical process, and none can doubt that the first-in-man study, and achieving an active Clinical Trials Exemption (CTX) or Investigational new drug application (IND) (or equivalent regulatory permissions in other countries; see Chapters 23, 25 and 26), are important milestones in the history of a drug. The essence of this crucial step of drug development is the making of valid predictions of *in vivo* drug effects from *in vitro* data.

The collection of *in vitro* data from animal materials and extrapolation: (a) from physical properties to *in vitro* data; (b) from *in vitro* data to non-human *in vivo* data; and (c) from non-human *in vivo* data to clinical *in vivo* responses, can be done more efficiently using on-line analysis and simulations. This chapter seeks to show how rapid progression may be achieved for new chemical entities through this process, using *in vitro* and *in vivo* data and advanced modeling procedures. This must be seen in the context of the entire drug discovery process, which, on a larger scale, is designed to find potent, safe drugs (in man), based on animal data (Figure 10.1). We anticipate a time when *in vitro* pharmacodynamic data will be routinely combined with *in vitro* drug metabolism data in a rational prediction of drug responses in healthy human volunteers, with consequent acceleration of the drug discovery effort, and therefore a general trend for more efficient use of resources in early clinical development.

Principles and Practice of Pharmaceutical Medicine. Edited by A. J. Fletcher, Lionel D. Edwards, Anthony W. Fox and Peter Stonier © 2002 John Wiley & Sons Ltd.

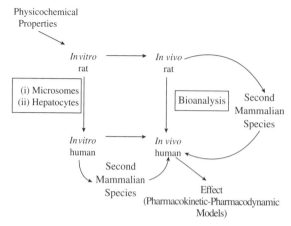

Figure 10.1   General scheme showing the pharmacokinetic prediction pathway from physicochemical properties to human drug response via *in vitro* and *in vivo* studies in laboratory animals

THE *IN VITRO/IN VIVO* PREDICTION

The challenge is to predict systemic clearance, volume of distribution, and oral bioavailability in man from a combination of *in vitro* and *in vivo* preclinical data. If this prediction can become reliable, then Phase I studies become more confirmatory. The use of human hepatocytes and isolated enzymes can form a critical part of the *in vitro* database.

Clearance of almost all drugs is by renal, metabolic, and/or biliary mechanisms. There are rare exceptions, such as anaesthetic gases that are exhaled unchanged. However, here we shall concentrate on the typical situation.

Physicochemical properties, especially lipophilicity, frequently govern the clearance route; lipophilicity is commonly measured as log $D_{7.4}$, where this variable equals $\log_{10}$ ([drug in octanol]/[drug in buffer]) at pH = 7.4, in a closed system at equilibrium. Generally compounds with a log $D_{7.4}$ value below 0 have significant renal clearance values, whereas compounds with log $D_{7.4}$ values above 0 will principally undergo metabolism (Smith et al 1996). Molecular size also has some effect on these clearance routes. For example, compounds with molecular weights greater than 400 Da are often eliminated through the bile unchanged, whilst smaller lipophilic compounds will generally be metabolized.

Elementary Aspects of Clearance

The common, clinical measurement of drug clearance involves taking serial venous blood samples. As time passes after dosing, drug concentrations are seen to decline: this is really merely the modeling of drug disappearance, and is essentially a descriptive process, requiring actual human exposures. First-order elimination, after equilibrium in the circulating compartment, has a constant (k) with units of h^{-1}, and plasma concentration (C) is then modeled by equations of the general form:

$$C = Ae^{-kt}$$

where A is the concentration of drug at time (t) = 0, assuming that there was instantaneous and homogenous equilibration of the dose into the circulating compartment. As the number of compartments increases, then so do the number of terms of the form shown on the right-hand side of the equation shown above.

The *elimination rate* always has units of (mass/time) for any elimination process. For first-order processes, the elimination rate is represented by a tangent to the elimination curve.

In contrast, zero-order elimination processes are occasionally encountered. These usually represent saturation by the drug of the elimination mechanism(s). These 'drug disappearance' curves are straight, and thus described simply, by:

$$C = A - bt$$

where the elimination rate (b) does not change with time or drug concentration. If followed for long enough, most drugs that are subject to zero-order elimination eventually fall to such low concentrations that the elimination mechanism becomes unsaturated, and first-order elimination then supervenes; good examples include ethanol and sodium dichloroacetate (Hawkins and Kalant 1972; Curry et al 1985; Fox et al 1996).

The elimination rate for zero-order processes may also be treated as a maximal rate of reaction (V_{max}), and thus this type of data may be subject to ordinary Michaelis–Menten analysis (see further, below). Note that first-order elimination curves are so common that 'drug disappearance' curves are routinely analyzed as semi-logarithmic plots (which linearizes the curve). The literature is sometimes ambiguous in its use of the term 'linear data', authors may or may not assume that the semi-logarithmic transformation is to be taken as read.

When the elimination rate is known, then clearance (Cl) is defined simply as:

$$Cl = elimination\ rate/C$$

where C is again drug concentration. Note that in first-order elimination processes, the elimination rate of the drug (with units of mass/time) changes with time (and drug concentration), and thus only instantaneous clearances, specifying time or drug concentration, can be stated.

Urinary clearance, obviously, may only partly explain the rate of drug disappearance from plasma. In any case, the urinary clearance of an agent may be found from the familiar equation:

$$Cl = (U \times V)/P$$

where U is the urinary concentration, V is the volume of urine excreted during a specified time period, and P is the average plasma concentration during that time period. Pharmaceutical physicians will remember that for inulin and sodium iothalamate, but not for creatinine or urea, the urinary clearance is a good measure of glomerular filtration rate.

These elementary aspects of clearance may be revised in any textbook (e.g. Curry 1980; Benet et al 1996). The purpose of the remainder of this section is to show how much more informative the concept of clerance may be, and to provide an illustration of its use.

Prediction of Human Drug Clearance

For those compounds predominantly cleared by metabolism, human blood clearance can be pre-dicted using simple enzyme kinetic data (Houston 1994; lwatsubo etal, 1996 Obach 1996a; Ashforth et al., 1995). These predictions may be strengthened by comparing preclinical *in vivo* data with the predictions made from *in vitro* data using tissues from the same preclinical species. Rane et al 1977 As an illustration, consider a novel compound currently in development, identified as Compound X. This compound has a molecular weight less than 400, and a log $D_{7.4}$ value of approximately 0.5, suggesting that it could undergo both renal and hepatic clearance. Preclinical *in vivo* studies indicate that Compound X is eliminated largely unchanged in the urine in the rat ($\sim 90\%$). Several oxidative biotransformation pathways have nonetheless been identified. In common with studies of Compound X clearance in humans, simple *in vitro* enzyme kinetic studies were used in conjunction with knowledge from rat *in vivo* data. The general strategy for prediction of kinetic studies, is shown in Figure 10.2.

Using liver microsomes from different species, the intrinsic clearance (Cl'_{int}) for each species can be determined, and then scaled to hepatic clearance. This is typically done by first determining *in vitro* K_m (the Michaelis–Menten constant) and V_{max} (the maximal rate of metabolism) for each metabolic reaction, using substrate saturation plots (using the familiar algebra and, because of enzyme saturation, finding that $Cl'_{int} = V_{max}/K_m$). However, for Compound X, the situation is more complicated because we know that the Cl'_{int} (drug disappearance) actually is due to several combined biotransformation pathways (i.e. Cl'_{int} (total) $= Cl'_{int\ 1} + Cl'_{int\ 2} + Cl'_{int\ 3} + \ldots$), thus complicating any K_m and V_{max} determinations from a simple substrate saturation plot.

To determine the Cl'_{int} of compound X, we are able to use the *in vitro* half-life method, which is simpler than finding all the component Cl'_{int} values. When the substrate concentration is much smaller

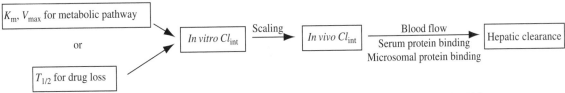

Figure 10.2 Strategy for the *in vitro–in vivo* scaling of hepatic clearance (see for example Iwatsubo et al., 1996)

than the K_m, the Michaelis–Menten equation simplifies from velocity $(V) = V_{max}([S])/(K_m + [S])$ to $V = V_{max}/K_m$, because ([S] is substrate concentration) becomes negligible. Furthermore, under these conditions the *in vitro* half-life ($T_{1/2} = 0.693/K_{el}$) can be measured, and this, in turn, is related to the Michaelis–Menten equation through the relationship velocity (V) = volume $\times K_{el}$ (where volume is standardized for the volume containing 1 mg of microsomal protein). When both V and V_{max} are known, then the K_m is also found. Although simpler than finding a complicated C_{int}, one caveat of the *in vitro* half-life method is that one assumes that the substrate concentration is much smaller than the K_m. It may be necessary to repeat the half-life determinations at several substrate concentrations, and even model the asymptote of this relationship, because very low substrate concentrations that are beneath biochemical detection may be needed to fulfill the assumptions needed to simplify the Michaelis–Menten equation.

Note that in this *in vitro* application, intrinsic clearance, like all conventional mathematical evaluation of clearances, has units of volume $\cdot$ time^{-1}. It is obtained from V_{max} and K_m measurements, where V_{max} has units of mass $\cdot$ time^{-1}. The definition of intrinsic clearance as $V_{max} \cdot K_m^{-1}$ should not be confused with the historically prevalent calculation of k_{el} (the first-order rate constant of decay of concentration in plasma), calculated from $k_{el} = V_{max} \cdot K_m^{-1}$, where V_{max} is the zero order rate of plasma concentration decay seen at high concentrations, and K_{max} is the concentration is plasma at half-maximal rate of plasma level decay.

Once the *in vitro* intrinsic clearance has been determined, the next step, scaling *in vitro* intrinsic clearance to the whole liver, proceeds as follows:

In vivo Cl'_{int} = *in vitro* $Cl'_{int} \times$ weight microsomal

protein/g liver

$\times$ weight liver/kg body weight

The amount of microsomal protein/g liver is constant across species (45 mg/g liver). Thus, the only species-dependent variable is the weight of liver tissue/kg body weight.

In vivo, hepatic clearance is determined by factoring in the hepatic blood flow (Q), the fraction of drug unbound in the blood (fu), and the fraction of drug unbound in the microsomal incubations ($fu_{(inc)}$), against the intrinsic clearance of the drug by the whole liver (the *in vivo* Cl'_{int}). The fu and $fu_{(inc)}$ are included when the drug shows considerable plasma or microsomal protein binding (Obach 1996b). Several models are available for scaling *in vivo* intrinsic clearance to hepatic clearance, including the parallel tube model or sinusoidal perfusion model, the well-stirred model or venous equilibration model, and the distributed sinusoidal perfusion model (Wilkinson 1987).

Thus far, for Compound X, we have obtained good results in this context with the simplest of these, the well-stirred model (see Table 10.1 for the equations, with and without significant plasma and/or microsomal protein binding). Using this well-stirred model, it has proved possible to predict the hepatic clearance from *in vitro* intrinsic clearance rates in the rat, dog and human (Table 10.2). The hepatic clearance value for the rat (0.972 ml$\cdot$min$^{-1} \cdot$mg^{-1} protein) was approximately one-tenth the actual clearance found *in vivo*; well in agreement with the observation that *in vivo* Compound X was eliminated by the rat, largely unchanged, by the kidneys ($\sim 90\%$).

To predict hepatic clearance of Compound X in man, human *in vitro* intrinsic clearance could then be scaled to hepatic clearance, using a technique that had been validated in the rat. Ashfortt et al 1995Renal clearance is subject to an allometric relationship and can generally be scaled across species (see below). The predicted *in vivo* renal Cl for the rat (estimated by multiplying the predicted hepatic Cl by 9) may be scaled allometrically to

Table 10.1 Equations for predicting hepatic clearance using the well-stirred model

In the absence of serum or microsomal protein binding	In the presence of significant serum protein binding	In the presence of both serum and microsomal protein binding
$Cl_{hepatic} = \dfrac{Q \times Cl'_{int}}{Q + Cl'_{int}}$	$Cl_{hepatic} = \dfrac{Q \times f_u \times Cl'_{int}}{Q + f_u \times Cl'_{int}}$	$Cl_{hepatic} = \dfrac{Q \times f_u \times Cl'_{int} \times f_{u_{(inc)}}}{Q + f_u \times Cl'_{int} \times f_{u_{(inc)}}}$

Table 10.2 Comparison of the predicted *in vivo* hepatic clearance and the actual clearance values for Compund X

	Predicted *in vivo* hepatic CL (ml min^{-1} kg^{-1})	Predicted *in vivo* renal CL (ml min^{-1} kg^{-1})	Predicted *in vivo* total CL (ml min^{-1} kg^{-1})	Actual *in vivo* CL (ml min^{-1} kg^{-1})
Rat	0.972	8.75	9.72	8.17–10.7
Man	0.223	1.93	2.15	1.87–2.45
Dog	0.463	3.74	4.20	21.2–22.5

Predicted values were scaled from *in vitro* half-life data using liver microsomes and the well-stirred model of hepatic extraction. Hepatic CL predictions were corrected for plasma and microsomal protein binding. Predicted total CL was obtained by adding in renal CL estimates which were, in turn, scaled allometrically ($Y = aW^{0.75}$).

obtain a prediction for human *in vivo* renal clearance. Total or systemic *Cl* in man can then be estimated by adding the two clearance parameters (hepatic and renal) together; in practice, for Compound X, later first-in-man data revealed an actual *in vivo* *Cl* nearly identical to the predicted total *Cl* (2.15 vs. 1.87–2.45 ml min^{-1} mg^{-1}, respectively; Table 10.2). Here, then, is a real-world example of, first, how rat *in vitro* and *in vivo* preclinical data were used to develop and validate a scaling method for Compound X in the rat; and second, how the scaling method successfully predicted *in vivo* overall drug clearance in man.

However, if the same methods are used for Compound X in the dog, things initially appear to be different. Scaling the *in vitro* intrinsic clearance to hepatic *Cl* using the rat-validated method, in conjunction with allometric scaling of renal *Cl*, resulted in a five-fold underprediction of total or systemic clearance *in vivo*. However, further metabolism studies in the dog *in vivo* revealed that Compound X undergoes significant additional biotransformation, particularly *N*-methylation, which is unique (as far as we are aware) to this species, and invalidates some of our *in vitro* assumptions. This canine biotransformation pathway was not detected by our initial microsomal studies because there are no *N*-methyl transferases in microsomes. Thus, although we did not successfully predict dog systemic clearance for Compound X, our scaling tactics did eventually teach us about a new clearance mechanism, and how important this was for the systemic clearance of Compound X in the dog.

This is an example of how *in vitro* studies can be combined with *in vivo* preclinical data, leading to useful prediction of human systemic drug clearance. Nonetheless, several caveats are encountered in such scaling exercises, which warrant restating.

The first caveat is that all clearance pathways (hepatic, renal, biliary, or other) must be taken into consideration. If a compound undergoes a high level of hepatic clearance, then *in vitro–in vivo* scaling may be used to predict the fraction of systemic clearance expected from this pathway. If a compound undergoes a high level of renal elimination, allometric scaling may be also used to predict the clearance attributed to this pathway.

The second caveat is that, in order to accurately predict hepatic clearance, the correct *in vitro* system must be chosen. If the candidate drug is primarily oxidatively metabolized, then liver microsomes will be sufficient. However, if the potential for nonmicrosomal biotransformation exists, then a different *in vitro* system, such as hepatocyte suspensions, should be used. In the illustration above, it turned out, as far as clearance of Compound X is concerned, man is specifically like a rat, and unlike a dog.

The third caveat is that one must consider the variability in the expression of metabolizing enzymes between individuals. Oxidative metabolism (seen *in vivo* and in microsomal enzymes), and especially cytochrome P_{450}s, vary tremendously between human individuals (Meyer 1994; Shimada et al 1994). Had we used a single donor microsomal sample, rather than pooled liver microsomes (a pool consisting of at least eight individual donors), to scale *in vitro* data to *in vivo* hepatic clearance, we might have made greatly misleading predictions (note that oxidative, initial drug metabolism is sometimes called 'Phase I metabolism' in the literature, causing ambiguity with the stage of drug development or type of clinical trial).

Volumes of Distribution

Review of Elementary Concepts

Volume of distribution is a theoretical concept that may or may not correspond to the anatomical compartment(s) which drugs or metabolites may access after dosing. When size of the dose (D) is known, and when drug concentration (C) may be found by sampling biological fluids, then, in the simplest case, the volume of distribution (VD) is:

$$VD = D/C$$

Clinical protocols can usually only prescribe the sampling of a subset of compartments when a drug is known to distribute widely in the body. For example, a lipophilic drug may penetrate lipophilic organs such as brain, and, obviously, brain sampling simply for pharmacokinetic purposes is usually possible only in animals. In such cases, blood concentrations fall far lower than if the dose had distributed solely into the circulating compartment; C becomes very small, and VD becomes correspondingly very large. The opposite effect would require the drug to be restricted to a fraction of the compartment that is sampled, essentially suggesting that too few compartments have been postulated, and is almost never encountered. Again, see Curry (1980) or Benet et al (1996) for expansion of these elementary aspects of volume of distribution.

Prediction of Human Volumes of Distribution

The free (not plasma protein-bound) volume of distribution of experimental drugs is generally considered to be constant for all species. Thus, the volume of distribution in man can easily be predicted through a simple proportionality between *in vitro* plasma protein binding data in man and in a preclinical species, and *in vivo* volume of distribution in that same preclinical species:

$$VD_{\text{human}} = \frac{VD_{\text{preclinical species}} \times fu_{\text{human}}}{fu_{\text{preclinical species}}}$$

Table 10.3 shows the predicted volume of distribution of a single intravenous bolus dose of Compound X in man; this is found by using the above equation, an *in vitro* estimate of protein binding data for rat and dog plasma, and the observed volumes of distribution for these two species *in vivo*. For man, VD_{human} was predicted to be 3.48–4.591 kg^{-1} using the rat data and 3.01–5.061 kg^{-1} using the dog data.

Elementary Aspects of Oral Bioavailability

The oral bioavailability (F) of a drug is dependent on (a) the absorption of the drug from the gastrointestinal (GI) tract, and (b) capability of the liver to clear the drug during its first pass through the portal venous system. Oral bioavailability may be described as the fraction of the total oral dose for which systemic exposure is achieved. It is a measurement of *extent* of exposure, and contrasts with the *rates* of absorption or elimination discussed above.

Clinically, F is found by comparing the systemic exposures that result after intravenous and oral doses of the same drug. Note that this comparison need not be for doses of the same size (an important consideration when the pharmaceutical physician assesses the tolerability aspects of a proposed normal volunteer study). It is, in fact, preferable to achieve concentrations in the same range from the two doses. Typically, C_{max} for a standard dose is going to be higher after bolus intravenous dosing (IV) than after oral administration (PO), and ad-

Table 10.3 *In vitro* plasma protein binding, *In vivo* volume of distribution and predicted volume of distribution in man

	Fraction of Compound X unbound in the plasma (f_u)	*In vivo* volume of distribution (l . kg)	Predicted volume of distribution in man (l . kg)
Rat	0.45	3.02–3.97	3.48–4.59
Human	0.52	–	–
Dog	0.66	3.82–6.43	3.01–5.06

verse effects of new agents are likely to be concentration-dependent. The relevant equation is:

$$F(\%) = [(AUC_{PO} \times Dose_{IV})/$$
$$(AUC_{IV} \times Dose_{PO})] \times 100$$

where AUC is the area under the time–plasma concentration curve after each of the respective administrations (the dose terms cancel when equally sized doses are administered by both routes of administration). A residual of less than 15% (sometimes 10%) of the total AUC is a commonly-used standard for timing the last plasma sample. These studies are usually conducted under standard conditions, and using crossover protocols, although, occasionally, a double-label study may be used to measure F instantaneously (see Chapter 12). Comparison of generic with innovator's formulations, and slow-release with rapidly absorbed formulations, may be compared using equations of the same form. Similarly, subcutaneous and intravenous injections can be compared. With very rare exceptions, the intravenous administration of a dose is assumed to be 100% bioavailable. For example, very short-acting drugs, e.g. some arachidonate derivatives, remifentanil, esmolol and adenosine, may be metabolized during their first return circulation after intravenous administration, and still not achieve 100% 'bioavailability'. Also, the concept is not applicable to topically-acting drugs. However, assessing the bioavailability of these drugs by any other route of administration is usually pointless, unless there is some highly specialized issue, e.g. absorption after intrathecal administration or potential for drug abuse.

Fluctuation of plasma drug concentration is an important aspect of the bioavailability of slow release formulations, which almost always have lower C_{max} values for a standard dose size than, albeit similar AUC to, a more rapidly absorbed tablet. Assuming that the assay can handle the inevitably lower plasma concentrations, then a useful measure of fluctuation, after the initial absorption phase of the curve, and during the next four half-lives of elimination, is:

$$(C_{max} - C_{min})/C_{avg}$$

where C_{avg} is the average concentration during the specified time period; whether to use the arithmetic or geometric average is a controversy, with respected protagonists on both sides.

Prediction of Oral Bioavailability

Oral bioavailability can be predicted using the following equation:

$$F = Fa \cdot (1 - Cl/Q)$$

where Fa represents the fraction of drug absorbed through the intestinal lining, Cl is the hepatic clearance (predicted from *in vitro* studies, see earlier section) and Q is the hepatic blood flow in man (see, for example, Rane etal., 1977). Octanol/water partitioning has traditionally been used to predict the fraction absorbed through the intestinal lining. Recently, Caco-2 cell permeability studies have replaced the use of octanol/buffer partitioning studies. Yee (1997) established a relationship between Fa and Caco-2 cell permeability, expressed as the apparent permeability constant (P_{app}), as follows:

$$P_{app} < 10^{-6}\,cm/s, \text{ then } Fa = 0 - 20\%$$
$$1 \le P_{app} \le 10 \times 10^{-6}\,cm/s, \text{ then } Fa = 20 - 70\%$$
$$P_{app} > 10^{-5}\,cm/s, \text{ then } Fa = > 70\%$$

The use of Caco-2 cell permeability studies has resulted in more accurate oral bioavailability predictions. Using the predicted hepatic clearance for Compound X in man (see above), estimating Fa by extrapolation from the Caco-2 cell P_{app}, and an assumed hepatic blood flow for man (see, for example, Rane et al., 1977) of 20 ml/min/kg, the human oral bioavailability of 69–98% for Compound X is predicted. This compares well with the known oral bioavailability of this compound in rats and dogs (83% and 72%, respectively).

PREDICTION FROM ANIMALS TO HUMANS *IN VIVO*

Elementary Aspects

Allometric scaling is an empirical method for predicting physiological, anatomical, and pharmacokinetic measures across species in relation to time and size (Boxenbaum 1982; Boxenbaum and DiLea 1995; Ings, 1990). Allometric scaling is based on similarities among species in their physiology, anatomy, and biochemistry, coupled with the observation that smaller animals perform physiological functions that are similar to larger animals, but at a faster rate. The allometric equation is $Y = aW^b$, and a log transformation of this formula yields the straight line:

$$\log Y = b \log W + \log a,$$

where:

$Y =$ the pharmacokinetic or physiological variable of interest
$a =$ the allometric coefficient (and log a is the intercept of the line)
$W =$ body weight
$b =$ allometric exponent (slope of the line)

One of the first applications of allometric scaling was the use of the toxicity of anticancer agents in animals to predict toxicity in humans. It was observed that the toxic dose of a drug is similar among species when the dose is compared on the basis of body surface area (Freireich et al 1966). For most vertebrate species, the body weight/volume ratio varies very little, but the surface area/volume ratio increases as species become smaller. Allometric correction of dose multiples in toxicology (compared with proposed human doses) is thus important, especially when small rodents provide the principal toxicology coverage.

Body surface area (Y) is related to body weight (W, in kg) by the formula:

$$Y = 0.1W^{0.67}$$

This allometric relationship between body surface area and species body weight then allows for a simple conversion of drug doses across species (Figure 10.3), and allometrically eqivalent doses of drugs (mg/kg) can be calculated for any species (Table 10.4). The conversion factor (km is simply the body weight divided by the body surface area. Thus, by using the km factors, the dose in Species 1 (in mg/kg) is equivalent to ($km_{species2}/km_{species1}$) times the dose in Species 2 (in mg/kg). For example, a 50 mg/kg dose of drug in mouse would be equivalent to a 4.1 mg/kg dose in human, i.e. approximately one-twelfth of the dose (Table 10.4). Likewise, the conversion factor can be used to calculate equivalent doses between any species. An equivalent dose in mg/kg in rat would be twice that for the mouse.

Allometric Approaches to Drug Discovery

Using limited data, allometric scaling may be used as a part of drug discovery. To do this we assume

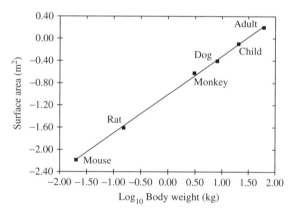

Figure 10.3   Allometric relationship between body surface area and species body weight on a log vs. log plot

Table 10.4   Equivalent surface area dosage conversion factors

Species	Body weight (kg)	Body surface area (kg/m²)	Factor (k_m)	Approximate human dose equivalent
Mouse	0.02	0.0067	3.0	1/12
Rat	0.100	0.0192	5.2	1/7
Dog	8.0	0.400	20	1/2
Monkey	2.5	0.217	11.5	1/3
Human	60	1.62	37	N/A

Dose in species 1 (mg/kg) = dose in species 2 (mg/kg) × (km₂/km₁).

that, for the formula $Y = aW^b$, the value of the power function 'b' (or slope of the line from a log vs. log plot) is drug-independent, unlike the intercept 'a', which is drug-dependent. By doing this we can use data from a single species (the rat) to successfully predict the pharmacokinetics of Compound X in humans and cats. This method could be expected to save time and money in the drug discovery process by enabling us to:

1. Select the correct dose in an animal model of disease. These studies are expensive and time-consuming. The selection of the wrong dose in an animal model, especially in a model in a larger species such as cat, could lead to invalid results, either through toxicity (if the dose is too high) or inactivity (if the dose is too low).
2. Provide confidence that the pharmacological model will predict efficacy in humans. If a drug is effective in therapeutic models using different species and these animals receive equivalent exposures (as measured by the maximum plasma concentration, C_{max}, or area under the plasma concentration curve, AUC), then the clinician can choose a dose for trials with confidence.
3. Eliminate unnecessary doses and plasma samples in the first trials in humans.

The discovery process for Compound X, which is efficacious in a number of *in vivo* models, is again an illustration of how allometric considerations can enhance the development process. The whole brain concentrations of this compound are in equilibrium with plasma concentrations within 5 min after dosing, and it is also eliminated from the brain in equilibrium with the declining plasma concentration. We also know that Compound X is ~80% orally bioavailable in rats and dogs (see above), and has linear (first-order elimination) and predictable pharmacokinetics in animals.

Next, this compound was tested in a model of excitotoxicity, in which the neurotoxin malonate was injected into the striatum of rats. A subcutaneous injection of compound X at 9 mg/kg caused an 80% reduction in the lesion activity produced by malonate. The C_{max} plasma levels of Compound X at this dose would be about 1500 ng/ml.

In a study using spontaneously hypertensive rats, a dose of 12 mg/kg of compound X was also

neuroprotective [these rats were subjected to 2 h of focal ischemia by occlusion of the right middle cerebral artery (MCA), followed by 22 h of reperfusion]. With the assumption of 100% systemic absorption, the expected plasma C_{max} at this dose was 2000 ng/ml. In this model, there was a significant reduction (greater than 30%) in cortical infarct volume, compared with saline controls, when the drug was given at the time of occlusion and at 0, 0.5, 1, and 1.5 h post-MCA occlusion.

Using the data from the neuroprotection models from rats, we then scaled a dose to the cat that was expected to achieve a neuroprotective plasma concentration of 1500 ng/ml. To do this, we predicted the volume of distribution (V_{1cat}) using data collected from the volume of distribution in rat (V_{1rat}). For our calculations we used a value of 0.938 for the power function b (see Ings 1990, Table 2). In doing this we made the standard assumption that in the formula $Y = aW^b$ the value of the power function b was compound-independent and that the function a was compound-dependent (Ings observed that the power function b is reasonably constant for each pharmacokinetic parameter). Substituting into the allometric formula, $\log(V_{1cat}) = b \log W + \log a$, we found:

$$\log 0.426 \text{ liters} = 0.938 \log 0.3 \text{ kg} + \log a$$

Thus:

$$\log a = 0.120.$$

By substituting back into the formula and using a cat weight of 4 kg, we found:

$$V_{1cat} = 4.8 \, l \text{ or } 1.21 \, l/kg.$$

Our formula for calculating the dose to be administered was:

$$Dose_{cat} = Dose_{rat}(V_{1cat}/V_{1rat})$$

The formula for predicting the plasma half-life was:

$$T_{1/2\,cat} = T_{1/2\,rat}(W_{cat}/W_{rat})^{y-x}$$

in which y is as defined earlier and x is a clearance parameter (Boxenbaum and Ronfeld 1983). The measured plasma half-life in the rat was 4.53 h.

Filling in the formula (Boxenbaum and Ronfeld 1983), we predicted a plasma half-life in the cat of 7.3 h ($= 4.53 \times (4/0.3)^{0.938-0.75}$). The measured plasma half-life in the cat was 6 h. We knew from data collected in the rat that a dose of 3.06 mg/kg administered over 15 min would give a plasma C_{max} of 1500 ng/ml of plasma. This equated to a dose in the cat of 2.6 mg/kg over 15 min or 175 μg/kg/min for 15 min.

When we performed studies to determine the C_{max} in cats following a dose of 2.6 mg/kg administered over 15 min, our predicted values were very close to the actual values, with a measured C_{max} of 1240 ± 100 ng/ml.

Data from the rat can also be used to predict the pharmacokinetics of Compound X in humans. As with the cat we made our predictions prospectively, by assuming, as stated earlier, that for the formula $Y = aW^b$, the value of the power function b (or slope of the line from a log vs. log plot) was drug-independent, and that the intercept function a was drug-dependent. We assigned values of 0.75, 0.938, and 0.25 for clearance, volume of distribution, and plasma half-life, respectively, using data taken from the literature and discussed above. The intercept function a was then determined for each parameter by substituting the pharmacokinetic data from rats, i.e. clearance = 0.54 l/h/kg, $V_1 = 1.42$ l/kg, $V_{dss} = 3.33$ l/kg. We estimated the pharmacokinetic parameters for humans by substituting the calculated intercept function back into the formula and solving for Y for a 70 kg human. The prediction of the plasma half-life in humans was determined by three separate methods. For our predictions, we also assumed that the protein binding was the same in rats and in humans and that the metabolism of Compound X was similar in both species. Clearly, approaches like this could be a routine part of drug discovery.

The values estimated by allometric scaling were compared with those observed in the single-dose human volunteer study (Table 10.5). We predicted that for Compound X in humans the plasma half-life would be 14.5 h, the plasma clearance would be 0.138 l/h/kg, and the V_1, V_{dss}, and $V_{dβ}$ would be 1.01, 2.37, and 2.56 L/kg, respectively. The predictions using rat data were within 15% of the actual mean values in human volunteers. A complex Dedrick plot of the rat and human data showed nearly superimposable concentration–time curves,

Table 10.5 Predicted and actual pharmacokinetic parameters for humans

Pharmacokinetic parameter	Predicted	Actual
Clearance	0.138 l/h/kg	0.123
Half-life[a]	14.5 h	13.6 h
V_1	1.01 l/kg	1.02 l/kg
V_{dss}	2.4 l/kg	2.1 l/kg

[a] Plasma half-life is the average from three values by three different methods: (a) $T_{1/2\,human} = (0.693 \times V_d)/Cl_p$; (b) $T_{1/2\,human} = T_{1/2\,rat} (W_{human}/W_{rat})^{y-x}$; and (c) $\log T_{1/2\,human} = \log a + b \log W_{human}$.

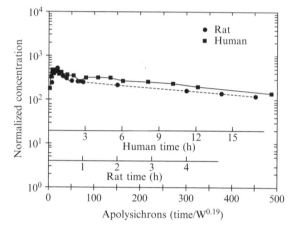

Figure 10.4 Complex Dedrick plot of rat and human data for Compound X

again showing very good scaling between rat and human (Figure 10.4).

This illustrates how allometric scaling is a useful part of the drug discovery process: we avoided studying irrelevant doses and saved time. Ideally, allometric scaling should be done using pharmacokinetic data from at least four species, even though accurate predictions can be made using data from a single species. If possible, information about differences in metabolism among species should be considered when making predictions.

PHARMACOKINETIC/ PHARMACODYNAMIC MODELS

Elementary Aspects

The possibility that time since lose changes the relationship between pharmacological effect size and drug concentrations in plasma has been known for a long time (Levy 1964, 1966; Levy and Nelson 1965; Wagner 1968; Curry 1980). The pioneering work was done by Levy and his colleagues in the 1960s on single dose–plasma level–effect relationships, and on the duration of action of drugs as a function of dose. Brodie and colleagues had shown even earlier how complicated the relationships are when drugs with multicompartment distribution are studied in this context (e.g. Brodie 1967). Lasagna and colleagues, using diuretics, found that depending on whether a cumulative effect (24 h urine production) or an 'instant' effect (rate of urine flow at a particular time) were measured, different relationships of response were possible (Murphy et al 1961). Nagashima et al (1969) demonstrated the relative time courses of anticoagulant concentration and effect. Thus, the relationship between effect size and concentration of drug in plasma should not be expected to be constant or simple, and can vary with time.

The objectives of modern analysis of drug action are to delineate the chemical or physical interactions between drug and target cell and to characterize the full sequence and scope of actions of each drug (Ross 1996). Preclinical models describing the relationship between the concentration of drug in blood or plasma, and drug receptor occupancy or functional response, provide clinically useful tools regarding *potency, efficacy*, and the time course of effect.

Potency is an expression of the activity of a compound, in terms of either the concentration or amount needed to produce a defined effect. E_{max} is the maximal drug-induced effect. EC_{50} is the concentration of an agonist that produces 50% of the maximal possible response. An EC_{50} can be described for drug concentrations using *in vitro* assays, or as a plasma concentration *in vivo*. IC_{50} is the concentration of an antagonist that reduces a specified response to 50% of its former value.

A measure of the tendency of a ligand and its receptor to bind to each other is expressed as K_d in receptor occupancy studies. K_d is the equilibrune contant for the two processes of drug-receptor combination and dissociation. K_d may be found for both agonists and antagonists, although sometimes the former poses more technical challenge, due to alterations to the conformation of the binding site. In contrast, *efficacy* is a relative measure, amongst different agonists, describing response

size for a standard degree of receptor occupation (Jenkinson et al 1995). When an agonist must occupy 100% of available receptors to cause E_{max}, its efficacy may be said to be unity. If occupation of all receptors achieves a response that is less than E_{max}, then the agonist's efficacy is less than one, and equal to the ratio of observed maximal effect/ maximal effect for an agonist with efficacy = 1 (we call these *partial agonists* or *agonist–antagonists*). Some agonists need occupy only a subset of the available receptors, in order to achieve E_{max}, and these have efficacy greater than unity. In the latter case, the concentration–response curve lies to the left of the concentration–receptor occupancy curve (e.g. Minneman *et al* 1983). Drugs with efficacy ≥ 1 are also called *full agonists*.

Below, we present some model relationships between observed concentration and effect size, as examples from a considerable volume of literature. The reader is referred to key texts for comprehensive coverage of this topic (e.g. Smolen 1971; Gibaldi and Perrier 1982, Dayneka et al 1993; Levy 1993; Lesko and Williams 1994; Colburn 1995; Derendorf and Hochhaus 1995; Gabrielsson and Weiner 1997; Sharma and Jusko 1997).

Pharmacokinetic–Pharmacodynamic (PK/PD) Modeling

Single-compartment, Time-independent PK/PD Models

The simplest model is where: (a) the drug distributes into a single compartment, represented by plasma; and (b) the effect is an instantaneous, direct function of the concentration in that compartment. In this situation, the relationship between drug concentration (C) and a pharmacological effect (E) can be simply described by the linear function:

$$E = S \cdot C$$

where S is a slope parameter. If the measured effect has some baseline value (E_0), when drug is absent (e.g. physiological, diastolic blood pressure, or resting tension on the tissue in an organ bath), then the model may be expressed as:

$$E = E_0 + S \cdot C$$

The parameters of this model, S and E_0, may be estimated by linear regression. This model does not contain any information about efficacy and potency, cannot identify the maximum effect, and thus cannot be used to find EC_{50}.

When effect can be measured for a wide concentration range, the relationship between effect and concentration is often observed to be curvilinear. A semi-logarithmic plot of effect vs. log concentration commonly linearizes these data within the approximate range 20–80% of maximal effect. This log-transformation of the concentration axis facilitates a graphical estimation of the *slope* of the apparently linear segment of the curve:

$$E = m \cdot \ln(C + C_0)$$

where m and C_0 are the slope and the hypothetical baseline concentration (usually zero, but not for experiments of add-on therapy or when administering molecules that are also present endogenously), respectively. In this equation, the pharmacological effect may be expressed, when the drug concentration is zero, as:

$$E_0 = m \cdot \ln(C_0)$$

As mentioned earlier, for functional data based on biophase, plasma or tissue measurements, we often represent potency as EC_{50}, and when two compounds are compared with respect to potency, the one with the lowest EC_{50} value has the highest potency. A general expression for observed effect, by analogy with the Michaelis–Menten equation (above) is:

$$E = \frac{E_{max} C}{EC_{50} + C}$$

There are various forms of this function for agonist (stimulatory) and antagonist (inhibitory) effects. For example, if there is a baseline effect (E_0), then this may be added to the right-hand side of the equation:

$$E = E_0 + \frac{E_{max} C}{EC_{50} + C}$$

Alternatively, the relationship between concentration and effect for an antagonist, including a baseline value, is:

$$E = E_0 - \frac{I_{max} C}{IC_{50} + C}$$

In the E_{max} model above, plasma concentration and EC_{50} are raised to the power of n (Hill factor) equal to 1. A more general form of the equation is the sigmoid curve:

$$E = \frac{E_{max} C^n}{EC_{50}^n + C^n}$$

where, by addition of a single parameter (n) to the E_{max} model, it is possible to account for curves which are both shallower and steeper than when $n = 1$ (i.e. unlike the ordinary E_{max} models). Note that the sigmoidicity parameter (n) does not necessarily have a direct biological interpretation and should be viewed as an extension of the original E_{max} model to account for curvature.

The larger the value of the exponent, the more curved (steeper, concave downwards) is the line. A very high exponent can be viewed as indicating an all-or-none effect (e.g. the development of an action potential in a nerve). Within a narrow concentration range the observed effect goes from all to nothing, or vice versa. An exponent less than unity (< 1) sometimes indicates active metabolites and/or multiple receptor sites.

The corresponding inhibitory sigmoid E_{max} model is functionally described as follows:

$$E = E_0 - \frac{I_{max} C^n}{IC_{50}^n + C^n}$$

In vivo, these models, analogous to the classical dose or log dose–response curves of *in vitro* pharmacology, are limited to direct effects in single compartment systems. These models make no allowance for time-dependent events in drug response.

Complex PK/PD and Time-dependent Models

The most common approach to *in vivo* pharmacokinetic and pharmacodynamic modeling involves sequential analysis of the concentration vs. time and effect vs. time data, such that the kinetic model provides an independent variable, such as concentration, *driving* the dynamics. Only in limited situations could it be anticipated that the effect influences the kinetics, for example, effects on blood flow or drug clearance itself.

Levy (1964), Jusko (1971), and Smolen (1971; 1976) described the analysis of dose–response time data. They developed a theoretical basis for the performance of this analysis from data obtained from the observation of the time course of pharmacological response, after a single dose of drug, by any route of administration. Smolen (1976) extended the analysis to application of dose–response time data for bioequivalence testing.

In dose–response time models the underlying assumption is that pharmacodynamic data gives us information on the kinetics of drug in the *biophase* (i.e. the tissue or compartment precisely where the drug exhibits its effect). In other words, apparent half-life, bioavailability and potency can be obtained simultaneously from dose–response–time data. Considering such a model, assuming (a) first-order input/output processes and (b) extravascular dosing, the kinetic model then drives the inhibition function of the dynamic model. It is the *dynamic behaviour* which is described by the response model. A zero-order input and first-order output governs the *turnover* of the response. This permits us to consider situations where the plasma concentration represents delivery of the drug to an effect compartment; the time course of drug concentration and of effect (both in the biophase), is different from that simply observed in plasma concentrations.

The amount of drug in a single hypothetical compartment after an intravenous (IV) dose is usually modeled with mono-exponential decline, and analogous to the 'plasma disappearance' curve (above):

$$X_{IV} = D_{IV}e^{-Kt}$$

The amount of drug in a single hypothetical compartment after an extravascular dose is then modeled with first-order input/output kinetics:

$$X_{po} = \frac{K_a F D_{po}}{K_a - K}\left[e^{-K(t-t_{lag})} - e^{K_a(t-t_{lag})}\right]$$

Concentration–time effect modelling is illustrated by the example which follows. This example was chosen to illustrate a single dose of drug causing the reversal of a symptom (pain). Many other types of examples exist.

The plasma kinetics of the analgesic were describable by the following expression after the intravenous bolus dose, with $C_0 = 45.0$ and $K = 0.50\,h^{-1}$:

$$C = 45.0\,e^{-0.50t}$$

In the same study, effect measurements were recorded during 80 min, as shown in Figure 10.5.

Often, drug effects do not parallel changes in plasma concentration. This can result from distribution phenomena, such as when the effect occurs outside the plasma compartment (e.g. the sedative effect of a dose of benzodiazepine, which occurs in the brain), or when the effect recorded reflects, for example, a chain of biochemical events triggered by the presence of drug (e.g. the aborting of a migraine attack by a serotoninergic drug). In relation to the first of these possibilities, a model sometimes called a 'link model' (also called the 'effect-compartment' or the 'effect-distribution' model) allows estimation of the *in vivo* pharmacodynamic effect from non-steady-state effect (E) vs. time and concentration (C) vs. time data, within which potential exists for observed E and C to display temporal displacement with respect to each other (Segre 1968; Wagner 1968; Dahlstrom et al 1978; Sheiner et al 1979). The rate of change of drug amount (A_e) in a hypothetical effect compartment can be expressed as:

$$\frac{dA_e}{dt} = k_{le}A_1 - k_{e0}A_e$$

where A is the amount of drug in the central compartment of a pharmacokinetic model, linked to the effect compartment, with first-order rate constants k_{le} and k_{e0}. The corresponding expression for the amount of drug in the effect compartment, for a one-compartment model with bolus input of dose (D) is:

$$A_e = \frac{k_{le}D}{k_{e0}-K}\left[e^{-Kt} - e^{-k_{e0}t}\right]$$

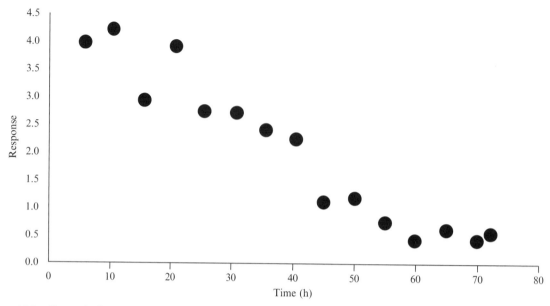

Figure 10.5   Observed effect-time data for an analgesic

where K is the elimination rate constant. The concentration of drug in the effect compartment, C_e, is obtained by dividing A_e by the effect compartment volume, V_e:

$$C_e = \frac{k_{le} D}{V_e(k_{e0} - K)} \left[e^{-Kt} - e^{k_{e0} t} \right]$$

At equilibrium, the rates of drug transfer between the central and effect compartments are equal:

$$k_{le} A = k_{e0} A_e$$
$$k_{le} V_c C = k_{e0} V_e C_e$$

If the partition coefficient, K_p, equals C_e/C at equilibrium (steady-state), then we can rearrange the above equation:

$$V_e = \frac{k_{le} V_1}{K_p k_{e0}}$$

Substituting for V_e in the above equation (i.e. $k_{le} = k_{e0}$) yields:

$$C_e = \frac{k_{e0} D K_p}{V_1(k_{e0} - K)} \left[e^{-Kt} - e^{-k_{e0} t} \right]$$

At equilibrium, C will be equal to C_e/K_p by definition, and thus:

$$C_e = \frac{k_{e0} D}{V_1(k_{e0} - K)} \left[e^{-Kt} - e^{-k_{e0} t} \right]$$

This is how the link-model relates the kinetics in plasma to the kinetics of drug in the effect compartment. When used together with the E_{max} model for estimation of the maximal drug-induced effect, the concentration at half-maximal effect (apparent EC_{50}), and the rate constant of the disappearance of the effect (k_{e0}):

$$E = \frac{E_{max} C_e^n}{EC_{50}^n + C_e^n}$$

Computer fitting of the equations to the effect data and estimation of the rate constant for the disappearance of the effect, k_{e0}, EC_{50}, and E_{max} follows, assuming the sigmoidicity factor (n) to be equal to unity.

At steady-state, C_e is directly proportional to the plasma concentration (C), since $C_e = K_p C$. Consequently, the potency (EC_{50}) obtained by regressing the last two equations, represents the steady-state plasma concentration producing 50% of E_{max}.

Note that the effect equilibration rate constant (k_{e0}) may be viewed as a first-order distribution rate constant. It can also be thought of in terms of the rate of presentation of a drug to a specific tissue, determined by, for example, tissue perfusion rate, apparent volume of the tissue, and eventual diffusion into the tissue. The results of the data fitting in this exercise with the analgesic are: E_{max} 4.5; EC_{50} 0.61 ng·ml^{-1}; and k_{e0} 0.07 h^{-1}.

Effect compartment or link models are limited by their applicability to situations in which the equilibrium between plasma and response is due to distributional phenomena. In reality, there is often a delay between occurrence of maximum drug concentration in the effect compartment and maximum intensity of effect caused by slow development of the effect, rather than by slow distribution to the site of action. In this situation, indirect or 'physiological substance' models are more appropriate (Dayneka et al 1993; Levy 1994; Sharma and Jusko 1997). Warfarin is a good example, where this drug inhibits the prothrombin complex activity (PCA) (inhibition of production of effect). This is illustrated by the following example, which relates changes in (s)-warfarin concentration to observed PCA. The dose was intravenous. The change in PCA is shown in Figure 10.6. The plasma

kinetics of (s)-warfarin were described by the following mono-exponential expression:

$$C_{w(s)} = 1.05e^{-0.0228t}$$

and the equation for the turnover of clotting factor [P] was:

$$\frac{dP}{dt} = k_d \left[\frac{P_0}{1 + \left[\frac{C_{w(s)}}{IC_{50s}}\right]^n} - P \right]$$

In this equation, k_d is the apparent first-order degradation rate constant (also called k_{out}). This constant can be obtained experimentally from the slope of a ln (P) vs. time plot, after administration of a synthesis-blocking dose of coumarin anticoagulant (Nagashima et al 1969; Pitsui et al 1993). P_0 is the baseline value of the prothrombin time, $C_{w(s)}$ the concentration of (s)-warfarin, and IC_{50s} the concentration of warfarin at 50% of maximal blocking effect. It was also possible to estimate the half-life of the apparent first-order degradation.

An alternative model, including a lag-time to allow for distributional effects embedded in the observed time delay of the onset of the effect after warfarin administration, was published by Pitsui et al (1993). Setting the baseline value of clotting factor activity in the absence of warfarin (P_0) to a fixed mean of three predose measurements, the program can estimate that parameter.

The model equations are as follows:

$$\frac{dPCA}{dt} = \frac{K_{in}}{I(C_{w(s)})} - k_d \times P$$

where $I(C_{w(s)})$ is the inhibition function of warfarin (see next equation). It is appropriate to substitute K_{in} with $k_d \times P_0$. Inhibition of synthesis (rate in) has an impact upon the peak (trough) level rather than the time to the peak. This is similar to a constant-rate of drug infusion into a one-compartment system. The time to steady state is only governed by the elimination-rate constant and not the rate of infusion. At steady state:

$$\frac{dR}{dt} = \frac{K_{in}}{I(C_{w(s)})} - k_{out} P = 0$$

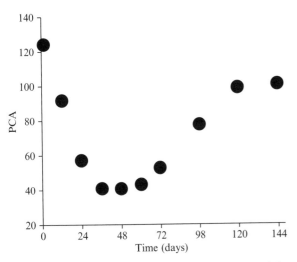

Figure 10.6 Observed PCA time course following the administration of an intravenous bolus dose of warfarin

If the baseline condition for *PCA* with no inhibition of drug is:

$$PCA = P_0$$

then the steady-state condition for the pharmacological response (PCA_{ss}) with drug present becomes:

$$PCA_{ss} = \frac{P_0}{I(C)} = P_0 \frac{1}{1 + \left[\dfrac{C_{w(s)}}{IC_{50s}}\right]^n}$$

and where $I(C_{w(s)})$ is a function of $C_{w(s)}$, n, and IC_{50s}, then:

$$I(C_{w(s)}) = 1 + \left[\frac{C_{w(s)}}{IC_{50s}}\right]^n$$

As stated before, the intensity of a pharmacological response may not be due to a direct effect of the drug on the receptor. Rather, it may be the net result of several processes only one of which is influenced by the drug. The process that is influenced by the drug must be identified and an attempt made to relate plasma drug concentration to changes in that process. Warfarin provides a good example of this, as the anticoagulant (hypothrombinemic) effect is an inhibition of the synthesis of certain vitamin K-dependent clotting factors.

Initial parameter estimates were obtained from the PCA vs. time data. The baseline value (120 s) was obtained from the intercept on the effect axis. This value is the ratio K_{in}/k_d. From the intercept and slope, K_{in} was calculated to be 3.5 s h^{-1}. The plasma concentration at the time of the trough of the effect corresponded approximately with the EC_{50} value. Thus, $IC_{50} = 0.35$ mg $\cdot$ l^{-1}, $k_d = 0.3$ h^{-1}, $n = 3.5$, $P_0 = 130$ s, and $t_{lag} = 0$ h. The computer fitting gave 0.262 ± 9.46 for the IC_{50}, 0.033 ± 17.9 for k_d, 2.68 ± 39.6 for n, and 121 ± 58 for P_0 (limits are CV%) with no lag time. Precision increased when a finite lag time was included in the fitting.

As stated earlier, these are two of many examples that can be chosen to illustrate principles. These two cases, however, are especially relevant to the relationship between animal work, and Phase I studies in which only the simplest effects, such as counteraction of a painful stimulus, or raising/lowering of a physiological parameter such as PCA, are likely to

be commonly measured. The reader is again referred to standard texts for more thorough treatment of models of this kind (Sharma and Jusko 1997).

COMMENTARY

We have not sought here to describe Phase I studies as such. This is a postgraduate textbook, and we wish to convey how *in vitro* and *in vivo* data of various kinds may be used to help extrapolate observed drug effects from simple experimental systems to more complex situation. The ultimate need is to obtain useful predictions of response in healthy human subjects (Phase I studies) from observed drug effects in animals or in the test tube.

What are the strengths and weaknesses of these approaches? The use of intrinsic clearance *in vitro* permits predictions between species for the particular enzyme/route of metabolism concerned. If humans have qualitatively different routes of metabolism for any particular compound, then this will weaken the predictive value of the *in vitro* observation. Similarly, allometric scaling works best for compounds with a high component of non-enzymatic elimination, such as our model compound with approximately 90% excretion as unchanged drug. This prediction weakens as variations in rates of enzymatic reactions become more important. The pharmacokinetic–pharmacodynamic modelling approaches use existing *in vivo* data to calculate constants which can be applied to other *in vivo* data, but does not, in its present form, link *in vitro* and *in vivo* data.

Significantly, none of these approaches uses drug-receptor binding data. Although K_d values are generated during initial screening of the scores of compounds emerging from medicinal chemistry laboratories, it has been a traditional problem that relative efficacy remains unknown (this does not detract from their value in chemical, structure–activity analyses). Neither do any of these approaches use results of *in vitro* functional assays which emerge from screening of the compounds in biochemistry laboratories. It should be added that there are exceptions, however: drug–receptor binding constants and EC_{50} values from *in vivo* studies in animals were used by Danhof and Mandema (1995) to model drugs effects at benzodiazepine receptors and effects on EEG (Figure 10.7). Row

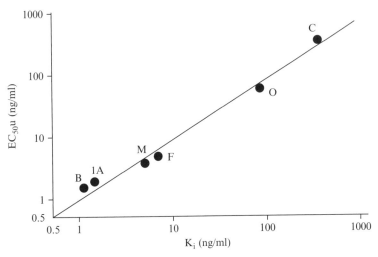

Figure 10.7 Correlation ($r = 0.993$, $p < 0.001$) between benzodiazepine free drug concentrations $EC_{50}u$) producing 50% of the maximal EEG effect (change in amplitudes in the β frequency band, as determined by aperiodic EEG analysis) and affinity to the GABA–benzodiazepine receptor complex (K_i). Binding to the benzodiazepine receptor was determined on basis of displacement of [^{3}H] flumazenil in washed brain homogenate at 37°C. (Reproduced with permission from Danhof and Mandema, 1995)

ley et al (1997) have taken a similar approach with NMDA antagonists.

Prospectus

In the future, models will exist which will link constants for *in vitro* binding to cloned human receptors (K_d), data from *in vitro* functional assays (IC_{50}), and animal and human *in vivo* EC_{50} values. A composite prediction matrix will be applied rapidly and accurately to the process of synthesis of new compounds for Phase I testing.

In the shorter term, what can we now do to expedite the drug selection process? Figure 10.8 represents a flow chart illustrating one form of metabolism/pharmacokinetics input into the drug discovery process. Arrows (indicating the flow of work and communication) pointing to the right represent perceived progress, whereas arrows pointing to the left represent 'disappointments' (and other feedback) leading to corrections and revisions. The numbered asterisks indicate continuations. The 'flow of time' is from left to right, and from the top panel to the bottom panel. The rectangles indicate tasks that are to be completed, and rectangles in a column within a panel represent work done by different departments which may

be simultaneous or not simultaneous but do not require much interaction between the investigators involved. Unlike the flow chart of a computer program, after which the diagram is modeled, most of the decisions are made in discussions among committee members, and may not necessarily be based on hard and fast criteria. Also, unlike a computer flow chart, the decision concerning a particular drug will usually be based in part on the results of work with other compounds that have the same indication.

In the boxes representing tasks to complete in the Phase I study in humans, we have used the symbol 1 to represent work that can be expedited by good validated preclinical data. The symbol 2 represents the tasks that can be expedited by on-line pharmacokinetic modeling. Among the pharmacokinetic questions that will be asked on-line in the Phase I trial are the following:

1. As the doses are escalated, do the kinetics of the drug appear to be linear or non-linear over the dose range?
2. With repeated dosing, is there any evidence of a change in kinetics, e.g. a higher elimination rate that might be indicative of autoinduction?
3. Does the drug accumulate in tissues more than predicted with repeated dosing?

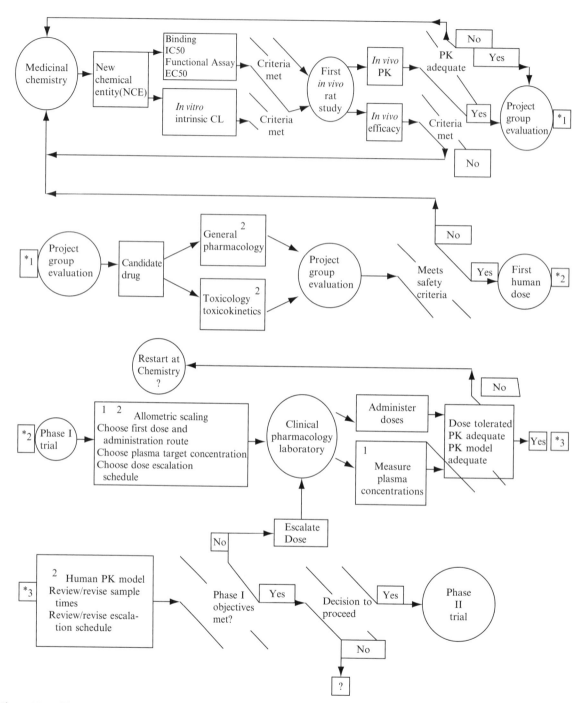

Figure 10.8 Flow diagram for involvement of pharmacokinetic and pharmacodynamic mode/computer-generated feedback into the iterative process of drug discovery from medicinal chemistry to the decision to enter Phase II trials. This is not a comprehensive flow diagram for all aspects of drug discovery—it is restricted to the components of the process discussed in this chapter. This flow diagram emphasizes efficient involvement of *in vitro* and *in vivo* experimental science and computer modeling, in review of data obtained in Phase I studies, in the decisions related to selection of the best compound for patient studies

4. If preclinical work identified metabolite(s) to measure in humans, are the pharmacokinetics of metabolite(s) linear and as predicted?
5. Does the relationship between concentration and effect change with dose, time and duration of treatment?

We expect that the task lists represented by some of the boxes will increase. For example, within the box including 'in vitro intrinsic clearance', there may be in vitro predictors of oral availability, and measures of potentially toxic metabolites. The 'in vivo pharmacokinetics' in rats may include an increasing number of compartments whose concentrations are measured by microdialysis, and may include measures of a few selected metabolite concentrations.

This diagram is not a comprehensive guide to drug discovery. However, it does show that the chemists discover new chemical entities with desirable properties. In vitro biochemistry is followed by initial in vivo work in the rat, which is conducted with pharmacokinetic support and in vitro drug metabolism in parallel. Compounds meeting prearranged criteria proceed through pharmacological screening to general pharmacology and toxicology, all with pharmacokinetic support, which involves the development of pharmacokinetic and pharmacodynamic models. As a chemical series develops, correlations such as that in Figure 10.6 are developed. Eventually, a compound or compounds is/are chosen for Phase I studies.

In this scheme, Phase I is influenced by pharmacokinetic and pharmacodynamic modeling. This modeling is used to refine the Phase I protocol, providing advice on sampling times, doses, and warning signs of difficulty if they occur, as well as permitting comparison of, for example, EC_{50} data from humans with EC_{50} data from animals, and in vitro/in vivo comparisons. The objective is expeditious choice of the best compound, with the ever-present limitations on information available. Note that this scheme can involve feedback from Phase I to renewed chemical synthesis, as well as choice of a second or third compound for human testing.

Currently, Phase I studies themselves tend to be quite straightforward and focus on single compounds. Typically, after adequate preclinical characterization of a candidate drug and 14 day and/or 3 month multiple-dose toxicology studies in two mammalian species, a very low dose is chosen for the first human exposure to the drug. In later exposures, the dose is escalated according to some prearranged criteria until the drug concentrations in plasma associated with undesirable properties in animals are reached, and/or until some other limiting response is threatened or observed in the human volunteers. Doses may be single or short multiple-dose series. Simple physiological and biochemical measurements are routinely made in order to monitor for safety. If possible, responses to the drug are also measured when relevant to the intended therapeutic use. A drug successfully passes to Phase II if, with appropriate plasma levels, responses are predictable, reversible, related to the known pharmacological mechanisms of the drug, and there is a viewpoint among the investigators concerned that the drug could safely be given in initial studies to patients from its target population. Hopefully, all or most of what is observed in Phase I is in line with predictions based on the pharmacokinetic and pharmacodynamic properties of the drug in animals.

Once Phase I is complete, the human becomes the first-choice test species, under all but the most specialized of circumstances (e.g. effects on reproduction). In this context, Phase I serves as the interface between preclinical research and clinical development, and the validity of the predictions from animals to man involved is of paramount importance.

We believe that with enhanced integrated study of animals and humans, and with data feedback based on computer models, the process of drug discovery from synthesis to proof of safety in humans could be dramatically improved in its efficiency. This is beyond what has traditionally been expected from departments of drug metabolism and pharmacokinetics (Welling and Tse 1995). The time saved could be used to permit a larger number of compounds with better prospects, from a single research program, to be compared in Phase I studies. Consequently, the extremely costly testing programs in patients which follow Phase I could be started sooner and conducted better.

REFERENCES

Ashforth EIL, Carlile DJ, Chenery R, Houston JB (1995) Prediction of in vivo disposition from in vitro systems: clearance of phenytoin and tolbutamide using rat hepatic microsomal and hepatocyte data. *Journal of Pharmacology and Experimental Therapeutics* 274: 761–6. (1995).

Benet LZ, Kroetz DL, Sheiner LB (1996) Pharmacokinetics: the dynamics of drug absorption, distribution and elimination. In Hardman JG et al (eds), *Goodman and Gilman's Pharmacological Basis of Therapeutics*, 9th edn. McGraw-Hill; New York; 3–28.

Boxenbaum H (1982) Interspecies scaling, allometry, physiological time and the ground plan for pharmacokinetics. *J Pharmacokin Biopharm* 10: 201–27.

Boxenbaum H, DiLea C (1995) First-time-in-human dose selection: allometric thoughts and perspectives. *J Clin Pharmacol* 35: 957.

Boxenbaum H, Ronfeld R (1983) Interspecies pharmacokinetic scaling and the Dedrick Plots. *Am J Physiol* 245: R768–74.

Brodie BB (1967) Physical and biochemical aspects of pharmacology. *J Am Med Assoc* 202: 600–609.

Colburn WA (1995) Clinical markers and endpoints in bioequivalence assessment. *Drug Inf J* 29: 917.

Curry SH (1980) *Drug Disposition and Pharmacokinetics*, 3rd edn. Blackwell Scientific: Oxford.

Curry SH, Chu P, Baumgartner TG, Stacpoole PW (1985) Plasma concentrations and metabolic effects of intravenous sodium dichloroacetate. *Clin Pharmacol Ther* 37: 89–93.

Dahlstrom B, Paalzow LK, Segre G et al (1978) Relation between morphine pharmacokinetics and analgesia. *J Pharmacokin Biopharm* 6: 41.

Danhof M, Mandema JW (1995) Modeling of relationships between pharmacokinetics and pharmacodynamics. In Welling PG, Tse FLS (eds), *Pharmacokinetics: Regulatory—Industrial—Academic Perspectives*, 2nd edn. Marcel Dekker: New York; 139–94.

Dayneka NL, Garg V, Jusko W (1993) Comparison of four basic models of indirect pharmacodynamic responses. *J Pharmacokin Biopharm* 21: 457.

Derendorf H, Hochhaus G (eds) (1995) *Pharmacokinetic/Pharmacodynamic Correlation*. CRC Press: Boca Raton, FL.

Fox AW, Sullivan BW, Buffini JD et al (1996) Reduction of serum lactate by sodium dichloroacetate, and human pharmacok9inetic-pharmacodynamic relationships. *J Pharmacol Exp Ther* 279: 686–93.

Freireich EJ, Gehan EA, Rall DP et al (1966) Quantitative comparison of toxicity of anticancer agents in mouse, rat, hamster, dog, monkey and man. *Cancer Chemother Rep* 50: 219–40.

Gabrielsson J, Weiner D (1997) *Pharmacokinetic and Pharmacodynamic Data Analysis: Concepts and Applications*, 2nd edn. Apotekarsocieteten: Stockholm.

Gibaldi M, Perrier D (1982) *Pharmacokinetics*, 2nd edn. Marcel Dekker: New York; 231–2.

Hawkins RD, Kalant H (1972) The metabolism of ethanol and its metabolic effects. *Pharmacol Rev* 24: 242–9.

Houston JB (1994) Utility of *in vitro* drug metabolism data in predicting *in vivo* metabolic clearance. *Biochem Pharmacol* 47: 1469–79.

Ings RMJ (1990) Interspecies scaling and comparisons in drug development and toxicokinetics. *Xenobiotica* 20: 1201–31.

Iwatsubo T, Hirota N, Ooie T et al (1996) Prediction of *in vivo* drug disposition from *in vitro* data based on physiological pharmacokinetics. *Biopharmaceut Drug Disposit* 17: 273–310.

Jenkinson DH, Barnard EA, Hoyer D et al (1995) International union of pharmacology committee on receptor nomenclature and drug classification. IX. Recommendations on terms and symbols in quantitative pharmacology. *Pharmacol Rev* 47: 225.

Jusko WJ (1971) Pharmacodynamics of chemotherapeutic effects: dose–time response relationships for phase-non-specific agents. *J Pharm Sci* 60: 892.

Lesko LJ, Williams RL (1994) Regulatory perspectives: the role of pharmacokinetics and pharmacodynamics. In Cutler NR, Sramek JJ, Narang PK (eds), *Pharmacodynamics and Drug Development: Perspectives in Clinical Pharmacology*, 1st edn. Wiley: Chichester.

Levy G (1964) Relationship between elimination rate of drugs and rate of decline of their pharmacologic effects. *J Pharm Sci* 53: 342.

Levy G (1993) The case for preclinical pharmacodynamics. In Yacobi A, Shah VP, Skelley JP, Benet LZ (eds), *Integration of Pharmacokinetics, Pharmacodynamics, and Toxicokinetics in Rational Drug Development*. Plenum: New York.

Levy G (1994) Mechanism-based pharmacodynamic modeling. *Clin Pharmacol Ther* 56: 356.

Levy G (1966) Kinetics of pharmacological effects. *Clin Pharmacol Ther* 7: 362.

Levy G, Nelson E (1965) Theoretical relationship between dose, elimination rate and duration of pharmacological effect of drugs. *J Pharm Sci* 54: 872.

Meyer UA (1994) The molecular basis of genetic polymorphisms of drug metabolism. *J Pharm Pharmacol* 46(suppl 1): 409–15.

Minneman KP, Fox AW, Abel PA (1983) Occupancy of α-adrenergic receptors and contraction of rat vas deferens. *Mol Pharmacol* 23: 359–68.

Murphy J, Casey W, Lasagna L (1961) The effect of dosing regimen on the diuretic efficacy of chlorothiazide in human subjects. *J Pharmacol Exp Ther* 134: 286.

Nagashima R, O'Reilly RA, Levy G (1969) Kinetics of pharmacologic effects in man: the anticoagulant action of warfarin. *Clin Pharmacol Ther* 10: 22.

Obach RS (1996a) Prediction of human pharmacokinetics using *in vitro–in vivo* correlations. In Schlegel J (ed.), *Pharmacokinetic/Pharmacodynamic Analysis: Accelerating Drug Discovery and Development*. Biomedical Library Series. International Business Communications: Southborough, MA.

Obach RS (1996b) The importance of nonspecific binding *in vitro* matrices, its impact on kinetic studies of drug metabolism reactions, and implications for *in vitro–in vivo* correlations. *Drug Metab Disposit* 24: 1047–9.

Pitsui M, Parker E, Aarons L, Rowland M (1993) Population pharmacokinetics and pharmacodynamics of warfarin in healthy young adults. *Eur J Pharm Sci* 1: 151.

Rane A, Wilkinson G, Shand D (1977) Prediction of hepatic extraction from *in vitro* measurement of intrinsic clearance. *J Pharmacol Exp Ther* 200: 420–24.

Ross EM (1996) Pharmacodynamics: mechanisms of drug action and the relationship between drug concentration and effect. In *Goodman and Gilman's Pharmacological Basis of Therapeutics*, 10th edn. Pergamon: New York.

Rowley M, Kulagowski JJ, Walt AP et al (1997) Effect of plasma protein binding on *in vivo* activity and brain penetration of glycine/NMDA receptor antagonists. *J Med Chem* 40: 4053–68.

Segre G (1968) Kinetics of interaction between drugs and biological systems. *Il Farmaco* 23: 907.

Sharma A, Jusko WJ (1997) Characterization of four basic models of indirect pharmacological responses. *J Pharmacokin Biopharmaceut* 24: 611–35.

Sheiner LB, Stanski DR, Vozeh S et al (1979) Simultaneous modelling of pharmacokinetics and pharmacodynamics: application to D-tubocurarine. *Clin Pharmacol Ther* 25: 358.

Shimada T, Yamazaki H, Minura M et al (1994) Inter-individual variations in human liver cytochrome P450 enzymes involved in the oxidation of drugs, carcinogens, and toxic chemicals: studies with liver microsomes of 30 Japanese and 30 Caucasians. *J Pharmacol Exp Ther* 270: 414–23.

Smith DA, Jones BC, Walker DK (1996) Design of drugs involving the concepts and theories of drug metabolism and pharmacokinetics. *Med Res Rev* 16: 243–66.

Smolen VF (1976) Theoretical and computational basis for drug bioavailability determinations using pharmacological data I: general considerations and procedures. *J Pharmacokin Biopharm* 4: 337.

Smolen VF (1971) Quantitative determination of drug bioavailability and biokinetic behavior from pharmacological data for ophthalmic and oral administration of a mydriatic drug. *J Pharm Sci* 60: 354.

Wagner JG (1968) Kinetics of pharmacological response: I. Proposed relationships between response and drug concentration in the intact animal and man. *J Theoret Biol* 20: 173.

Welling PG, Tse FLS (eds) (1995) *Pharmacokinetics: Regulatory–Industrial–Academic Perspectives*, 2nd edn. Marcel Dekker: New York.

Wilkinson GR (1987) Clearance approaches in pharmacology. *Pharmacol Rev* 39: 1–47.

Yee S (1997) *In vitro* permeability across Caco-2 cells (colonic) can predict *in vivo* (small intestinal) absorption in man—fact or myth. *Pharm Res* 14: 763–6.

11

Phase II and Phase III Clinical Studies

Anthony W. Fox

EBD Group Inc., Carlsbad, CA, USA

THE PHASES OF DRUG DEVELOPMENT: AN OBSOLETE MODEL?

In former times, it was assumed that development of drugs proceeded in step-wise fashion from Phase I, through Phase II, to Phase III, prior to filing a Product Licence Application (PLA) or new drug application (NDA). Phase I was conducted in 'normal volunteers' (although some medical students might hardly characterize this term!). Phase II trials were initial studies in selected patients, and Phase III trials were seen as wide-scale studies in broader patient populations. After approval, certain studies to find new indications, address special patient subpopulations for marketing purposes, or otherwise broaden product labeling might or might not be conducted. All post-approval studies were termed Phase IV.

In modern practice, the distinctions between Phases I, II, III, and IV are very often blurred. Three principal, and interlocking, pressures have caused this blurring: time, finance, and an evolving regulatory environment.

Of these three pressures, the most important is time. Strategies such as the overlapping of development 'phases', as well as the use of early dose-ranging studies as pivotal, and choosing doses based on surrogate end-points, are technical responses to this challenge. Financial pressures, even for the largest pharmaceutical companies, are generally much greater than in the past. The technical response is to maximize resources, avoiding any and all redundant clinical studies.

The regulatory pressures come both from the regulatory authorities and from within the pharmaceutical companies themselves. Regulatory authorities have increased in their scientific sophistication during the last 30 years. The questions that are now asked of companies, and the earlier stages of drug development when these questions are asked, have driven change in clinical study design. Increasingly sophisticated data are now developed at earlier and earlier stages of drug development.

In the later stages of the development of successful drugs, the interval between PLA or NDA filing and product launch is not wasted. The term 'Phase IIIb' has been invented for the conduct of Phase IV-type studies during the pre-approval period. Furthermore, in some companies, the old 'Phase IV', is now divided into Phases IV and V, without any generally agreed definitions except, perhaps, that the studies are run by different teams.

Quite apart from these general trends blurring the distinctions between Phases I, II, and III, there are (and always have been) sound medical or pharmacological reasons for doing so. Good examples might be:

- It would be unreasonable to study the pharmacokinetics of relatively toxic agents, at potentially therapeutic doses, in normal volunteers due to the near-certainty of the adverse events. Typically, this information can be gained in patients with diseases potentially responsive to these agents. Thus, the first-in-man studies in this case are 'Phase II', using the classic nomenclature. Cytotoxic and antiviral drugs are two important classes of agent where this is commonly the case.
- There is little point in testing the tolerability of drugs in normal volunteers, when only patients with the disease of interest are able to demonstrate a relevant pharmacodynamic effect. The doses at which tolerability must be confirmed are unknown until the exposure of patients can indicate the doses that may be effective. The

Principles and Practice of Pharmaceutical Medicine. Edited by A. J. Fletcher, Lionel D. Edwards, Anthony W. Fox and Peter Stonier © 2002 John Wiley & Sons Ltd.

development of potent opioids, such as alfentanil, sufentanil and remifentanil, as anaesthetic
agents, are a good example.

- There are some diseases which have no animal
  model or relevant pharmacodynamic or surrogate end-points in normal volunteers. Such diseases may also alter the pharmacokinetics of
  the drug, thus invalidating anything that
  might be learned from normal volunteers. A
  good example is the migraine syndrome. No
  animal species has migraine, and normal volunteers cannot report an antimigraine effect.
  Nausea, vomiting, and gastric stasis are common
  during migraine attacks and may be expected
  to alter the pharmacokinetics and effectiveness
  of oral therapies.

There is nonetheless little hope that the Phase I, II
III aphorism will die. Nevertheless, it is quite
wrong to assume that these 'classical' terms and
definitions still apply to how drugs are developed
according to modern practice. The classical four-
phase strategy of drug development is far too
stereotyped, simplistic and pedestrian to have survived into the modern era of drug development.
None of today's successful companies actually use
such a strategy. We are simply shackled with an
outmoded terminology.

CONCEPTS OF BIAS AND STATISTICAL NECESSITIES

Bias is a general consideration in clinical trial
design, regardless of the type of trial being conducted. It is considered here as an overarching
issue, to be applied to the systematic description
of the types of study design, as considered below.

The word 'bias' has many definitions, but in this
context it is best described as a distortion of, or
prejudice towards, observed effects that may or
may not truly be due to the action of the test
drug(s). Many things can distort the true measurement of drug action, and bias is the trialist's most
unremitting enemy, which comes from many quar-
ters (Table 11.1). The clinical trialist must be sufficiently humble to realize that he/she, him/herself,
may be a source of bias.

The pharmaceutical physician may not be
expected to be a specialist statistician, and statistics
are not the subject of this chapter. However, the
ability to talk to and understand statisticians is
absolutely essential (sine qua non: involve a good
statistician from the moment a clinical trial is
contemplated). Furthermore, the pharmaceutical
physician should be confident of a sound understanding of the concepts of type I and type II error,
and the probabilities α and β (e.g. Freiman et al.

Table 11.1   Some example sources of bias in clinical trials

- Poorly matched placebos
- Subtle or obvious non-randomization of patients
- Failure of double-blinding, e.g. when pharmacodynamic effects cannot be controlled
- Prompting of prejudiced subjective responses
- Non-uniform medical monitoring
- Protocol amendments with unequal effects on treatment groups
- Peculiarities of the study site itself (e.g. psychotropic drug effects in psychiatric institutions which fail to predict effects in outpatients)
- Differing medical definitions across languages, dialects or countries (e.g. 'mania')
- CRF with leading questions, either toward or away from adverse event reporting
- Informal, 'break the blind' games played at study sites
- Selective rigour in collection and storage of biological samples
- Selectively incomplete data sets for each patient
- Inappropriate use of parametric or non-parametric statistical techniques
- Failure to adequately define end-points prospectively, and retrospective 'data dredging'
- Acceptance of correlation as evidence of causation
- Averaging of proportionate responses from non-homogenous treatment groups, also known as Simpson's paradox; see Spilker (1991)
- Unsceptically accepting anecdotal reports
- Tendency to publish only positive results

CRF case report form; the term 'controlled' is used in its technical sense (see section on Bias and Statistical Necessities, this chapter).

1978). This is one of your best defences against bias.

PROSPECTIVE DEFINITIONS: THE ONLY WAY TO INTERPRET WHAT YOU MEASURE

It does not require a training in advanced statistics to hold a commonsense and accurate approach to creating clinical hypotheses, translate them into the precise quantities of a measured end-point, and then interpret the results. Whilst the finer points of statistics are presented in Chapter 19, it is commonsense that the only way to interpret what you measure is to define this whole process, *before* the experiment starts.

Thinking carefully about what might actually constitute an observed response *before* you measure it removes at least one important source of bias. That bias is the clinical trialist him/herself. There has been too little emphasis in recent years on the fundamentals of end-points, their variability and how they are measured. Furthermore, the relationship between what is measured and its clinical relevance is always debatable: the tendency is to measure something that *can* be measured, rather than something that *needs validation as clinically relevant*. Good examples include rheumatological studies: counts of inflamed joints before and after therapy may be reported, but do not reveal whether the experimental treatment or the corresponding placebo caused some of the patients to recover the ability to write or others the ability to walk (Chaput de Saintonge and Vere 1982).

Most clinical trialists experience the urge, especially in early studies, to collect every piece of data that they possibly can, before and after every drug exposure. This urge comes from natural scientific curiosity, as well as a proper ethical concern, because the hazard associated with clinical trials is never zero. It behooves us to maximize the amount of information gained in return for the risk that the patient takes for us, and for medicine in general.

Consequently, large numbers of variables are typically measured before and after drug (or placebo) administration. These variables all exhibit biological variation. Many of these variations have familiar, unimodal, symmetrical distributions, which are supposed to resemble Gaussian (Normal), Chi-squared, f, binomial, etc., probability density functions. An intrinsic property of biological variables is that when measured 100 times, then, on the average and if Normally distributed, 5% of those measurements will be more than ± 2 standard deviations from the mean (there are corollaries for the other probability density functions). This meets a typical, prospective, '$p < 0.05$, and therefore it's significant' mantra. It is also true that if you measure 100 different variables, on two occasions only, before and after administration of the test material, then, on the average, 5% of those variables are going to be significantly different after treatment (this masquerades sometimes in findings among 'selected secondary end-points'). A sound interpretation, of course, is based upon only those end-points that were selected before the experiment began, and comparing these with those for which no such statistical differences were found.

HISTORICAL CLINICAL TRIALS

Any general work must include these classic bits of history. Perhaps unusually, clinical trials appear to be a European scientific invention. There is no evidence that either the ancient world or the mediaeval Arabs carried out prospective studies (although there are some anachronisms in recent fiction). It is generally accepted that the earliest clinical trial was held by James Lind.

Thomas (1997) has pointed out that sailing men-of-war frequently went many months without docking, e.g. Nelson spent 24 unbroken months on HMS *Victory* while blockading French ports, and it is said that Collingwood once went 22 months without even dropping anchor. Scurvy was rampant in the Royal Navy, often literally decimating ships' crews. Sailors survived on the poor diets carried aboard for long months, with water-weevils and biscuit-maggots constituting important dietary protein! Before Lind's time, the Dutch had already learned to treat scurvy by replenishing their ships at sea with fresh fruit and vegetables. This was also known by Cook: when in command of HM Barque *Endeavour*, men were flogged for not eating their vegetables.

Lind had been pressed into the Royal Navy, as a surgeon's mate, in 1739, and with some experience as an apprentice surgeon in Edinburgh. It is a nice irony that the first prospective clinical study was actually conducted by a surgeon!

The clinical trial was held at a single site, HMS *Salisbury*, a frigate in the English Channel, during the early summer of 1747 (Lind 1753; Frey 1969; Thomas 1997). The experimental controls included that all 12 patients met the same inclusion criteria (putrid gums, spots on the skin, lassitude, and weakness of the knees). All patients received the same diet, except for the test materials. All treatments were administered simultaneously (parallel group). Compliance with therapy was confirmed by direct observation in all cases. The trial had six groups, with $n = 2$ patients per group. The test medications were (daily doses): (a) cider, 1 quart; (b) elixir of vitriol, 25 drops; (c) vinegar, two spoonfuls plus vinegar added to the diet and used as a gargle; (d) seawater, 'a course'; (e) citrus fruit, two oranges, plus one lemon when it could be spared; and (f) nutmeg, a 'bigness'. Lind noted, with some disdain, that this last treatment was tested only because it was recommended by a surgeon on land. The famous result was that within 6 days only 2 of the 12 patients had improved, both in the citrus fruit group, one of whom became fit for duty, and the other at least fit enough to nurse the remaining 10 patients.

We should note the absence of dose-standardization and probably of randomization, because Lind's two seawater patients were noted to have 'tendons in the ham rigid', unlike the others. However, the result had been crudely replicated by using $n = 2$ in each group. If we accept that the hypothesis was that the citrus-treated patients alone would improve (Lind was certainly skeptical of the anecdotal support for the other five alternative treatments), then, using a binomial probability distribution, the result has $p = 0.0075$. But statistics had hardly been invented, and Lind had no need of them to interpret the clinical significance of this brilliant clinical trial.

Lind was not quick to publish his most famous treatise reporting this clinical trial (Lind 1753). Indeed, in 1748, his Edinburgh MD thesis was on an entirely unrelated subject. Subsequently, Lind was Treasurer of the Royal College of Surgeons of Edinburgh, and then appointed physician to the Royal Naval Hospital, Haslar (one-fifth of his first 6000-odd admissions were for scurvy). He

subsequently developed a large private practice, but little fame amongst his peers, and was buried at Gosport in 1794. The Royal Navy was even slower to act on his findings, and did not introduce citrus juice in sailors' diets until the year after Lind's death, following much administrative resistance but no scientific controversy (Bardolph and Taylor 1997). The British, especially those in the Royal Navy, are still known as 'limeys', which is the unique example of a national nickname based on a therapy proven by clinical trial.

Thus, Lind illustrates some other aspects of clinical trials: first, he had little academic kudos, although he was clearly qualified by experience and training (a requirement of trialists by law in the USA). Second, he did not publish his results rapidly. Third, his results were not implemented promptly in the interests of the public health. It is important to realize that these undesirable aspects of clinical trials persist to this day.

LIMITATIONS OF CONTROLLED CLINICAL TRIALS

Progress in therapeutics has not always arisen from controlled clinical trials. Chance observations have historically led to huge advances. Today's three most commonly used cardiovascular drugs are good examples: digoxin is a component of digitalis (famously reported by Withering after observing the treatment of a dropsical lady by a gypsy); aspirin is derived from the willow tree bark, first reported by the Reverend Edmund Brown to treat his own malarious fevers; and warfarin is the result of a University of Wisconsin investigation into a hemorrhagic disease of cattle. Lest we forget, Jenner's experiments would be ethically impossible today: they included deliberate exposure to smallpox, and aspirin is a drug that would probably fail in a modern preclinical toxicology program due to chromosomal breaks and gastrointestinal adverse effects due to systemic exposures in rodents. Modern clinical trials are therefore not necessarily the Holy Grail of therapeutic progress.

Statistical theory must also be held not only with respect but also with healthy skepticism (although this is really the subject of Chapter 19). It should be remembered that the development of statistics, as they have come to be applied to clinical trials, has arisen from a variety of non-mammalian biological sources. Experimental agriculture stimulated the early giants (Drs Fisher, Yates) to explore probability density functions. While epidemiological studies have confirmed much that is similar in human populations, it is unknown whether these probability density functions apply uniformly to all disease states. Any statistical test that we employ makes assumptions that are usually not stated.

THE CLINICAL DEVELOPMENT PLAN

It is impossible to consider clinical trial protocol design in isolation. All clinical protocols should be written after a clinical development plan has been agreed by the diverse membership of the clinical development team. The clinical development plan should itself follow the construction of an hypothetical drug label (see Chapter 29). The goals of such a plan might be as limited as to provide for the start of Phase II, or as complex as mapping an entire route from first-in-man studies to product registration. The path from the present status to the overall goal can then be understood. It may be added that, within a large company, this is also a good way for clinical and marketing departments to communicate.

PROTOCOLS, CASE-REPORT FORMS, AND INVESTIGATORS' BROCHURES

Chapters 23–26 describe the regulatory governance of clinical trials, and little needs to be added here. These clinical trial documents are central to these processes. Equally the regulatory requirements (which still vary from country to country), and the documents needed to support them, must be taken into account when constructing the clinical development plan.

OBJECTIVES AND PREREQUISITES OF PHASE II STUDIES

Gallenical Forms

A good rule of thumb is that pivotal clinical trials for registration purposes ought to be conducted

with the same formulation and manufacturing process that is proposed to be taken to market. While the nuances of pharmaceutical constructs are described in Chapter 5, it is important to understand the sometimes grave consequences when this rule of thumb is not observed.

Most regulatory authorities will want reassurance that the pharmacokinetic properties of the marketed product closely resemble those in which the pivotal studies are carried out. This is not unreasonable: if the pharmacokinetic (PK) properties differ, then so may dose size and frequency. Occasionally, a Phase III study will be 'bridged' to the marketed formulation by the demonstration, for example, that two different tablets have the same PK profile. However, the risk is that different formulations will not turn out to possess the same PK profile: either new pivotal studies will have to be conducted with the new formulation, or registration will be delayed until the new formulation is adapted so that it does match the Phase III test material. For inhaled drugs, this is especially difficult. Time and money is often lost in both cases. It is a risky gamble to leave development of the final formulation until the end of a clinical development plan.

Informed Consent

This is considered in detail in Chapter 7. The clinical trialist should remember, however, that he/she ultimately carries the ethical responsibility for this document, regardless of what corporate lawyers and others may wish to do with it. Typically, institutional review boards in the USA are more likely to be tolerant of long forms than ethics committees in Europe.

Toxicological Coverage

This is covered in more detail in Chapter 6. However, the clinical trialist is encouraged to consider this for every protocol. A useful method is to start with the general case: what is the relationship between duration and dose sizes of animal studies and the clinical protocol-specified dose size and duration? This exercise ought to be conducted using methods that standardize for both body weight and body surface area across species. Next, review closely all the prior human exposure to the test drug (if any) to see whether any unexpected signals for investigation may be found. Last, consider from the known pharmacology of the drug whether there are likely to be any particular tolerability issues for which special monitoring methods are needed, and *think laterally*.

For example, what is likely to be the adverse effects of a potassium channel-blocking drug being investigated for a central nervous system indication? The answer may lie in all the excitable tissues that contain potassium channels. Is there is any preclinical evidence that the drug discriminates between potassium channels in different tissues? Are there changes in the EEG or ECG that may be found in the non-human database or among prior human exposures to the test agent, that escaped being reported because 'not thought to be clinically significant'?

COMMON PHASE II/III STUDY DESIGNS

Many initial studies are conducted in an uncontrolled fashion. Eminent professors will treat a few of their patients with a test medication (perhaps under an investigators' IND in the USA) and form opinions about the worth (or otherwise) of a new therapy. While this may be grist for the mill of press releases and fund-raising for small companies, these uncontrolled observations often mistakenly become a cast-iron credo for the sponsoring company. An observed effect, any effect, is viewed as better than none, and the relative lack of scientific controls permits large biases to arise.

The first risk from this haphazard start to clinical development is that potentially good options for a test compound may be needlessly rejected. The professor's patient population may not include a disease state or disease subtype for which the new drug is actually well-suited. Equally, efficacy and tolerability may be dose-dependent, and this can only be assessed when studied in a systematic fashion. Lastly, most drugs are just one of a series of compounds which share closely related properties in preclinical testing. It is impossible to know which of these is the most promising, when only one has been tested.

Assuming that reasonable tolerability, reasonable understanding of pharmacokinetics and (preferably) a relevant pharmacodynamic effect has been observed in normal volunteers (see Chapter 10), then the first task is to reassess all of these in a relevant disease state. This is slower and uses more patients than the professor's uncontrolled observations. But at the end of a small number of such small studies, there ought to be good information about the feasibility of a pivotal clinical trials program, and, if not, then the feasible course corrections (e.g. alternative indications). Note that one such course correction may be ceasing to develop the drug, and switching to another member in the series. Arguably, the appropriate 'killing' of drugs is the most valuable thing that a Phase II program can accomplish, before too much time and money has been wasted.

When choosing a clinical trial design (Table 11.2), economic factors include numbers of patients, time that will elapse, drug supply and total cost. While these economies are important and relevant in all design choices, they should also be factored against the end-points that may or will be measured. The relevance of an end-point, and its sensitivity to detect a drug-related effect may be primarily dependent upon the duration of patient exposure, e.g. a short period of observation is unlikely to detect a difference in time to next seizure in a study of an anti-epileptic drug with an add-on design in patients who are only moderately disabled by epilepsy. On the other hand, the identification of a PK interaction between a new and an established therapy in the same population may only require very short observation periods.

There are several common classes of study design. These classes apply to almost all phases of drug development. No list of trial designs can be exhaustive, because almost all clinical trials are different. What follows is an attempt to briefly review the classes of clinical trial design that will encompass a large majority of studies, and to comment on their economy and end-point possibilities.

Parallel-group Studies

These are typically thought of as the most straightforward design case. In fact, a bewildering array of variations exist within this class.

In the simplest case of parallel-group study, a group of patients presenting sequentially are

Table 11.2 Basic trial designs and the factors that are suited and unsuited to each

Trial type	Factors suited	Factors unsuited
Parallel-group, single treatment	Episodic disease Imperfect placebo matching Blinding difficult (e.g. surgical procedures, psychtropic drugs)	Rare disease
Parallel-group, chronic treatment	Stable disease state	Unethical to use active comparator or placebo
Cross-over with washout	Stable disease state Ethical to use placebo after active	Untreated washout not ethical
Sequential	Rare disease Homogenous disease state Urgent need to save life	Complicated tolerability profile Many concomitant disease factors
'n of 1'	Stable disease state	Few or no feasible alternative therapies
'Large simple'	Very common disease Easily measured end-points Well-understood drug	Tolerability issues not closely related to efficacy variable
Open label	Tolerability issues only	Spontaneous adverse event frequency high
Within-patient dose ranging	Stable disease state Intolerable high initial dose	Drug tolerance
Combination therapy	*A priori* reason to expect favourable drug interaction	Unethical to use single therapy

randomized to one of two equally-sized treatment groups, until a prospectively determined total number of patients has been recruited. All these patients are followed for a predetermined period of time, or until some end-point is achieved. The database is quality assured and locked before the randomization code is broken. The patients are then sorted according to their treatment, the end-point measurements are subjected to a statistical test, and an interpretation of the effect (or absence thereof) of the drug is made. What could possibly go wrong?

The answer is that little can go wrong when there are ample patients, plenty of drug available, the choice of dose size has been perfect, the end-points are incontrovertible, the measurements are possible using a ratio or absolute scale, there is ample toxicological coverage for all the dose sizes employed, and the trialist has an unlimited budget! This combination of utopian conditions never exists.

The Ascending Dose-ranging Cohort Design

This is one variant within the parallel-group class. It is best suited when there is no cast-iron assurance of tolerability for all the dose sizes of interest.

Patients are randomized in cohorts to either active or placebo treatment; frequently there are fewer placebo-treated patients in each cohort. The objective is to accumulate tolerability experience as dose size gradually increases. If the treatments in the first cohort prove to be well-tolerated, then the next cohort is randomized in the same way except that the active-treated patients receive a larger dose size. Note that this judgment can be made without breaking the blind. A comparable number of placebo-treated patients to any single active-treatment group can be accumulated across several cohorts, each cohort having fewer placebo treated than active-treated patients. This economizes on patient numbers in comparison to randomizing each cohort in a 1:1 fashion, and may also economize on both drug and patients if two doses are found to be similarly effective and well-tolerated, albeit not the highest dose that was projected.

Sequential cohort designs do not usually economize on time. Treatment codes can be broken at the end of each cohort (and not introduce bias into observations of succeeding cohorts). Sometimes this can lead to early closure of the study when the desired pharmacodynamic effect is observed at a lower dose than the maximum projected by the study. However, the deliberations of safety committees at the end of each cohort can often be time-consuming.

Within-patient Dose Titration Designs

These may be conceptualized as the application of an ascending dose cohort design within a single patient. The advantages of such designs are when immediate high-dose therapy is contraindicated for tolerability reasons, and when there are likely to be large variations *between patients* in the tolerability and efficacy of the test drug.

Patients are reviewed during and after completion of a course of therapy, which may include programmed changes in dose size. If the drug was well-tolerated, they may progress to a course of therapy at higher dose. A prospective limit on dosing and the number of courses of treatment is made (e.g. according to toxicology coverage). Dosing may be curtailed at any time when either there is unreasonable intolerance of the drug, or when acceptable efficacy and simultaneous tolerability has been observed. This is not unlike the approach to therapy under ordinary clinical circumstances. For example, patients with epilepsy are often treated by dose alterations. Another advantage of this design is that at the end of the study, the range of tolerated and efficacious doses can be examined among all treated patients in comparison to demographic factors, disease subtypes, etc.

The greatest difficulty with ascending-dose, within-patient designs is usually in treatment-masking. Double-blind requirements have to take into account a wide variety of dose sizes, and that contemporaneous placebo formulations will be needed. Some studies of this type are hybridized with a cross-over strategy (see below). Dose-tailing at the end of the study may be viewed as the same procedure in reverse, although may be conducted open-label and more rapidly (guided by suitable PK information) than when therapy is being introduced.

Sources of bias in this study design arise from the exposure of patients to lower doses first. Patients obligatorily must tolerate, and fail to respond to, lower doses before being exposed to higher doses. Any degree of treatment familiarization, tachyphylaxis, or patient withdrawal rate biases dose–response curves to the right (i.e. tend to overestimate the ED_{50}) in comparison to a parallel-group study in the same patients with the same endpoints.

Cross-over Studies

Generally, cross-over studies are more complicated than parallel-group designs. Patients are exposed to more than one test medication, in sequential treatment periods, perhaps with periods of no therapy intervening between those of active therapy. Active therapies may be different drugs, or different doses of the same drug, or, in complicated studies, both.

The most famous problem is eliminating carryover effects ('washout'). Ideally, end-points should be measured and unambiguously attributable to one of the test regimens. This requires no residual effects of the previous regimen(s) (see Laska et al 1983). If this involves intervening placebo-treatment periods in between test medications, then clearly this approach is not possible when placebos are ethically unjustifiable.

Usually, patients are randomized to a particular treatment order, and all patients are eventually exposed to the same variety of treatments. Large numbers of treatment periods, assigned using a Latin square, have been reported; however, the logistics and patient retention in such studies is usually difficult, and these ideal designs are likely to be successful only when treatment periods are short; ideal designs are commonest for normal volunteer studies (e.g. Amin et al 1995).

In later-phase studies, if there are still numerous treatments or dose sizes that need to be tested, then partial cross-over designs can be used. These expose patients to a random subset of all the study treatments, again in a random order. Partial cross-over designs necessarily require the availability of large numbers of patients. However, there can be economies of the amounts of test drug needed, and in the time needed to conduct the study in comparison to an equivalent, complete, cross-over design. Shorter durations of patient participation are also usually associated with fewer missing data and fewer patients lost for administrative reasons. Overall patient recruitment is more efficient.

Pharmaceutical physicians should be wary of using randomized, cross-over designs when there are likely to be appreciable numbers of patients who are withdrawn before completing the study. This can cause serious imbalance among treatment groups and seriously jeopardize the likelihood of achieving a statistically robust result. Cross-over studies with three or more periods have a substantial advantage over two-period designs, when the amount of missing data is likely to be large, and statistical salvage is necessary (Ebbutt 1984).

MINIMIZATION TRIALS

Less common are trial designs that specifically and adaptively minimize the number of patients needed, while preserving design integrity for appropriate statistical analysis. Early 'evolutionary' designs are now being succeeded by independent treatment allocation, in pursuit of this goal. All minimization designs involve arduous statistical planning, and the pharmaceutical physician should seek expert help from the outset.

Evolutionary Designs

These were devised by Dixon and Armitage. Although the statistical analysis is rather different,

they have the same objective, which is to detect a treatment effect at the earliest moment possible, using the fewest possible patients, while retaining statistical robustness. Both types are suited for exploratory clinical research, and both types are suited for diseases which are rare.

The Dixon 'Up–Down' Technique

This was first described in the statistical literature in 1947. It is designed to estimate an ED_{50} in clinical trials or toxicological tests, when a quantal response is measured (see Figure 11.1). However, it should be remembered that continuous responses can be converted into quantal responses with appropriate, prospective efficacy criteria, e.g. blood pressure is a continuous variable, but a drug may be deemed effective or ineffective by stating prospectively that a desired response is quantal-positive after a 15 mmHg fall in diastolic blood pressure within 60 days of commencing therapy. Theoretically, this strategy can be implemented with groups of patients treated in the same way instead of individuals. Sometimes this technique is termed an 'adaptive' trial design, because dose size is adapted according to the response of the previous patient or group of patients.

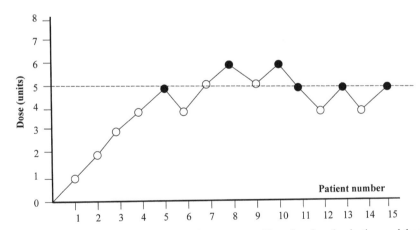

Figure 11.1 Illustration of the Dixon 'up–down' method. Patients are treated in order of randomization, and the size of each test dose is determined by the response of the previous patient. In this example, patients who do not respond (O) are followed by a patient treated at the next higher dose size; vice versa, patients who do respond (●) are followed by a patient treated at the next lower dose. When the line has changed direction at least six times, the mean effective dose is about the EC_{80} (in this case, 5 u, broken line). There are many, often more sophisticated, variants of this basic technique

The Armitage Technique or 'Sequential Analysis'

This technique was originally employed in the testing of explosive ordnance. Patients or groups of patients are paired, and then treated with alternative therapies. A control chart is developed that records the result of each comparison with time, and crossing a boundary on the chart, after an unpredictable number of paired comparisons, gives the trial result. For a trial of a new therapy that can both benefit and harm the patient, a typical probability control chart forms a 'double-triangle' pattern, as shown in Figure 11.2.

The original methods have been extended in many ways. The design of control charts is always prospective, and their shape depends upon the *a priori* expectations of the development team. For example, when it is important to test only the tolerability of a compound, the chart can have an 'open top': this is when it is important to the development team to detect drug toxicity early, but not efficacy. Similarly, depending upon the hypotheses under test, control charts can be rhomboidal, parallelogram-shaped, or many other shapes. Whitehead (1999) is the best entry to the literature on this specialized topic.

Contemporaneous Independent Treatment Allocation

Taves (1974) has described a study design that requires an independent coordinator who allocates each patient, as he/she is recruited, to one or other treatment group. The independent coordinator allocates each patient so as to minimize the difference between the two treatment groups, according to prospectively defined patient characteristics, e.g. age, sex, genotype, disease state or stage, or concomitant therapy. This allocation is therefore also based upon the accumulating characteristics of the treatment groups, as has developed during the study to date. Patients are therefore not allocated to a treatment group by the chance of a randomization schedule.

Bias in minimization trials can be avoided when three conditions are met. First, those performing the clinical trial itself, i.e. administering test medications and measuring end-points, should be double-blind and unaware of which treatment the patient has received. Second, the independent coordinator need only allocate patients to anonymous groups A or B, and the study pharmacist need be the only person who knows which treatments these codes represent. Third, the criteria for which

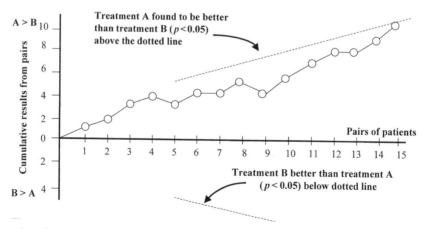

Figure 11.2 Illustration of the Armitage 'sequential analysis' study design. Patients are paired, and one of each pair receives each alternative treatment. If the patient receiving treatment A does better than the one receiving treatment B (A > B), then the line moves upwards; vice versa, if the patient receiving B does better than the one receiving A (B > A), then the line moves downward. If the treatments cannot be distinguished within a pair of patients, then the line moves horizontally. The critical boundaries (broken lines) are computed from prospective measures of α and β (e.g. $p = 0.05$ and 80% power, respectively). The technique derives from an engineering control chart and, once again, can be adapted to more sophisticated forms, including limits on the study size for indeterminate results

the treatment groups should be balanced must be prospectively identified and rigidly adhered to, using a recorded, quantitative system of scoring the factors.

In its simplest form, this class of minimization designs usually results in treatment groups of nearly equal size. By equitably assigning patients to three or more treatment groups, and yet having identical treatments for two or more of these, un-balanced sample sizes can be created. This is of use when, for example, it may be desirable to expose fewer patients to placebo than to active therapy, especially when conducting a trial of compounds whose properties are fairly well known or may be predicted with some confidence.

Note that minimization trials can only alter power calculations when assumptions of the size of worthwhile differences in effect are also pro-spectively defined. For example, from a clinical point of view, a small-sized improvement in out-come (perhaps a few per cent of patients more than that observed for placebo treatment) may be viewed as very worthwhile in an extremely heterogenous patient population when subjected to multivariate analysis (this is common in large, simple studies; see below). On the other hand, when designing a mini-mization study, the assumption is that the treat-ment groups will be devoid of relevant differences in baseline characteristics, and therefore clinical significance might only be assumed to follow from a large-sized difference in patient response. The size of the difference that is assumed to be of interest, as it increases, may compensate for the reduction in variability amongst study group samples, and thus have less than expected impact on the sample sizes needed to conduct the clinical trial.

Minimization designs are probably under-used by the pharmaceutical industry. This approach is not well-designed for pivotal clinical trials, or for diseases with large numbers of prognostic factors, where, in any case, large numbers of patients are needed for a tolerability database. If the controlled clinical trial is a gold standard, then it would be wrong to assert that the independent treatment al-location design is the 'platinum standard' (*pace* Treasure and MacRae 1998). The interested reader is referred to a good published example (Kallis et al 1994), and to more detailed statistical treatments (Pocock and Simon 1975; Freedman and White 1976).

THE 'LARGE, SIMPLE STUDY' AND STRATIFICATION DESIGNS

These similar classes of study require large numbers of patients. The choice between them lies in being able to 'hedge one's bets' with a partial indication approval, vs. 'all or nothing' with huge logistical costs and potentially huge rewards.

Stratification Studies

In pivotal studies, large numbers of patients are studied so that their diverse clinical characteristics can imitate better the ordinary patient population than in earlier, more selective, trials. When a var-iety of concomitant factors (e.g. other diagnoses, wider degree of disease severity, concomitant medi-cations, etc.) are suspected, and may interact with drug tolerability or efficacy, then patients may be stratified into randomization groups according to the presence or absence of such factors. For example, patients with Crohn's disease might be stratified according to whether or not they also have cutaneous manifestations, and each stratum then randomized to active or placebo for a total of four treatment groups, although only two test treatments. Separate statistical analyses for the strata can then be planned, and the study size adjusted accordingly. The efficacy of the new drug may be found to be restricted to one or more particular patient subset(s). Regulatory authorities will often approve indications with caveats based on such subsets. For example, in the USA, one indication for aprotinin is '... to reduce periopera-tive blood loss ... in selected cases of primary cor-onary artery bypass graft surgery where the risk of bleeding is especially high, e.g. impaired hemo-stasis, presence of aspirin, or coagulopathy of other origin'. The risk of stratification studies is that conservative regulatory authorities will want to see statistical significance in all patient subsets before allowing a short, broad indication in labeling.

The 'Large, Simple Study'

This is a recently recognized alternative to strati-fication, pioneered by Peto. Large numbers of unselected patients are subjected to a single randomization. If enough patients are recruited, and if the randomization is truly unbiased, then the large sample sizes will allow all the potentially interacting variables (concomitant drugs, concomitant diseases, demographic variables, etc.) to balance out between the treatment groups.

The 'simple' part of this approach is that, in fundamental terms, the case report form can be very short. There is no need to collect lots of information about the patient's clinical condition because there is no use for these data. Trials of cardiovascular drugs, on an almost epidemiological scale, have been the most significant examples of this alternative approach. Literally tens of thousands of patients have been recruited under these protocols with case report forms having fewer than 10 pages for each patient. Dr Robert Temple (1997; Director of the Office of Drug Evaluation I, at FDA) has commented that it may even be possible to conduct large simple studies in treatment investigative new drug application (IND) situations, thus permitting the generation of efficacy data outside of orthodox 'Phase III' clinical trial programs. However, in this case the end-point would have to be just as simple, e.g. survival or death of the patient, during a documented period of observation; Kaplan–Meier analysis and other epidemiological approaches may also be applied to such databases.

Whilst the conditions under which large simple trials can provide efficacy data are fairly well worked out, it is important to consider whether (or which) tolerability issues can be precisely addressed in this way. If a tolerability factor (adverse event) relates to the efficacy variable of interest (e.g. a fatal adverse event in a patient survival study), then a simple case report form may provide relevant information. However, if the adverse event type is rare or unanticipated (e.g. the test drug causes unanticipated, significant anemia in 0.1% of patients, and the protocol and case report form do not collect hemoglobin values before and after treatment), then it is very likely that the adverse event will be missed. Large simple studies can thus create undue confidence in product tolerability ('thousands of patients were exposed to the agent during clinical trials').

TREATMENT WITHDRAWAL AND OTHER SPECIALIZED DESIGNS

There are rare cases where established treatments are without strong evidence-based support. Two good examples exist for digoxin: the treatment of mild heart failure, and the treatment of cardiac asthenia, a diagnosis that is especially common in Europe, and for which relatively small doses are prescribed. When the effect of such treatments on the natural progression of disease is unknown, it can then be ethical to recruit patients into a study with inclusion criteria that include that they are *already* being treated with the drug of interest. Almost any of the designs discussed above may then be used, where patients are randomized either to remain on the treatment of interest or to be withdrawn from that treatment. All the usual needs for precisely defined prospective end-points and sound statistical advice before starting the study apply.

Early-phase clinical trials in patients with cancer often use a two-stage design that has been promoted by Gehan and others (Gehan 1979; Ellenberg 1989). With progressive, fatal diseases, the problem of preventing an untoward number of patients from being treated with a useless therapy increases. These two-stage designs usually include a small number of open label-treated patients (usually $n \leq 14$) in the first stage. The proportion and degree of tumor responsiveness is then used to fix the number of patients in the second stage of the design, which may use an active comparator or no therapy as the alternative treatment, depending upon whether an active comparator therapy can be identified. Such studies cannot produce fundamental evidence of efficacy but, in the hands of experienced statisticians and development teams, can predict whether wider trials are justified.

STOPPING CLINICAL TRIALS

Safety Issues

Stopping a clinical trial because of an emergent safety problem, either by a medical monitor or by a safety committee, is always a unique situation. Little useful, generalizable guidance can be provided here. These are decisions that are always taken in consultation, and the safety of potential future trial recruits must be the paramount concern (including the abrupt cessation of therapy). Trial suspension is usually the best immediate option, allowing time for collective thought, notification of regulatory authorities and wider consultations as appropriate.

Efficacy Issues

Pocock (1992) has succinctly summarized most of the situations that obtain when it is considered whether to stop a clinical trial. Efficacy, like safety, can cause ethical concerns to the pharmaceutical physician when he/she suspects that patients will be exposed to alternative therapies that are sub-optimal.

Interim Efficacy Analyses

These usually make a mess! They require either that the overall size of the trial has to be greater than if no interim analysis was performed, or that a smaller α must be accepted as indicating statistical significance at the end of the whole study.

Pharmaceutical physicians will hear loud complaints about these drawbacks of interim analyses, especially from senior management with purely commercial backgrounds. Everyone will want to know as soon as possible whether 'the drug is working', but lax scientific thinking is behind these complaints. Common statements are: 'We don't want to stop the study at the halfway stage, we just want to see how it is going'. When asked why, the answer is usually something like, 'There would be no point in spending more money on the study if there is no chance of achieving a statistically significant result'. This is a popular misrationalization: the decision not to stop a study is a decision to allow it to continue. Any interim decision introduces a bias on the dataset that is eventually analysed.

Spectacularly effective drugs may achieve a very small α at the time of the interim analysis. Stopping the trial by reason of the unethical basis for treating the patients with anything else is a rare and pleasant event for the clinical trialist. However, in that spectacular success, the pharmaceutical physician

should ask whether a minimization design would have achieved the same thing with even fewer patients, and thus actually feel chastened.

It is not the purpose of this chapter to delve into the mechanics of statistics. However, a few comments about the relationships between values for α at the stage of an interim and complete statistical analysis of a clinical trial may be in order. There are several statistical points of view on this subject, and regulatory authorities have a habit of believing only the most conservative.

At the time of writing, the O'Brien and Fleming rule is becoming an acceptable standard. As a rule of thumb, pharmaceutical physicians should expect statisticians to provide alternatives that obey a simple subtraction rule. For example, clinicians might agree that the study should stop due to great efficacy when $p = 0.01$ at an interim analysis, when sufficient patients (power of 0.8) to detect such a difference have been recruited. In that case, if the study continues after the interim analysis fails to achieve $p < 0.01$, then it will be required to achieve approximately $p < 0.04$ for the whole patient population in the final statistical analysis in order to demonstrate the efficacy of the test drug. Even so, Pocock and Geller (1986) have shown that trials stopped by reason of efficacy at an interim stage are likely to have exaggerated the size of the difference between treatment groups. Marketing departments should be aware of this error in their extrapolations to the commercial worth of the product.

Bayesian Trial Designs

A typical Bayesian design might be where, for example, there are several drugs with preclinical rationale for the treatment of cancer; since none are clinically proven, one of the test treatments is placebo. Patients are then recruited sequentially into the study, and the results (e.g. tumor size reduction) are recorded. After a while, the proportions of patients responding to each treatment are compared using a sophisticated probabalistic method which takes into account the uncertainties associated with small and unequal treatment group sizes. The randomization code is then adjusted to favor more patients being allocated to the treatments that have started out looking better than the others, while very poor, placebo-equivalent, treatments might be dropped altogether. Eventually, the several test therapies are reduced to two and a definitive demonstration of superiority or non-superiority for that pair of treatments can be reported.

The difficulties with interim analyses do not arise when a Bayesian approach to the original design has been taken (Berry 1985). The Bayesian methodology essentially revises the proportionate patient allocation among the test therapies according to the latest and best information available (e.g. Berry 1995): essentially, after some minimum number of patients have entered the trial, an interim analysis is done every time another patient completes the trial. The important distinction between Bayesian and sequential designs (above) is that although the number of patients required to complete a sequential design study are undefined at the beginning, the treatment allocations are nonetheless according to a fixed randomization schedule. Thus, the sequential designs are still, essentially, a frequentist methodology, and not Bayesian.

Bayesian approaches currently find little understanding on the part of regulatory authorities, and thus are, probably unduly, little utilized by generalist pharmaceutical physicians. However, Bayesian methods are finding increased uses in specialized areas, e.g. trials of cancer chemotherapy, and studies in rare diseases. The potential benefits of Bayesian methods include the use of fewer patients to demonstrate efficacy, as well as potential seamlessness of Phase II and Phase III development when the number of drugs or dose sizes of interest has been reduced during the trial from several to one or two; patients recruited after this transition may be regarded as patients in a pivotal trial by an enlightened regulatory authority.

The general pharmaceutical physician cannot be expected to be able to generate Bayesian statistical plans for him/herself. These require an experienced statistician and, it may be added, a statistician who is not, him/herself, philosophically opposed to Bayesian rather than frequentist thinking. The decision to employ a Bayesian design for a clinical trial will be viewed as courageous in most companies, and there will be many clinical trials for which an orthodox, frequentist approach will be selected, for several good reasons. Overall, the general pharmaceutical physician should be advised that, when considering a new trial, he/she should at least consider whether a Bayesian approach might help. If this option is rejected, then that is fine, but the brief consideration, as a matter of routine, might occasionally lead to a superior trial design.

SERIES OF PUBLISHED CASES

Some diseases are so rare that the prospects of conducting a clinical trial are remote. It is unlikely that enough patients could ever be collected at any reasonably small number of study sites for any useful randomization. These diseases may be found in the literature as case reports. In these cases, probably the best that can be accomplished is to collect and retrospectively analyze as many such cases as possible. If the drug of interest has been used in a sufficient number of patients, then retrospective risk ratios for benefit and harm can be calculated. This may be the strongest evidence that can ever be collected about a particular drug under these rare conditions, albeit never as strong as a controlled clinical trial. One example is the effectiveness of dantrolene in malignant hyperthermia (Strazis and Fox, 1993).

OBJECTIVES AND PREREQUISITES OF PIVOTAL CLINICAL TRIALS

Licensing requirements typically are greater than reporting data from by multicenter Phase III studies. Special populations may require small-scale studies to supplement a traditional two-study, large-scale registration development scheme. Similarly, if (in the USA) the proposed indication has an approved orphan drug designation, then small-scale Phase II-type studies may be all that is possible due to disease rarity (see Chapter 16). Furthermore, even for conventional indications, the resource implications of pivotal studies are usually much greater than any earlier phase of development, and efficient resource utilization becomes exponentially more important than before. The incorporation of pharmacoeconomic and humanistic outcomes alongside the primary registration end-points is becoming essential, and preparatory work is best done in conjunction with the smaller, earlier studies, and must also factor treatment compliance.

BENEFIT–RISK ANALYSIS

The accumulation of all the data from the clinical trials of a new drug product, assuming a fairly orthodox regulatory strategy for a typical dossier or NDA, will form the largest fraction of the application. However, these data are also needed for derivative documents within the application, one of which is a benefit–risk analysis, which forms the last part of an integrated safety summary (Section 9 of the NDA), and is a central objective of the Expert Report in European applications. These benefit–risk assessments must be derived from the clinical study reports and summaries elsewhere in the applications.

All clinicians constantly weigh benefit–risk in their daily practice. Their assessment of this 'ratio' in everyday practice, using approved drugs, is usually not as numerical as it sounds. In practice, clinicians make prescribing decisions based upon: (a) a subset of the published information that might be available about the drug (labeling, drug representatives, comments from colleagues, etc.); (b) their current and prior experience with this particular patient; and (c) prior experience with other patients. This prior experience, even if personal, may or may not be consciously recalled. Furthermore, we all operate algorithms taught us by others whom we respect, and thus we use others' experience with drugs and patients, quite apart from the often hard-learned lessons from our own therapeutic adventures (*pace* 'evidence-based medicine').

Clinical trialists also weigh benefit–risk, every time a protocol is written. Often, unlike for approved drugs, there is much less information to go on. In early clinical development, extrapolations are obligatory. However, unlike in general medical practice, these extrapolations are often not from clinical experience, but rather from pharmacokinetic models or animal data, or at best from patients who are clearly dissimilar from those proposed in the new trial. This is obligatory: if the answers to the clinical trial questions were known, then there would be little point in doing the trial.

There are highly mathematical approaches to benefit–risk assessment. When a single (binary) end-point of interest can be balanced against a single adverse event of concern, then the number of patients required, and the number of required therapeutic events, can be defined, and the confidence intervals can be calculated, in order to examine what the true benefit–risk ratio might be, e.g. for the global utilization of streptokinase and t-PA for occluded coronary arteries (GUSTO; Willan et al 1997). The number needed to treat, number needed to harm (and corresponding reciprocals) can be used to compare drugs for this purpose. However, this is an highly unusual and artificial situation, and the sophisticated statistical answers that result are unlikely to have more that a partial impact on the more non-numerical approach taken by clinicians.

Usually, however, the clinical trialist has to stick out his/her neck, based upon an highly personal, non-numerical assessment of benefit–risk. The highly mathematical approaches usually work best in retrospect, and this is not the situation of the clinician who must decide whether to prescribe, or the clinical trialist who must decide whether to commit patients to a particular study design, both being prospective decisions. Furthermore, both in clinical trials and general medical practice, it is a rare situation where the benefit to the patient arises from a single binary variable, and there are no drugs which possess a single type of adverse event, whose probability may be confidently, prospectively estimated for any given patient. Even the simplest case, a drug with substantial history and experience, cannot fit the contrived mathematical approach described above. Penicillin has three adverse events of primary interest (anaphylaxis, bacterial drug resistance, and sodium load at high doses). The mechanism by which infection recedes, if it is to recede, is only partly due to the action of the drug, because the extreme variability introduced by the concomitant condition of the patient. Whether to prescribe penicillin is a common decision for doctors and dentists: the mathematical analysis of the benefit–risk 'ratio' is unlikely to affect most prescribing decisions.

The informed consent document is where we ask patients to make their own benefit–risk assessments, albeit with some guidance (Marsh 1990). Certainly, the mathematical approach cannot be expected on the part of the patient, neither will it be useful in a balanced and fair communication with the patient about the nature of the clinical trial.

Benefit–risk, then, is a central part of the practice of pharmaceutical medicine and its regulation. It can almost never be reduced to a numerical exercise. Benefit–risk assessment of clinical trials data is an important part of all new drug applications. Good people will differ in their benefit–risk assessment, even when using the same body of clinical trials data.

SUMMARY

This chapter has attempted to provide a philosophy of clinical trials. The place of clinical trials in the overall development plan and what the pharmaceutical physician must *know about* rather than be able to actually implement him/herself, has been emphasized. Almost all clinical trials are unique because of the infinite combinations of hypothesis to be addressed, pharmacological properties of the drug under investigation, the types of patients that are likely to be available, and likely users of the resulting data. The major categories of trial designs have been surveyed in some detail; it is hoped that, when challenged with testing any clinical hypothesis, a good pharmaceutical physician would consider all these broad categories, select that most relevant to the clinical situation, and then refine the proposed trial design from that point. Some of the subtle interactions between statistical, financial and psychological aspects of trial design have been hinted at. The pharmaceutical physician will only really grow in this discipline through experience and good mentorship.

REFERENCES

Amin HM, Sopchak AM, Esposito BF, Henson LG et al (1995) Naloxone-induced and spontaneous reversal of depressed ventilatory responses to hypoxia during and after continuous infusion of remifentanil or alfentanil. *J Pharmacol Exp Ther* 274: 34–9.

Bardolph EM, Taylor RH (1997) Sailors, scurvy, science and authority. *J R Soc Med* 90: 238.

Berry DA (1985) Interim analyses in clinical trials: classical vs. Bayesian approaches. *Stat Med* 4: 521–6.

Berry DA (1995) Decision analysis and Bayesian methods in clinical trials. *Cancer Treat Res* 75: 125–54.

Chaput de Saintonge DM, Vere DW (1982) Measurement in clinical trials. *Br J Clin Pharmacol* 13: 775–83.

Ebbutt AF (1984) Three-period crossover designs for two treatments. *Biometrics* 40: 219–24.

Ellenberg SS (1989) Determining sample sizes for clinical trials. *Oncology* 3: 39–42.

Freedman LS, White SJ (1976) On the use of Pocock and Simon's method for balancing treatment numbers over prognostic factors in the controlled clinical trial. *Biometrics* 32: 691–4.

Freiman JA, Chalmers TC, Smith H, Kuebler RR (1978) The importance of beta, the type II error and sample size in the design and interpretation of the randomized control trial. *N Eng J Med* 299: 690–4.

Frey WG (1969) British naval intelligence and scurvy. *N Eng J Med* 281: 1430–33.

Gehan EA (1979) Clinical trials in cancer research. *Environ Health Perspect* 32: 31–48.

Kallis P, Tooze JA, Talbot S, Cowans D et al (1994) Pre-operative aspirin decreases platelet aggregation and increases post-operative blood loss: a prospective, randomized, placebo-controlled double-blind, clinical trial in 100 patients with chronic stable angina. *Eur J Cardiothor Surg* 8: 404–9.

Laska E, Meisner M, Kushner HB (1983) Optimal crossover designs in the presence of carryover effects. *Biometrics* 39: 1087–91.

Lind J (1753) *A Treatise of the Scurvy*. 460 Edinburgh.

Marsh BT (1990) Informed Consent. *J R Soc Med* 83: 603–6.

Pocock SJ (1992) When to stop a clinical trial. *Br Med J* 305: 235–40.

Pocock SJ, Geller NL (1986) Interim analyses in randomized clinical trials. *Drug Information J* 20: 263–9.

Pocock SJ, Simon R (1975) Sequential treatment assignment with balancing for prognostic factors in the controlled clinical trial. *Biometrics* 31: 103–15.

Spilker B (1991) *Guide to Clinical Trials*. Raven: New York; 1156 pp.

Strazis KP, Fox AW (1993) Malignant hyperthermia: review of published cases. *Anesth Analg* 77: 297–304.

Taves DR (1974) Minimization: a new method of assigning patients to treatment and control groups. *Clin Pharmacol Ther* 15: 443–53.

Temple R (1997) Public hearings on Myotrophin: Peripheral and Central Nervous System Drugs Advisory Committee, May 8, 1997.

Thomas DP (1997) Sailors, scurvy and science. *J R Soc Med* 90: 50–4.

Treasure T, MacRae KD (1998) Minimisation: the platinum standard for trials? *Br Med J* 317: 362–3.

Whitehead J (1999) A unified theory for sequential clinical trials. *Statist Med* 18: 2271–86.

Willan AR, O'Brien BJ, Cook DJ (1997) Benefit–risk ratios in the assessment of the clinical evidence of a new therapy. *Control Clin Trial* 18: 121–30.

12

Phase IV Drug Development: Post-marketing Studies

Lisa R. Johnson-Pratt

Merck & Co. Inc., North Wales, PA, USA

OBJECTIVES OF THE PHASE IV CLINICAL DEVELOPMENT PROGRAM

While the earlier phases of drug development (I, II, III) are geared toward demonstrating safety and efficacy and obtaining regulatory approval, Phase IV clinical trials are usually conducted after regulatory approval. Often, however, these trials are started prior to approval (despite risks that the drug or one of its indications may not be approved) to try to gain a competitive advantage.

While Phases I, II and III have regulatorily-determined functions and goals Phase IV trials are much more flexible and cover a variety of purposes (e.g. support label changes or demonstrate cost–effectiveness). Depending on the organization, Phase IV trials may be conducted by the clinical research team that conducted the original NDA or by a separate research team. If the latter, communication links between the two research teams must be established early in the clinical program, to provide information necessary to the conduct of later trials and to advise the marketing department and corporate affairs during the launch and post-approval life of the drug.

The objectives of the Phase IV program (see Tables 12.1 and 12.2) include further safety evaluation, comparative safety and efficacy vs. other products, discovery of new indications, and market expansion. Phase IV trials are not restricted to randomized, double-blind, placebo-controlled trials, but may include other study formats, such as open-label trials and case control and cohort studies.

Table 12.1 Typical goals and tactics of Phase IV clinical trials

Extension of tolerability information	Broader range of patients than in NDA/PLA
	Larger numbers of patients (to detect rarer adverse events)
Competitive efficacy claims	Active comparator studies
New indications	Supplemental efficacy studies
Market expansion	All of the above
	'Formulary tests'
Ethnopharmacology	Ethnic minority or overseas studies
Outcomes assessment	Pharmacoepidemiology
	Pharmacoeconomics

TYPES OF PHASE IV TRIALS

The scope and goals of Phase IV clinical trials are broader than Phases I–III. In general, the trials are larger (often having up to several thousand patients), the inclusion/exclusion conditions are less restrictive, and the end-points may be less objective (e.g. 'quality of life').

As the market becomes more congested and products compete for position on formularies and for reimbursement, additional data of use to consumers and health organizations may become critical. Unless the product is novel, sponsors can no longer be satisfied only with data from Phase III trials demonstrating efficacy superior to placebo. Sponsors must now demonstrate superiority (or at least equivalence) to competing products, and meaningful and sustained efficacy, together with acceptable long-term safety and tolerability.

Principles and Practice of Pharmaceutical Medicine. Edited by A. J. Fletcher, Lionel D. Edwards, Anthony W. Fox and Peter Stonier © 2002 John Wiley & Sons Ltd.

Table 12.2 Practical aspects and problems of Phase IV clinical trials

Active comparators	Obtaining competitor's drug
	Blinding, reformulation and bioequivalence
	Giving new ideas to competitor's marketing department
	Placebo groups must be ethically justifiable
	Dose ranges must be appropriate for both drugs
Equivalence trials	Useful when superiority is unlikely to be demonstrated
	Scientific problem of proving a negative
	Large sample sizes
	Standards of care not previously studied
Megatrials	Unusual statistical strategy
	Few inclusion/exclusion criteria
	Representativeness to marketing target only known at end of study
Open-label studies	Patient-introduced bias
	Non-random designs possible
	Scientifically limited
Safety surveillance studies	Few options for control groups
New indication	Similar to NDA efficacy studies
Dosage form comparisons	Patient satisfaction end-points
Special patient populations	See Chapter 14–16
Drug interaction studies	Almost infinite set of alternatives

Comparative Superiority Trials

In comparative superiority trials, the test drug is typically compared with a drug that is the standard of care or is the class market leader. The goal is to demonstrate superiority in efficacy, cost-effectiveness, patient satisfaction, quality of life, or another parameter that may be helpful in increasing market share. The aim is to publish the trial (preferably in a peer-reviewed journal) and use the data in a promotional campaign. Although historically such studies were often of poor design (e.g. inadequate sample size; inappropriate end-points) to obtain a superiority claim for use in promotional pieces, the FDA now requires two adequate and well-controlled clinical trials or one study large enough to detect clinically useful differences. These studies must have well-defined end-points that are relevant for both products and include a range of doses for each product to ensure an optimal response. Double-blind and, if necessary, double-dummy studies are generally favored over open-label trials. A placebo group is often added to minimize an active control bias (Spilker 1991).

One of the difficulties in conducting double-blind comparative trials is acquiring suitable supplies of the comparison drug. The sponsor can request supplies from the competing sponsor or purchase the product on the open market and modify it (e.g. encapsulation; reformulation) or, via new packaging technologies, mask the identity of the product. These options increase the time and costs associated with the trial. Modifying the product requires the development of a pharmaceutical process and evidence of bioequivalence. This may be particularly difficult for a product with a unique dosage form (e.g. wafer or patch). There is also a risk that the competing sponsor will challenge the study results, citing formulation differences that may affect product efficacy.

Although obtaining clinical supplies from the competing sponsor is scientifically the best option, requests for such supplies may not be handled quickly or may be denied altogether. A study synopsis is usually required by the competing sponsor, so that the design and hypotheses can be evaluated for scientific rigor. The synopsis also alerts the competing sponsor to the ultimate aims of the study, giving their marketing group time to respond to potentially damaging data. As the marketplace becomes increasingly competitive, companies are less willing to provide supplies for comparative studies, so that alternatives should always be explored.

Equivalence Trials

Sometimes, it is not possible to demonstrate superiority but may be sufficient to demonstrate efficacy and safety equivalence, particularly if the marketing strategy is based on price.

Equivalence trials usually require very large sample sizes due to small efficacy differences between the two treatments. Equivalence trials typically do not include a placebo group; therefore, both treatments should have previously demonstrated superior efficacy to placebo, which may be difficult to achieve when the standard-of-care drug has not been stringently evaluated for efficacy and is used to treat a condition for which it is not approved (Makuch 1989). In addition, equivalence trials require the trialist to choose a clinically relevant treatment difference to determine the appropriate sample size, which is often difficult to do (Makuch 1986).

Megatrials

Megatrials are commonly used to establish small differences of new drugs over existing drugs, e.g. the global utilization of streptokinase and t-PA for occluded coronary arteries (GUSTO) study. Thus, they can be important marketing tools and can justify the use of the new and usually more expensive agents instead of older therapies of proven value (Hampton 1996).

Unlike conventional randomized clinical trials, megatrials do not usually attempt to control for confounding variables—rather, their goal is to distribute bias evenly between groups of subjects. The group, rather than the individual, is the subject of analysis. Megatrials appear to have had their biggest impact when used to compare different allocated protocols with respect to a selected outcome. These trials consist of large numbers of patients (up to tens of thousands) and typically have very loose entry criteria, although the ideal megatrial study population should be representative of the target population and have rigorous diagnostic criteria for entry (Charlton 1996).

Open-label Trials

In an open-label trial, both the subject and the investigator know the treatment being adminis-

tered. In the earlier phases of drug development, open-label trials are rarely appropriate, except for very early safety and efficacy (e.g. dose-ranging) studies. Open-label studies are often useful in the later phases of drug development and when conducting 'real-world' safety/efficacy trials, particularly when treatment will be prolonged and when cost or utilization data are required by purchasers of health care.

Open-label studies may be conducted using a longitudinal trial design, in which a subject's treatment data may be compared to his own baseline data or those of a treatment group may be compared to those of a control group. Longitudinal designs are often used in epidemiologic studies, such as the famous Framingham study, but can also be used in drug studies where the effects of treatment on various variables (e.g. pharmacoeconomics, quality of life) can be assessed over a finite time period. Since subjects are enrolled in a non-randomized manner, some of the ethical issues inherent in randomized trials, in which subjects have no choice as to which treatment group they are allocated, can be avoided. Criticisms of this approach include the following (Friedman 1985):

- The cohort being followed may not be representative of the larger population for whom the drug is intended.
- It is difficult to obtain comparable treatment groups, since patients are typically only matched on one of many possible variables.
- Subjects may be inadvertently assigned to treatment groups based on characteristics that can influence the outcome.

Further problems are that open-label studies may result in increased patient dropouts, from patients being randomized to receive an agent they view as less beneficial and that is not viewed as favorably by the medical community or by regulatory authorities.

On the positive side, open-label studies are usually administratively easier to conduct, offer investigators more comfortable decision-making if they know which treatment the subject has received, and may be the only option when blinded study supplies are not available (Friedman 1985).

SAFETY SURVEILLANCE

Once a product is released onto the market, the number of patients exposed to it increases significantly. As a result, the sponsor has an opportunity to identify adverse drug reactions that are rare or idiosyncratic. The sponsor does this in two ways: by monitoring spontaneously reported adverse events and by conducting large clinical trials (postmarketing safety surveillance studies). These trials, which may be mandated by the regulatory agency in order to gain approval, are usually conducted under the Phase IV development program in an unblinded manner and under normal-use conditions.

SEARCHING FOR NEW INDICATIONS

Once a drug is approved for an indication, many years of its patent life have usually expired. Information gathered from Phase III clinical trials or from use of the drug under normal conditions (postmarketing) may suggest alternative indications that may extend the patent life. For an invention to be patented in the USA, it must be a new and useful improvement and not obvious (see also Chapter 35). Patentable categories in drug development include pharmaceutically active compounds, processes for making compounds, and compositions comprising an active compound and a pharmaceutical carrier (Hammer 1990). New formulations may satisfy these criteria and extend the patent life, e.g. minoxidil (originally used orally as an antihypertensive agent) as a topical preparation for the treatment of hair loss. New indications also help to keep up the 'noise level' for the product, enabling the marketing team to capitalize on new information that could potentially expand the market for existing indications.

The independent investigator can play an important role in identifying new indications by identifying and studying a particular drug effect. When published, such findings may lead to widespread use of the product for a new indication and, ultimately, adoption by the medical establishment. This process can occur without the intervention of the product sponsor or any formal clinical development program. However, generally new indications are evaluated in a formal trial and submitted as a supplemental NDA (sNDA). To assist independent investigators with this process, many large pharmaceutical companies have set up investigator grant programs.

NEW DOSAGE FORMS

In a clinical development program, initially one lead dosage form is typically taken through full development. The chosen form usually represents the most easily developed, stable and marketable form that is suitable for adults. For some products, the initial form is found to be suboptimal and alternative forms are introduced early in the clinical development process. For other products, the need for multiple forms is not recognized until future competitors are found to have a more acceptable or a unique formulation that may lead to a greater market share.

In other cases, a new dosage formulation is required to satisfy a new market segment. Oral solutions and chewable tablets are beneficial for a pediatric population. A slow-release preparation (such as percutaneous patches) may be preferred in elderly patients taking multiple drugs if it allows once-daily (or less frequent) dosing. Trials demonstrating safety and efficacy of new formulations are often conducted in Phase IV and typically act as the supporting information for an sNDA.

Developing Dosage Forms to Improve Patient Compliance/Satisfaction

Although there are numerous reasons for lack of compliance (e.g. lack of perceived benefit of treatment, few disease symptoms), the sponsor may be able to improve compliance by developing formulations that are more acceptable to the patient (e.g. once-daily rather than q.i.d. regimen, oral rather than injectable form). Dosage forms can also influence overall patient satisfaction, which can be useful in achieving market expansion or patient product switches.

If the sponsor has developed a new, more acceptable dosage form and can demonstrate improved patient satisfaction, patients may switch products and demand that the new drug be placed on a formulary. Dosage forms may be evaluated in a Phase IV comparative trial and may require the use of a double-blind, double-dummy technique.

Role of New Dosage Forms in Maintaining Formulary Status

Multiple dosage formulations of a drug give a sponsor a significant advantage over other products in its class. Not only can the sponsor reach groups of patients that may have not accepted a particular formulation (e.g. bulky tablet for a pediatric population), but in the formulary wars, a drug with multiple formulations is generally considered a better choice because different subgroups of patients can be treated with the same product. Additionally, patients may be able to switch formulations, depending on their medical requirements, e.g. as they move from an inpatient (i.v.) to an outpatient (oral) setting without changing products. This obviates the need for the pharmacy to make multiple product purchases in a particular drug class, simply to accommodate patient needs.

USE IN SPECIAL POPULATIONS

The entry and exclusion criteria for Phase I–III trials are usually very strict, eliminating as many opportunities for confounding of data as possible. As a result, patients with multiple medical conditions are routinely excluded from these trials. In addition, entire classes of patients are excluded because of ethical or liability concerns and recruitment difficulties. These patients include women of childbearing potential, children and adolescents, the elderly, and ethnic minorities (see also Chapters below). Since these patient subgroups will undoubtedly use the product, trials are conducted in Phase IV to evaluate the safety and efficacy in these populations. The goal is to gather information that will supplement information in the label and instruct physicians on any differences in pharmacokinetics/dynamics in the special population, compared to the Phase III population. This information may also be used to expand the potential market by broadening the population for whom the drug is indicated.

EVALUATING DRUG INTERACTIONS

Rarely is a drug devoid of potential for drug interactions. A sound early clinical development program is used to assess such interaction potential, typically with drugs that are expected to be used concomitantly with the investigative drug, or with those that may have a significant effect on the pharmacokinetics of the drug (e.g. the effect of oral contraceptives on the pharmacokinetics of a drug that will be used by women of childbearing potential).

After the drug is marketed, and more patients use the product under a multitude of conditions with a higher degree of concomitant medication use, the potential for drug interactions can be more fully assessed. Potential interactions are usually reported via the spontaneous reporting system, and can result in further evaluation in large Phase IV post-marketing safety surveillance trials. If a beneficial effect of concomitant medication use is anecdotally reported, such concomitant usage can be formally explored in a Phase IV clinical trial.

CLINICAL–LEGAL INTERFACE: IMPROVING AND CLARIFYING THE LABEL (TACTICAL ASPECTS)

In the USA, the concern regarding product liability has led arguably to an ultra-conservative approach in labeling, advertising and promotion, and compensation for investigators and patients in clinical trials. This conservatism is expressed not only in the development of the original label that is submitted for approval by the regulatory agency, but also in requests by the legal department to improve the label after marketing to minimize risk of liability. On occasion, clinical trials are conducted to evaluate specific risks. This may be in response to pharmacodynamic effects seen in Phase III or to serious adverse events reported spontaneously. Results from these trials will then be used to add to or clarify information in the label, to encourage safer use of the drug. Phase IV trials that are used for this purpose include: large safety surveillance trials (e.g. to assess rare serious adverse events or pregnancy outcomes); additional dose-ranging studies (e.g. to assess a reduction in dose on the risk–benefit profile); double-blind placebo-controlled trials, that assess effects on a target organ (e.g. using angiography or cognitive function tests); or pharmacokinetic trials (e.g. assessing the effect of alcohol or food on drug concentration).

The impact of anticipated study results on labeling should be evaluated carefully prior to initiating a trial. Although the ultimate goal of such labeling changes is to convey important, clinically useful information to the physician and patient (via the Patient Package Insert) to allow better clinical decisions, haphazard label additions purely to decrease legal liability may confuse rather than assist the prescriber.

CLINICAL/MARKETING INTERFACE: EXPANDING THE MARKET

Conduction of Studies to Promote Local Operating Company Needs

To obtain reimbursement and formulary acceptance as health-care dollars become scarcer, the sponsor at launch or soon after should be able to demonstrate cost–effectiveness, superiority, convenience, and patient satisfaction, usually through data from Phase IV pharmacoeconomic trials (see also Chapter 19).

Choosing Investigators: Advocate Development

When selecting investigators for the pivotal Phase III clinical trials, the sponsor typically searches for physicians who are well-known specialists in a particular therapeutic area. These physicians are typically referred to as 'thought leaders' or 'opinion leaders' and include editors and authors of major textbooks or other publications and leaders in important medical societies. They may also be representatives on advisory committees to the FDA or other regulatory agency who will ultimately determine whether the drug is approved for marketing.

One goal of Phase IV studies is to expand the numbers and types of physicians who are using the product. While a few 'thought-leaders' may lend credibility when attempting to get a manuscript published in a key journal, they represent an extremely small percentage of physicians who will actually be prescribing the product. Physicians chosen for participation in Phase IV studies are those who can potentially increase market share by serving as regional and local advocates for the products, and are commonly referred by the business group. These are the physicians who may sit on formulary committees of hospitals, develop local treatment guidelines, see high volumes of patients, are active in local medical societies, and serve as consultants to the sponsor. In the USA, with increased use by managed-care organizations of a 'gatekeeper' generalist physician, use of family practitioners, general internists and gynecologists as clinical trial physicians may prove to be extremely beneficial for ultimate product acceptance. Generalists are often the physicians who will most prescribe a product and therefore should be given the opportunity to test it in phase IV trials.

CONCLUSION

Phase IV clinical trials are the next step in drug development after completion of pivotal safety and efficacy trials. No longer viewed as, Phase IV clinical trials are becoming an increasingly integral part of the overall development program. The questions they are designed to answer are those asked by the purchasers of pharmaceuticals, with goals of demonstrating the overall benefit of using a product and distinguishing it from its competitors in terms of pharmacoeconomics, safety, and efficacy. These trials can provide timely data to respond to a rapidly changing market place and fill information gaps that might otherwise preclude successful market penetration.

REFERENCES

Charlton BG (1996) Megatrials are based on a methodological mistake. *Br J Gen Pract* 46: 429–31.
Friedman LM, Furberg CD, DeMets DL (1985) *Fundamentals of Clinical Trials*. Mosby-Year Book: St. Louis, MO.
Hammer CE (1990) *Drug Development*, CRC Press: Boca Raton, FL.

Hampton JR (1996) Alternatives to mega-trials in Cardiovascular Disease. *Cardiovasc Drugs Ther* 10: 759–65.

Makuch RW, Johnson MF (1986) Some issues in the design and interpretation of 'negative' clinical studies. *Arch Intern Med* 146: 986–9.

Makuch, RW, Johnson Mary F (1989). Issues in planning and interpreting active control equivalence studies. *J Clin Epidemiol* 42(6): 503–11.

Spilker B (1991) *Guide to Clinical Trials*, Raven: New York, NY.

13

The Unique Role of Over-the-counter Medicine

Paul Starkey

Formerly Vice-President, Smithkline Beecham Healthcare, Parsippany, New Jersey.

THE EXPANDING PLACE OF SELF-MEDICATION

In recent years, the role of over-the-counter (OTC) medication in the overall health system has increased dramatically. The increased interest in and availability of OTC medications is being driven by several factors:

1. There is a growing recognition of the capability of patients to treat themselves in a rational and safe manner. The older authoritarian model of medicine is being gradually replaced by a more participative model.
2. There is an increasing desire by patients to participate in their own medical care. This is not just a result of changes in philosophy but also of the dramatic increase in average educational level over the past half-century. The world increasingly possesses a well-informed and intellectually capable population that demands an active and inclusive role in its own health care.
3. The quantity of information now available to the average person, both through formal education and through the media, has increased enormously, giving increasing awareness of treatment options.
4. There is a growing need to contain medical costs. OTC drugs are not only cheaper than prescription drugs, due to their simpler and more efficient distribution channels, but they also eliminate the need for an expensive visit with the doctor for each episode of illness. The professional intervention required to prescribe pharmaceuticals represents the dominant cost in the handling of many common types of illness.
5. There is a need to increase treatment effectiveness, which is not ordinarily considered an advantage of self-medication. The increase in effectiveness depends on the generally more rapid availability of OTC medications than prescription medications, so that treatment may begin sooner. This can significantly shorten the total length of suffering, especially when the natural course of a disease is brief or when severe discomfort makes prompt therapy especially helpful.

An example of this last phenomenon is in the treatment of vaginal candidiasis. Prior to the OTC availability of topical antifungals, it was often necessary for a woman who had already recognized the symptoms of the disease to call and arrange a physician's appointment. This often took several days. Delaying treatment caused much unnecessary suffering and encouraged disease progression. Many physicians, recognizing these difficulties, would prescribe over the phone, based solely on the woman's description of symptoms. Research has shown that the accuracy of the physician's diagnosis in this setting is no better than that of the woman herself. This constituted an ideal situation for the switching of an important class of drugs from prescription to OTC status. The patient obtained equally accurate diagnosis and far more rapid treatment for a disease that is very uncomfortable. Severe cases of vaginal candidiasis with heavy discharge are now much less common.

A second example is in the treatment of the common cold. Anti-cold medications have been

Principles and Practice of Pharmaceutical Medicine. Edited by A. J. Fletcher, Lionel D. Edwards, Anthony W. Fox and Peter Stonier © 2002 John Wiley & Sons Ltd.

available OTC for many years, because of the compelling need for rapid treatment. A cold evolves quickly, the entire illness lasting only a few days. A delay of only a day or two in seeing the physician for a prescription may eliminate any possibility of obtaining effective treatment for at least half of the duration of the illness. The prompt availability of self-medication improves treatment efficacy, while reducing costs and enhancing patient satisfaction with the medical system.

The above factors have combined to greatly increase public awareness of the importance of self-medication in the total health care scheme. The pharmaceutical physician should recognize the opportunities for OTC use of medications and the advantages and pitfalls attendant upon such use. As self-medication becomes a central part of the health care system, the skillful and appropriate movement of pharmaceuticals from prescription to OTC availability will increasingly become a vital role of the pharmaceutical physician in optimizing the nation's health.

CRITERIA FOR OTC USE OF MEDICINES

The criteria by which a drug may be judged as suitable for self-medication are never absolute. A drug's 'OTC-ness' is always a matter of careful judgment. The Food and Drug Administration (FDA) has lessened the requirements for OTC use substantially in recent years. In time, it may dramatically shift the standards for conditions and drugs considered suitable for self-medication. The old tendency to restrict OTC treatment to conditions of short duration and primarily to symptomatic therapy is rapidly disappearing. Neither is the suitability of a medication for OTC use solely the result of its pharmacologic characteristics. Appropriate labeling and advertising of the medication can have a major impact on the extent to which patients understand its proper use. An OTC product should be envisioned not just as the drug but as the complete package of drug, labeling, and advertising, designed to encourage safe and effective self-medication. With this is mind, several vital considerations concern suitability of a drug for OTC marketing.

Self-diagnosis

Surprisingly, the first of these considerations has nothing to do with the drug itself but rather with the condition it is to treat. Self-treatment implies self-diagnosis. Only diseases that can be made self-diagnosable through appropriate labeling can be considered for OTC treatment.

Fortunately, there are many common conditions that are self-diagnosable. Indeed, it should not be assumed that a diagnosis made by the patient is necessarily inferior to that made by the physician. The patient can actually feel the symptoms as well as observe the signs of a disease—a real advantage in the diagnosis of conditions where symptoms predominate.

Of course, disorders vary in the extent to which laboratory tests and other sophisticated techniques are important in their diagnosis. If these are a major factor, a satisfactory patient diagnosis is unlikely, no matter how skillfully written labeling may be. At the other extreme are many conditions whose diagnosis rests primarily on history and symptoms, where a patient may be educated to give an equal or better diagnosis than that of the physician.

An example of this is headache, where the diagnosis rests largely on history and symptoms. The patient has lived the history and experienced the symptoms. The physician has at best a description of these symptoms, which a patient may be able to communicate well or poorly. Even with the most skillful physician eliciting the history, there is a degradation of information as it moves from patient to physician. If patients can be educated about the criteria for diagnosis, they may be as capable of rendering the diagnosis as accurately as the physician.

Even when a fully adequate description of symptoms and signs is not practicable for patient labeling, this barrier may be surmounted by limiting use to patients who have previously had the condition and been diagnosed by a professional. Once some diseases have been experienced, they are unmistakable. This approach emphasizes the need for the pharmaceutical physician to think creatively in evaluating whether or not a disease can be made self-diagnosable.

Differential Diagnosis

Once a condition is established as self-diagnosable, a related consideration is the differential diagnosis—the potential consequence of confusing the disease with other similarly presenting ones, possibly resulting in a major delay in treatment. This consideration can often be a dominant factor in determining whether a condition is safely self-treatable. In conditions where minimal consequences are likely from a misdiagnosis, a modest level of diagnostic inaccuracy is tolerable to obtain the benefits of self-medication. If the major downside of misdiagnosis is simply the persistence or modest worsening of symptoms without serious health consequences, even more difficult self-diagnoses may reasonable. However, it is usually wise to place a time limit on the length of self-treatment without a satisfactory response.

Drug Safety

When evaluating the safety and tolerability of a drug for possible OTC use, one must first consider the quality of available information. Many drugs, particularly those used for a long time as prescription medications, have extensive safety databases. However, some do not, particularly older drugs that predate modern research standards and newer drugs with insufficient usage. Also, with some drugs, the tolerability of one formulation may differ greatly from that of another. One example is benzyl peroxide, in which formulations may very greatly, even at the same strength but with different excipients. Where such problems mean that there is an inadequate database for an intended OTC formulation, clinical testing will be needed before launch.

Safety is usually the controlling factor in determining suitability for OTC use, and involves several factors:

- The therapeutic index (the ratio of therapeutic dose to toxic dose), which varies widely for both prescription and OTC drugs and is often less of a safety determinant than might be supposed. For example, the prescription drug sucralfate

for the treatment of ulcers has extremely low toxicity, whereas OTC systemic decongestants typically have a lower therapeutic index than have most prescription drugs.
- The effects and consequences of toxicity and overdosage.
- The ease of recognition of early signs of toxicity to allow reduction in dosage or professional assistance.

Safety (negative propensity to cause harm) must be distinguished from tolerability (negative propensity to cause annoying side effects). Tolerability can limit OTC, use even when safety is good. This is particularly true for topical agents such as anti-acne preparations, most of which are of little safety concern but can produce very substantial irritation.

However, the effect of a drug on the general population is only part of the story. The acceptability of a drug for market, particularly an OTC drug without a physician intermediary, is often determined by its effect on special populations, including those patients who are particularly sensitive to its effects. Care should be taken to examine atypical patients in a study population, as well as individual adverse reaction reports. Precautions may be required in the labeling for populations at particular risk.

The conclusion that a drug is not acceptable for OTC use based on safety should be reached only after determining that satisfactory labeling cannot be developed. The pharmaceutical physician must weigh safety and tolerability against efficacy, both in the general population and in special populations. Here the responsibility rests directly on the pharmaceutical physician, since there will be no other medical professional between the drug and the patient using it.

Efficacy

Efficacy is a central issue with all pharmaceutical products, and especially with OTC drugs. In the context of self-medication drugs, it is traditional to accept a somewhat lesser degree of efficacy in order to improve the safety profile. Also, a lesser standard of efficacy is normally expected by the patient, since OTC medication tends to be a first step in therapy. Failure to obtain satisfactory efficacy typically results in the patient seeking professional advice, at which point more potent treatments can be utilized. This does not mean, however, that OTC drugs should not be effective for the conditions they treat.

Dosage Selection

The extent of efficacy will depend considerably on dosage. In the past, there was an automatic tendency to reduce the dosage to half or less of prescription strength. Today, it is widely realized that dosage should not be reduced simply as a matter of course; rather, a considered judgment on optimum dosage should be made. It is being progressively appreciated by both the pharmaceutical industry and the regulatory agencies that inappropriate reduction of dosage can result in reduced efficacy with little or no safety and tolerability benefits, thus leading to needlessly ineffective treatment. The goal is to provide the lowest *effective* dose. It is vital to retain medically meaningful efficacy that will provide patients with satisfying results if self-treatment is to fulfill its proper role in the medical care system.

THE UNIQUE CHARACTERISTICS OF THE OTC FIELD FROM THE PHARMACEUTICAL PHYSICIAN'S VIEWPOINT

The role of the pharmaceutical physician in the OTC division of a major pharmaceutical company is substantially different from that played in the research or medical affairs departments dealing with prescription drugs. One might assume that OTC work is simpler and less involved than that related to prescription medications. In many ways, the opposite is true.

The OTC pharmaceutical physician must be a generalist, requiring a broad expertise in medicine, toxicology, and regulatory affairs. The OTC physician deals with a vast variety of drugs from many different areas of medicine, including some that are little taught in formal medical education. This contrasts with research on new chemical entities, where the physician generally focuses on a single therapeutic area, enjoys a large support staff that provide him/her with in-depth assistance, and uses a limited number of research protocols and techniques that can be thoroughly mastered. In contrast, the OTC physician must be an expert on smoking cessation one day, gastroenterology the next, and dermatology the next. The OTC physician must also be concerned with detailed issues of formulation and manufacturing.

The regulations governing OTC medications are substantially different from those in the prescription field, and the OTC physician is typically more involved in regulatory matters than his/her non-OTC colleagues.

Because staff are fewer and the hierarchy simpler, the OTC physician has much more general authority, with broad responsibility for in-line, new, and forthcoming products. On the prescription side, this would not be true of any job short of the Vice President of Research.

Another difference concerns marketing. Typically in the prescription area, interaction with the marketing department is infrequent, although sometimes intense. In the OTC area, it is constant. The physician educates the marketing department on medical issues surrounding a particular drug and on the opportunities and limitations that these present. In particular, the physician must understand the needs of the brand managers and be able to offer guidance. For instance, when difficulties occur in the implementation of marketing plans, the physician must be able to assist in developing alternative strategies. An OTC business is subject to intense market pressures. The physician must help the marketers deal with them effectively by frequently playing the roles of educator and creative thinker as well as medical expert.

One of the most surprising aspects of the pharmaceutical physician's role in OTC medication is the very high degree of creativity required of the physician. With prescription medication, one must work with whatever compounds have been previously developed by chemistry and toxicology. These are brought to the physician for clinical testing. There is seldom any input by the physician into drugs he/she will select to work on. Sometimes the project on which the physician will be spending years of his/her life is of considerable medical interest, in other cases it is not. No matter what the case, the physician will be able to exercise only minimal control over what compounds he/she is working on at any given time. While it is possible for the clinical development of a new chemical entity to be poorly handled, it is not possible for the clinical researcher to add any characteristic that the particular chemical entity did not possess when it was synthesized.

In contrast to this, in the OTC area, the physician is actually in a position to greatly influence the choice of compounds on which he/she and the company will do research. He/she can even creatively discover new indications suitable for OTC therapy. The OTC physician typically enjoys major input into all decisions involved in the company's commitment to particular compounds and formulations. This is true for OTC switch and for new formulations of older products. The formulators in an OTC operation seek extensive input from their medical colleagues and the corporation looks to the physician for more than just straightforward opinions. Creativity is required and he/she has an opportunity to devise concepts that are actually developed by the company.

Since the development cycle of OTC drugs is much shorter than that of prescription compounds, the physician is often able to see an idea of his/her own brought to fruition in the form of an actual product. Typically, it requires only 3 years or less for the development of an OTC drug, as opposed to 7–10 years for a new chemical entity. The skillful use of medical knowledge and its creative application to new products can make all the difference in the medical and business success of an OTC company.

The extent to which the OTC physician is a key decision-maker is especially clear in dealing with the release to market of new formulations of drugs that have monograph status. Here the pharmaceutical physician makes direct judgments on the safety and marketability of products without the intervention of a regulatory agency. The US Food and Drug Administration has provided for the direct marketing of a wide variety of OTC drugs which it has pre-approved in the so-called 'monograph' system. The underlying concept of this system is that there are many drugs that have long been on the OTC market and for which abundant information already exists. Therefore, it would be redundant and wasteful for a new NDA to be submitted

each time a new formulation of one of these compounds is to be brought to market. The FDA has provided a series of numerous monographs, each one of which deals with a particular narrow therapeutic area, ranging from acne and anthelminthics to hormones and weight control. The therapeutic area is discussed in some detail and specific requirements for well-established drugs in that area are set forth. As long as a new formulation remains within the exact requirements set forth in the monograph for type of drug, dosage, indication, and labeling statements, a compound may be formulated and marketed on the judgment of the company alone. No further pre-approval or examination of any application to the FDA is necessary. However, if the requirements set forth in the monograph for a particular compound are to be changed in any way by a different dosage, a new indication, or by changes in labeling, the formulation no longer is covered by the monograph and it is necessary to submit a full NDA. As long as the monograph requirements are strictly met, the physician in charge will make the final judgment on whether a new formulation is satisfactory for market. This system exists only in the USA and it provides for a striking amount of speed and flexibility in the OTC marketing of products.

However, it also places a very substantial amount of responsibility on the OTC physician. You can never appreciate the value of having a regulatory agency review your work and make the final decision to allow marketing until you don't have them and must take the responsibility yourself. This is particularly true with regard to the tolerability of new formulations. It is unlikely that major safety problems will arise with well-known drugs dosed at well-known levels for indications that are thoroughly understood. However, with topical drugs, where irritation and allergenicity are a problem, the judgment of suitability for market can be difficult. These drugs tend to be very dependent on the details of individual formulations and you want to be sure that you have enough information before you release them to market.

The need for specific clinical testing must be determined by the physician in each individual instance. A wide variety of situations may arise, varying from those in which no particular testing is required to those in which an extensive series of tests is needed before full confidence can be felt in a formulation. In short, the American monograph system provides unparalleled speed and flexibility of drug development for those compounds which come under it, but it requires particular vigilance on the part of the OTC physician. For all the delay and difficulty involved in obtaining approvals from FDA, it does have the major advantage that it provides a second source of learned judgment prior to the marketing of products. Even in the limited scope of monograph drugs, the physician can often find it necessary to use all his/her abilities to ensure that adequate testing is done and that careful judgments are made before individual formulations are allowed to reach the marketplace.

Because of the monograph system, one of the more striking features of OTC drug development is the speed with which new formulations may be moved from the conceptual stage to actual product realization. This contributes in a major way to the job satisfaction of the pharmaceutical physician, but it also creates a need to act with much more speed in advancing one's own portion of the development efforts. There is a need for the physician to participate in every phase of early planning of a development program. This is the only way to ensure that it is properly handled and can be quickly executed. Frequently, several companies will be moving forward with similar projects. Both commercial and personal success rely on being the first to market. Thus, the program must be planned for success on the first try. If major delays in research occur, the product will usually be so far behind competition in reaching the market that it will have little commercial value.

Several factors accelerate the entire process of research in the OTC area. Since it is much quicker and simpler for a product to remain within the monograph requirements, every effort is made to do so if it is possible. For research with monograph drugs, it is perhaps surprising to learn that an investigational new drug (IND) exemption is not always required prior to undertaking research. This is only logical, however, since for a monograph drug there is pre-approval from the FDA to actually launch the product into the market. It would not be sensible to require special pre-approval to perform human research via the IND system. This considerably speeds and simplifies the course of the research effort but again results in greater responsi-

bility for the OTC physician. The physician must ensure that the research undertaken will be complete and adequate for both safety and efficacy determination purposes and must make a solo judgment as to the safety of the research subjects involved, with no FDA oversight.

The details of the clinical research process are little different for OTC and prescription work. What changes most is the role of the pharmaceutical physician. This role is greater in scope and responsibility in the OTC area and everything must be done with greater speed.

PRESCRIPTION-TO-OTC SWITCH

One of the most dynamic areas in the pharmaceutical industry today is the prescription-to-OTC switch, commonly called the *Rx-to-OTC switch.* This is the process by which a drug that has previously been used only by prescription is converted to self-medication status. We have already considered the criteria for OTC use of medications and these criteria represent a sound guide to determining what drugs are suitable for switching. There are no hard and fast guidelines for determining which drugs may become suitable for OTC switch, but a consideration of self-diagnosability of the disease state to be treated, the general safety and tolerability of the drug, its ability to show efficacy in the hands of non-professionals, and a relative absence of problems with masking of symptoms all contribute to making a drug more OTC-able.

The first question that arises when considering the possibility of an OTC switch is, why has the drug not been available OTC before and what can be done to remove the obstruction? It is possible that a drug may simply not have had adequate prescription experience in the past. It takes time to accumulate a substantial use database of real-world experience. This is essential to make it possible to form a judgment about safety in prescription use and, therefore, projected safety in OTC use. What constitutes substantial use is always a relative matter. Typically, at least 3 years of data accumulation with a widely marketed drug is required to be able to feel some security in making judgments from the adverse reaction database accumulated. For small selling drugs, this can easily take 10 years or more. The fewer problems this database reveals, the better the drug will be as a switch candidate.

It is sometimes possible to accelerate the accumulation of data for a promising OTC candidate by specialized Phase IV studies. These studies accelerate the process of data collection by conducting what amounts to a survey amongst physicians using the drug on a prescription basis. Since the sole interest is the gathering of adverse reaction data, with special emphasis on rare and serious events, record forms are kept very minimal, often to a single page. The study design consists simply of a survey, done without control groups. Hundreds of physicians, or even thousands, must be contacted to participate in the survey by submitting brief record forms on patients they treat in their usual manner with the prescription drug. Such a survey can rapidly provide a much more reliable database than spontaneous reporting. With a survey, you get both a frequency of the various side effects and a reasonable estimate of the number of patients treated, which permits the calculation of accurate rates for the adverse effects observed. This is in marked contrast to the data obtained from an entirely spontaneous adverse reaction database, where it is impossible to determine what the efficiency of reporting is. Therefore, it is extremely difficult to estimate correct rates of occurrence of individual adverse effects. The spontaneous databases are more useful for the qualitative evaluation of what can happen with a drug than for the quantitative evaluation of its true frequency. This type of adverse reaction survey study can pave the way for a switch effort in much less time than needed if reliance is placed solely on spontaneous reports for collection of data.

If the principal barrier to switch has been a lack of clinical experience with a drug, this can be remedied by the collection of a large adverse reaction database. Once this is done, it is usually straightforward to establish that the drug is safe in prescription use. This is a major advance on the road to OTC approval, but it certainly does not yet prove that the drug will be safe and effective in the hands of consumers without the benefit of a learned intermediary. In order to establish this additional point, it is almost always necessary to supplement the analysis of adverse reaction databases with clinical studies in realistic conditions, using the labeling composed for the OTC product.

We will discuss the peculiar aspects of the design of clinical studies suitable for such purposes later, but for now it is sufficient to note that they may usually proceed with the objectives of establishing efficacy and common side effects only, and that very rare side effects have already been evaluated in the prescription use setting.

Regardless of the reasons underlying a drug's prescription-only status, once a decision is taken that a drug should be moved OTC, it is extremely important to get early interaction with the regulatory agencies. This can establish at an early stage whether or not they have concerns that the company has not yet considered. The obvious concerns of safety and efficacy are not always the principal issues obstructing a switch. It is possible in some cases that FDA has no concerns in these two areas, but that self-medication use is prevented by some other peripheral but still highly important consideration. Examples of such problems are indications which the FDA does not regard as self-diagnosable, and such problems as spread of antibiotic resistance by OTC use of an antibiotic that might adversely affect the overall public health picture.

It should be remembered that FDA's principal concern in considering an Rx-to-OTC switch is from a public health perspective. This is in contrast to the usual viewpoint of the pharmaceutical companies, which tends to be focused on the treatment of the individual patient. The FDA's positions may be better understood by remembering that they tend to take the big picture, whereas the pharmaceutical company tends to concentrate on narrower issues. There is nothing that will facilitate the Rx-to-OTC switch of a drug more powerfully than convincing the Agency that its OTC availability will benefit public health.

Other issues that may concern the FDA far more than the industry, are precedent-setting issues. The FDA functions in an environment in which they have ongoing responsibility for the approval and switch of many different types of drugs. They may feel that the precedent set by a particular switch could be damaging in terms of their overall policy posture, even though they have relatively little concern about the switch itself. If this is the situation, careful negotiation with the FDA and care in how the switch is presented to minimize setting an awkward precedent can often resolve the issue.

Another broad-scale public health concern which may worry the FDA is the implied message given to the consumer by the OTC availability of a particular compound. This concern is illustrated by the situation with soluble fiber cholesterol-lowering agents of the psyllium type. These agents have been shown to lower cholesterol, but only to a very small degree. It was felt by the FDA that, if they become established with claims of cholesterol reduction, the population may be misled into feeling that they have made major inroads into their cholesterol problems when, in fact, they have not. The message communicated to the consumer by making these compounds available constituted a barrier to this use.

Early negotiation with the FDA will assist in identifying their concerns and will help in obtaining their insight into the types of studies required to resolve the difficulties presented by any given case. The skill of the regulatory department in structuring and presenting a switch proposal is vital to its success.

The timing of an Rx-to-OTC switch project is always a major contributor to its success. The timing is influenced by both regulatory and commercial considerations. The completeness of the available database is critical and can set the timing of a switch. Often, however, the key factor in deciding when a switch effort should begin will be commercial. This involves the major benefits to a company in moving a drug to OTC status at approximately the same time as its patent expires. By doing this, the company may greatly mitigate the loss of patent protection. A switch can offset the precipitous decline in the innovator's share of the Rx market. At this difficult time for a company, nothing is welcomed more than the rapid growth of an OTC market that, in some cases, can be even larger than the original prescription sales. Typically, once a drug has gone OTC, it is sold at a lower price with smaller profit margins, but the total volume tends to increase several-fold. The result can be a highly favorable economic situation for the company.

Unfortunately, in many cases, a switch at the time of patent expiration does not occur and a long delay intervenes before OTC status is reached. This is generally due to the tendency within companies to seriously examine the need for an OTC switch only a year or two before patent expiration looms. This

will be too late to complete the necessary studies and regulatory applications in time for a smooth transition. In order to make a seamless transition at the time of greatest opportunity for a company, it is necessary to plan for the OTC switch many years in advance. Nothing can substitute for an awareness of the OTC potential of the company's portfolio of drugs so that suitable programs can be designed and put into action on a timely basis.

There are two fundamentally different types of Rx-to-OTC switches from the standpoint of the scope of the research program required. Switch programs can vary from large NDA programs as extensive and expensive as anything found in the new chemical entity development, to programs consisting of little more than a single study. What influences the basic size and expense for an Rx-to-OTC switch is whether or not you propose to change either the indication or the dose of the drug when you bring it into the OTC market. If the indication or the dose is to be changed, you will be involved with an entirely new NDA, which is needed to show the fundamental efficacy and safety of the drug, either at its new dose or in its new indication. Such a program obviously will require several years and involve extensive expenditure. In startling contrast to this are the programs of modest size often required for the switch of drugs that will be taken into the OTC market at their existing prescription dosage and for their existing prescription indications. Here, the regulatory agencies will generally accept the concept that there is no need to prove again the basic safety and efficacy of the drug, because this has already been done in the primary new chemical entity NDA. Such a repetition would not provide useful new data. What will be required is an actual use study, to show that the proposed labeling for OTC use is effective in enabling patients to use the drug properly. Also, it may be necessary to address whatever specific factor it is that has been previously obstructing the drug from OTC use. For example, if there is a question as to whether the prescription indication that will now be taken OTC is self-diagnosable, then a study of self-diagnosis will be required. This occurred with the vaginal anti-fungal compounds, which were long kept on prescription status because of questions as to whether women could effectively diagnose vaginal candidiasis themselves. Only a single study was required to resolve this issue. It was extremely unusual for the pharmaceutical industry, in that it involved no drugs of any kind. It was simply a study of women's ability to self-diagnose but it resolved the one outstanding issue that had blocked OTC approval.

The time required to carry out studies on such special questions can vary, considerably depending on the complexity of the question. However, it is typically a brief program and its budget is commonly small by the standards of the pharmaceutical industry. It is obvious that in the planning and preparation of a switch program, it is essential not to assume that a full safety and efficacy program will be required. Rather, early communication with the regulatory agencies is needed in order to establish what barriers actually exist.

SPECIAL STUDY DESIGNS FOR THE OTC AREA

The philosophy for OTC study design is significantly different from that of prescription medication studies. With prescription medications, you are typically striving to answer the basic scientific questions of 'can this drug work effectively?' and 'is it safe to administer to people?'. Therefore, it is appropriate to study these new chemical entities primarily in controlled settings with extensive inclusion and exclusion criteria. This provides increased safety for the study participants, who will be using a drug of relatively unknown toxicity, and allows a reduction in the inherent variability of the study population, so as to obtain a clearer scientific answer to the questions of basic safety and efficacy. Every effort is made in studies of this type to control for all possible variables and to reduce random real-world circumstances to a minimum.

In the case of drugs being prepared for the self-medication market, just the opposite sort of philosophy applies. In this situation, a great deal of evidence is already available about the abstract safety and efficacy of the drug. Its basic ability to function has already been well established or it would not have been approved in the first place. The key issue in the switch of drugs is to establish whether the drug can work in the real-world context, with all the inherent happenstance and randomness that implies.

Realism is the key to OTC research design. The best OTC studies are often called 'slice-of-life' studies. This communicates effectively the idea that you want to get a realistic real world impression of what the drug will do when subjected to all the variables of an actual use setting. In order to achieve this, selection criteria should be minimized rather than maximized. You want to study the same kind of population that will come into drug stores and even into supermarkets and actually buy this drug. Eliminating large segments of this population by strict admission criteria will only produce a result that is redundant of what has been previously demonstrated and which is not relevant to the actual conditions of use the drug will encounter. Every effort should be made to simulate the way in which patients will actually use the drug. In some cases, it is even known to go so far as to actually have patients pay for the drug in order to obtain the motivational factors associated with a purchase. This illustrates the degree to which some studies go to ensure that they're actually studying the conditions of use and not some artificial situation which is set up for the study and may give seriously misleading results. In the same philosophical vein, it is important to design the study for minimum interference with the patient. He/She must be left free to act, guided only by the labeling. Excessive intervention by the investigator will distort the results.

Some may react to studies of this type by feeling that they are unscientific. Actually, they are just addressing a different question. What is important to remember is what hypothesis is being tested. At the stage where a drug is being considered for a switch, the question is, 'What impact will this drug have on the public health as it will really be used by the lay public?'. This is the question that the FDA needs answered. Excessively controlled study designs will only detract from the studies' relevance.

These studies are tests of the labeling as much as they are tests of the drug itself. It is essential that the combination of the drug and its OTC labeling work closely together to enable patients to self-medicate effectively. One should never study an OTC drug as the pharmaceutical substance alone, but always as the combination of the labeling and the pharmaceutical. It follows, then, that the development of this labeling is very important for OTC use. It may, in fact, make the entire difference between a drug being a switch candidate and remaining on prescription status indefinitely. Not only is a great deal of creativity necessary in developing effective labeling but appropriate label comprehension studies are also important in ensuring that the best labeling is obtained.

Research has shown that patients by and large do read labeling and they do heed it, particularly with new drugs that they have not used before. Prior to any program being advanced to the stage of the definitive clinical studies, it is wise to develop a variety of different versions of the proposed labeling, so that these versions can be tested in label comprehension studies. These studies are sometimes organized by the medical department and sometimes they are carried out as market research, since they need not involve actual ingestion of drug. They consist of comparative studies in which patients in a realistic setting read the proposed labeling and then are quizzed on their comprehension of it. In this way, it is possible to see whether they understand how the drug ought to be used and whether they have understood key precautions. It is best to check both short-term and long-term comprehension to see how well the patients are able to remember what they have learned. This sort of pre-screening of labeling can be absolutely essential to success and it has saved many careers by avoiding disasters in large-scale definitive studies.

MARKET SUPPORT STUDIES

In addition to the Rx-to-OTC switch, a second type of study is very prominent in the OTC area. This is the market support study. These are clinical studies intended to demonstrate particular advantages of one company's drug over another's, or of one particular formulation of the same drug over other competitors. Opportunities for demonstrating such advantages depend on locating genuine differences that can be successfully studied. While anything can be tried in a clinical study, only authentic differences will emerge as successful claims at the end of the study process. Locating such possible advantages can be done through careful attention to feedback from actual users of the drug. Usage and attitudes (U and A studies) studies done by the

marketing department and focus group sessions can be invaluable in discovering the possible existence of advantages for a particular formulation over its competitors. Careful review of the pharmacologic literature is another way in which differences can be detected. Even small differences may be quite meaningful to patients, even though they may appear minor to the pharmacologist, who is not actually using the drug him/herself. In the case of an anti-nausea drug, for example, a difference in onset of action of 10–15 min can be highly significant if you're the one suffering from the nausea. Therefore, a careful review of literature can often find pharmacokinetic and other differences that can be more meaningful than they at first appear. Any difference that is not meaningful to the patients will not produce much difference in sales. In selecting market support opportunities for study, it is important to manage expectations so that the marketing group can understand that only real differences that are meaningful to the patient and can be demonstrated with reasonable certainty in clinical trials are worth pursuing. If expectations are allowed to grow out-of-hand, one will find oneself designing studies for the most bizarre purposes and encountering a very high rate of failure, because you're chasing after advantages that never existed in the first place.

Once a probable new claim has been identified and the chances of its being scientifically valid have been assessed, you must carry out actual studies to support the claim. In most situations, two-good quality studies are necessary to support an advertising claim, even though these are not necessarily regulated by the FDA. In some special situations, a single study may be enough. Guidance on this issue may be taken from the company's legal department.

To understand what will be needed to support a claim, it is important to understand how the advertising and marketing of OTC drugs is regulated. Typically, after a brief initial period, the FDA does not take a primary role in such regulation. Rather, this duty passes to the Federal Trade Commission and, much more importantly, to the federal courts. The OTC industry's advertising claims tend to be self-enforcing. The companies maintain a close vigilance on each other's advertising and tend to be eager to sue their competitors in the federal courts if any unsupportable advertising claims are suspected. The possession of scientifically sound studies is of great value in preventing lawsuits and ensuring that if they do occur, they will be won.

Although the pharmaceutical physician rarely pictures him/herself as a person testifying in lawsuits, this is not an uncommon experience for the OTC medical director. This need not be viewed with any particular trepidation if you have been careful to prepare a satisfactory scientific basis for the advertising claims that you have approved.

In summary, the role of the OTC physician is significantly different from that of the pharmaceutical physician working in any other area of the industry. It requires a greater degree of creativity and independence. It features a different kind of responsibility, since there is no other physician between you and the patient to share that responsibility with. One is more completely on one's own and called upon to utilize an expertise which is broader than that required of the physician in virtually any other area of pharmaceutical development.

Section III

Special Populations

Introduction to section III

Lionel D. Edwards

Pharma proplus INC and Novartis, New Jersey, USA

In 1993, the US Food and Drug Administration (FDA), Europe's Committee for Proprietary Medicinal Products (CPMP) and Japan's Ministries of Health and Welfare (MOHW) issued regulatory requirements for testing and labeling in a 'special population', namely the elderly. These were not promulgated in isolation but after consultation with academia and industry. In the USA, initially this was done under the auspices of the American Society of Clinical Pharmacology and Therapeutics. Industry was allowed to participate and was largely credited with aiding the process. The First International Conference on Harmonization (ICH) held in Europe (November 5–7 1991), again involved the regulators and the regulated and, for the first time, involved Japan as a major contributor. As a result of pre-, during-, and postconference discussions, success was achieved. The 'elderly' drug guidance was the forerunner of many future tripartite agreements in the clinical area.

The special populations covered in the following chapters include the four major demographic segments: the elderly, women, children and major ethnic groups. While any smaller grouping of people or diseases may be labeled 'special', such may be better described as 'orphan' populations, which are the subject of discussions elsewhere in this book (see Chapter 16). The four major demographic segments were designated 'special populations' because, despite the large size of each segment (globally, women constitute 51% of the population), pharmaceutical research has been sparse in these groups. The basis for this is multifactorial. Different responses to needs and medicinal interventions, compared with that in the white male population, have been only sporadically addressed by the research, academic, and industry pharmaceutical development communities.

In general, globally and especially in the USA, legislation controlling food and drugs (including devices and biologics) has been stimulated by therapeutic disasters. This, in the USA, caused the implementation of the Food, Drug and Cosmetic Act of 1906, which outlawed the practice of embalming meat for consumption. Further disasters triggered subsequent multiple amendments to the Act.

In special populations, perceived omissions of research and development have also resulted in specific amendments to this Act. On occasion, these amendments have been due to political pressure from special advocate groups, rather than due to a specific therapeutic disaster.

Why did industry ignore these special populations, which represent major markets? First, the costs of additional research would add to the already enormous cost of drug and devices research. Second, the ever-present fear of litigation resulting from perceived exploitation, coercion, and vulnerability of these special populations discouraged industry and the FDA from policies of inclusion.

Other influences determining research directions in drugs and devices were paternalism (protectionism) and the money available for grant projects, guided by the numerical male dominance in the reviewing process of research priorities.

For the pharmaceutical industry, it is ironic that attention to these special populations is now proving 'good business', either because of an extension of protected patent life, or because of the development of special business units. These units have increased market penetration and retention of drugs for third-party reimbursement and allowed niche dominance. The latest of the four major special populations rulings by ICH, the final rule on Acceptability of Foreign Data, was implemented in July 1998. While it is the latest, it will not be the last—the future impact of the genome project on each of these major demographic segments, and its influence on genomic pharmacology and gene therapy with regard to these 'special populations', has yet to be felt.

Each chapter will give a limited historical context. The chapters dealing with drug development in women (chapter 15) and ethnic populations (chapter 29) explore issues of physiology and metabolism in detail, because of the societal sensitivity and because of a relative paucity of data in the literature.

The chapters on geriatrics and pediatrics (chapters 14 and 16) focus mainly on the evolution and requirements of the drug development process, because data on the physiology and metabolism of these groups are both widely known and available in the literature.

14

Drug Research in Older Patients

Lionel D. Edwards

Basking Ridge, NJ, USA

DEMOGRAPHICS

The elderly (over 64 years old) comprise 12% of the US population and 17% of Sweden and Japan. This sector continues to grow. In the USA it, is estimated that the elderly population will grow to 14% by the year 2010 and reach 17% by 2030 (US Bureau of the Census 1996). This, together with their known sensitivity to medications (Everitt and Avorn 1986), contributed to acceptance by industry of additional requirements for testing in the elderly.

The US Bureau of the Census, International Database (1996) (National Center for Health Statistics 1996) projected that, for the year 2020, the less developed countries would contain only 16.4% of the world population compared to 27.1% in 1996, and that by 2020 the mean age of the population in more developed countries would be 42 years, up from 36 years in 1996. In developed regions, the elderly would outnumber young children by 8:1, e.g. in Italy, based on current fertility and survival rates, only 2% of the population would be 5 years or younger, but 40% would be 65 years and older.

There were even more startling projections by the United Nations International Population Division (1996). They projected life expectancy in the 'developed' countries to reach 81 years by 2050. For less developed countries, this would still reach 76 years. However, this increase in the global elderly population would be proportionally offset by a decrease in fertility rate, now under way, from 1.7 births/woman down to 1.4 in the Western world. This is below the replacement rate. For Second World regions, the rate of about 3.3 births/woman would decline to 1.6. Even in the least developed (Third World) countries, 5 births/woman would fall to 2 by 2050. Thus, the whole world would actually start to 'depopulate' in 40 years.

The social and healthcare impact of these demographics in the USA and globally will lead to an increased demand for better medicines directed at a healthy old age. This elderly population have more income than average per capita income. In addition, with more time on their hands to lobby, they are more likely to vote, and can be expected to use their political muscle to make demands on their governments. The governments will respond in the usual knee-jerk reaction—'more regulations and controls' on industry—while increasing funding for academic research aimed at improving the quality of life and the prolongation of active old age. It will be interesting to see whether a more extended life expectancy, over and above the current projections, will reverse the depopulation trend.

IMPACT ON SOCIETY OF AN AGING POPULATION

In developed countries, by 2020, the working population aged 15–65 years will fall from 22% in 1996 to 16%. Those aged 65 years and over will increase to 20% from 16% (US Bureau of Census 1996). In the USA, 60 years ago, the retirement age for Social Security 'pension' was designed for an expected average lifespan of 65 years. Already this has been pushed back to 67 years by year 2004, and additional legislation will probably push the age requirements back to 70 in 10 years' time, when the 'baby boomers' swell the retired population.

To encourage the healthy older person to continue working beyond 65 years, legislation was passed to remove the penalty (in workers 65–70 years) of the loss of $1 for every $3 earned from Social Security benefits in the US. In 1999 it was

Principles and Practice of Pharmaceutical Medicine. Edited by A. J. Fletcher, Lionel D. Edwards, Anthony W. Fox and Peter Stonier © 2002 John Wiley & Sons Ltd.

proposed that, because of the high cost of medication and because the older people were the greatest
users, they be eligible for drug cost reimbursement
under Medicaid. This would give the US Government reimbursement control on over 58% of drugs
prescribed and the power to 'set prices', as in other
countries (e.g. Canada, the UK, France, Italy, Germany). This has sent a chill through the US
pharmaceutical industry.

Of great concern is the social and financial
impact of Alzheimer's disease, whose incidence
per capita increases to 32% of the surviving population at ages 80–85 (and declines rapidly after age
85). Many live with this disease for 5–8 years before
succumbing. This causes enormous detriment to
the surviving spouse and family and to family
finances, and must eventually impact Medicaid
and Medicare Federal and State budgets. The duration of financial burden of terminal care is 1–4
months in general (1–18 months for Alzheimer's
patients) and, even with what would normally be
an adequate pension, this burden can financially
ruin the surviving spouse.

Immigration from the Third World to the developed countries will increase as countries of
aging populations try to replace the loss of their
labor pool. This is already happening in Europe
and in the USA. This again will put further pressure on Medicare and Medicaid, as many of these
immigrants will suffer from tuberculosis, hepatitis,
and intestinal disease, endemic to many of their
home countries. In 1997, 39% of tuberculosis
cases in the USA were in foreign-born parents; in
California this rose to 67% (Satcher, 1999) and the
annual cost of diagnosis and treatment of the 1 million immigrants was $40 million (Muenning et al
1999). This will cause further competition for available health dollars.

PRESCRIBING AND ADVERSE EVENTS

Studies of drug utilization in the elderly showed
that older people receive disproportionate amounts
of medication (Rochon and Gurwitz 1995). A
study in rural persons 65 years or older showed
that, of 967 interviewed, 71% took at least one
prescription drug and 10% took five or more prescription medications. Again, women took more
medications than men, and in both groups the

number of drugs increased with age. The elderly
comprised 18% of the population but received 45%
of all prescription items (Lassila, Stoehrt Gangula
1996).

One in 10 admissions to acute geriatric units were
caused or partly caused by adverse drug reactions.
The drugs involved most commonly were benzodiazepines, warfarin, digoxin, and non-steroid anti-
inflammatories (Deaham and Barnett 1998). Tamblyn (1996), in his review article, cited reports of
adverse events causing 5–23% of hospitalizations,
nearly 2% of ambulatory visits and 1 in 1000 deaths
in the general population. These rates increase in the
elderly. Errors in prescribing accounted for 19–36%
of hospital admissions due to drug-related adverse
events.

To compound this worrying situation, there is
the concomitant use of over-the-counter (OTC)
non-prescription drugs. Only 50% of physicians
or health workers ask about OTC drug use, yet
40% of all drugs used by the elderly are non-
prescription drugs. In all, 69% of the elderly use
OTC drugs and 70% take at least one prescription,
as described earlier. In addition, 31% take alcohol
frequently (Conn 1992).

This new potential for adverse drug interaction is
enormous. NSAIDs and aspirin interact with anticoagulants such as warfarin or coumadin, can increase the bleeding tendency, and not just from the
stomach. Antacids can decrease the excretion of
antidepressant tricyclics, quinidine, pseudoephi-
drine and indomethacin. They can also reduce the
absorption of digoxin and β-blocker hypertensive
medication. These are only a few of the multitude
of interactive drug effects. This is imposed upon the
reduced efficacy of hepatic metabolism and elimination, and renal excretion in the elderly; thus, drug
OTC use can add to the recipe for toxic drug accumulation and, in the latter case of antacids, cause
further damage to the kidney by loss of blood
pressure control and worsening cardiac failure.

PRACTICAL AND ETHICAL ISSUES OF DRUG RESEARCH IN OLDER POPULATIONS

Traditionally, elderly subjects were frequently excluded from clinical drug development (unless the
disease being treated was more prevalent in that

age group). The reasons given were that the elderly suffer from too many other diseases, require concomitant medicines, are more frail, and are more vulnerable to adverse events. All these can cause 'static' in the interpretation of the data, and give undue weighting to adverse events in the labeling and product package insert.

In addition, the elderly can exhibit differences, both physiologically and pathologically compared with the younger population; the contrast in speed of disease progression of prostate cancer in the 'younger elderly' compared to the slow rate in the 'older old', is an example.

The elderly are often confused or demented, making informed consent and their continuation in a study questionable. Lastly, because the elderly indication may represent only a small use of a drug, it is uneconomic to include the elderly in a drug's development program. These are often the perceived concerns of both investigators and pharmaceutical firms.

What is 'geriatric'? Strictly defined, it describes a person aged 65 years or over, but aging is neither a homogeneous nor a linear process. There are very fit 80 year-olds who climb mountains, and young children dying from genetic advanced aging (progeria). The elderly therefore cover a spectrum of fitness. So many of the above concerns can be reduced by selecting 'uncomplicated, healthy' older patients in Phase I studies, who are increasingly available due to the success of medicines and preventative medicine.

However, there is a need to know how medicines behave in the real world—not just their interactions with other medicines, but in other disease states suffered concurrently, which is often the case in a geriatric population and less so in younger age groups.

For the elderly, of equal importance to life extension and cure is improvement or preservation of their activities. Thus, the results of quality of life, disease outcomes and pharmacoeconomic studies are of even greater relevance to this special population and to third-party payers.

REGULATORY RESPONSE

By the 1980s, most of the new medicines still had little or no information on elderly dosing or contained disclaimers. As a result of this, and the fact that 30% of prescription drugs by then were consumed by just 12% of the population (those over 65 years), a new guideline was issued. Thus, the FDA *Guideline on Drug Development in the Elderly* (1990) recommended that, if a drug was likely to have significant use in the elderly, then studies should be done in an elderly population. These studies should look at effectiveness and adverse events by age. In addition, other studies should determine whether older people handle the new drug differently (a 30% decrease in renal excretion and liver metabolism is normal in a healthy elderly person). This guideline also required studies of the pharmacokinetics and, where possible, pharmacodynamic studies of the new drug in the elderly. The *Guideline* also urged the study of possible drug interactions with drugs commonly used concurrently in this age group. Digoxin was given as an example. Looking even further forward to the future, the *Guideline* encouraged the inclusion of patients over 75 years.

Medicines in the elderly had become a world issue and, in 1994, the FDA implemented the ICH tripartite guidance, *Studies in Support of Special Populations: Geriatrics* (*Fed Reg* August 1994). The agency followed up with specific requirements on content and format of labeling for human prescription drugs; addition of a 'Geriatric Use' subsection in labeling (*Fed Reg* August 1997). This set out priority implementation lists of drug categories for information in geriatric population and gave the industry 1 year to comply. It also set out the specific content and format of wording to be used.

OVERVIEW OF INTERNATIONAL HARMONIZATION CONFERENCE GUIDELINES

This guideline was very similar to the 1990 FDA guideline in intent. It requested that:

1. Studies should be done in new molecular entities (NMEs) or new chemical entities (NCEs) likely to be used in the elderly, either to treat a disease of aging or because the disease is also common in the elderly.

2. Studies should include patients 65 years and older, and preferably patients aged 75 or older, and advised against arbitrary age cutoff (patients aged 60–65 are not considered elderly).

3. Meaningful numbers, especially in Phase III: a minimum of 100 patients was suggested for a non-geriatric specific disease (e.g. hypertension).

4. Analysis of the database for age-related differences of efficacy, adverse events, dose, and (gender) relationships. A geriatric database may contain data from the main Phase II, III studies or from a geriatric-specific study.

5. Pharmacokinetic studies (PK), either formal pharmacokinetic studies or on a population basis. For the latter, a blood sample is taken from many patients on up to four occasions. The time of dosing is recorded, and the time of samples. The patients must be at 'steady state'. This way, an adequate population PK plot can be built.

6. Pharmacokinetic studies in renal impaired patients if the drug or metabolites are renally excreted. If the NME is excreted and/or metabolized by the liver, a hepatic-impaired study should be undertaken. These studies do not have to be done in elderly patients (they are usually done on a new NME anyway).

7. Usually, differences in the therapeutic response or adverse events are too small to detect at an equivalent plasma level between ordinary adult and elderly patients to make this a requirement. However, separate studies are requested of sedative hypnotic psychoactive drugs or drugs having a significant CNS effect, and, similarly, if Phase II, III studies are suggestive of an age-related difference.

8. Drug interaction studies should be done on digoxin and oral anticoagulants, for these drugs have a narrow therapeutic range and are commonly prescribed in the elderly. These drugs frequently have their serum levels altered by other drugs. Where drugs are heavily metabolized by the liver, the effect of drug enzyme inducers and inhibitors should be explored. Similarly, drugs which will share the same cytochrome P450 enzyme pathways should be tested. Ketoconazole, macrolides, and quinidine are given as examples. Finally, other common drugs most likely to be used with the test drug are recommended to be explored for possible synergistic or antagonistic drug interactions.

INDUSTRY RESPONSE

A survey conducted by the FDA in 1983 (Abrams, 1993) showed that, for 11 drugs recently approved or awaiting approval of New Drug Applications, in seven applications 30–36% of patients were aged over 60. In one application, a study on a drug for prostate cancer, 76% of patients were, not surprisingly, over 60 years old (Everitt and Avorn 1986). An additional survey by the FDA in 1988 of 20 NDAs showed similar results but, in addition, analysis by age and pharmacokinetic studies in the elderly were frequently included. A survey by the Pharmaceutical Research and Manufacturers of America (PhRMA) (Mossinghoff, 1995) showed that 132 medicines were being studied for potential use in the elderly in 157 indications.

A private survey of 19 pharmaceutical companies operating in the USA (Chaponis, 1998) ranked cardiovascular, depression, Alzheimer hypertension, rheumatoid arthritis osteoarthritis, and oncology as the most important therapeutic areas in their company. All of these are commonly found in the elderly. Why did companies target these therapeutic areas in the geriatric population? This drew the response: 'It's a growing population,' from 77% of respondents, and 'increasing market size' from 58% of the 27 company respondents. Companies were asked which types of geriatric-based clinical trials they conducted. Safety, efficacy, pharmacokinetic- and drug interaction studies were quoted in that order of frequency, which, because of the introduction of the guidelines, is to be expected. However, the next most frequent studies were quality-of-life, pharmacoeconomic, drug disease (outcomes) and patient satisfaction studies. The later studies reflect the elderly and third-party payers' influences (Chaponis 1998). In its 1999 survey, PhRMA reported that over 600 medicines were then being developed for diseases of aging. This reflects the increasing importance of medicines for the graying population of America.

ISSUES OF DISEASES IN THE ELDERLY

Heart failure is a leading cause of hospitalization of the elderly. About 5 million Americans suffer from this disease, which has a high mortality rate. Control of blood pressure, use of β-blockers, ACE inhibitors, and now spironolactone (Pitt et al 1999) will result in further improvement of mortality which have started to fall from 117 per 110 000 in 1988 to 108 in 1995, according to the Center for Disease Control and Prevention (CDC).

Because of its severity, patients are on many concomitant medications apart from the aforementioned drugs, such as diuretics, digoxin, potassium supplements, medicines to improve pulmonary function, and antibiotics to control frequent infection in edematous and often emphysematous lungs. Measurements of heart function, and the long duration of these studies and large patient numbers required for mild to moderate heart failure (endpoint death), make these very challenging and expensive studies.

Hypertension affects about 50% of the elderly population. There is also a unique form called isolated systolic hypertension, which affects 9% of the geriatric population and is growing as the population ages. The challenges of doing studies in this area increase with the age of patients admitted, which correlates with increased concomitant medications and illness and compliance, but otherwise relates well to study designs in the younger age group.

Stroke thrombotic or hemorhagic is the third leading cause of death, killing 160 000 persons in the USA each year, Seven out of 10 victims are aged 65 or older. Of those that survive, one-third will be permanently disabled. Some improvements in these figures are hoped for, with earlier use of thrombolytics in case of cerebral thrombosis. As of 1999, over 20 new drugs were in development to treat this condition.

Arthritis causing inflammatory and degenerative changes around joints affects 43 million in the USA, and CDC projects that this will rise to 60 million by 2020. It can be caused by over 100 different diseases, but the commonest is osteoarthritis and rheumatoid arthritis. New medications, such as the antitumor necrotic factor α-blockers, raise fresh challenges to clinical study methodology because of limitations on non-clinical toxicity predictors and the application of biologic measurements on a traditional drug appraisal system.

The new non-steroidal anti-inflammatory drugs, including the Cox II inhibitors, because of the vast range of arthritic diseases, require that careful selection of indications for initial product approval must be undertaken. Rarely do companies have the time or money to develop all the pain indications (acute, chronic use) or to study arthritic diseases prior to product launch. As with hypertension, the numbers of patients required in the database will be large for product approval, especially for safety.

Depression is a frequently missed diagnosis in the elderly. The Alliance for Aging Research says that 15% of Americans aged 65 years and older experience clinically relevant depression. It can amplify the underlying disabilities in stroke, arthritis, Parkinson's disease, slow or prevent recovery from hip fracture and surgery, and be mimicked or masked by an underactive thyroid. The latest receptor-specific medicines have a very much reduced potential for adverse events and drug interactions. Difficulties can arise from confusion, memory impairment and disorientation, which are common in the depressed elderly. This brings challenges of ensuring both drug compliance and follow-up attendance in clinical studies. It also may require guardian co-signature for informed witnessed consent.

Parkinson's disease affects more than 1 million Americans and about four in every 100 by 75 years of age. Ten new drugs are under development. The patients may become very physically disabled but still retain a clear sensorium until the very end stages of the disease. Thus, drug compliance and follow-up visits are easier to achieve than with Alzheimer or depressed patients.

Alzheimer's disease is the eighth leading cause of death in the elderly and already affects some 4 million Americans. The incidence rises from 2% at 65 years to 32% at age 85. The National Institute of Health estimates that at least half of the people in nursing homes have this disease. A small study of donezil showed that this treatment avoided the need for home nursing care by half compared to those who did not receive the medicine (Small, 1998).

Clinical studies in this disease are very expensive, often requiring several collaborating disciplines at each investigative site. A gerontologist, a neurologist, a psychologist and a psychiatrist may be required, in addition to the usual support staff. Multiple cognitive tests and behavioral ratings of the patient often involving primary caregiver ratings, will be required—all this in addition to the basic Alzheimer's Disease Assessment Scale (ADAS–COG). These studies at present require large numbers of patients to show the often small improvement, as well as months of observation to detect a slowing of progression.

ISSUES IN THE CONDUCT OF CLINICAL STUDIES IN THE ELDERLY

Informed Consent

In general, the principles are no different with the elderly than with other adult persons; the elderly are just as subject to the relationship to the researcher if the clinician and researcher are one and the same. Not wishing to offend (by refusal) is very strong in the elderly, and also they are also subject to 'therapeutic fallacy', i.e. they find it hard to accept that, despite repeated descriptions of risks and possible benefits, the treating physician could be really offering them treatment of uncertain benefit or risk. The elderly are more likely to have cognitive impairment or mild dementia, and to be living alone, in poverty, or under institutional care. They are also vulnerable to caregiver abuse, often because of indifference, anger, or physical abuse triggered by the patients' behavior and difficulties derived from their disease.

Hearing or vision problems must be expected; bright light and large print, together with honest and simple language, much used for eliciting the informed consent. Research subjects, whether elderly or not, should be able to understand the informed consent process, feel free to refuse or to withdraw from the study without reprisal, and understand the uncertain outcomes of the new drug, the use of placebo and the random allocation of treatment.

The most vulnerable elderly population is found in nursing homes or mental institutions and frequently comprises persons of diminished or fluctuating mental ability. Ironically, regulations governing research in these patients were proposed but never voted upon. The NIH established a policy which allowed a patient, when he/she was still in good cognitive condition, to appoint a 'Health Care Agent'.

For industry, prior written agreement of a family member with the potential subject to act as 'guardian' is preferred but not always attainable. It is best for the researcher him/herself to meet with relatives, nursing staff, and residents and fully explain to them the study purpose, benefit and risks, as well as to the patient. Not infrequently, any of these persons may feel protective of the patient and undermine the research objective. It is wise that all family members who are not involved be sent a letter explaining the research, including a form to be completed if they wish to prevent the patient being involved in research.

Compliance

Compliance in the elderly in general is similar to that of the general population. If more than six drugs are prescribed long-term, or more than three doses/day are required, then compliance will suffer (Blackwell, 1979; Gately, 1968). These factors are more common in the elderly. Recommendations for improving compliance in older patients are similar to any other studies, except for one—that the physician should set priorities for which medications are critical to patients' health in a polypharmacy setting. The medication regimens should be as simple as possible; the caregiver and patient should be educated about the name, dose, and reason for all medications. Patients should be given simple instructions on cards, together with suggestions on how to remind themselves—'tick-off cards on fridge', 'diary notes' on bathroom mirror for morning dose, or on pantry door 'with food', etc. Patients and their caregivers should be given educational pamphlets about their diseases. They should be encouraged to ask questions or report possible adverse events or strange feelings. Patients should be asked to repeat back instructions. Lastly, there are telephone call services which will call and remind patients to take the medicine, or help organize cabs or transport for follow-up visits, either to the laboratories for blood work, etc., or to the investigator appointments.

Screening and Recruitment

The Chaponis (1998) survey of 19 USA-based companies reported also that 32% reported difficulty in finding suitable investigative sites for geriatric patients. In addition, those respondents involved in Phase IV outcomes, quality-of-life and pharmacoeconomics studies, etc., said that the lack of 'in-company' geriatric expertise and resources was a barrier. Locating suitable investigative centers for geriatric studies is only part of the solution and works well for the smaller elderly experience studies. Nonetheless, in clinical studies undertaken for specific diseases in aging, much larger numbers of patients must be enrolled.

Even the large resources of the NIH can be strained. The Systolic Hypertension in the Elderly Person (SHEP) investigation recruited 4736 patients aged 60–96 years (average 72). The patient screening and selection was organized from 16 sites but took 31 months to complete, which had initially been projected to be 24 months. Nearly 450 000 patients were screened (SHEP Cooperative Research Group 1991).

Hall (1993) reported on 15 cardiovascular studies funded by the National Heart and Lung Blood Institute (NHLBI) over 10 years. All overran their projected recruitment times by an average of 27%. Over-optimistic projections are the norm, and this norm has been called 'Lasagna's Law' (Spilker and Cramer, 1972). For pharmaceutical clinical physicians and their staff, similar overruns are not excused by management, and raise the temptation to 'move the target' by closing recruitment at a lower level. This solution compromises the statistical robustness of the study; both the problem and this solution are career busters. Better to project realistically and plan recruitment and fallback strategies. Hall (1993) also varied the recruitment strategies used; the most successful was community screening. This can be done through appeals to senior centers, churches, shopping centers and major industrial sites (Melish 1982). Medical chart review is also productive if the condition has a International Classification of Disease (ICD) code and charts are available to the investigators.

For large studies, mass-mailing to registered voters, members of organized groups such as AARP, or members of a disease association can be helpful, with 7–12% response rate (McDerman and Bradford 1982). Use of media campaigns can result in up to 11% of first protocol visits (Levenkrow and Farquhar 1982). These need at least 3–6 months of planning for resources to respond to the initial wave of inquiries. The approach can be a newspaper article and advertisements in regional papers, TV and radio. Appeals to community physicians for referrals are usually disappointing, possibly caused by the physician believing that he/she will lose a paying patient to a research clinic.

CONCLUSION

The growth of the aging population, regulatory overview and increased business opportunities will ensure the growth of clinical research in the elderly. Recent reports of the high level of seniors' adverse events, many leading to deaths, both in and outside hospitals, will force more monitoring systems for medications. Soon, plastic medicine card chips with imprinted medication recorded by the pharmacist will be required by third-party insurers. This would ensure that all current concurrent medications are captured.

There is a shortage of geriatric specialists, which will take time to be corrected if the 600 drugs under development are to be adequately researched. The rapid growth of sheltered self-care communal housing for active seniors, which guarantee health care up to terminal status, illustrates that seniors wish to stay out of nursing homes. Their expectation of the pharmaceutical industry is that it should provide them with medications which allow for an active old age. The industry has heard.

REFERENCES

Abrams WB (1993) Food and Drug Administration Guideline for the study of drugs in elderly patients: an industry perspective. In Wenger NK (ed.), *Inclusion of Elderly Individuals in Clinical trials*. Marian Mennel Dow: 213–17.

Blackwell B (1979) The drug regimen and treatment complications. In: Haynes RB, Taylor DN, Sackett DL (eds), *Compliance in Health Care* John Hopkins University Press; 144–56.

Chaponis R (1998) Geriatic-based research in the pharmaceutical industry. Private survey (personal correspondence).

Conn VS (1992) Self-management of over-the-counter medications by older adults *Publ Health Nursing* Mar 9(1): 22–8.

Denham MJ Barnet NC (1998) Drug therapy and the older person; the role of the pharmacist. *Drug Safety* 19(4): 243–50.

Everitt DE, Avorn J (1986) Drug prescribing for the elderly. *Arch Int Med* 146: 2393–6.

Fed Reg (1994) Studies in support of special populatons: geriatric *Fed Reg* August 2, 1994, 59 FR: 390–398.

Fed Reg (1997) Specific requirements of content and format of labeling for huma prescription drugs: addition of 'Geriatric Use' subsection (1997) *Fed Reg* 62 (166), August 45313–26.

Fed Reg (1999) Guidelines for the study of drugs likely to be used in the elderly *Fed Reg* March 55 FR: 7777.

Gately MS (1968) To be taken as directed. *J R Coll Geriat Pract* 16: 39–44.

Hall WD (1993) Screening and recruitment of elderly participants into large-scale cardiovascular studies. In: Wenger NK (ed.), *Inclusion of Elderly Individuals into Clinical Trials.* Marian Mennel Dow; 67–71.

Lassila HC, Stoehr GP, Ganguli M, *et al* (1996) Use of prescription medications in an elderly rural population. *Ann Pharmaco-other* 30 (6): 589–95.

Levenkrow JC, Farquhar JW (1982) Recruitment using mass media strategies. *Circulation* IV: (suppl IV) 32–6.

McDermon M, Bradford RH (1982) Recruitment by use of mass mailings. *Circulation* 66(6 pt 2): 27–31.

Melish JS (1982) Recruitment by community screenings. 66 Circulation IV: (suppl IV) 20–3.

Mossinghoff GJ (1995) Survey of new drug development in the elderly. **www.phrma.org** (under Publications).

Muenning P Pallin D, Sel RC, Chan MS (1999) The cost of effectiveness of strategies for the treatment of intestinal parasites in immigrants. *N Eng J Med* 340 (10): 773–9.

National Center for Health Statistics (1996) US Department of Health and Human Services (data from 1996)

PhRMA (1999) Survey of new drug developments in the elderly. **Web www.phrma.org** (under publications).

Pitt B, Zannad F, Remme WJ et al (1999). The effects of spironolactone on morbidity and mortality in patients with severe heart failure. *Engl J Med* 2341(10): 709–17.

Satcher D (1999) Global health at the cross-roads: Surgeon General's report to the 50th World Assembly. *J Am Med Assoc* 281: 942–3.

SHEP Co-operative Research Group (1991) Prevention of stroke by hypertensive drugs treatment in old persons with isolated systolic hypertension: final results of the Systolic Hypertensio in the Elderly Program (SHEP). *J Am Med Assoc* 265; 3255–64.

Small J (1998) An economic evolution of donepezil in the treatment of Alzheimer's Disease. *Clin Ther* 20(4): 838–50.

Spilker B, Cramer JA (eds) (1972) *Patient Recruitment in Clinical Trials.* Rowen: New York.

Tamblyn R (1996) Medical use in seniors: challenges and solutions. *Therapy* 51(3): 269–82.

United Nations International Population Division (1996).

US Bureau of the Census (1996) current population report series.

15

Drug Development Research in Women

Lionel D. Edwards

Basking Ridge, NJ, USA

BACKGROUND

The pharmaceutical industry is in the business of developing, manufacturing and selling drugs, vaccines, and devices. Although basic research has become more important in recent years, it is not the primary aim of industry. However, increasingly and usually dictated by opportunity, industry is investing in a highly targeted fashion in some aspects of basic research, but the development of a product is always to the fore.

This thrust, however, need not exclude the gathering of basic data, which may prove invaluable to the research process. Regrettably, these data were frequently inaccessible, in some instances owing to the needs of confidentiality, product protection, or even legal concerns, but by far the greatest reason is that such data are regarded as a by-product, almost 'waste data', for they are not part of the mainstream of product development. Such data are recorded but rarely utilized, frequently residing in notebooks, case records, mainframe databanks, statistical reports, or data tabulations in the back of appendices of regulatory submissions.

So it is with gender data: it is collected, analyzed and tabulated by each study and by each drug, but data on drugs of the same class and between each government agency handling multiple applications are virtually inaccessible. Mining this data requires more creative solutions than 'regulations'. This is now happening.

It has been estimated that the cost of developing a new medicine is now $350–550 million (Arlington, 2000). This estimate mostly comprises costs in development, but includes the loss of other revenue if the development money had instead been invested cumulatively. These costs are passed directly on to the consumer.

Drug costs have risen slowly compared to other health costs, when adjusted for inflation. When compared to other health costs, in 1965 the drug/device cost was less than a dime per health dollar and in 1999 is less than a nickel (Health Care Financing Administration). Drug cost is, and must remain, one of the most affordable aspects of treatment. A large component of drug development cost is caused by regulatory needs to test for drug safety and efficacy, both for the USA and foreign agencies. Clearly, the cost of any additional regulation imposed on top of the current burden will also be directly reflected in the eventual cost to the consumer.

Women comprise 51% of the population of most nations; in Western countries, 54% of women are of child-bearing potential (15–49 years). Women account for 57% of physician visits (National Disease and Therapeutic Index, 1991). In the age group 20–39 years, women were found to be the biggest users of anti-infectives, especially ampicillin and amoxicillin; antidepressants are prescribed twice as often to women as to men (Stewart, 1998); and of some concern was that tetracycline, a known teratogen, was the eighth most prescribed drug in this group most likely to bear children (FDA, 1986).

As major users, it might be postulated that women, including those of child-bearing age, should be *the* group on which Phase I and Phase II dosing (early efficacy and safety) should be based. Why is this not so? Critics of the industry, and indeed of the wider research process, claim that it is entrenched discrimination by males, which is disguised as 'concern and gallantry'. Critics also point out that both medicine and research are dominated by males, who place research into women's diseases on the back burner of their male priorities

Principles and Practice of Pharmaceutical Medicine. Edited by A. J. Fletcher, Lionel D. Edwards, Anthony W. Fox and Peter Stonier © 2002 John Wiley & Sons Ltd.

and only see data, even on women, from a man's point of view. They point to a report by Coale (1991) on the 'missing 100 million women' in Asia and the Indian subcontinent, whom are speculated not to exist becaues of abortion and medical and nutritional neglect. They also point to the misuse of science (ultrasound or amniocentesis) for sex determination.

While these are extreme examples of societal attitudes, it is true that women have been excluded from many large, well-published studies, such as the Physicians' Health Study of aspirin in cardiovascular disease (Hennekens, 1989). It is also true that many early studies of drugs in Phases I and II were conducted in healthy white males 18–40 years old and the results then extrapolated to women in Phase III studies, primarily aimed at expanded efficacy and safety. Only recently, Paul Williams (1996) confirmed that exercise raised HDL cholesterol in women, many years later than reported in men. It is, however, in most cases, grossly naive to attribute this to deliberate 'male discrimination' to exclude research on women.

It is also frequently mentioned that fear of embryonic malformation, whether or not drug-related, and subsequent litigation is *the* major determining factor for exclusion of females from therapeutic and basic research projects. This overly simple explanation covers up other difficulties, such as methodology, lack of relevant baseline information, and biochemical variables, both hormonal and gender-related. It also ignores the use of information derived from other groups of women, those of no child-bearing potential, sterile or postmenopausal, the elderly, or children just entering puberty, where the risk of fetal exposure is nonexistent or minimal.

THE DILEMMAS

Do women respond to medications differently to men? If so, in what ways and how frequently are these changes clinically meaningful? Review of the literature shows some examples of differences between the sexes in drug handling, particularly with certain classes of drugs. These will be dealt with later, but it is important to bear in mind that, despite some detectable differences, usually no therapeutically significant differences are seen

(Edwards, 1991). This is unlikely to be due to lack of compliance, as women are generally more reliable than men, although compliance does fall off to 67% over a few weeks for both genders (Cramer et al, 1990). This does not exclude self-adjustment of dose by female patients, a phenomenon seen in both sexes and probably much more common than reported.

It has also been claimed (because gender data are rarely mentioned in clinical studies, papers or reports) that gender differences are not sought. This presupposes that data are neither collected nor examined. In fact, the opposite is much more likely: 94% of surveyed pharmaceutical firms were found to collect gender data in their studies (Edwards, 1991). The reality is that findings of *no differences* are rarely reported, but sometimes this finding may just be a function of small sample size for each individual study or the small degree of difference to be found. It must also be recognized that many drugs were introduced into medicine prior to the current modern-day comprehensive testing programs. Nonetheless, after many years and millions of prescriptions, it is of reassurance that few have shown significant clinically important gender-related differences.

Differences in Disease Presentations

A report from the *National, Heart, Lung and Blood* Institute (NHLBI, 1996), showed that the age and incidence (1988–1993) of onset of heart disease between genders were different; 24% of the 65–74 year-old males compared to about 18% of females in the same age group. This incidence rose in both genders at 75–84 years to about 28% males and 30% females.

Not only do women develop heart disease later, but they also present differently. The signature symptom of a heart attack, severe chest pain, is often absent in women, and pain in the upper back or neck, or breathlessness and nausea, may present either as a single symptom or as multiple symptoms. The American Heart Association states that 44% of women are likely to die in the first year of their heart attack, compared to 27% of men.

It is not surprising that heart attack and angina are misdiagnosed more commonly in women than men during emergency room visits. The range between hospitals of misdiagnosis was 0–11%, with an average 2.3% for angina and 2.1% for heart attacks. The diagnosis was missed in 7% of women under 55 years (Pope, 2000).

What's Representative?

An additional dilemma is, what population is 'representative' for female dose and efficacy determination? Women of child-bearing potential (54%)? These will have possible hormonal cycling changes and those on contraceptive hormones will have even greater changes, added to a possible basic gender difference, either amplifying or even suppressing effects.

The needs of women aged 66 years or over are already represented in regulatory drug testing guidelines in the elderly Federal Register (1990), but women 50–65 years old also can lay claim to special consideration, given the special problems associated with combined hormonal loss and age changes (e.g. osteoporosis, loss of possible cardiac estrogen protection and changes in body fat composition and its distribution). Pregnant women, already isolated from drug development by fear of legal tort laws and, indeed, by their physicians' reluctance to even prescribe in early pregnancy, can also stake a claim to require additional studies. Finally, when studying females of child-bearing potential, should we include patients on oral contraceptives, with their large levels of regulated fluctuating but synthetic hormones, or rely on females not taking oral contraceptives? The latter option will increase the risk of potential fetal exposure.

It must now be apparent that the female population (51%) contains *many* potential subgroups, none truly 'representative', for all have major physiological differences from each other. For industry to study all groups would be impractical, uneconomical and would gravely slow the drug development process and compromise the number of agents placed into development. To include all groups within one all-encompassing study, unless extremely large, offends a basic research nostrum—i.e. 'stabilize, reduce or remove all the variables except the one to be measured', or the signals many be lost in the static. This is especially true in Phase II studies.

THE PHANTOM FETUS

Teratogenic Issues

The term 'phantom fetus' has been used to describe the current apprehension regarding the use of drugs in women of child-bearing potential. This apprehension has dominated industrial, and institutional, and private research. The thalidomide tragedy of the 1960s—the 10 000 or so deformed children now grown to adults—continue to haunt us. It must be recognized that, despite careful animal testing, the full potential for teratogenic activity of any drugs in humans will only come to light once the drug is in the marketplace, and then only when sufficient multiple exposures have occurred in pregnant patients and their fetuses. It is extremely unlikely that deliberate drug testing in pregnant women will ever become routine. However, in special circumstances, such as HIV-infected pregnant women, it is justified to include them in appropriate clinical studies. Current predictive animal screening cannot give complete assurance that the potential for teratogenicity will be uncovered in all cases. It must be remembered that the then-current 1956 screens did not discover the teratogenicity of thalidomide, nor the 16-year delayed hyperplasia and neoplasia effects on the cervix and uterus of female adolescents exposed to stilbestrol (given to prevent miscarriages during their mothers' pregnancies).

Both historically and currently, the major determination of teratogenicity is made from findings from animal screening; many agents have been eliminated from further development, and only rarely does teratogenicity become uncovered in the marketplace. Nonetheless, it requires large numbers of exposures before the more subtle embryotoxic or teratogenic effects are found, as was demonstrated most recently by the ACE inhibitors, which had passed all the screens. Indeed, these events may never be exposed. How could this be? One must take into account the 'background noise' level, the so-called 'natural' incidence of cogenital abnormalities. By far the commonest is Down's syndrome, whose incidence is known to increase with the age of the mother, although nearly all other abnormalities appear *not* to increase with maternal age, according to a recent report (Wilson, 1973). Thus, a higher incidence of 'typical' drug-induced teratogenic effects serve as an early alert. The commonest abnormalities most frequently associated with drug exposure in the first trimester are neural tube defects, cardiac and renal anomalies, shortening of limbs and digits, and failure of closure of the palate and upper lip. More subtle changes associated with exposure to drugs occur in the third trimester, with hearing and eye abnormalities predominating (Wilson, 1973). Any such determinations require many, many thousands of exposures before they become apparent.

However, many millions of women become pregnant before being aware of their pregnancy and have been exposed to environmental chemicals (most of which have never been tested), as well as OTC drugs and prescription drugs. Also, a number of embryos are spontaneously aborted and a delay to the menstrual period of perhaps two or three weeks passes unremarked or sometimes unnoticed in a background of a national miscarriage rate of 1 in 3 pregnancies (Yoder, 1984). Teratologists have concluded that there is a threshold dose for any drug before it shows potential teratogenicity (in other words, enough must be given), and the effect tends to increase with the duration of exposure, with higher concentrations in the plasma or tissues, and with the timing of the developing fetal tissues and organs (Wilson 1973). In the first 7–8 days, the embryo is refractory to any teratogenic effect but is most *susceptible* 20–55 days after conception. Of some reassurance is that most drugs prescribed to women of child-bearing age are antibiotics and tend to be for relatively short durations. But the tetracyclines and anti-epileptic drugs are known to have effects on the developing fetus and are frequently prescribed to women (Stewart, 1998).

It is an irony that the normal tenet of US and UK law that an individual is 'innocent until proven guilty' does not apply to prescribed pharmaceutical products or devices. They must be proven safe and efficacious before they are approved; in other words, they must be *proven to be innocent*. Thus, it comes as no surprise that industry and other research groups tend to avoid the potential exposure of women of child-bearing age in the early clinical development of pharmaceuticals or devices, for many experimental drugs (perhaps 9 out of 10 tested in man) will never achieve the marketplace.

The Potential for Pregnancy While on a Trial Drug

What is the risk of pregnancy occurring in a study participant while a new drug is being developed? The author is not aware of any published figures, but from the author's experience in industry and from questions to colleagues, pregnancy does occur during drug development, even in those patients apparently taking *adequate* contraceptive precautions. A typical NDA database for most drugs will involve between 2000–4000 patients, of which perhaps one-third are female and exposed to study medication. It is not surprising, therefore, that given an average failure rate of the contraceptive pill of 2%, or even with the most stringent compliance, a failure fate of 0.5/100 women years will result in occasional pregnancy (Trussell et al, 1990). Other methods, such as the diaphragm, condoms and IUDs, can carry even higher failure rates, depending on whether 'usual' or 'perfect compliance' calculation of 18–6%, 12–2% and 3–0.5%, respectively, are used (Trussell et al, 1990). If we assume an average NDA database of 4000 patients, one-third or more female, it is likely that half of these will be females of child-bearing potential (the other half being post-menopausal or elderly). Thus, approximately 660 females of child-bearing potential may be exposed to the drug, the comparator, or a placebo. In the best circumstances of perfect contraceptive compliance, in a 1-year exposure and at a 0.5% failure fate, 3.3 fetuses are likely to be exposed. With a 'typical compliance' of the contraceptive pill, a 3% failure rate would leave about 19 fetuses exposed to experimental entities, one-third of which would be lost due to spontaneous miscarriage.

Few patients would be exposed for a full year, but more typically probably only to between 2 weeks to 3 months of study medication. Given all the above assumptions, between 0.8 and 5 early embryos will be exposed in a full drug development program. From the author's personal experience of over 27 years in industry, an average of two children are born exposed to a new chemical entity. This is most likely to occur in Phase 3 studies, which have many more patients and are often of longer duration. Currently, pharmaceutical firms, with the agreement of the FDA, follow up all possible exposures until any resultant child is 12–14 years of age, and a full medical examination (including a full neurological work-up) is done at yearly intervals.

The Potential for Teratogenic Damage during Drug Study Programs

As previously mentioned, the best sources for the actual figures for the above calculations resides within the FDA but may, as I alluded, be inaccessible. In recent years, figures given by the Agency, e.g. in elderly drug-testing studies, appear to have been hand-tallied rather than garnered from composite computer access. However, the agency is now involved in a large effort to 'mine' data across therapeutic classes, some of which, with meta-analysis, will provide data which individual drug programs never could, nor were designed to show. In time, the ability to access data across drugs and across drug classes will grow as more firms put in computer-assisted NDAs (CANDAs) in appropriate and compatible programs and formats.

What is the risk of a fetus being damaged during an 'average' NDA drug development program? Obviously small. Clearly, toxic but 'life-saving' treatment will carry a *heavy* embryotoxic risk; anticancer, anti-AIDS drugs, and fetal intrauterine surgical procedures are obvious examples, but the clear-cut risks involved are usually deemed acceptable. A more subtle judgment call involves the development of anti-epileptic drugs. Let's look at two examples. It has been estimated that exposure of pregnant women to normal therapeutic doses of valproic acid may give rise to 1% fetal abnormality rate involving the neural tube (Lindhaut and Schmidt 1986)—10 times the natural incidence. Many of these defects are correctable with modern surgical techniques. Exposure to phenobarbitone also has a reported higher incidence of cleft lip and palate defects (Frederick, 1973): most are surgically correctible. If used in combination, the incidence of anticonvulsant teratogenic effects are increased (Lindhaut et al 1984). Would either of these drugs be developed in today's litigious atmosphere? I doubt it. But both drugs are valuable in many circum-

stances; they may be the only drugs suitable for some patients and, indeed, frequently can be life-saving. Certainly status epilepticus is very injurious to the fetus, often resulting in miscarriage or premature birth.

The incidence of neonatal abnormalities in mothers taking anticonvulsant treatment is 70/1000 live births (Frederick, 1973). This is 2.4 times the 'spontaneous rate' in the general population (29 abnormalities/1000 live births). Thus, even using a known 'low-incidence' teratogen could cause 40 additional cases/1000 live births, but to determine that accurately would require many thousands of female patient exposures to be detectable against the 'spontaneous' background incidence.

So, back to the opening question. What is the likelihood of detecting low-incidence, drug-induced congenital effects in a drug development program? With our presumed database of 4000 patients, only 0.8–5 fetuses would be exposed to a background 'spontaneous' risk of 2.9%. Each program could carry a 1 in 33 to 1 in 6 chance of a single 'spontaneous' abnormality occurring. If the drug or procedure should have low teratogenic activity (at the level of an anticonvulsant), this risk rises to 1 in 14 to 1 in 2.5 that a child will be born with a congenital abnormality in any drug development program. Both 'spontaneous' or drug-induced abnormalities may occur, e.g. a neural tube defect. Thus, on a single-case basis, the abnormalities will be indistinguishable for drug causality. This in turn can lead to litigation, and certainly to a reference in the package label insert.

Wilson has estimated that both drugs and environmental chemical exposures only account for 2–3% of developmental defects in man (Wilson, 1972).Thus, a product-label reference of such an occurrence will be undeserved at least 97% of the time, but also may be the first signal of a teratogenic risk. It may now be appreciated why this 2–3% risk is termed the 'phantom fetus' and also why the difficulty in *disproving liability* dominates the mainstream concerns of research, regulatory authorities, and industry alike. This 'ghost risk' creates 'discrimination' against female patients in drug research. This 'ghost' must be exorcised and contained; possible solutions will be discussed later.

INDUSTRY PRACTICE: FACTORS IN PHASE I AND EARLY PHASE II TESTING

Medical journalist Paul Cotton (1990) asked, in a thought-provoking article, is there still too much extrapolation from data on middle-aged white men? Inspection of the demographics of recent NDAs will give us numbers to debate; however, these data are not readily accessible. Most Phase I testing is still undertaken in healthy young males, and even for Phase I testing of new contraceptives hormonal for women. Why this occurs is multifaceted.

Timing of Mutagenicity Fertility and Teratogenicity Testing

The complete battery of tests with full histology and the development of a final report can take as long as 2 years. In general, only some of the mutagenicity studies are completed, and perhaps 1–3 month reports of animal testing are available when male Phase I dosing volunteer studies commence. All animal studies do not commence at the same time but are usually sequential. Some, such as postexposure weaning and subsequent second-generation drug effect studies will be time-consuming and expensive. Often, if mutagenicity tests, e.g. Ames' test or mouse lymphoma test, are positive (Ames test has 30% false-positive rate), then females will be excluded until more data is collected. Thus, only limited data are available prior to the first human exposure. (For further reference *Fed Reg* 1994, 1996).

Volunteer dose-ranging studies will, by design, include high enough doses to provoke unpleasant adverse effects; also, information on 'target organs' (organs likely to be most affected or harmed) is usually predictable but unconfirmed at this point. Generally, as a result of animal studies, it is thought that the effect of drugs on reproductive function in males is less than that in females and only affects the sperm viability or, rarely, the size and function of the testicles, which is usually reversible. This is unduly optimistic, as one report by Yazigi et al (1991) suggests that spermatozoa may not be immobilized or destroyed by cocaine, but may interact, and the spermatozoa themselves have

the potential to act as an active transport mechanism for drugs, pesticides and even environmental chemicals to the unfertilized ovum. They may also alter the genetic make-up of either spermatozoa or ovum. In addition, spermatozoa can be made sluggish by calcium channel blockers, leading to male infertility while on medication. Hence, the European guidelines call for male animal testing prior to start of Phase 2.

The blastocyst (early embryo) is relatively resistant to damage in the first 7 days, for up to 75% of cells can be destroyed before tissue differentiation and the embryo can still survive. What might happen if garden pesticides, or house builders' formaldehyde containing glue and chemicals, are combined into the genetic material? If it is ever confirmed, then we may have the inkling of what makes up the 65% of the 'unknown' causes of developmental defects mentioned by Wilson (1972). If it could be shown that the synthetic chemicals are incorporated into the blastocyst, the field of male Phase I testing would be transformed, as would that of genetic counseling.

Testing Facilities

Largely because early testing of drugs occurred in males rather than females, for reasons discussed above, most commercial and hospital units devoted to human pharmacology testing were set up to deal with a unisex population. They ran one gender study at a time, usually male, in 1993. Sleeping and bathroom facilities in the units' dormitory accommodations did not provide for mixed gender groups. These were minor but not inexpensive attentions but were quickly adopted following the publication of the *FDA Guidelines for the Study and Evaluation of Gender Differences in the Clinical Evaluation of Drugs* (Fed Reg, 1993).

Standardizing for the Menstrual Cycle (Phase I and Early Phase II)

Of much greater concern is the issue of standardizing the drug administration to the menstrual cycle. Women of child-bearing age do not all have cycles for the same length of days; variations of 24–36 day cycles are not unusual between and within the same women. Thus, unless controlled by oral contraceptives (OC), women volunteers could not start and finish in a study all together. Indeed, if OC were used to standardize cycles, the issue of how really representative of *all* women of child-bearing age this artificial hormone-boosted group might be would be debatable. Evidence suggests that even low-dose contraceptives can affect metabolism (Abernathy and Greenblatt, 1981). The logistics of running Phase I single-dose and multiple-dose ranging studies while controlling for a natural menstrual cycle are truly horrendous, both for the Phase I testing units and for the volunteer. The duration of any study would be extended by at least 1 month (the time required for the last patient's cycle to start), and each patient volunteer would have to be measured separately because of the different days of her cycle. A small but frequently argued point is timing. Which is the preferred day in the cycle for single-dose studies? And for a multiple-dose study (usually only 10–14 days long), which segments of the cycle should be covered? This may seem academic, but in those clinically significant drug classes where womens' responses to drug handling are different to those of men because of biochemical hormone effects (not just gender), then the timing of drug dosing and measurement would be critical.

Too Many Young Volunteer Studies

Many volunteer studies, especially at commercial, academic and university clinical units, are frequently young people of college age. Both males and females will volunteer since financial remuneration, and a free medical check-up and medical care play their part in motivation. The young also have less career and family commitments interfering with their motivation. Time for studying, reading and relaxation within an atmosphere of camaraderie also contributes to the availability of younger volunteers, who, because of their age, also tend to be very healthy. It will readily be appreciated that most drugs or devices are not unique or life saving but hopefully an improvement on existing agents, and indeed this applies to most basic research experiments. Nearly all drug studies in Phase I are aimed at gathering data on a potentially safe and possibly efficacious dose range. As a result, it is often hard to recruit older, more mature women for these basic types of essential drug development programs.

What Is a Representative Female Population in Phase I?

It has been stated that large numbers of mature women are volunteering for the new lipid, heart risk, osteoporosis and arthritis studies, due to their concern that women have been represented so poorly as subjects in the past. Phase I studies are of short duration (1–2 weeks), but usually require confinement of the volunteers to the clinical unit for that time. Because of this time commitment, far fewer mature women volunteer, due to career conflicts or because they are often burdened unequally with family management. Those that do volunteer are generally unattached young female students. Thus, most female volunteers may not be typical of a 'representative', mature, child-bearing population (if this can ever be defined).

One alternative, a study design of stratification by age and sex, would lead to inordinately long study recruitment times, because the last 'cell' (group) always takes a disproportionately long time to fill. The most obvious way out of the quandary for Phase I testing would be to maintain a special cadre of 'safe, standard' volunteers. How 'representative' these much-used 'new-drug volunteers' would become is debatable. For example, studies in arthritic patients show that these 're-tread' volunteer patients will differ in their tolerance to pain and in their judgment of efficacy and severity of adverse events, when compared to drug-study 'naive' patients (Coles et al 1988). This 'training effect' increases with multiple drug exposure.

By far the biggest issue of undertaking additional dosing Phase I studies on women is expense. Most of these studies cost $100–250 thousands each. Altogether, single, multiple, and multiple-dose ranging studies, with food effect studies and extra staff costs, could add $1 million to development costs and very rarely show a difference which would prove clinically relevant. Indeed, the difference may not show up at all in Phase I or II gender-to-gender studies, due to other variables, e.g. small numbers, estrogen-cycle levels and oral contraceptive levels and drug polymorphism.

DRUG HANDLING DIFFERENCES BETWEEN MALES AND FEMALES

Due to space limitations this subchapter cannot discuss the many reports of apparent gender differences of psychology, different anatomic brain location of functions, skeletal build and muscle-to-fat mass ratios which might have marginal impact upon drug activity.

The Weight/Dose Problem

A casual appraisal of ideal weight-for-height tables for males and females (Metropolitan Life Insurance, 1999) shows clear differences between males and females. The mythical 'average' 70 kg (154 l) male would be 5'10" in height and his female counterpart 5'4" and weigh 130 lb. This is a 28% difference in weight. This mythical male is often used to calculate dose ranges for 'optimal' dose determinations, around which Phase II and Phase III efficacy and safety studies evolve. Even more striking is the *range* of *normal* heights and weights, remembering that the *same* dose is usually prescribed to individuals across the range. In males, this varies from 5' at 106 pounds to 6'8" at 226 pounds; in females, it varies from 85 pounds at 4'9" to 185 pounds at 6'5"; yet all are ideal weights for the respective heights. For both sexes this represents a 46% differential in healthy weight while taking the same dose of medication. Why should these great disparities be tolerated by the research community, industry and agencies? Because most drugs work—even over these ranges. First, the majority of the population falls towards the middle of the height–weight levels, rather than the extremes. Second, most drugs have a wide range where which they exert therapeutic effect before efficacy levels off. Third, the level of unacceptable adverse events generally occurs at much higher doses than the therapeutic level for most drugs (there are some notable exceptions, e.g. lithium, digitalis, warfarin etc.).

For lipophilic drugs, the composition of mass to fat/total body water is a further variable, increasing in women after puberty. The composition of 'good fat and bad fat' changes with age, both in increased fat, increased bad fat and its relocation to the fat around the heart. The quantity and distribution differs between genders. This may have an effect on lipid-soluble drugs, regarding the level, the time to achieve steady-state, and the time to eliminate the drug and its metabolites from such fat storage depots.

Different Gastric Emptying Time

Some studies have shown that women demonstrate greater duration in the gastric residence time of medications, which is reflected in an increased lag time of absorption, compared to men. This effect is increased when medication is taken with food, even when adjusted for the timing of the menstrual cycle (Majaverian et al, 1987). This was consistent with other reports that men had faster emptying times for both liquid and digestible solids than women (Majaverian et al, 1988; Wright et al, 1983). The length of time and variability of gastric emptying in women was also reported by Notivol et al (1984) to be altered in relation to the menstrual cycle and was shortest at mid-cycle (MacDonald 1965; Booth et al 1957).

These changes can affect the amount of drug in the blood. Miaskiewicz et al (1982) showed that, after a single dose of sodium salicylate, absorption was slower and achieved a lower level in women. This has also been shown for ibuprofen. The T_{max} was observed to be more than 54 min in females, compared to a T_{max} of 31.5 min in males. Majaverian even showed a delay of 9.5 h before absorption occurred in one woman (Majaverian et al, 1987). Sex differences in plasma salicylate albumin binding capacity have been reported (Miaskiewicz et al, 1982) and, for other agents (Allen and Greenblatt, 1981), γ-globulin transport systems have been reported to be altered with the menstrual cycle.

Some effects on absorption can be subtle, such as the greater absorption of alcohol in women due to their reduced gastric mucosal and liver alcohol dehydrogenase activity compared to men. This results in higher circulating levels of alcohol, in spite of body weight corrections (Frezza et al, 1990), with obvious implications. Odansetron, on the other hand, is more slowly metabolized by women and thus may be more effective.

Metabolic Gender Differences

Propranolol is still one of the most frequently used β blockers (National Prescription Audit, 1989), but Walle et al (1985) reported that women had higher plasma levels of propranolol than men following single oral dosing and, in an additional study, showed that on multiple dosing, propranolol steady-state (trough) plasma levels were 80% higher than in men (Walle et al, 1985). This is probably because propranolol is metabolized through three pathways, but in women, the P450 cytochrome oxidation pathways are less effective than in men (Walle et al 1985).

Methaqualone metabolism has been shown to be significantly increased at the time of ovulation (day 15), almost double that of day 1, and this was reflected in an area under the curve (AUC) reduced by half on day 15. It is of interest that men, used as a control, only sustained levels at the level of day 1 in women (Wilson et al 1982).

Differences between males and females in the amount of free drug found in plasma, and of protein binding, have been reported for diazepam (Greenblatt et al, 1979; Abel et al, 1979) and for imipramine (Kristensen 1983). In the latter instance, a direct correlation was found with differences in lipoprotein and orosomucoid protein (1-a-acid glycoprotein) fractions (Greenblatt et al, 1980). In women, oxazepam has been found to be eliminated at a slower rate, about (10%), and for temazepam about (25%) (Diroll et al, 1981). Chlordiazepoxide was also found to be less bound to protein and this was even further reduced if women were also on estrogen oral contraceptives (Roberts et al, 1979). Free lignocaine levels in women were 11% higher in estrogen oral contraceptive users and 85% of this effect was due to the reduction of the orosomucoid protein fraction (Routledge et al, 1981).

Circulating hormones, such as aldosterone and renin have long been known to fluctuate with the menstrual luteal phase. If an amenorrheic cycle occurs, these changes are not seen (Michelakis et al, 1975). If oral contraceptives are given, then an increase of these hormones is also seen in the first part of the cycle (M'Buyamba-Kabunga et al, 1985). Androgens transported on the β-globulin and albumen fraction are influenced by estrogen, which increases their binding. This effect is enhanced by the use of oral contraceptives (Clark et al, 1971).

In animals, estrogen has been shown to influence the effect of antidepressants on the brain. Wilson showed that estradiol increased the binding of imipramine to the uptake of serotonin at membrane sites. Estrone had no effect, but the addition of progesterone to low doses of estrogen increased this effect. In all, the greatest effect seen was about a 20% enhancement of imipramine binding (Wilson, 1986).

For low-therapeutic/toxic drugs such as lithium, this might prove to be an explanation of the reduction in efficacy seen at the end of the menstrual cycle, when these hormone levels fall (Conrad and Hamilton 1986). It might also explain the reduction in efficacy of other central nervous system drugs, such as antiepileptics (Shavit et al, 1984; Rosciezewesta et al, 1986) and antimigraine medications, seen with the fluctuation of the menstrual cycle (Gengo et al, 1984).

Young women appear to be the group most at risk of developing extrapyramidal reactions when taking the antinausea drug metoclopramide. This appears to be strongly age- and gender-related (Simpson et al, 1987). Another age/gender-related effect is seen in older women who have become newly postmenopausal and who are still taking antipsychotic medications, because the symptoms of tardative dyskinesia may appear or even worsen (Smith and Baldossarini, 1973). This is perhaps another example of the loss of estrogen protection.

Many of the examples quoted involve central nervous system drugs. This is very important, for gender-related prescription *usage* is heavily weighted in this area towards women. The FDA 1985 drug utilization report showed that for benzodiazepines, the increased usage in women outnumbers men by 2:1 (339 vs. 171 prescriptions/1000 women and men, respectively). Twice as many women are treated for depression and anxiety neurosis than men, first described by Raskin (1974), and confirmed by Weissman and Klerman (1977). It is by no means certain that this is solely due to biochemical differences, for women are more likely to seek help than men. Of importance from the prior discussion is that, if women are the greatest users of these medications, should not study recruitment members be biased in their favor? However, some of the psychotropic CNS drugs also have animal data—and a few, even some human data—suggesting an increased teratogenic potential (Physician's Derk Reference, 1991; Jefferson et al, 1987). There is no consistent evidence of class teratogenicity (Elia et al, 1987), but there is a high association of fractured hips with the use of psychotropic medicines, even when corrected for women's greater age-related hip fracture rate (Ray et al, 1987). One of the commonest causes of the elderly being admitted to institutional care is urinary incontinence. Women have been found to be more susceptible than men to medications that can cause incontinence to occur (Diokuo et al, 1986).

Adverse Event Differences

One of the most striking differences between male and female responses to drugs is the finding reported by Martin et al (1998) in 513 608 patients with serious adverse events, which occurred in 43.2% males and 55.7% females when adjusted for age. In women of all ages, Tran et al (1998) also reported that, in findings from records of 2367 patients, female patients were at twice greater risk of adverse reactions than males. More than one agent was reported to be responsible in 50% of female patients vs. 33.1% of all male patients. Drug doses in both genders most likely to cause an adverse event were anti-infectives (60.4%) and nervous system agents (21.5%) (Martin et al, 1998). The commonest events were skin-related reactions (49%). It is possible that bare arms and exposed legs in women may cause more phototoxic reactions than in men; nonetheless, this cannot be said of nervous system agents. Clearly, these two classes of agents need special gender exploration in clinical development.

GOVERNMENT AGENCY AND INDUSTRY ACTIONS ON GENDER-RELATED RESEARCH

The Public Health Service Task Force on Women's Health Issues (1985) and the National Institutes of Health (NIH) Guide (1989) both recommended that biomedical and behavioral research should be expanded to ensure emphasis on conditions unique to, or most prevalent in, women of all age groups: 'in addition, studies are needed to study the metabolism and disposition of drugs and alcohol by age and gender'. The National Institute for Drug and Alcohol Abuse (NIDAA) (1990) policy provides detailed, almost affirmative-action instructions for the inclusion of women and minorities into study designs, according to their prevalence in the diseases being studied.

Since 1988, the FDA has requested tabulations of gender, age, and racial distributions in NDA submissions. Many of their senior officials, e.g. Drs. Peck and Temple, had forcefully stated that women should be included in drug development studies. Indeed, the 1977 guideline, *General Consideration for the Clinical Evaluation of Drugs*, included a policy for the inclusion of women of child-bearing potential in clinical trials but excluded them, in general, from Phase I and early Phase II studies, with exceptions for life-saving or life-prolonging treatments. Child-bearing potential was strictly defined as 'any woman capable of becoming pregnant', including women using reversible contraceptive precautions and those with vasectomized partners.

The FDA issued new guidelines in 1993 (*Fed Reg* 1993), perhaps spurred by its own findings in 1989, and confirmed by the General Accounting Office (GAO), that in only 50% of submissions were gender analysis discussed in NDA submissions. Temple (1992) reported that two FDA surveys demonstrated that women were included routinely and in proportion to the presence in the treatment population, and young women in large numbers (Bush et al, 1993). Not recorded were his concluding remarks, in which he said many NDAs did not adequately discuss gender difference, which would be addressed in the new amended guideline. The FDA, in its discourse in the 1993 guidelines, *Revised Policy on Inclusion of Women of Childbearing Potential in Clinical Trials*, mentions that it was swayed by a legal precedent. In 1991 the US Supreme Court found on behalf of the plaintiff workers union that their pregnant members had been unfairly excluded from jobs by the Johnson Control Company, because the working conditions exposed their fetuses to potential risk. The court wrote: 'Welfare of future children should be left to the parents... rather than to employers who hire them'. While not quite the same circumstances, the FDA were of the mind that this opinion would also apply to pregnant (informed) women, giving them the right to enter drug trials irrespective of phase of development.

The FDA revised guidelines on this and ethnic differences which appeared in July 1993 in the *Federal Register*, in essence abolished the prior ban on women of childbearing age from Phase I and Phase II studies, and stipulated additional topics, including the embryotoxic and teratogenic risk potential, to be covered in the patients' informed consent.

Earlier, the NIH had issued its own guidelines to its staff, grant applicants, and academic centers it supported. It called for *all* research on human subjects concerning drugs, devices, epidemiology, non-drug device studies and treatment outcomes, to include both genders and minority representatives whenever possible. In Phase III studies, 'women and minorities and their subpopulations in sufficient numbers should be included, such that valid analyses of differences can be accomplished'. It stipulated that 'cost was not an acceptable reason for exclusion, and that programs and support for outreach efforts to recruit these groups be undertaken'. (NIH, 1986). Failure to ensure adequate effort to implement could be reason for grant rejection or loss of financial support.

To amplify the female view both the FDA and NIH during the last decade have appointed women to significant roles. Dr Bernadette Healy headed the NIH and created the Office of Research in Women's Health; Dr Henny led the FDA until 2001 and within the FDA, Dr Janet Woodcock and Dr Kathy Zoon were appointed to head CDER (drugs), and CBER (biologics), respectively, two of the largest centers perhaps partly in response to an article by LaRosa and Pinn (1993), both women bemoaning exclusion of women in decisions of research.

The industry is now encouraged by the FDA to include women earlier in the clinical development program, but there are also still good reasons why the FDA might deny inclusion of women of child-bearing potential—insufficient toxicology data; a disagreement over the interpretation of such data; agency knowledge of another company's confiden-

tial data indicating a potential risk with a drug class-related compound; and, finally, an FDA reviewer's individual comfort level with 'high-risk population exposure'. Such an event has now become rarer.

Pharmaceutical Industry Practice

In July 1991, a survey was completed by this author for the Pharmaceutical Manufacturers Association (PMA), Special Populations Committee on the current practice of the industry in handling gender and minority data (Edwards, 1991). Vice-Presidents of headquarters, clinical and regulatory affairs were contacted at 46 companies; 33 companies responded (nearly all the major companies). All 33 responding companies collect gender-related data on the participant patients in clinical studies. Over three-quarters of the companies reported that they deliberately recruit 'representative' numbers of women. It should be noted that the term 'representative' has not been defined by the FDA or by industry. However, only 10 companies (30%) frequently or usually collected data on menstrual cycle; 56% replied that the FDA at some time or other had requested the *inclusion* of women in trials. When women of child-bearing potential were included in protocol proposals, 21% of the respondents said that the FDA never disagreed, but 79% had experience of some FDA reviewers at one time or another excluding women *of child-bearing potential*. When excluded, this was usually in the Phase I and Phase II trials, 58% and 45%, respectively, correspondents reported.

While this survey was qualitative rather than quantitative, the results should not be dismissed lightly; because the survey was confidential, no respondents or their firms were exposed to open criticism. Because of their experience and senior positions, respondents had reviewed many different drugs and NDA applications. The survey replies were therefore likely to be reliable and provide a good approximation of the then-current industry gender practices and the frequency of clinically meaningful differences.

When gender differences in safety or efficacy were found to be clinically significant, most respondent companies (94%) opted to put the data in the product label, the *Physicians' Desk*

Reference and the product literature (72%), and to publish in the medical journals (69%). Presumably, the two companies that did not amend their labels acted thus because the products were only intended for one-gender use. By December 1999, there were 348 medicines in development for diseases only in women or where women are disproportionately affected (Holdin 2000). Not only has industry stepped up its research efforts, but many large firms have units devoted to women's health care.

Finally, correspondents were asked how frequently gender differences were found; 73% said 'occasionally', 3% said 'frequently' and the rest said 'never'. Of those who saw differences, only one-third found these differences to be *clinically* significant 5% of the time, while 17% of respondents said that significant differences occurred 10% of the time. This was more than expected, and provides further justification for gender testing.

POSSIBLE SOLUTIONS

This author must stress that the opinions and the suggestions that follow are personal, based on 27 years in industry, over Phase I–IV study experience, with five large international pharmaceutical firms.

Women's Inclusion as Drug Research Subjects

Women should be and, indeed, are included into new drug and device development programs when not specifically excluded due to male-only disease or existing pregnancy. If it is predictable that a drug or device will be used in women (though they may not be the majority users), then a 'reasonable number' should be included into Phase II and Phase III studies. If the disease occurs more frequently in women, e.g. rheumatoid arthritis, then women should be involved in Phase I studies. The reality is that of the many hundreds of drugs and devices approved for use today, very few show major gender-related differences in either side effects or efficacy. Clearly, in the drug classes that have been shown to demonstrate significant gender clinical differences, 'specific' gender-related studies should be included for investigation drugs and

devices. These could be similar to those now undertaken in the elderly. First, a single-dose study should be undertaken. If important differences are found compared to men, a multiple-dose study ought to be undertaken, and then a shorter duration efficacy and safety study in women. Such studies can be conducted later, perhaps concurrently with Phase III of the development program.

What do we mean by 'a reasonable number'? 'Reasonable' is that number which would be expected to show a significant gender *clinical* difference if a real difference is present, and probably will only apply to efficacy and adverse events 5% or larger, because a difference in low-incidence adverse events will not show up until the drug is on the market. This would mean at least 300 women exposed to the new drug. The number of patients should be based on what is judged to be a clinically significant percentage loss or enhancement of efficacy, e.g. 30%, dependent on the disease or symptoms.

Representative Population of Women

This can be based on the incidence of disease proportional to gender distribution and can be studied when drug development and toxicity are well-enough advanced, usually by Phase III. Women of child-bearing age must be represented if the disease is prevalent in the age group 15–50 years. Indeed, diseases such as endometriosis can only be studied in such a population, whereas drugs to treat urinary incontinence would be better undertaken in older patients.

In some diseases, such as hypertension, where both sexes are similarly affected, balanced numbers of male and female patients in Phase III would not seem out of place, although many investigators are finding recruitment of sufficient numbers of female patients increasingly difficult.

In diseases such as osteoarthritis, where women patients outnumber males (80%), a legitimate case can be made for a 'female-weighted database', and also when women are the majority *users* for medicines, such as psychotropic agents (although they are not necessarily the majority of sufferers). Provision and timing of adequate animal toxicology and fertility data is critical to avoid expensive delays and to allow adequate female recruitment, so this animal data may be advanced on an 'at-risk basis', depending on the drug's clinical significance and its market potential. A list of diseases more prevalent in women is provided in *New Medicines in Women* (Holden, 2000).

The Potential Child-bearing Population

The probability of potential early embryonic exposure occurring in a drug development program must be expected and confronted because, despite careful pregnancy testing and adequate contraceptive precautions being undertaken, it happens. Levine (1975) in his book suggested that, in the consent form, there should be 'a statement that the particular treatment or procedure may involve risks to the subject—(or to the embryo or fetus if the subject is or may become pregnant) which are currently unforeseeable'.

When a woman of childbearing age participates in a research procedure in which there is a risk to the fetus, the nature of the risk being either known or unknown, she should be advised that, if she wishes to be a subject, she should avoid becoming pregnant. Her plans for avoiding conception should be reviewed during consent negotiations. At times, if her plans seem inadequate and she does not consent to the investigator's suggestions, it will be necessary to exclude her from the research. She should be further advised that if she deviates from the plans discussed at the outset, she should advise the investigators immediately.

Halbreich and Carson (1989) made the point that not to include women of child-bearing age could even increase liability:

The general policy of an academic institution should be to favor the conduct of research involving women and children in testing of new drugs with potential for major therapeutic value to those populations. Such research may expose the institution to risk of liability for damage to subjects; however, that is inherent in research involving human subjects anyway, and there are many ways of minimizing such risks. Not to do such research, while it may serve to protect the interests of the institution as narrowly conceived, would involve a failure to serve the public interest in a much more serious manner by exposing classes of persons to knowable but unknown risks, through

the practice of clinical medicines using drugs not thoroughly tested and understood, and withholding drugs that may be of benefit.

It has been suggested that members of female religious orders, women who have had tubal ligation or lesbians could provide a 'no-risk pregnancy' pool of volunteers. While possible, this is not generally a widely applicable solution, because geographic, environmental and volunteer numbers now become added variables.

Should women on oral contraceptives (OC) enter studies, could the high level of artificial hormones could confound the results? Female oral contraceptive users make up 28% of the potential child-bearing population (Ortho, 1991), and these hormone concentrations (10–20 times higher than the natural hormone levels) may cause drug interactions which cannot occur during ordinary menstrual cycling. Intra-uterine devices are currently regaining popularity, subdermal implants have had little influence on contraceptive practice at the epidemiological level.

Liabilities for Fetal Damage

Given all of the above reasons for including women of child-bearing potential, the issue of the chilling effect of legal liability for fetal damage on firms and institutions is still present, and the necessary addition to the patient's informed consent does not help. The Supreme Court in 1992 rejected an attempt to cap the amount juries could award in damages as 'unconstitutional', i.e., would require a constitutional amendment. This is highly unlikely to occur. The consequence of litigation, particularly in obstetrics, was a dramatic increase in caesarean section (18–20% of live births; this level was even higher in 1999), resignation from this specialty, and a broader rejection of 'high-risk' or Medicaid patients (O'Reilly et al, 1986; Bello, 1989). A possible solution might be to follow the example of the National Vaccine Injury Act of October 1988, where a trust fund was set up derived from an excise tax imposed on each vaccine. The funds, through an arbitration panel, are used to compensate persons injured by vaccination. It should be noted that a Drugs in Pregnancy Registry has been set up to follow up early embryonic exposure to the anticonvulsants and antiviral drugs acyclovir and retrovir. This is administered by the American Social Health Association (ASHA), Center for Disease Control (CDC), and Glaxo-Smithkline. One wonders if it could be expanded (with suitable support) to cover additional agents.

Data Gathering

Gender data are collected by major pharmaceutical companies; few, however, record the menstrual dates. Frequently, no drug-handling differences between the sexes is detected; much less commonly is the absence commented upon in reports or publications. It is suggested that LMP dates could be included in case report forms, and that publications and reports should contain statements on the presence or absence of gender differences, also giving the patient gender numbers and p values. This would allow for later meta-analysis. Both of these suggestions would be inexpensive to implement.

Gender-related data from the FDA is more readily available as the FDA continues to increase its computer ability and pharmaceutical firms utilize computer-assisted NDAs and increase their efforts to adequately power the studies to find differences. Unified systems and formats would enhance this. The information is included in the Summary Basis for Approval or in the Medical Reviewer's Report. Either should be available through the Internet at www.fda.gov./cder under 'New Approvals'.

CONCLUSION

Gender-related differences do exist in drug handling, but in general are relatively clinically insignificant. Theoretically, because of weight differences, women may receive more medication than men for a standard dose when converted to mg/kg. Greater effects might be expected from the range of normal weights rather than from the effects of gender.

Clinically significant gender effects have been reported with CNS, anti-inflammatory and cardiovascular drugs. It is suggested that women continue to be enrolled into most drug study programs,

but that greater thought be given to obtaining 'representative' numbers in the early program planning stage. For drugs intended mainly or entirely for women, even Phase I testing in women should be usually considered. Single-dose testing, even in women of child-bearing potential, poses minimal risk if done early in the cycle, with adequate precautions and 'consort' consent to short sexual abstinence. Alternatively, women with tubal ligation could be enrolled for these small studies.

'Representative' could be twofold: a reflection of the percentage of women suffering from the disease, or a 'reasonable or sufficient' number to show clinically significant differences in efficacy or safety in the main efficacy and safety studies; alternatively, conducting at least one study just in women in Phase III. What is a 'clinically significant effect' would depend on the drug and disease, but effects with a less than 15% difference get harder to detect and generally will be less meaningful. Again, women of child-bearing potential could be included, depending on the age/prevalence of the disease. Women using oral contraceptives may be compared not only with males but also with non-OC users. OC and drug interaction studies are currently required for most drugs.

Early embryo drug exposure and the potential liability for any damage continues to influence industry, agencies, and some research workers. It must be recognized that, if an agent has human teratogenic potential, it is better to detect this before it achieves the marketplace. Unfortunately, this is unlikely to be detected because the small numbers of women becoming pregnant in any NDA program make it impossible to detect drug-induced effects from spontaneous birth defects. Data in women are needed and the possibility is suggested of an expanded National Register along the lines of the International Clearing House for Birth Defects Monitoring to follow up the expected small number of embryos exposed and a Compensation Panel in the event of proven damage, funded by an excise tax, as with vaccines.

Finally, with all the great strides being made to unravel the human genome and determine the gene structures and their influence, we are much nearer to tailoring drugs to match male and female differences, and with enhanced computer power, this chapter may become moot.

ACKNOWLEDGMENTS

The author wishes to acknowledge that much of this chapter was supported by a grant from the NIH branch, Office of Protection from Research Risks.

RECOMMENDED READING

Mastroianni AC, Faden R, Federman D (eds). (1994) *Women and Health Research: Ethical and Legal Issues of Including Women in Clinical Studies* Academy Press.

REFERENCES

Abel JG, Sellers EM, Naranjo CA, et al (1979). Inter and intrasubject variation in diazepam free faction. *Clin Pharmacol Ther* 26: 247–55

Abernathy DR, Greenblatt DJ (1981) Impairment of antipyrine metabolism by low dose oral contraceptive steroids. *Clin Pharm Ther* 29: 106–110.

Allen MD, Greenblatt DJ (1981) Comparative protein binding of diazepam and desmethyldiazepam. *J Clin Pharmacol* 21: 219–23.

Arlington S (2000) Pharma 2005 (Industry Trends) *Pharmaceut Exec* 20(1): 74–80.

Bello M (1989) Liability crisis disrupts, distorts maternity care. *National Research Council New Report* 39: 6–9.

Booth M, Hunt JN, Miles JM, Murray FA (1957) Comparison of gastric emptying and secretion in men and women with reference to prevalence of duodenal ulcer in each sex. *Lancet* 1: 657–9.

Bush JK, Cook SF, Seigel E (1993) Issues of special populations in drug developments. *Drug Inf J* 27: 1185–1193.

Clark AF, Calandra RS, Bird CE (1971). Binding of Testosterone and 5-dihydrotestosterone to plasma protein in humans. *Clin Biochem* 4189–96

Coale AJ (1991) Population and development review. *J Population Council NY*.

Coles SL, Fries JF, Kraines RG, Roth SH (1988) Side effects of non-steroidal antiinflammatory drugs. *Am J Med* 74: 820–828.

Conrad CD, Hamilton JA (1986) Recurrent premenstrual decline in lithium concentration: clinical correlates and treatment implications. *J Am Acad Child Psychiat* 26(6): 852–3.

Cotton P (1990) Medical news and perspective. *J Am Med Assoc* 263 (8): 1049–50.

Cramer JA, Scheyer RD, Mattson RH (1990) Compliance declines between clinic visits. *Arch Intern Med* 150: 1509–10.

Diokno SC, Brock BM, Brown MB, Hertzog AR (1986) Prevalence of urinary incontinence and other urological symptoms in non-institutionalized elderly. *J Urol* B6: 1022–5.

Divoll M, Greenblatt DJ, Harmatz JS, Shader RI (1981) Effect of age and gender on disposition of temazepam. *Pharm Sci* 70: 1104–7

Edwards LD (1991) Summary of survey results on including women in drug development. PMA. In Development Series, *New Medicines for Women*, Dec. 1991; 22–8.

Elia J, Katz IR, Simpson GM (1987) Teratogenicity of psychotherapeutic medications. *Psychopharmacol Bull* 23: 531–86.

FDA (1986) *Drug Utilization in the US 1986*—Eighth Annual Review. FDA: Washington, DC.

Fed Reg (1990) Guideline for study of drugs likely to be used in the elderly. *Fed Reg* 55: FR 7777; (1997) Labeling: subsection, geriatric use. 21 CFR Pt 201.

Fed Reg (1994). Detection of toxicity to reproduction for medicinal products. ICH Guideline SSA (59 Fed Reg: 48746)

Fed Reg (1996). Detection of toxicity to reproduction for medicinal products. Addendum an toxicity to male fertility. ICH Guideline 553 (61 Fed Reg: 15360)

Fed Reg. (1993). Guideline for the study and evaluation of gender difference in the clinical evaluation of drugs. (58 Fed Reg: 39406–16)

Frederick J (1973) Epilepsy and pregnancy: a report from the Oxford Record Linkage Study. *Br Med J* ii: 442–8.

Frezza M, DiPadova C, Pozzato G et al (1990) High blood alcohol levels in women. The rate of decreased gastric alcohol dehydrogenase activity and first-pass metabolism. *N Eng J Med* 322: 95–9.

Gengo FM, Fagin SC, Kinkel WR, McHugh WB (1984) Serum concentrations of propranolol and migraine prophylaxis. *Arch Neurol* 41: 1306–8.

Greenblatt DJ, Divoll M, Harmatz JS, Shader RI (1980) Oxazepam kinetics: effects of age and sex. *J Pharmacol Exp Ther* 215: 86–91

Greenblatt DJ, Harmatz JS, Shader RI (1979). Sex differences in diazepam protein binding in patients with renal insufficiency. *Pharmacology* 16: 26–9

Halbreich U, Carson SW (1989) Drug studies in women of childbearing age: ethical and methodological consideration. *J Clin Psychopharmacol* 9: 328–33.

Health Care Financing Administration US Health and Human Services. www.hcfa gov/stats/stats.htm

Henrekens CH et al (1989) Steering Committee of the Physicians Health Study Research Group Final report on the aspirin component of the ongoing Physicians Health Study. *N Engl J Med* 321: 129–35.

Holden A (2000) New medicines in development for women: a 1999 survey. Pharmaceutical Research and Manufacturers' Association. **www.pharma.org/pdfw99**.pdf, 29–36.

Jefferson JW, Greist JH, Ackerman DL (eds) (1987) *Lithium Encyclopedia for Clinical Practice*, 2nd edn. American Psychiatric Press: Washington, DC. 640–45.

Kristensen CB (1983) Imipramine serum protein binding in healthy subjects, *Clin Pharmacol Ther* 34: 689–94

LaRosa GH, Pinn VW (1993) Gender bias in biomedical research. *J Am Med Womens Assoc* 48(5): 145–51.

Levine RJ (1975) *Ethics and Regulations of Clinical Research*, 2nd edn.

Lindhaut D, Happener RJ, Meinardi H (1984) Teratogenicity of antiepileptic drug combinations with the special emphasis on epoxidation of carbamazepine. *Epilepsia* 25: 77–83.

Lindhaut D, Schmidt D (1986) *In utero* exposure to valproate and neural tube defects. *Lancet* i: 1392–3.

MacDonald I (1965) Gastric activity during the menstrual cycle. *Gastroenterology* 30: 602–7.

Majaverian P, Rocci MC, Connor DP et al (1987) Effect of food on the absorption of enteric coated aspirin correlation with gastric residence time. *Clin Pharm Ther* 41 (1): 11–17.

Majaverian P, Vlasses PH, Kellner PE, Rocci ML (1988) Effects of gender posture and age on gastric residence time of an indigestible solid: pharmaceutical considerations. *Pharmaceut Res* 5(10): 639–44.

Martin RM, Biswas PN, Freemantle SN, Pearce GL, Minow RD (1998) Age and sex distribution of suspected adverse drug reactions to newly marketed drugs in general practice in England. *Br J Clin Pharmacol* 46(5): 505–11.

M'Buyamba-Kabunga JR, Lijen P, Fagard R, et al (1985). Erythrocyte concentrations and transmembrane fluxes of sodium and potassium and biochemical measurements during the menstrual cycle in normal women. *Am J Obstet Gynecol* 151: 687–93

Metropolitan Life Insurance (1999). Height – weight trades. www.indexmedico.com.

Miaskiewicz SL, Shively CA, Vesell ES (1982) Sex differences in absorption kinetics of sodium salicylates. *Clin Pharmacol Ther* 31: 30–37.

Michelakis AM, Yoshida H, Dormois JC (1975) Plasma renin activity and plasma aldosterone during the normal menstrual cycle. *Am J Obstet Gynecol* 123: 724–6.

National Disease and Therapeutic Index 1991 Plymouth Meeting, PA IMS 1991 America 1978–1989

National Institutes of Health Guide, vol 15. (1986) National Institutes of Health: Bethesda, MD; 14.

National Prescription Audit 1991 Plymouth Meeting, P. A., IMS America, Ltd. 1964–1989.

NIH/ADAMHA (1990) Policy concerning inclusion of women in study populations PT 343, 11: KW 1014002, 1014006. *NIH Guide Grants Contracts* 19: 18–19.

Notivol R, Carrio I, Cano LE, Storch M, Vilardell F (1984) *Scand J Gastroenterol* 18: 1107–14.

O'Reilly WB, Eakins PS, Gilfix MG, Richwald GA (1986) Childbirth and the Malpractice Insurance Industry. In Eakins JNP (ed.), *The American Way of Birth*. Temple University Press: Philadelphia, PA; 195–212.

Ortho (1991) 23rd Ortho Annual Birth Control Study. Survey by Ortho. Rariton, NJ.

Physician's Desk Reference Montvale, New Jersey: 56th Edition Medical Economics.

Pope J, Aufderheide TP, Ruthazer R, Woodard RH et al (2000) Missed diagnoses of acute cardiac ischemia in the emergency department. *N Engl J Med* 342 (16): 1163–71.

Raskin A (1974) Age–sex differences in response to antidepressant drugs. *J Nerv Ment Dis* 159: 120–30.

Ray WA, Griffin MR, Schaffner W et al (1987) Psychotropic drug use and the risk of hip fractures. *N Engl J Med* 316: 361–9.

Report of the Public Health Service Task Force on Women's Health Issues (1985) *PHS Rep* 100: 73–105.

Roberts RK, Desmond PV, Wilkinson GR, Schenker S (1979) Disposition of chlordiazepoxide: Sex differences and effects of oral contraceptives. *Clin Pharmacol Ther* 25: 826–50

Roscizieweska D, Buniner B, Guz I, Sawisza H (1986) Ovarian hormones anticonvulsant group and seizures during the menstrual cycle in women with epilepsy. *J Neurol Neurosurg Psychiat* 49: 47–51.

Routledge PA, Stargel NW, Kitchell BB, Barchowski A, Shand DG (1981) Sex-related differences in plasma protein binding of lignocaine and diazepam. *Br J Clin Pharmacol* 11: 245–50

Shavit G, Lerman P, Konczyn AD et al (1984) Phenytoin pharmacokinetics in catamenial epilepsy. *Neurology* 34: 959–61.

Simpson JM, Bateman DN, Rawlins MD (1987) Using the adverse reactions register to study the effects of age and sex on adverse drug reactions. *Statist Med* 6: 863–7.

Smith JM, Baldessarini RJ (1973) Changes in prevalence, severity and recovery in tardise dyskinesia with age. *Arch Gen Psychiat* 29: 177–89.

Stewart DE (1998) Are there special considerations in the prescription of serotonin reuptake inhibitors for women. *Can J Psychiat* 43(9): 900–904.

Tran C, Knowles SR, Liu BA, Shear NH (1998) Gender differences in adverse drug reactions. *J Clin Pharmacol* 38(1): 1003–9.

Trussell J, Hatcher RA, Cates W, Stewart FH, Kost K (1990) Contraceptive failures in the United States—an update. *Stud Family Planning* 21(1).

US Public Health Services Office of Womens Health (1996). Heart disease and stroke in women. Report on data collected by the National Heart, Lung, and Blood Institute. Chart Book: Bathesda, Maryland.

Walle T, Byington RP, Furberg CT et al (1985) Biologic determinants of propranolol disposition. Results from 1308 patients in the β-blocker heart attack trial. *Clin Pharmacol Ther* 38: 509–18.

Walle T, Walle U, Cowart TD, Conradi EC (1989) Pathway selective sex differences in metabolic clearance of propranolol in human subjects. *Clin Pharm Ther* 46(3): 257–63.

Weissman MM, Klerman GL (1977) Sex differences and the epidemiology of depression. *Arch Gen Psychiat* 34: 98–11.

Williams PT (1996) High density lipoprotein cholesterol and other risk factors for coronary heart disease in female runners. *N Engl J Med* 334 (20): 1298–1303.

Wilson JF (1973) *Environment and Birth Defects*. Academic Press: New York.

Wilson JG (1972) Environmental effects on development—teratology. In Assali NS (ed.), *Pathophysiology of Gestation* vol 2. Academic Press: New York, 269–320.

Wilson K, Oram M, Horth CE, Burnett D (1982). The influence of the menstrual cycle on the metabolism and clearance of methaqualone. *Br J Clin Pharmac other* 14: 333–9.

Wilson MA, Dwyer KD, Roy EJ (1986). Direct effects of ovarian hormones on antidepressant binding sites. *Brain Res Bull* 22: 181–5

Wilson MA, Roy EJ (1986). Pharmacokinetics of imipramine are affected by age and sex in rats. *Life Sci*, 38: 711–8.

Wright RA, Krinsky S, Fleeman C et al (1983) Gastric emptying and obesity. *Gastroenterology* 84: 747–51.

Yacobi A, Stoll RG, Di'Sanio AR, Levy G (1976) Intersubject variation of warfarin binding to protein in serum of normal subjects. *Res Commun Chem Pathol Pharmacol* 14: 743–46.

Yazigi Odem RR, Polakoski KL (1991) Demonstration of specific binding of cocain to human spermatozoa, *J Am Med Assoc* 266 (14): 1950–60.

Yoder MC, Belik J, Lannon R, Pereita GR (1984) Infants of mothers treated with lithium (Li) during pregnancy have an increased incidence of prematurity. *Pediat Res* 18: 163A.

16

Clinical Research in Children

BACKGROUND

The world population reached 6 billion in June 2000, and half of the world's population (3 billion) are less than 15 years old. Sadly, the mortality rate of children in Third-World countries is 10 times higher than in the developed world. Before 1850, half of the children born in the USA died from infections before 5 years of age. The introduction of sanitation, antiseptics and, in the last century, vaccines, and lately medicines, have made such early deaths in the USA now very uncommon.

Today, accident is the largest killer of children, accounting for 2500 deaths in children under 5 years old; this compares to 700 deaths from congenital abnormalities, 518 from cancer and 473 from murder. AIDS is the leading infectious cause of death in the under–5 year-olds (200). The major causes of death in the 5–14 year-olds are accidents (3500), cancer (1053) and murder (570). Again, in this age group, AIDS is the leading infectious cause of death (National Center for Health Statistics 1996).

Many of the childhood cancers are hematologic, and great improvements in survival have been achieved. For example, the acute leukemia survival rate in children has risen from 53% in 1970 to 80% by 1989 (American Cancer Society); and new surgical techniques and new devices are improving and sometimes correcting (even by intrauterine surgery) many previously fatal congenital abnormalities, e.g. hypoplastic heart.

In June 1998 (Holmer 1998), the Pharmaceutical Research Manufacturers' Association (PhRMA) reported, from their survey of pharmaceutical companies, that 187 medicines or vaccines were in development for children. This was an increase from 146 the previous year. In addition, 20 new medicines were approved and made available for children. Together, they included 44 new agents targeting cancer, 14 for cystic fibrosis, 13 for asthma, nine for epilepsy, and 23 potential vaccines.

This chapter will focus on the current regulatory requirements, their background, the clinical study, challenges and the clinical issues of drug research in the pediatric population.

Gordon Still has estimated that over 2500 studies in the FDA's pediatric subgroups may need to be conducted over the next 3 years (Still 2000). This includes completion of pediatric studies on the FDA priority list of marketed products. Estimates of the annual cost to the industry of these studies vary. The FDA estimated in 1994 that $13.5–20.9 million/year would be spent by industry (Fed Reg 1998). At a press conference, Christopher Jennings, President Clinton's principal health care advisor, said that pediatric label studies would only be about 1% of the development cost of a drug. Dr Henry Miller (1997), a former FDA Director of the Office of Biotechnology, said that applying Jennings' figure will mean an industry cost of $200 million (1% of the $20 billion spent on R&D). Dr Gordon Still, presenting at the 36th Drug Information Association (DIA) Annual Meeting (1999), estimated the cost at $892 million if all five pediatric subgroups were to be studied (based on 1999 study costs).

These additional costs for pediatric studies may be justified if these studies satisfy all global markets. Macleod (1991) estimated that 'developing countries' by the year 2000 will comprise 36% of the total pharmaceutical market and that half of their populations are children (accounting for 18% of the market). In the developed countries, children under 18 years account for 20% of the market. It would seem that the 38% pediatric share of the global market is worth an extra effort.

Principles and Practice of Pharmaceutical Medicine. Edited by A. J. Fletcher, Lionel D. Edwards, Anthony W. Fox and Peter Stonier © 2002 John Wiley & Sons Ltd.

CHILDREN, THE THERAPEUTIC ORPHANS

The Food, Drug and Cosmetic Act, first passed in 1906, was dramatically altered by the 1962 Kefauver–Harris amendments as a direct result of the thalidomide tragedy. This amendment required that drugs must be both safe and effective before marketing approval could be given. In addition, adequate animal, toxicology and fertility testing had to be concluded prior to the first dose in humans. Substantial additional testing in animals and in humans was required prior to marketing approval. This led to the era of the Science of Clinical Trial Design. Regrettably, the testing of drugs in children did not advance at a similar pace, and most drugs (unless specifically intended for children) were never tested in children by the sponsors of new medicines.

Physicians were thus forced to use most drugs 'off-label' and extrapolate the child dose on a comparative weight basis from that in adults. This often involved parents splitting or crushing tablets, hiding medication in spoonfuls of honey, or sprinkling a crushed tablet onto a meal. Each time this happened, a little more confidence in and knowledge of the drug was gained, but each child was a 'one-off experiment' and only provided a learning curve for the individual physician. Eventually, academia would publish a series of cases, so giving guidance on dosing and likely toxic effects. Even so, the average pediatrician and family practitioner felt uneasy and legally vulnerable about off-label use.

A few drugs were developed for children in such categories as antibiotics, antihistamines, and antiepileptics. But otherwise, few firms undertook studies to develop full pediatric label instructions or even pediatric formulations. Liquid formulations did exist for some drugs, but mainly for use in the elderly. In 1975, Wilson surveyed the 1973 Physician's Desk Reference for labeling instructions for pediatric patients and pregnant or breast-feeding women. He found that 78% of listed drugs either had no information for pediatric dosing or contained a disclaimer. A subsequent survey by Gilman (1992) showed that this situation had not improved qualitatively and had also risen to 81%. Eventually, the FDA issued the 1994 rule, which sought to strengthen the 1979 guideline on pediatric labeling requirements (Fed Reg 1994).

The Pediatric Use Working Group, chaired by Miriam Pina (1995) (FDA Division of Pulmonary Drugs), examined data that the FDA had acquired on 1994 pediatric prescriptions from IMS. From these they identified the top ten drugs used 'off label' in children: Albuterol, Phenergan, Ampicillin i.m. or i.v., Auralgan otic solution, Lotison, Prozac, Intal, Zoloft, Ritalin (under 6 years old) and alupent syrup (under 6). A combined total of over 5 million of these 10 products were prescribed in 1994.

Clearly, firms needed further encouragement to submit additional pediatric data, so in 1997 Congress passed the FDA Modernization Act (FDAMA). This called for firms to submit data on children to support labeling for a new pediatric subsection before the drug could be approved. This applied to drugs that could be projected to provide therapeutic benefit to substantial numbers of children. In exchange, Congress felt that an inducement was required and wrote into the Act provision for an extension of a drug's patent life by 6 months if pediatric studies were done. For a $2 billion drug such as Claritin (Loratidine) 6 months' extra exclusivity is not 'small change'. The FDA was requested to provide guidance and, in December, 1998, it issued the Final Rule Amendments to the Pediatric Subsections to be implemented April 1999, governing the need for pediatric studies, and extending the requirements to biological drugs and already-marketed drugs. The FDA identified drugs for which supplemental data was still needed for pediatric labeling. The FDA has issued an annual list of 'priority drugs' for which additional pediatric information may be 'beneficial'.

FDA chose to interpret the patent life extension as applying to all indications, not just to pediatric use. As might be expected, the generic companies are appealing this interpretation of the pediatric rule.

1994 AND 1998 FINAL RULES ON PEDIATRIC STUDIES (*FED REG* 1994, 1998)

Products Subject to the Rule

For drugs that are new molecular entities (NMEs), a determination should be made by the sponsor of the potential usefulness of the new drug in a pediatric population. If it is likely to generate over 100 000 prescriptions/year, this would indicate the need to develop a pediatric formulation and suitable pediatric studies. If it is likely to generate less than 50 000 prescriptions/year, the sponsor may be granted a waiver by the FDA for pediatric data, and a disclaimer statement allowed. Either way, in a children's disease, if less than 200 000 patients/year may benefit, then orphan-drug status with seven/year exclusivity may be applicable. This would then apply only to that pediatric indication.

The requirements of the Pediatric Final Rule now includes marketed drugs and biologics. The FDA has already listed products affected and sent pediatric data requests to firms. The firms had until April 2001 to provide the extra data.

Data to Be Provided

If considerable data exists, or is planned, for same indications in adults, it may be appropriate to extrapolate safety and efficacy from adults to children. But pharmacokinetic studies to determine dosing and, if possible, pharmacodynamics data, will usually be required for children. Discussion with the FDA is recommended early on, to establish whether pediatric data will be required and which of the five groups should be covered (preterm, neonate 0–1 month, infants 1–2 years, children 2–12 years and adolescents 12–16 years). One or more adequately sized efficacy and safety studies may be required, especially if the drug or disease behaves differently in children, or the drug uses different metabolic pathways. This may occur if the particular adult enzyme is not present in children, or is only present in low quantities. If a different indication to that in adults is being sought, then one or two sizable safety and efficacy studies, in one or more age groups, are likely to be required. This is in addition to pediatric pharmacokinetic data. Sponsors should also plan for the major ethnic groups to be represented in these studies.

Frequently, the FDA may allow approval of a drug with incomplete pediatric data and defer the completion to a Phase IV commitment, especially when the product is life saving and the only treatment available.

MAJOR PHYSIOLOGIC VARIATIONS IN PEDIATRICS

In the past, the statement that 'children are not little people' dominated research thinking. In general, both in children and in the elderly, drugs and biological products behave similarly to that in the 18–65 year-old population, although this expectation must be adjusted for age-related differences in pharmacokinetic variables, such as immature or aging enzyme metabolism systems as well as elimination rates affected by immature or aging organs of excretion.

In neonates, the gastric pH is biphasic, being high in the first few days after birth and decreasing by day 30, but it takes 5–12 years for the adult pattern and value to emerge (Signer and Fridrich 1975). On the other hand, the methylation pathway, unimportant in adults, is well developed in children. Furthermore, acetaminophen is less toxic to children than to adults, probably because it utilizes the sulphate metabolic pathway (Rane 1992).

Most infants are slow acetylators and may accumulate toxic levels of those drugs that are metabolized by this second phase of metabolism route. Renal perfusion and glomerular filtration rates (GFR) vary: for the premature, 2–4 ml/min; for neonates, 25 ml/min; and by 1–1.5 years old, 125 ml/min, which is equivalent to adult clearance rates (Arant 1978). The potential toxic implication of renal metabolites and elimination of unchanged drug in the very young are obvious (Stewart and Hampton 1987).

Dosing

Without pediatric pharmacokinetic data, dosing in children has depended on extrapolations from the adult data, either by weight or by body surface area. Using weight may result in overdosing neonates but underdosing infants and children. Using body surface area may be better because of its linear increase with age and its good correlation with cardiac output, renal flow and glomerular filtration rate—more so than weight. Neither method compensates for the varying metabolism aforementioned, nor for differences in drug disposition between children and adults.

Concerns in Formulations for Pediatrics

If a drug is to be given by injection, i.m. or i.v., this may require only volume variations. But most drugs developed for adults are given by the oral route, as tablets, capsules or caplets. The adult formulation is usually determined by marketing considerations. Invariably, for children, especially under age 7 years, liquid or syrup must be formulated. Most drugs taste bitter or unpleasant (which is why most tablets are sugar-coated). Sometimes, it may be impossible to completely mask the taste. A commitment to a pediatric formulation requires a whole gamut of testing and the development of specific product specifications. If the liquid formulation changes the bioavailability (faster or slower absorption), then further efficacy and safety studies may be required. A further concern is that liquid formulations often have a shorter shelf life than tablets. Finally, stability characteristics or other factors may make it impossible to make a liquid or syrup or glycolated elixir, sprinkle beads or powder sachets, and split or crushed tablets may be a last resort. In the later two cases, an even distribution of active compound and other inactive excipients must be demonstrated. In addition, a lack of effect an bioavailability must be proved if such advice is to appear in the dosing instructions.

Toxicology

The plastic nature of immature organs such as kidney, liver, brain and lung may indicate the need for more animal toxicology. Frequently, neonatal acute and subacute toxicology studies are undertaken in two animal species. Because of the small size of both mouse and rat pups, this may prove a challenge to administer the active drug. The common 'mixing with chow' is inappropriate in neonates. Dog pups usually provide one of the two species, so a special liquid formulation for

animals may be required (if the product is intended for oral delivery), and given by dropper gauage.

CLINICAL STUDIES

Pharmacokinetic

The traditional pharmacokinetic (PK) study volunteer study in healthy children has proved very hard to set up, because of the attitude of many parents and overviewing independent review boards (IRBs). Even in pediatric patients, the frequency and total volume requirements for samples for conventional PK studies can cause the same refusals. However, there are pediatric research units that specialize in these studies, with minimum needle sticks, minute blood volumes, and IRBs sympathetic to the needs of the pediatric community. The National Institute of Child Health and Human Development has set up a 'network of pediatric pharmacology units', usually in academic regional centers, now numbering 13 units. There are other non-governmental specialized units also available for pediatric PK work.

An alternative method of getting pharmacokinetic data is to take a small extra sample of blood (and urine) at a child's regular scheduled visit when blood is drawn for routine blood work. The time of day of this sample is predetermined by the time of the administration of the medicine. If samples are obtained from many children, a weight–age-corrected, scatter-plot graph can be constructed and a pharmacokinetic profile be calculated. This is the 'pharmacokinetic screen' method. A version of this method is also utilized to gather ethnic data for labeling in adults as well as children, and is called 'population pharmacokinetics'.

Recruitment

One of the major problems in running pediatric clinical trials is the availability of pediatric patients, who tend to be scattered, because they are numerically less likely to have diseases (other than asthma and the usual childhood illnesses). This affects the logistics of screening and subsequent clinic visits.

Another hurdle is finding trained pediatric investigators or pediatric pharmacologists, and overseas they are even harder to find. In Europe, there is collaboration between the USA-based Pediatric Pharmacology Research Units (PPRU), the European Society of Developmental Pharmacology, and the European Network for Drug Investigation in Children (ENDIC). For diseases of children, there are often self-help organizations who can prove invaluable in recruiting children and in reassuring their parents.

A large package of data, and two well controlled pivotal studies of safety and efficacy are rarely required, with the exception of diseases specific to childhood, such as surfactant studies in respiratory Distress Syndrome. This is especially the case if the drug has similar effects in both adult and pediatric populations e.g., antihistamines.

However, if a disease or drug behaves in different ways in children compared with adults but a large body of safety data exists in adults, then usually only a single efficacy and safety study is required.

Ethical Concerns

The American Academy of Pediatrics formed a Committee on Drugs to examine ethical issues of pediatric studies for its members and for the guidance of IRBs dealing with pediatric studies. The Committee released its report in 1995. This report (Committee Drugs, American Academy of Pediatrics) is very comprehensive, but amongst its many recommendations the following areas are highlighted, as follows.

Vulnerability

In this special population, there is a special duty to avoid (unintended) coercion of the patient, parent or guardian. This coercion may arise because the investigator is usually also the treating physician. It would be better to have a colleague explain and obtain the informed consent. There are varying degrees of vulnerability. Patients handicapped either mentally, emotionally or physically are frequently institutionalized and may be supervised

as Wards of Court or by a social welfare agency. These patients should be rarely used, unless the treatment is for serious disease specific to institutional settings and no other treatment is available.

Emergency situations can arise where it may be impossible to obtain written informed consent from a parent or guardian. Medications for this type of problem will require intense IRB review and overview; only in special circumstances will informed consent be waived, and then it must 'not adversely affect the rights and welfare of the subject'. (Abramson et al 1986). The last category is the use of a research medicine in a child close to dying who has either no response to standard therapy or where no alternative therapy exists. The agent to be considered must have some evidence of efficacy (animal proof of concept or clinical data and a good chance of a beneficial result). The risk of unintended coercion of desperate parents is especially to be guarded against.

IRBs' Special Emphasis

IRBs have a duty to make sure the study is of value to children in general and in most cases to the patient him/herself; is robust enough to give answers; and attempts to minimize risk and maximize benefit. In reviewing the protocol, the IRBs should involve health care specialists who are aware of the special medical, psychological, and social needs of the child, and the disease as special medical, psychological and social needs of the child, and the disease as might be impacted by the study.

In studies conducted on diseases mainly affecting pediatric patients, the development will be entirely in pediatric patients. However, in addition to the appropriate usual toxicology and neonate animal toxicology, the first-in-humans studies for toxicity and safety are usually done in healthy adult volunteers. Clearly, however, drugs such as the surfactants would yield no useful data from adult testing. For these unique pediatric situations, new measurements and endpoints may need to be developed and validated. Frequently the FDA will involve an advisory panel to help determine what these might be.

The Use of a Placebo Control

Placebo control is desired whenever possible if using a placebo does not place the pediatric patients at increased risk. The AAP Committee on Drugs (1995) outlined other circumstances:

- No other therapy exists or is of questionable efficacy, and the new agent might modify the disease.
- If the commonly used therapy has a high profile of adverse events and risk greater than benefits.
- When the disease fluctuates frequently from exacerbations to remissions thus the efficacy of the (new) treatment cannot be evaluated.

CONCLUSION

The ICH draft guidance on pediatric issues has been published in the *Federal Register* (2000), but at this point of writing has not been issued as a final rule. This guidance covers pediatric formulation, development, ethics, regional and cultural issues, regulatory expectations, duration and type of studies, and age ranges to be studied. The guidance is similar to the FDA Final Rules (*Fed Reg* 1994, 1998) with the addition of a fifth group, preterm newborn infants. It also seems better organized and informative, but then, hindsight is always helpful.

The face of pediatric pharmacologic medicine has been changed. In future, for pediatricians there will be less uncertainty and better predictive information available; for children, safer and more effective dosages will result. For the industry, the added cost of research will be more than recouped in a new global market to which previously they could not promote their products. This is supported by the 1998 survey by PhRMA, which showed that medicines and vaccines in development for children were up 28% from the previous year.

REFERENCES

Abramson VS, Meisal A, Sufar P (1986) Deferred consent—a new approach for resuscitation research on comatized patients. *J Am Med Assoc* 225: 2466–71.

Arant BS (1978) Developmental patterns of renal function maturation compared to the neonate. *J Pediat* 92: 705–12.

American Cancer Society.

Committee on Drugs, American Academy of Pediatrics. Guidelines for the Ethical Conduct to evaluate drugs in Pediatric populations. Pediatrics 95: 286–94.

FDA (1997) Food and Drug Administration Modernization Act. Pub. Law 105–115 (1997) Nov. 21), USDC 355a, 111 Stat. 2296.

Fed Reg (1994) Specific requirements on content and format of labeling for human prescription drugs revision of 'pediatric use' subsection in the labeling (1994) *Fed. Reg.* 59(238): 64240–50.

Fed Reg (1998) Final rule regulations requiring manufacturers to assess the safety and effectiveness of new drugs and biological products in pediatric patients (1998) *Fed Reg* 63: 66632.

Fed Reg (1983), 16d.

Fed Reg (2000) International Conference on Harmonization: clinical investigation of medicinal products in the pediatric population (2000) *Fed Reg* 65 (71): (draft).

Gilman JT, Gal P (1992) Pharmacokinetic and pharmacodynamic data collection in children and neonates. *Clin Pharmacokinet* 23: 1–9.

Holmer AF. (1998) Survey or new medicines in children (1995) *Pharmaceutical Research and manufactures of America.* http://www.phrma.org.

MacLeod SM (1991) Clinical pharmacology and optimal therapeutics in developing countries: aspirations and hopes of the pediatric clinical pharmacology subcommittee. *J Clin. Epidemiol* 44(suppl II): 89–93.

Miller telephone interview (1997) Script No. 2260, Aug. 22, 1997.

National Center for Health Statistics (1996) Based on data from US Dept. Health and Human Services.

Pina LM (1995) Drugs widely used off-label in pediatrics. Report of the Pediatric Use Survey Working Group of the Pediatric Subcommittee.

Rane A (1992) Drug disposition and action in infants and children. In Yaffe SJ, Arand AJV (eds), *Pediatric Pharmacology, Therapeutic Principles in Practice*. Sanders: New York; 10–12.

Signer E, Fridrich R (1975) Gastric emptying in newborns and young infants. *Acta Paediat Scand* 64: 525–30.

Stewart GF, Hampton EM (1987) Effect of maturation on drug deposition in pediatric patients. *Clin Pharm* b: 548–64.

Still JG (2000) The pediatric research initiative in the United States: implications for global pediatric research. *Drug Inf J* 35: 207–12.

Wilson JT (1975) Pragmatic assessment of medicines available for your children and pregnant or breast-feeding women. In Morsell PL, Garattini S, Serini F (eds), *Basic Therapeutic Aspects of Perinatal Pharmacology*. Raven: New York.

Section IV

Applied Aspects of Drug Development

Introduction to Section IV:

Anthony W. Fox

President, EBD Group, Carlsbad, California.

Having covered in Sections II and III the strictly clinical, more orthodox aspects of drug development, we now turn to some applied aspects. In general, these reflect relatively modern sophistications in the development process, compared with, for example, many types of clinical trial design, which have been available for decades.

These modern aspects of drug development are rarely optional. All are crucial for the success of a product in the marketplace. Several of the next chapters describe methodologies that teach us, on new dimensions, about properties that are intrinsic to drugs. Some (e.g., pharmaceoeconomics) are also becoming of increasing importance in the regulatory approval process.

17

Biotechnology Products and Their Development

David Shapiro and Anthony W. Fox

Scripps Clinic, La Jolla, CA, and EBD Group Inc., Carlsbad, CA, USA

The objectives of this chapter are to describe what biotechnology products are, and how their regulation is similar to, or differs from, small molecule drugs. It is a common assumption that biotechnology has sprung from nothing, *de novo*, within a small number of recent years. This is not the case, and we shall show how the recent growth of this field actually has a basis which is, in many ways, common to and interconnected with the development of all other types of drugs.

Definition: Biotechnology products are those that are prepared using biological, rather than chemical synthetic, processes. Biological processes may be manipulated *in vivo*, *ex vivo* or *in vitro*.

The list of types of biotechnology products is quite long: peptides, organisms (living, dead or attenuated), gene 'constructs', any type of fermented product (even when these may also be synthesized chemically), and antisense compounds. To date, peptides have been the largest of these product groups, and themselves comprise such diverse biological agents as hormones, antibodies, cytokines (including interferons), and immune adjuvants (including non-mammalian examples, such as keyhole limpet hemocyanin).

Biological products have a longer and more illustrious history that is generally assumed: at one time smallpox accounted for 10% of deaths in some countries, but today this is the only infectious disease ever to have been eradicated from our planet; the development of cow pox vaccination was in 1796, while the last case of the disease occurred in 1979 following a laboratory accident. The Variocella vaccine may yet not be redundant in combatting bioterrorism.

It is beyond the scope of this chapter to discuss all potential applications and all present technologies associated with biological drugs. We merely provide an overview. We shall not cover orthodox vaccines, fermented products (e.g. for antibiotics), blood products, tissue-extracted hormones, diagnostic products (e.g. antibody-based assay systems), and devices utilizing biotechnology products, which are not themselves used therapeutically. These are, technically, biotechnology products, but here we wish to concentrate on the newer technologies.

There are approximately 1250 biotechnology companies in the USA and Canada, about half this number in Europe, and a few more throughout the rest of the world. Many of these companies are small organizations. Small companies' research activities may be restricted to the preclinical discovery and investigation of compounds; therefore their business environment and practices differ from large, fully integrated 'pharmaceutical' companies. On the other hand, the less numerous but much bigger pharmaceutical companies are all engaged in biotechnology. Somewhat arbitrarily, we shall use the term 'biotechnology company' rather loosely in this chapter to mean the typical small organization. The term 'biotechnology products' refers to the compounds themselves, regardless of the size of the organization developing them.

Principles and Practice of Pharmaceutical Medicine. Edited by A. J. Fletcher, Lionel D. Edwards, Anthony W. Fox and Peter Stonier © 2002 John Wiley & Sons Ltd.

REGULATORY CONSIDERATIONS

In most countries regulation of drug and biological compound development and marketing has usually derived from governmental response to crisis.

USA Perspective

The Kefauver–Harris Act in the USA, after the thalidomide catastrophe, is a good example of response to crisis. Such *post hoc* legislation results in differential oversight of different types of agents.

The initial legislation affecting biologics was the Safe Vaccines and Sera Act of 1904, the focus of which was the development of safe, pure, and potent vaccination preparations. This was somewhat superseded by the Public Health Service Act (1944), written with blood products and prevention of the transmission of disease by infusion in mind. All the previous drug legislation had been supervised by the Department of Agriculture. It was not until 1972 that orthodox drugs and biologics were brought under the same regulatory umbrella. The Food and Drug Administration (FDA), a single branch of the Public Health Service, then accepted the responsibility for biologics, transferred from the Department of Agriculture.

Similar historical events stimulated other models in other countries. In spite of the modern uniformity of regulatory authority that exists in the USA, much of the legislation has not been repealed or replaced, and inconsistencies between the regulations relating to biologics, drugs, and devices illogically persist. In the USA, regulatory oversight of therapeutic biological compounds (i.e. applicable to the prevention, treatment, or cure of disease or injuries of man) includes:

- Viruses.
- Therapeutic sera, toxin or antitoxins.
- Vaccines.
- Blood and its components and derivatives.
- Allergenic products.
- Arsphenamine and derivatives.

However, 'jurisdictional challenges' (i.e. regulators' turf battles) continue for various compounds and combination of drugs, biologics, and devices. For no biological reason, it has been agreed, for example, that hormones are always 'orthodox' drugs, while HIV diagnostics are 'biologicals'. 'Blood-devices' and 'blood-drugs' are handled by both the drug and biological divisions within FDA.

However, regulators' approaches and practices for drugs and biologics are slowly converging. In the USA and elsewhere, evidence of this convergence may be found in:

- Common IND regulations (there are no unique regulations for biologics undergoing experimental study).
- Good clinical practices (GCP).
- International harmonization.
- Good manufacturing practice (GMP).
- 'Fast-track' designation for accelerating review and approval.
- Treatment INDs.
- Compassionate (emergency) INDs.

However, illogicalities persist, particularly with new Congressional Acts. For example, the Waxman–Hatch legislation gave authority for generics and provided patent term exclusivity for drugs, but not for biologics licensed prior to 1972. Similarly, the pediatric 'exclusivity' that the Act initiated also only pertained to drugs with unexpired patent or Orphan Drug exclusivity. Another example: the Centers for Disease Control remains involved with some compensation issues for pediatric vaccines, a unique administrative arrangement.

BIOTECHNOLOGY VS. CONVENTIONAL DRUG PRODUCTS

There is a widespread, but largely unreasonable, perception that biotechnology products differ in their properties to conventional small molecules drugs. For example, it is widely believed that simple pharmacokinetic models cannot adequately describe the behavior of biological agents *in vivo*. However, Table 17.1 lists the factors that need to be considered when modeling pharmacokinetic–pharmacodynamic (PK–PD) relationships for gene therapy products, and most of these have correlates with the behaviour of orthodox drugs. While quantitative data relating to the intracellular distribution of these agents may not be known or

Table 17.1 Pharmacokinetic considerations for gene therapy agents

Pharmacokinetic Property	Gene Therapy Property
Absorption	DNA vector distribution
Distribution	Vector fraction target cell uptake
Distribution	Genetic material traffic in organelles
Metabolism	DNA degradation
Metabolism	mRNA production
Metabolism	Protein production—quantity
Excretion	Protein production—stability
Metabolism, excretion	Protein production—compartmentalization
Excretion	Protein production—secretory fate

Adapted from Ledley and Ledley, (1994).

easy to measure, the underlying principles of absorption, distribution, metabolism and excretion (ADME) are quite constant, even though new paradigms and models are required to describe the properties of biological compounds.

Most biotechnology products have complicated PK–PD relationships. However, this can also be the case for orthodox drugs. Consider, for example, antidepressant therapies, where 3 weeks or more is usually needed before any therapeutic response may be seen. Again, angiotensin-converting enzyme (ACE) inhibitors are characterized by prolonged activity in chronic therapy, yet these drugs are still antihypertensive, even after ACE activity has compensated and been restored. Corticosteroid therapy requires access to the cell nucleus, as do many gene therapies. Among biotechnology products, antibody complement fixation and cellular attack may be an all-or-none phenomenon, DNA lysis in sputum may not actually require drug absorption at all, and clot lysis may depend on a wide range of endogenous plasma proteins, each with its own concentration–response relationships. The problems and analysis of tachyphylaxis are therefore common to both orthodox and biotechnology products.

MANUFACTURING ISSUES

Manufacturing changes are more like to affect the clinical profile of biological compounds than small chemical entities. Small changes in the three-dimensional folding, post-translational modification, or glycosylation of proteins can significantly alter biological activity. The potential for the replication of viruses or bacteria in fermenters, and their persistence in finished drug product raise additional safety concerns about the manufacturing process for such compounds. For the clinical trialist, this leads to a generality: when studying biologicals, there is usually a greater need for early-stage test medications to be as similar as possible to the marketed product than for 'orthodox' small chemicals.

PRODUCT CLASSES AND RESULTANT CLINICAL TRIAL ISSUES

Many of the principles outlined in other chapters for Phase I and II studies of these compounds are equally applicable to the testing of most biotechnology products. The same basic principal of demonstrating clinical tolerability as a priority over proving efficacy must apply. Other chapters also discuss some specific toxicology and drug discovery aspects of biotechnology products.

The design of a development program for a biological product has the same principles as for ordinary drugs, and this should be familiar to the competent clinical trialist. The development program should be determined by the nature and needs of the disease; often the pharmacological activity of a biological product is likely to be very precise, e.g. an antibody will bind to a previously identified, narrow range of antigens, and the pathogenesis or source of antigen presentation will have a fixed relationship to a well-described disease or set of diseases. Equally useful in the case of biologics is to begin development with an agreed, desirable package insert or product information leaflet. That document can then be used to define the development strategy. Only those tactics (i.e. clinical trial designs, milestones, and product-killing findings) that are justified or validated by that strategy should be implemented. The nature and seriousness of the disease being treated is just as important as in more orthodox clinical trials—the degree of lethality or morbidity associated with the disease treated with existing therapies is correlated positively with the degree of intolerability of the test agent that may be accepted.

Likewise, the trialist who switches to a biological product will find it very familiar to prove efficacy by comparing study medication to active or placebo comparative agents. With 'breakthrough' agents that offer the potential for a new type of therapy, clinical trials can be conducted, comparing the trial agent to a placebo. As usual, the central ethical consideration is whether standard treatment is being withheld from patient, and the debate should not be about the use of placebo in an absolute sense. Dose–response relationships need to be evaluated for biological agents prior to approval, even when the biological response is a 'all-or-nothing' type of response (e.g. serological conversion). It should be remembered that dose-response relationships must be understood for populations, as well as within individuals. Therapies like vaccines need to be evaluated in different racial populations.

Peptides

For a long time, interest in biotechnology centered on the production and properties of administered hormones ranging from tripeptides, e.g. corticotrophin releasing factor (CRF); through nonapeptides, such as vasopressin analogues; to longer polypeptide chains, e.g. insulins and growth hormones. As the length of the molecule increases, the three-dimensional structure becomes an important determinant of *in vivo* activity and properties.

However, there are also important freedoms that an increase in protein size can bring. Single-peptide mutations become less important as protein size increases. The scope for post-translational modification is also greater in large polypeptides than in small ones. Good examples of this are the large qualitative changes in pharmacology of the single amino acid that distinguishes arginine-vasopressin (the human antidiuretic hormone) from human oxytocin, or the marked differences in pharmacodynamics between calcitonin and calcitonin gene-related peptide (CGRP), which are both encoded by the same gene.

In comparison with non-peptide, non-nucleic acid drugs, the principal specific adverse events associated with peptides may be viewed as the sum of two processes: immunological and physiological changes. The former is non-specific and familiar to most physicians, the latter is usually specific to the known function of the hormone or enzyme. Immunologic adverse events can, in turn, be viewed as either active or passive: what the drug does to the patient (histamine release, B lymphocyte proliferation, etc.) and what the patient does to the drug (enhanced clearance, peptide cleavage, etc.). The clinical correlates of these cellular processes then range from a need for ever-increasing doses to maintain biological effect, to the acute emergencies of anaphylaxis. For example, around 13% of patients given aglucerase used for Type 1 Gaucher's disease develop IgG antibodies to the enzyme; approximately 25% of these have symptoms of hypersensitivity.

Clinical trialists should be careful not to ignore the toxicological potential of the often large amounts of vehicle (ionic strengths, buffering materials, extreme pH) that may be required to maintain complex peptides in a stable form. These can include unanticipated allergens, nephrotoxins and hepatotoxins.

Historically, insulin is an early and classic example of a biotechnology product, illustrating the general problems that are associated with peptide drugs and how modern technology leads to improved therapy. Prior to the production of human insulin by cell-based fermentation processes, treatment was with pancreatic extracts of porcine or bovine origin. Insulin resistance correlated with effective, specific antibody responses in many diabetics, who had a 'career' of increasing insulin dose, punctuated by hypoglycemia when changing from one animal source to another without changing dose size. Some patients became so competent at clearing bovine or porcine insulin that they needed extracts from exotic species such as whales. The modification of recombinant chimeric or pure cell lines to secrete human insulin, the development of large-scale fermenters to multiply such cultures, and the ability to purify cell-free insulin from other materials in the broth, has led to a sufficient supply of exogenous, but human, insulin. Now in use by almost all diabetics in the Western world, immune responses to this homobiotic molecule are very rare, and dose sizes remain more stable than before.

We shall now consider the principal subsets of peptide therapeutic classes within the context of similarities to, and differences from, orthodox small molecules of purely chemical synthesis.

Hormones

In addition to insulin, various other hormones made by recombinant methods have been approved or are under development. The most commonly prescribed examples at present include growth hormone (somatrem, Protropin™, Genentech, Inc.) or erythropoietin (epoeitin α, Epogen™; Amgen Inc.).

Enzymes

There are a few peptide drugs that act as enzymes. Dornase alpha (Pulmozyme®; Genentech Inc.) is an example; in both adult and pediatric patients with cystic fibrosis, the rate of DNA release from dead and dying lymphocytes is sufficient to significantly increase sputum viscosity. The enzyme (inhaled through a nebulizer) digests this released DNA, liquifies the sputum, enhancing its expectoration, and thus improves the management of chest infections and pulmonary function in these patients.

The clinical trials of this product were of generally orthodox design. The fact that the product is made by fermentation of genetically engineered Chinese hamster ovary cells, containing DNA encoding for the native human protein, deoxyribonuclease I (DNAase), was essentially irrelevant to the design of the clinical trials program. Placebo-controlled trials were conducted, and dose–response relationships were evaluated.

Significant other enzymes in common clinical use, made using similar processes, including tissue plasminogen activator, other thrombolytic agents, and aglucerase (Ceredase™, Genzyme Corp.) for Type 1 Gaucher's disease, illustrating the diverse clinical applications that enzymes may find.

Antibodies

Since antibodies, by their nature, bind to antigens, their function is often to augment intrinsic clearance mechanisms, as well as potentially exerting definitive therapeutic effects themselves. It is not surprising, therefore, that the therapeutic targets for antibody therapy are extremely broad, ranging from anti-tumor therapy to specific immunological diseases, e.g. the prevention of rhesus immunization in the perinatal period.

Therapeutically, antibodies may be targeted against a variety of antigens or a single specific antigen. As an example of a broad-spectrum antibody therapy, WinRho® may be used to prevent rhesus immunization in an Rh-negative mother *post partum*. There are at least 60 known epitopes of the rhesus D antigen, and the product, which is made from pooled plasma of rhesus-immunized, Rh-negative volunteers or patients, binds to red cells from 99.7% of all Rh-positive blood donors.

In contrast, rituximab (Rituxan®; IDEC Pharmaceuticals) is a highly targeted antibody that binds principally with CD-20-positive B lymphocytes implicated in one form of non-Hodgkin's lymphoma. Muromonab-CD3 (Orthoclone OKT3; Ortho Pharmaceuticals), used to reverse acute rejection of transplanted kidneys, is another example of the specific type of therapeutic antibody. Specific antigens are far more common as therapeutic targets.

Specific targeting of single, infrequently expressed antigens forms the basis of the large number of monoclonal antibody therapies that are either in development or on the market. These are generally manufactured by mammalian cell fermentation process, as described above (see Chapter 6 for issues relating to the manufacturing process and viral contamination of these products). The presence of single-antigen targets in or on tumor cells can be further exploited by conjugating the antibody to a radioactive or cytotoxic molecule. For example, human milk fat globule I monoclonal antibody, complexed with ^{90}Yttrium (Theragyn™), is under development for the treatment of ovarian carcinoma by Antisoma, PLC.

Cytokines

Fundamentally, cytokine responses to infection or tumors are biologically the most primitive form of immune response. Cytokines are generated in response to antigen challenge. However, unlike antibodies, the cytokine response is non-specific, and its principal biological effect is to enhance general, lymphocyte-mediated attack on the antigen-bearing cell.

Cytokines include the large and ever-increasing set of interleukins, various interferons, and numerous other factors, e.g. tumor necrosis factor, angiogenesis factor II, and various growth factors. Granulocyte macrophage colony stimulating factor (GMCSF; sargramostim, Leukine™; Immunex Corp.) is used for myeloid reconstitution after bone marrow ablation, exploiting its eponymous property initially identified *in vitro*. Interleukin 2 (IL-2; aldesleukin, Proleukin™, Chiron Corp.) is approved in the USA for the treatment for renal carcinoma and metastatic melanoma. Platelet-derived growth factor can be used to heal diabetic foot ulcers, presumably by imitating normal physiology that is blunted in patients with diabetes (gel becaplermin, Regranex®; Ortho-McNeil/Chiron Inc.).

Since cytokines have non-specific effects, existing drugs are likely to find additional indications. Similarly, their adverse effects also reflect their non-specificity, with symptoms such as fever, myalgias, flu-like symptoms and rhabdomyolysis.

Immune Adjuvants

Immune adjuvants can be classed as:

- Non-specific, e.g. BCG vaccine for bladder cancer.
- Specific, e.g. Salk vaccine for polio prevention.
- Genetic, to elicit cytokine responses (*vide infra*).

Vaccines, used widely in medicine since Jenner's pioneering work in preventing small pox by inoculating intradermal cow pox virus, are probably the best examples of the broad application of biotechnology products prior to the twentieth century. Traditionally, vaccines have been directed against the prevention of specific infectious diseases. Attenuated live and killed microrganisms are used as antigens to elicit cellular and humoral responses. They may be viewed as adjuvants, because it is the enhanced endogenous physiology that protects against the pathogen, and not the material in the vaccine itself.

The potential for preventing infectious disease is far from complete, and there is a continuing need for worthwhile research programs. Current challenges include HIV and prion-mediated disease, although the latter may (controversially) also be regarded as 'autoimmune' or 'congenital' when it is due to the derepression of prion genomes, which lurk dormant in many normal mammals. The numerous diseases that plague tropical countries and the developing world provide much scope but little financial incentive to the traditional pharmaceutical industry. Drug resistance, occurring in numerous microorganisms ranging from staphylococcus to malaria, is another field that could conceivably be conquered by taking the adjuvant approach.

Not surprisingly, there is considerable interest in using adjuvant tactics for the prevention or treatment of non-infectious disease. Spontaneous tumor regression (although rarely observed clinically) and the development of rare tumors in immunocompromised patients (such as Kaposi's sarcoma in patients with AIDS) are both consistent with the usefulness of endogenous host mechanisms to either prevent or retard cancer. Tumor-specific antigens may be used as therapeutic targets for exogenous therapy.

There is a broad range of mechanisms against these targets, such as specific cytokines, tumor cell expression of rejection antigens and inducing lymphocyte co-stimulatory molecules on tumor cells (*vide infra*). Non-specific approaches also exist, e.g. Bacille Calmet–Guerrin vaccine (BCG), which elicits a T lymphocyte cell-mediated immune response, can be used not only to prevent tuberculosis but also to (non-specifically) prevent the recurrence of bladder cancer.

Antisense Drugs

Antisense drugs are exogenous oligonucleotides that bind to specific endogenous nucleic acid sequences. Binding to mRNA prevents the construction of proteins by ribosomes and similarly, binding to specific gene sequences on DNA prevents both RNA coding and protein production. The application of antisense technology is broad, since this approach can be used to inhibit the production of a wide range of proteins, including stimulatory and inhibitory molecules.

While the synthesis of antisense molecules using modern combinatorial chemical approaches is easily automated, the delivery of these molecules to the appropriate intracellular and intranuclear sites is more difficult. The first antisense drug to be approved (ISIS Pharmaceutical Inc.) was for the treatment of cytomegalovirus retinitis in patients with AIDS. The route of administration of this drug is unique: direct intraocular injection. While this does deliver sufficient drug to the appropriate site, it illustrates well the ADME problems associated with antisense drugs.

To date, most regulatory authorities have treated antisense drugs in the much same way as any other biological product. The additional constraints that apply to gene therapies (for example) have not been imposed. Since these oligonucleotides have specific binding activities, safety considerations are usually dependent on the potential for non-specific effects of protein synthesis inhibition. At present, with the current limited experience, there would appear to be sound *in vitro* methods for the testing of the specificity of antisense drugs to be predictive for their tolerability in man. Furthermore, when the properties of the protein that is inhibited are discrete and consistent across individuals, then it is likely that the potential adverse effects will be predictable.

Gene Therapy

Gene therapy may be defined as the administration of exogenous DNA, in the form of intact gene or genes, for therapeutic purposes. Gene therapies usually have two major components, the DNA-containing molecule itself (the 'construct'), and an administrating adjuvant (the 'vector'). Vectors are usually necessary because genes are large, hydrophilic molecules that do not readily cross lipid membranes, although in some cases constructs are injected directly, without a vector (termed 'naked DNA').

Vectors may be viral or non-viral. Viral vectors include:

- *Potentially pathogenic DNA viruses*. These include adenoviruses and pox or vaccinia viruses. Both virus types can replicate in mammalian cytoplasm, whether or not the host cell is in mitosis or quiescent, and usually elicit a host immune response.
- *Herpes simplex virus I (HSV1)*. This also contains double-stranded DNA, but replicates in the nucleus of cells that are successfully infected, which need not themselves be dividing.
- *Non-pathogenic adeno-associated viruses*. These parvoviruses carry single-stranded DNA and are able to integrate into a broad range of non-dividing cells.
- *Retroviruses*. These RNA-containing viruses exist in an envelope derived from host cell membrane, and thus do not usually elicit vigorous immune responses. Retroviruses also tend to replicate only in dividing cells.

It is perhaps surprising that naked DNA can cause gene expression. Current examples where this concept has been proven include genes injected into skeletal and smooth muscle. Gold-coated DNA containing gold particles may also be inserted into cells by a 'gene gun', where electrostatic or gas pressure-powered displacement from a plastic matrix occurs.

Liposomal envelopes can also transport substances across cell membranes which would otherwise be repelled by the hydrophilicity of the gene construct. Liposomes may be constructed that are either anionic or cationic, and can also be coated with antibodies that will target specific antigen-presenting cells.

DNA protein conjugates are again without a vector. These act as ligands for specific cell surface receptors. Some cell types will then convey the gene construct during the ordinary processes of endocytosis.

Two-stage delivery systems are also under development, often manipulating somatic tissue *ex vivo*. A good example would be following the biopsy of some bone marrow from a patient. The gene therapy can be introduced into the biopsy material, using either a viral or a non-viral vector *in vitro*, until expression has definitely been established. Thereafter, the biopsy may be used as an autologous bone marrow transplantation, with the intention of its proliferation and generation of the desired protein product.

Early human gene transfer experiments in lymphocyte marking studies began in 1989. These early studies showed that gene transfer was feasible and could be well-tolerated, although there was no demonstrable therapeutic benefit. The first human gene therapy clinical trial was in 1990, in a patient with adenosine deaminase (ADA) deficiency; initial responsiveness proved not to be uniform when the series of cases was extended, possibly due to the fact that the disease phenotype could be elicited by a variety of genotypes.

There are some *a priori* characteristics for diseases that are likely to be attractive targets for gene therapy. There is a fundamental contrast between the gene therapy of inherited and acquired disorders. For inherited disorders, the absolute or relative deficiency of a particular protein needed for health may be correctable, e.g. the enzyme needed to reverse Gaucher's disease.

However, theoretically, there may be congenital disorders involving relative deficiencies of a particular protein, where therapeutic-induced overexpression is as likely to be as harmful as underexpression. Controlling gene expression is likely to be more difficult than merely inducing it. The thallassemias are *a priori* a good example of this problem. Overproduction of the missing haemoglobin chain is unlikely to be helpful to the patient. Similarly, when the principal desired target for gene therapy is a specific target organ, then overexpression of genes in other tissues may create tolerability problems.

The pharmacokinetics of gene therapy, and its relationship to dynamic effects, are very different form the orthodox pharmaceutical situation (Table 17.1). Ledley and Ledley (1994) have proposed a corollary of traditional PK–PD modeling, predicated upon the specific events in the cellular response to gene uptake and activation. These authors have developed a six-compartment model, which appears to have general applicability, to evaluate the apparent kinetic properties of a therapeutic gene product. This leads to the possibility of designing dosing regimens and relating them to measurements of expression and efficacy responses.

Acquired disorders are likely to have alternative therapeutic approaches. An increase in the production of some cytokine that is a normal response to a tumour might be a fairly direct strategy. On the other hand, some other biochemical process that indirectly compensates for a disease or injury could be another. A good example might be the differential sensitization of cells in a tumor to a particular cytotoxic drug, thus obtaining enhanced therapeutic response, permitting the use of lower doses of cytotoxic, and minimizing dose-limiting systemic adverse effects.

There are two areas of specific tolerability concerns associated with gene therapies, related to the expressed gene product and the vector. Both are immunological in nature, and may lead to therapeutic ineffectiveness.

If the gene therapy causes the production of a protein that was previously absent in the body, then an immune response is likely. This is simply analogous to patients who used to become resistant to xenobiotic insulins, and has also been demonstrated in the case of human factor VIII in some hemophiliacs. Escalating doses may be needed to maintain efficacy, or efficacy may be eventually lost. Furthermore, viral vectors are liable to replicate and also to elicit immune responses, just as for any vaccination, creating many of the same problems. Resistance to way gene therapy can result from immunization against either the construct or the vector.

One approach has been to develop strains of many of the viruses listed above as 'replication-defective' or 'replication-incompetent'. These viruses are cultured initially in conditions that provide some nutrient or element of the replicating machinery exogenously. Spontaneous mutations then create strains of virus that cannot replicate unless the crucial element is provided, and it is assumed that after human administration this will be the case. There is always the concern that, after injection, the virus will find some way to overcome its incompetency, e.g. by recruitment of the host cell machinery for this purpose. Similarly, non-viral vectors may offer an advantage by presenting the patient with less foreign antigen.

SAFETY ISSUES IN PRODUCT DEVELOPMENT

While issues surrounding sterility, mutagenicity, stability and carcinogenicity, and the attendant GLP and GMP issues, are much the same for gene and orthodox therapies in principle, there is often greater complexity associated with the former. These complexities include a triple effort on preclinical toxicology and the potential for germ cell line incorporation.

First, the toxicology of any gene therapy needs to be considered as a combination of three products: the construct; non-genetic elements in the construct (e.g. pharmaceutical adjuvant stabilizing materials); and the vector.

Second, there is a need to test in animals the possibility of incorporation of the therapeutic gene into the germ cell line. Many constructs contain multiple genes: not only is the therapeutic gene present, but also genes to assist in manufacturing, e.g. those conferring antibiotic resistance to the microorganism that is being used for production, or a gene for a marker enzyme. All of these genes require toxicological assurance that they do not incorporate into the germ cell line, and thus will not be replicated in the offspring of the treated patient. This is a special field of toxicology that is in its infancy; in some cases clinical trials have to be restricted to surgically sterile patients in the absence of this information.

REGULATORY ISSUES

In the USA, gene therapy protocols attract an additional degree of regulatory review. Not only must an IND be approved by the US FDA, but also the protocol must be approved by the Recombinant DNA Advisory Committee of the National Institutes of Health (the 'RAC'). To date, many dozens of such protocols have been approved, with the largest group for therapies that are designed to increase production of a specific cytokine in a specific tissue location. In Europe there is no RAC-equivalent, and regulatory requirements are handled within the national regulatory authorities, reviewing research protocols for investigational agents, and the EMEA and CPMP, reviewing the final product licence applications (see Chapter 28).

CELL AND TISSUE PRODUCTS

As before, cell and tissue biological products are not such modern inventions as is commonly perceived. The history of blood transfusion is beyond the scope of this chapter, but was responsible for establishing some of the fundamental concepts in this area. Organ transplantation is both routine and seriously limited in its capacity by the paucity of available organs. The implantation of cultured tissues may be a means of circumventing some of these practical limitations, and extending these therapeutic tactics.

There are various clinical conditions where administration of cultured whole cells or organ tissue may be desirable. The sources of these tissues are as diverse as the disease targets. For example, cultured fibroblasts from human prepuces are being developed as 'artificial skin' for the treatment of leg ulcers and burns (Advanced Tissue Sciences, La Jolla, CA; Organogenesis, MA). Other companies are developing an artificial pancreas from isolated pancreatic islet cells. Unlike matched transplantations, such therapies may involve treatment of large numbers of patients from a limited or sole initial human source, or may be autologous, albeit after some *ex vivo* manipulation and culturing of the cell mass before reimplantation.

Ex vivo therapeutic strategies may take different forms. Chronic lymphocytic leukemias have been treated for long periods of time by using cell separators to reduce the burden of lymphocytosis, and permit red cell transfusion. Laser-directed cell sorters may be used to select appropriate subpopulations of lymphocytes, which are then transfected with an appropriate gene product *ex vivo* and returned to the patient, where these cells will hopefully target some diseased tissue, such as widespread melanoma. Expense, availability of therapy, and the duration and specificity of effect may currently limit the widespread application of these approaches.

ETHICAL ISSUES

The modern advances of biotechnology create numerous ethical issues. Care should be taken in directly relating the therapy type and the ethical issue: it is an easy extrapolation for those without technical training to extrapolate that *all* biological products have the same range of ethical issues that actually only affect *some* of these therapies.

For example, the recent cloning of sheep (Roslin Therapeutics, Scotland) and mice (University of Hawaii) force the consideration of cloning of humans. On the one hand, much of this technology can also be used for genetic screening of fetuses with an inherited disease. On the other hand, the same techniques can probably be used to provide parents with a deliberate choice of the sex of their next baby. This is one example that is typical in this field: there is an ethical continuum, without absolute limits or lines of demarcation. Science is likely always to be ahead of the lay public and politicians in creating these dilemmas in the absence of agreed guidelines or consensus.

However, it should be clear that it is the ethical dilemma that is the central difficulty, and that there are analogies in the pregenetic engineering era of medicine. Consider, for example, the parents of a child who needs a kidney transplant, and who find themselves without any suitable living donor. Without any modern technology at all, they may choose to have another baby with the hope or intention that the new child can become the suitable donor. In this case, tissue proliferation *ex vivo* and implantation seems to be a simpler ethical situation than parents having offspring by entirely ordinary means. Consensus guidelines are needed: but in our opinion they must remain flexible in order to deal with technological innovation that is not going to stop, and they must also be consistent with guidelines that have wide acceptance in other areas of medicine.

INFORMED CONSENT

More prosaically, the difficulties of explaining the nuances of biotechnology products to potential clinical trials subjects may be more difficult than for orthodox small molecule drugs. Often these patients will have life-threatening diseases, and the apparent novelty of, say, a gene therapy, could, under the wrong conditions, create undue hope and bias in deciding to provide what should be truly informed consent. It is crucial that the same principles apply for biotechnology as for conventional drugs; the protocol and therapy must still be clearly explained in a non-coercive manner that does not raise false hopes in the patient.

ACKNOWLEDGMENTS

The authors thank David Feigal, MD, MPH, Medical Deputy Director of the Center for Biologics Evaluation and Research of the USA Food and Drug Administration for providing us with information relating to the regulations of drugs and biologics and the current regulatory issues.

REFERENCES

Ledley TS, Ledley FD (1994) Multicompartment numerical model of cellular events in the pharmacokinetics of gene therapies. Hum Gene Ther 5: 679–91.
Ernst & Young (1998) New Directions '98: the Twelfth Biotechnology Industry Annual Report. New York.

APPENDIX

Table 17.2   Biotechnology industry statistics

($ billions)	1997	1996	Growth (%)
Number of companies	1,274	1,287	−1
Number of employees	140,000	118,000	19
R&D expenses	$9	$7.9	14
Product sales	$13	$10.8	20
Revenues	$17.4	$14.6	19
Market capitalization	$93	$83	12
Net loss	$4.1	$4.5	−9

Table 17.3   Product sales by market segment

Average company	Average 1997 sales/company ($)	Increase over 1996 (%)
Diagnostic	21 605 000	9
Therapeutic	29 882 000	20
Agricultural biotech	56 198 000	30
Supplier	31 679 000	15
Chemical, environmental and services	178 430 000	23

Market definitions: the diagnostic and therapeutic categories include human health care products; the agricultural category includes microbial crop protectants, plant genetics, food processing and animal health; the supplier category includes instrumentation, laboratory supplies, reagents and other similar products; and the chemical, environmental and services category includes fine chemicals and bioremediation. Except as otherwise noted, all data in the State of the Industry Section are derived from Ernst and Young (1998).

BIOTECHNOLOGY INDUSTRY PATENTS

Between fiscal years (FY) 1994 and 1995, biotechnology patent applications submitted to the US Patent and Trademark Office (PTO) increased by

13%. This is almost double the 7% increase in overall patent applications submitted to the PTO between FY 1993 and FY 1994. The PTO has responded to the growing demand for patents by the biotechnology industry by increasing the number and sophistication of biotechnology patent examiners. In FY 1988, the PTO had 67 patent examiners. By 1998, the number of biotech examiners more than doubled to 184.

FY 1997 Biotechnology Patent
   Application Submissions   10 500
FY 1996 Biotechnology Patent
   Application Submissions   8 860

FY 1995 Biotechnology Patent
   Application Submissions   15 652
FY 1994 Biotechnology Patent
   Application Submissions   13 600
Average pendency time for a
   biotechnology patent (FY 1997)   27.1 months
Average pendency time for a
   biotechnology patent (FY 1996)   26.2 months
Average pendency time for a
   biotechnology patent (FY 1995)   21.6 months
Average pendency time for a
   biotechnology patent (FY 1994)   20.8 months

Source: **Bio-http://www.bio.org/library/welcome.dgw**

18

Orphan Drugs*

Bert Spilker

Phrma, Washington DC, USA

A 'rare disease' is defined in the USA as one with a prevalence of less than 200 000 patients (currently less than 0.08% of the population). Other countries generally use prevalence criteria of 0.1–0.5%, although may also accord 'orphan' status to any untreatable disease (e.g. in Europe) or when there is proof of non-profitability regardless of disease prevalence (e.g. the USA). A rare disease may also be termed an 'orphan disease', and drugs solely for its therapy termed 'orphan drugs'. In the USA, closely related subsets of patients must also be considered because orphan drug designation cannot be obtained if the drug can be used by such subsets in addition to those with the orphan disease; FDA aggregates such subsets and will not designate a drug when the total of the subsets exceeds the 200 000 patients per annum limit. Worldwide, the legislation is intended to incentivize pharmaceutical company sponsors to research small patient populations.

Depending upon the prevalence criterion used, there are an estimated 4000–8000 rare (or orphan) diseases. Many involve genetic problems and often are related to birth defects that are poorly characterized or involve permanent defects of nerve, muscle, or bone that cannot be corrected with drugs. Almost all marketed drugs are used to treat some rare diseases. A few examples among the largest selling drugs in the world include: propranolol, which is used to treat idiopathic hypertrophic subaortic stenosis (in addition to hypertension and angina); cimetidine, which is used to treat Zollinger–Ellison syndrome (in addition to duodenal ulcers); and antibiotics, all of which are used to treat rare as well as common bacterial infections. Pharmaceutical companies have always developed orphan drugs. The Orphan Drug Act, passed in 1983 in the USA, did not initiate, but rather stimulated, the development of such drugs.

PRINCIPLES

One of the most important principles about orphan drugs is that they form a very heterogeneous group, for the reasons given in Table 18.1.

Orphan drug status can supplement patent protection, because a successful NDA for an orphan product garners 7 years' exclusivity, regardless of any other intellectual property rights. Thus, patents threatened by limited coverage, few years before expiry, non-patentability (e.g. a natural product), interference from wealthier competitors, etc., may not offer as much protection as Orphan Drug designation by the national drug regulatory authority.

Table 18.1 Reasons why orphan drugs are a heterogeneous group

Orphan drugs differ according to:

1. Medical value
2. Patent status
3. Investigational or marketed status
4. Availability in a generic equivalent form
5. Use for a common disease too
6. Costs of development
7. Commercial (and profitability) potential
8. Disease prevalence (stable, increasing or decreasing)
9. Availability of alternative therapies
10. Manufacture by conventional or biotechnology methods

---

* This chapter contains material originally published in Spilker (1996a, 1996b), Copyright Prous Science Publishers. Editorial assistance and updating of this version was kindly provided by A.J. Fletcher and A.W. Fox. Reprinted with permission.

The regulatory processes for investigation and approval of orphan drugs are substantially similar to non-orphan drugs. After designation, orphan drugs are investigated under orthodox INDs, and the drug approval process is by filing orthodox NDAs, PLAs, or BLAs. The numbers of patients in licensing applications may, however, be fewer than is typical, usually because of the life-threatening nature of the treated disease, and the scarcity of patients available for study.

Development costs, time to market, and commercial potential vary enormously among orphan drugs, as with all drugs. It is usually pointless to develop an orphan drug if a generic version of the same compound is already marketed or shortly will be (i.e. before the company can launch its product). Such a generic may not be indicated for the rare disease, but it is likely that it will be dispensed for the treatment of the rare disease.

CLASSIFICATION OF ORPHAN DRUGS

While several classifications of orphan drugs have been proposed, no single one has been universally accepted (Spilker 1991). This section briefly mentions the criteria on which a classification scheme could be based, followed by a proposal for a simple classification based on combined economic and medical value. The major criteria that may be used to create a classification for orphan drugs include the following:

- Therapeutic or disease area of the drug.
- Whether the drug is marketed or investigational.
- Patent status of the drug (e.g. patent issued and in force, patent expired, nonpatentable, patent pending).
- Generic drug status (whether or not marketed, whether the same dosage form, strength, excipients, etc.)
- Size of patient population worldwide.
- Whether drug development costs can be recovered through sales.
- Availability of alternative treatments (e.g. none exist, all alternatives are highly toxic, very expensive, limited in availability, only work in a few patients).
- Medical value of the drug. In the author's opinion, this is the most important criterion.

- Potential use in a more common disease, as well as in a rare disease. This is often difficult to know at the outset of development, but almost every drug that reaches the market is tested by the medical community in many other diseases to evaluate its efficacy.
- Whether biologically or chemically synthesized.
- Existence of a patient support group.

THE ECONOMIC–MEDICAL INTERFACE

There are four situations where legislators are keen to give incentive to product sponsors, but where the latter may assess development potential differently.

1. *Drugs with moderate or high commercial potential and high medical value.* Drugs in this category usually find a sponsor easily. This category excludes those drugs with generic equivalents (see above).
2. *Drugs with little commercial potential, but with high medical value.* The commercial value may be such that the product is expected to lose money and never pay back its development costs. Usually, only very large and profitable companies, wishing to perform a community service, or having reasons other than profitability, will undertake the development of such a money-losing drug.
3. *Variable commercial potential and low medical value.* Most orphan drugs, at an early stage of their development, are of this type because the clinical efficacy and safety profiles are not well understood. One exception to this principle is drugs that are developed in a new dosage form, but whose activity and safety are well known, where there is usually more certainty about the medical value. 'Me-too' drugs are usually of low medical value as candidates for orphan designation and are rarely developed for rare diseases.

The medical value of a drug may be independent of the efficacy and rarity of the disease. For example, in Wilson disease there are several effective products on the market, yet additional ones are still being developed. Penicillamine is often effective, but often causes serious adverse reactions. Zinc acetate and trientine are newer products and molybdenum is being evaluated for the same indication.

4. *Variable commercial potential for both a rare and common disease*. Virtually every pharmaceutical company that develops an orphan drug hopes that the drug will be found useful in treating a more common disease. This seldom occurs for a truly novel drug.

THE INTERESTED PARTIES

There are eight principal stakeholders in orphan drug development. Note that many can be either public or private institutions, as well as either individuals or larger groups. These stakeholders often have different motives.

Legislatures

National, provincial, and other levels of legislature are involved in orphan drug development, primarily through creating new legislation. They define the incentives. Incentives typically include product exclusivity, tax relief, grant awards, waiving of application and user fees, or *quid pro quo* arrangements of other types.

Regulatory Authorities

These authorities are primarily motivated to improve and protect the public health of the community they serve through approval of effective and safe new drugs. This includes underserved patient populations, however small, and orphan drugs. Regulatory authorities are influenced by their perception of a drug's medical value, and their obligations to supervising legislatures.

Patient Associations

These groups typically focus primarily on one specific disease or type of disease process (e.g. inborn errors of metabolism, muscle disease, glycogen storage diseases, autoimmune diseases). Occasionally, they may serve as umbrella organizations for larger numbers of rare diseases, in order to achieve a critical mass required for advocacy purposes, e.g. National Organization of Rare Disorders (NORD) in the USA. Their motives include anything that may stimulate the discovery and development of new treatments for their diseases of interest. Another important function of many of these groups is to provide patient information to their members, and often also to the public.

Pharmaceutical Companies

The motivation of these organizations is not solely profit-orientated in most cases, as they usually accept social responsibilities for the patients they serve with their more profitable drugs (see above). In addition to the small amount of profit they may make on orphan drugs, there is an enhancement of the company's image.

Trade Associations

Professional trade associations usually represent pharmaceutical companies or distributors. These are concerned with the image of the industry, as well as providing social benefits through publicizing the products of their members.

Patients and Families

The motivation of those with the disease or with affected relatives is clear—they want better treatments that are affordable and will improve quality of life for the patient.

Physicians and other Health Care Providers

The motivation of these people is also clear—they seek better treatments for their patients and are often willing to test new drugs in clinical trials.

Academicians

Orphan drugs offer research opportunities for scientists and academic clinicians, together with career enhancement opportunities.

SPECIFIC SOURCES OF INFORMATION ON ORPHAN DRUGS

The Food and Drug Administration (FDA) publishes an annual list of Orphan Drugs that have been either designated or approved for marketing. This is now available on the worldwide web (see www.fda.gov).

Most specific disease organizations, as well as umbrella disease organizations, provide information of relevant diseases for members and sometimes for researchers, and the public. These groups may also provide current scientific information. Again, most of these organizations have websites that are easily located by commonly used search engines when the disease of interest is used as the search term.

DISCOVERY, DEVELOPMENT, MARKETING AND DISTRIBUTION OF ORPHAN DRUGS

The process of *discovering* new orphan drugs is not different from that used to discover drugs for more common diseases (Spilker 1994); earlier chapters of this book are equally applicable to orphan drugs.

The processes of *developing* orphan drugs, in principle, also do not differ from those used to develop drugs for more common diseases in terms of strategies created, methodologies used, and criteria for success. However, quantities of data may differ. If there are only 500 patients with a specific disease, it is probably impossible to have two randomized, well-controlled placebo trials. However, it is interesting to speculate that NDA populations for orphan diseases might deviate from the general population less than for more conventional drug development programs. This lesser deviation is almost automatic when an NDA contains a greater proportion of all the patients for whom the drug is likely to be prescribed.

While the same *marketing* tools are available for orphan drugs and non-orphans, they are usually far too costly for small returns likely from the former. Large company might occasionally allow its sales representatives to discuss both the orphan drug when making calls about non-orphans. However, this is often compensated for when a patient

advocacy group exists. The word usually spreads far and fast among these end-users when a new orphan drug is approved.

Distribution methods differ more between orphans and non-orphans more than the other categories discussed in this section. Conventional drugs are generally sold through wholesalers and directly to institutions. Orphan drugs more often use 'alternative distribution techniques'—these include mail order pharmacies and direct sales to patients, physicians, and institutions.

MARKETING BENEFITS IN SELLING ORPHAN DRUGS

Most pharmaceutical companies that market their own products can benefit from also marketing orphan drugs, for the following reasons:

1. Sales representatives can use orphan drugs as an entrée to see physicians. In this busy world, physicians want new and important medical information and are less willing than previously to see sales representatives.
2. Products can be bundled more easily as comprehensive portfolios in a given therapeutic area. Several companies that have merged in recent years initially considered divesting or dropping some of the smaller products from the portfolio. However, they soon realized that there was value in even these smaller products, and that the sum of their value was much greater than the sum of their sales, particularly if the company approached managed care or other groups (with formularies) with a wide selection of products.
3. The company will probably enhance its image through development of drugs for rare diseases. Reporters can easily write heartwarming stories of patients with rare diseases who are helped by orphan drugs; word of mouth and other public relations methods can also disseminate such information.

Note that companies seeking an orphan approval, while hoping (or even encouraging) off-label use for a more common disease are usually treated to strong regulatory backlash.

Benefits of Orphan Drugs from a Development Perspective

The most obvious benefit for a company is that the number of clinical trials and the quantity of clinical data required for marketing approval will usually be less for an orphan drug, primarily based on the limited number of patients available for clinical trials. However, even though the numbers are fewer, the data must be convincing and the standards of trial design are often unchanged. Such standards may be modified for extremely rare diseases, where a company may be limited to obtaining a number of individual case studies. A further possible benefit in some drug development programs is that less toxicology data may be required later on, when there is already substantial human experience with the drug.

Standards of manufacturing and quality control for orphan drugs are generally identical to those of non-orphan drugs. Sometimes, fewer validation batches may be required, and stability tests may occasionally be allowed to continue while the drug is being evaluated by the regulatory authority or, in exceptional cases, even after the product is on the market. Thus, the time to develop the chemistry and technical package of data for the regulatory submission may or may not differ from that needed if the drug was for a common disease.

DISINCENTIVES AND OBSTACLES FOR ORPHAN DRUG DEVELOPMENT

There is no limit to the number of disincentives and obstacles that could be described for developing orphan drugs. Many have already been mentioned. Selected commonly encountered examples are described below.

1. The tax credit offered in the USA for developing orphan drugs is not much more than the tax credit for research and development of any new pharmaceutical.
2. Resources of the company could be applied to developing more profitable drugs (opportunity costs).
3. Orphan drug development may not be required if the drug is already marketed for a more common use. This implies off-label orphan use.
4. Because the safety and quality standards of manufacturing are the same, creation of a special formulation for orphan use may create too many technical problems and costs.
5. The medical need for the drug may not be great and/or the clinical effectiveness of the drug may not be strong.
6. The regulatory authority may require more data than the company thinks is warranted.
7. The liability risks may be unacceptably high. A drug that causes a serious adverse effect used to treat patients with a rare disease could increase the exposure of the company to a major court suit in return for minimal revenues.
8. There are difficulties in finding a small number of patients widely dispersed through the USA (or other countries) for conducting clinical trials or for marketing products.

US ORPHAN DRUG ACT OF 1983

The US Orphan Drug Act was passed by Congress in 1983, and signed into law by President Reagan during the first few days of 1984. In its original form, the Act provided for the following:

1. A 7 year period of exclusivity for designated drugs.
2. Establishment of the Orphan Products Board within the US government.
3. Tax credits for certain expenses in clinical trials.
4. A grant program that included medical foods and medical devices, although medical foods and medical devices could not obtain orphan designation (Spilker 1994).
5. Assistance by the FDA to corporations and academic investigators.

The Act was originally designed for unprofitable and unpatentable medicines only, and there was originally no disease prevalence criterion.

Amendment to the Act, both refining its scope and increasing its incentives, followed quite quickly. The 1984 amendment provided an additional way to justify designation, introducing the 200 000 patient per annum criterion, and making unprofitability an optional, rather than a compulsory, alternative. The

1985 Amendment to the Act specified that patented and patentable medicines could receive orphan drug designation. In 1988, a further Amendment established the time period for filing for orphan drug designation, introducing the commonsense requirement that designation must occur prior to filing a new drug application (NDA).

Next, in 1990, came the first of several failed amendments to the Act. the US Congress approved a fourth amendment that would have allowed shared exclusivity for companies that developed the same orphan drug simultaneously. However, this amendment was vetoed by President George H. Bush, for its anti-competitive nature. A 1991 amendment would have established a sales cap, after which an orphan drug would lose its exclusivity. This, and other minor amendments to the Act in 1992 and 1994, did not pass Congress.

Currently, the law provides three major direct benefits in the USA:

1. The 7 year period of marketing exclusivity.
2. The tax benefits on clinical trials between the date of orphan drug designation and NDA approval.
3. The FDA's Office of Orphan Products Development grants to support clinical trials on orphan drugs (although this is a relatively small amount of money each year).

Unintended Consequences of the Orphan Drug Act

When Congress passed the Act, there were several different factions, and all sides had to make compromises. Everyone accepted that some incentives had to be given to pharmaceutical companies for the Act to influence behavior. Nonetheless, the incentives worked too well in some people's opinion, in that some loopholes were exploited or were found to benefit companies in unintended ways.

For example, companies with orphan drug protection sometimes charge very high prices, which may not be always appropriate. In situations where the medicine had a reasonably strong patent, such as with Retrovir (zidovudine), the orphan drug designation and exclusivity was not of consequence to the company, at least not for market protection. For drugs such as growth hormone, erythropoietin,

pentamidine, and Ceredase, orphan drug designation and resultant exclusivity on FDA approval was essential. However, to some people, the high prices of these drugs represented an abuse of the Act.

An important issue for politicians was that the Medicare and Medicaid programs had to pay large sums of money for protected medicines. One final issue was the inability of a second company to market an approved orphan drug, although this was the obvious consequence of marketing exclusivity granted by the Act.

A current trend is that increasing numbers of biological products are applying for orphan drug designation. The main reason is that patents for biological proteins are are very difficult to obtain; orphan drug protection is valuable while inventors wait to see if a strong patent will be issued.

ESTABLISHING PREVALENCE OR INCIDENCE OF A DISEASE

The FDA recognizes any authoritative evidence to support the prevalence of 200 000 patients in the USA. The major sources of evidence include the following:

1. Peer-reviewed literature.
2. Textbooks.
3. Surveys by patient support groups.
4. Data from the National Disease and Therapeutic Index.
5. Hospital discharge data based on ICD codes or other clear classifications.
6. Data from the Centers for Disease Control.
7. Data from the National Center for Health Statistics.
8. Data from IMS or other reliable market data organizations.
9. Sales data of companies.
10. Testimony of a few experts, based on evidence from their (or other) hospitals or practices. This represents the weakest data.

ESTABLISHING DIFFERENCES AMONG MEDICINES

It is often important to establish that a company's medicine, for which it desires an orphan drug designation, differs from another medicine. There are a number of principles that will help a company establish such a difference:

1. *Different chemical structures*. If it is unequivocally shown that two structures differ and this makes a biological or clinical difference, both will be given orphan drug designation. However, if the chemical difference is minor (e.g. one amino acid difference in a protein or the terminal carbohydrate portion of a large molecule) and no clinical differences can be shown, they will usually be viewed as the same product.
2. *Differences in clinical effects*. This is often a very difficult criterion to demonstrate.
3. *Contribution to patient care*. If a marketed dosage form is unsatisfactory for certain patients, then a new dosage form suitable for them may be eligible for orphan drug designation.
4. *New production methods to purify a drug*. If such methods lead to a difference in safety or efficacy, this would qualify for orphan drug designation. A real example is a recombinant vs. extracted Factor IX.
5. *New excipients*. Differences in excipients that lead to a difference in clinical safety or efficacy would qualify for orphan drug designation.

It is obvious that arthritis, epilepsy, depression, asthma, and other similar diseases are not rare and drugs to treat them do not qualify for orphan drug designation. But would a medically plausible subset of each disease qualify as an orphan indication if there were fewer than 200 000 patients with, for example, a severe form of the disease? The FDA's principle in addressing this common question is to ask the question: 'Could (and would) patients with less severe forms of the disease also use the new treatment?' If so, then the FDA says that the indication is not a true orphan and usually denies the application for orphan designation.

A rare variant of depression, asthma, or other common disease might qualify as an orphan indication if it is deemed to be a medically plausible separate indication, and the company might receive the designation. However, the reviewing division of the FDA might impose much higher standards for regulatory approval of an orphan drug if they believe it will be widely used in medical practice. For example, a drug to treat a rare rheumatological disorder that could also be useful in rheumatoid arthritis would likely require much more data for approval than if the drug were limited to treating a very small patient population. On the other hand, a toxic but effective medicine that could only be used to treat severe cases of patients with a common disease (because of benefit–risk considerations) could receive orphan designation and regulatory approval for marketing as an orphan drug, with relatively little data.

RATING THE EFFECTS OF THE ORPHAN DRUG ACT IN THE USA

With over 650 active designations and now about 275 orphan drugs approved for the market (and even one medical device), plus numerous grants awarded since 1983, the Act has clearly been a success. Let us not forget that nothing in the Act creates compulsion, and that voluntary participation, as measured by applications for designation submitted, increase year by year.

The fact that some high priced blockbuster drugs have been approved under this legislation remains a controversial topic; probably these are an evasion of the intent of Congress.

The tax credit for clinical trial costs has been very modest and does not represent a significant sum of money to most companies; however, neither does it represent much lost to the US Treasury.

EUROPE

Orphan Drug legislation in Europe is more recent. A similar two-stage designation and approval system was established by EC Directive 141 in the year 2000. By early 2002, this had led to 131 European orphan drug designations, and three orphan drugs have been licensed for marketing. Among the designations are 20 drugs that are not so designated in the USA.

The regulation of European orphan drugs is by the Committee for Orphan Medical Products (COMP), which is separate from the Committee for Proprietary Medical Products (CPMP). All approvals are through the EMEA centralized process; there is neither country-by-country, nor concertation procedures for orphan drugs. The prevalence criterion is 0.05% of the population of the European Union (EU); this offers flexibility under conditions in which the EU is expected to grow with further recruited nations from about 320 millions (2001) to 415 millions by 2004. Significantly, in Europe, an investigational agent for any untreatable disease (regardless of prevalence) can receive orphan drug designation. An appeals procedure against unfavourable COMP decisions has been provided.

Europe offers the advantage, however, that incentives can be both community-wide and national. Community-wide incentives are provided by the Directive; most importantly, these include a 10 years' market exclusivity for first to market (not first to designate). As in the USA, designation in Europe also provides submission fee waivers, and small amounts of research grant money are available. National incentives vary: France provides genomics support and tax relief; Germany offers streamlined review of investigational applications (which remain nationally-based for all drugs); and The Netherlands offers both tax relief and has created a national coordination center.

REST OF THE WORLD

Orphan Drug legislation has been passed in Australia and Japan, and is currently under consideration in a number of other Asian countries. In general, prevalence criteria have trended towards that used by the EU, and that in the USA remains relatively liberal. However, the use of a fixed number of 200 000 cases causes a progressive decrease in the prevalence criteria when the denominator is a growing US population (Fox 2002).

WHAT HAS BEEN LEARNED?

First, there is no doubt that the major incentive that governments can provide is a period of exclusivity for marketing. Other incentives are secondary and not really necessary for legislation to be successful.

Second, abuses of the law by the pharmaceutical industry must be prevented if orphan drug privileges are to survive. Politicians may well wish to establish sales caps in the future, and legislate that market exclusivity must disappear when the cumulative sales of a drug reach a predetermined level. The sales cap should represent a fair incentive to the companies, yet protect the government or other groups from excessive payments.

There are now several millions of American patients who have benefited from the Orphan Drug Act (Haffner 2002). There is every indication that the same will shortly be true in Europe and the rest of the world.

REFERENCES

Fox AW (2002) Erosion of the scope of the United States Orphan Drug Act. *Int J Pharmaceut Med* (in press) [a response from Dr Haffner accompanies this article].

Haffner M (2002) Orphan drug product regulation—United States. *Int J Clin Pharmacol Ther* (in press).

Spilker B (1991) *Guide to Clinical Trials*. Raven: New York.

Spilker B (1994) *Multinational Pharmaceutical Companies: Principles and Practices*, 2nd edn. Raven: New York.

Spilker B (1996a) *Orphan Drug Challenges for Pharmaceutical Companies*. Drug News Perspect 9(7): 399.

Spilker B (1996b) *Orphan Drug Act of 1983*. Drug News Perspect 9(8): 460.

19

Pharmacoeconomics: Economic and Humanistic Outcomes

[1]Raymond J. Townsend and Jane T. Osterhaus, [2]J. Gregory Boyer

[1]Wasatch Health Outcomes, Park city, Utah, USA and [2]Pharmacia Corporation, Stokie, Illionrs, USA

For most of the past 25 years, the development of most pharmaceutical products has followed a predictable path from discovery to preclinical and clinical development, approval and marketing. With the onset of increased competition, decision makers want to hold down healthcare costs while maintaining or increasing quality. This has dictated changes in the traditional drug development path. To maximize the commercialization and clinical use of a product, successful drug development today must now also focus on measuring other outcomes of a pharmaceutical intervention.

Decisions, both large and small, relating to healthcare are now made based on information gathered from economic and humanistic outcome evaluations. The information gained from valid outcome measures can be used on a national level to allocate expenditures for treating various sectors of the population (e.g. the elderly, neonates, etc.) or to determine which programs will receive financial resources (e.g. vaccine programs vs. acute influenza treatments). Outcome information can be used to help make decisions regarding the inclusion or exclusion of drugs on formularies. Complete information about the economic, humanistic and clinical impacts that medications have on specific patients can help healthcare providers make better prescribing decisions.

Decision makers, including prescribers, providers, payers and patients, all want to maximize the clinical value received for the money spent. Value to a prescriber might mean achieving a desired clinical impact for the cost of drug; value to a payer could mean spending more for a drug that reduces the number of days in a hospital, thus reducing the total economic impact of a condition. Value to a patient or employer might also be making sure that the drug prescribed maintains quality of life or worker productivity. To be successful, the pharmaceutical developer must address the needs of all these decision makers. To do this, it is imperative that drug development programs today include quantitative measures of economic, clinical and humanistic value of the drugs they develop. It is never too early to begin to think about how the value of a product will be demonstrated.

The intent of this chapter is to help pharmaceutical developers and researchers understand how to document the value of pharmaceuticals through appropriate pharmacoeconomic development programs.

OUTCOMES, HEALTH ECONOMICS, AND PHARMACOECONOMICS

Outcomes research is the study of the end-results of medical interventions—does the healthcare intervention improve the health and well-being of patients and populations? The field of outcomes research emerged from a growing concern about which medical treatments work best and for whom. Outcomes span a broad range of types of intervention, from evaluating the effectiveness of a particular medical or surgical procedure to measuring the impact of insurance status or reimbursement policies on the outcomes of care. Outcomes research touches all aspects of healthcare delivery, from the clinical encounter itself to questions of the organization, financing, and regulation of the

Principles and Practice of Pharmaceutical Medicine. Edited by A. J. Fletcher, Lionel D. Edwards, Anthony W. Fox and Peter Stonier © 2002 John Wiley & Sons Ltd.

healthcare system. Each of these factors plays a role in the outcomes of care or the ultimate health status of the patient. Understanding how they interact requires collaboration among a broad range of health service researchers, such as physicians, nurses, economists, sociologists, political scientists, operations researchers, biostatisticians, and epidemiologists (Foundation for Health Sciences Research 1993).

Health economics offer basic tools and criteria with which to analyze issues of efficiency and the distribution of healthcare. These tools include techniques of optimization and the determination of equilibrium situations (e.g. predicting change in demand for services). The set of criteria is used to determine whether someone is better or worse off as a result of a particular action. Health economics tools are often used to evaluate how much money should be allocated to a healthcare program or service. To the extent that health economic analyses can clarify the costs of alternative medical treatments and make the values underlying those alternatives explicit, it is a useful approach to the study of medical care (Feldstein 1983). Health economics focuses on all aspects of healthcare and as such can be very useful for generating data to make policy decisions involving multiple healthcare programs and systems. While some health economists take a 'big-picture' or macro-view and focus on issues involving healthcare policy, others may focus specifically on pharmaceutical industry issues such as drug pricing, or the cost of drug development.

In recent years pharmacoeconomics has been used as a term to describe the identification, measurement and comparison of the costs and consequences of pharmaceutical products and services (Boótman et al 1996). As such, pharmacoeconomics focuses primarily on pharmaceuticals, and attempts to evaluate the economic and humanistic impact of drug therapy. Pharmacoeconomic tools are derived from a variety of sources, including the fields of economics and outcomes research. Quite often the pharmacoeconomist will bring to the development team skills and experience in quality of life, patient satisfaction and other patient-centered measures. Health economists and a pharmacoeconomists differ (while the terms are sometimes used interchangeably), in having stronger backgrounds in the theoretical and applied aspects of health economics, respectively. A researcher with solid

pharmacoeconomic skills may not be a very good health economist, and vice versa. When hiring a pharmacoeconomist or health economist, first determine what they will do, then evaluate their skills and experiences to make sure that they will be able to deliver what is needed for your specific drug development program.

NEW PARADIGM: THREE-DIMENSIONAL OUTCOME ASSESSMENT

Healthcare used to be constrained mainly by the technology available to assist in delivering care. That technology is becoming increasingly sophisticated and the cost of such technology is potentially outpacing the resources available to pay for such care. How should healthcare be allocated, or in some cases rationed? Which patients should get which treatment?

Health outcomes are the end result of a medical intervention. They represent what happened to the patient. Being cured of an illness is an outcome, as is death due to an illness (not all outcomes are positive). The simplest outcome evaluation would characterize people as being alive or dead. This gross distinction tells very little about the current functional status of the patient. Being alive but relying on a respirator to breathe is very different from being alive and fully functional. Additionally, intermediate outcomes (e.g. alleviation of pain or other symptoms of arthritis) are sometimes as important an outcome as the final outcome.

The measurement of outcomes is critical to the conduct of pharmaceutical research. Clinical outcomes (efficacy and safety) are the hallmarks of Food and Drug Administration (FDA) approval of a product for marketing. Clinical outcomes are necessary but no longer sufficient as a sole consideration in weighing decisions, and for reimbursement in socialized healthcare systems (where reimbursement essentially governs marketability). Patients have become more involved in their own healthcare decisions, and economic considerations have increased in importance. All have contributed to the movement to extend outcomes measured beyond the traditional clinical outcomes associated with pharmaceutical research. Healthcare decision makers are pressed to know more than simply the safety and efficacy parameters of an intervention.

It is important for them to know how a specific intervention will impact budgets and use of other resources, and how it will impact the patient from the patient's perspective.

Pharmacoeconomic information demands are often not anticipated early enough in the clinical development program. For example, several million people in the USA are taking antihypertensive medications to lower their blood pressure, something we would generally think of as good, since the medications can possibly extend life by reducing the risk of stroke and coronary artery disease. However, in some cases the potential benefits of antihypertensives may not outweigh the negative effects of the drugs on quality of life; one study reported that the health of a person treated with antihypertensive medication is comparable to that of an otherwise similar person 5–15 years older. Clearly trade-offs between the side-effects and benefits of the medications should be presented to patients so they can make informed decisions about treatment (Lawrence et al 1996).

If a pharmaceutical company is developing a new antihypertensive medication targeted for chronic use, then preparing a submission with a goal of having the drug prescribed is an accomplishment. But it is also necessary to convince the patient to take the drug on a regular basis, as well as to ensure that the patient understands the pros and cons of taking the medication from their quality of life perspective. An astute pharmacoeconomic researcher incorporates a quality of life component into appropriate comparative studies, so that patient-derived and patient-reported aspects of treatment are considered in addition to the management of physiological symptoms such as blood pressure reduction.

While clinical outcomes are critical, they are no longer the sole factor reviewed in making a decision to use an intervention. Just as the information requirements increased from safety, to safety and efficacy in the 1960s, the bar has been raised once again, and these requirements now include not only clinical (safety and efficacy), but also economic and humanistic outcomes. This paradigm shift has been represented in a model termed the ECHO (economic, clinical and humanistic outcomes) model, described by Kozma et al (1993). Economic outcomes include direct medical resources used to provide a service or achieve an outcome, including

Table 19.1 Examples of outcomes

Type of outcome	Examples
Clinical	Symptoms, diagnosis
	Adverse events
	Drug interactions
Economic	Hospitalizations
	Physician visits
	Prescription drugs
	Productivity
Humanistic	Quality of life
	Satisfaction with treatment
	Preference for one treatment vs. another

healthcare providers' time, laboratory services, and diagnostic procedures. Patient productivity is also an economic outcome. Humanistic outcomes include health-related quality of life, patient satisfaction with interventions and patient preferences.

Under the new paradigm for decision making, all decision makers will increasingly be forced to take into account the perspectives of the other players affected by their decisions. Prescribers will no longer consider just the clinical impact, but also the economic impact their decision will have on the payer, and the quality of life impact the decision will have from the patient's perspective. The payer and patients will need to consider the impact of their decisions on the rest of the system. Successful drug developers now evaluate three-dimensional outcome data as early as possible in the product development life cycle. This information will also be useful to investors who are making decisions regarding the ultimate potential for success or failure of a newly discovered therapeutic product.

Table 19.1 provides examples of clinical, economic and humanistic outcomes. Each outcome type is not mutually exclusive, e.g. pain could be a clinical or a humanistic outcome, but only needs to be measured once in a study.

PHARMACOECONOMICS IN DEVELOPMENT PROGRAMS: ADVANTAGES, DISADVANTAGES AND CHALLENGES

Pharmacoeconomic tools will not *make* a decision, but are useful as an aid to decision makers regarding the appropriate use of a product. While typically considered to aid the end-user, they also have great applicability at the drug development level. This is not an entirely altruistic concern for the pharmaceutical company: if incorporated early into the development of a drug, a strategic advantage due to a more complete package of outcomes information is available at the time of product approval.

Pharmacoeconomic tools can also assist in selecting an area of preclinical exploration, choosing which drugs should move forward into man, and whether to progress a drug from Phase II to Phase III research. An understanding of the current burden of the illness or condition, in terms of its natural history, resource use, and quality of life profile, can help a research team put the estimated development costs and the desired return on investment in proper perspective. A drug that 'cures' an illness that is common but not very debilitating is not likely to be seen as worthy of a premium price by many formulary committees. This does not mean that the drug should not be developed, but the expected return on the drug must be put in the appropriate context. Early research can also identify targets for comparative studies; a must under the new paradigm. If research is conducted in the most severe patients with a particular condition, but they constitute only 5% of the treatable population, then the perspective of those patients needs to be put in context with other patients who suffer a less severe form of the same condition. This will help to demonstrate how they might respond to treatment and to determine what the impact of the condition is on their quality of life.

A perception exists that disadvantages of incorporating pharmacoeconomic parameters into the development program include the idea that additional measures will delay the filing of a new drug application (NDA), delay the approval of an NDA, and may not generate data that will be 'useful'. However, the same statements could apply to any clinical measure, and every efficacy endpoint is carefully considered before incorporation into a study or program. Similarly, not every program requires all conceivable pharmacoeconomic components. Acute treatments (e.g. antibiotics for otitis media) may not require quality of life components; 'me-toos' (e.g. a new β-blocker or a NSAID) may only require a simple cost comparison study. Yet, a drug that is targeted for chronic use should be considered as a prime target for pharmacoeconomic study. If a disease is not going to be cured, and the patients are expected to take a product for the rest of their lives, there should be some message that can be provided to the patient that will support their use of the product in a compliant fashion for a number of years.

If Phase III studies are already completed by the time pharmacoeconomic components are considered, the likelihood of having any outcomes data beyond traditional safety and efficacy at product launch is small. A strategic advantage for the product will have been lost; one of the most frequently requested pieces of information by formulary committees and reimbursement agencies is, 'What is the impact on my budget?', and from patients is 'What will be the impact on me? Will I feel better?'

It is tempting to ignore pharmacoeconomics under the guise of 'it is not required by the agency' or 'it will slow things down'. The challenges associated with successfully incorporating pharmacoeconomic components into a clinical development program include making sure the right people are involved early enough, so that delays do not occur. Pharmacoeconomic components to clinical studies do not have to be rate-limiting, but will be so when the project team fails to bring the pharmacoeconomist into the project at an early stage, i.e. Phase I. Early involvement will enable the pharmacoeconomist to understand the characteristics of the investigational drug and the targeted conditions, and as the trials program is laid out, pharmacoeconomic components can be selected that are the most appropriate for the studies in the program. A thoughtful and documented pharmacoeconomic development plan should be available at the same time as the clinical and marketing development plans. Only then will all three plans must be coordinated and support one another.

VALUE-ADDED VS. TRADITIONAL CLINICAL DEVELOPMENT PROGRAMS

The magnitude of the challenge of incorporating pharmacoeconomics into a traditional clinical development program will be a function of the type of program being studied, the willingness of the

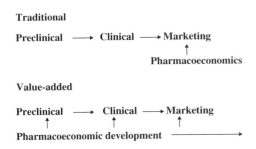

Figure 19.1 The difference between 'traditional' and 'value-added' development programs

research team to be open to new types of outcome measures, and the sophistication of the pharmacoeconomist. As research-orientated companies avoid 'me-too' products, and forge new areas of unmet medical needs, the need for value-added development programs with scientifically valid pharmacoeconomic outcome data will increase (Figure 19.1). The need to demonstrate value has been discussed long enough, so that there is an expectation that new programs will include some pharmacoeconomic parameters; in many cases there may need to be a reason to *exclude* pharmacoeconomic measures as opposed to a reason to *include* them.

The training and experience of the pharmacoeconomist will impact the conduct of how well value is added to a drug development program. Does the pharmacoeconomist understand the clinical trial process? Is the goal to have a pharmacoeconomic message that will be useful to marketing? Do they understand what messages a sales representative can communicate and what materials can be disseminated as promotion? Has the scientist interacted with the FDA and other regulatory agencies? Will he/she be able develop a pharmacoeconomic strategic plan that will complement the clinical and marketing plans and fullfill the goals of the company? These questions should be asked before hiring a staff pharmacoeconomist or consultant and embarking on a value-added development program.

PHARMACOECONOMIC BASELINE

The important first step in developing a pharmacoeconomic strategic plan is to start by finding out what is currently known about the disease and the economic and humanistic burden that it has on patients, payers and providers. The best place to start is with a review of the literature to determine what has already been accomplished. This may entail a review of the epidemiology and clinical aspects of the condition to verify that pharmacoeconomic components would be a worthwhile addition to a clinical program. After reviewing the literature (and other sources such as the Internet), the pharmacoeconomist should then formulate how to integrate which economic and humanistic outcome measures into the full development plan.

If adequate baseline measures do not exist, then an important part of the strategic plan will be to research and document the baseline burden of illness as it is currently being treated (or not treated, if this is the case). This can be done separately from the clinical trials that are taking place, although placebo-treated patient measures may also be important in finding this baseline. The goal is to identify a benchmark, documenting the *status quo*. This baseline is critical to being able to show the impact (improvement) that the new drug will have.

Table 19.2 lists some of the important questions to consider when documenting the baseline burden of illness. Answers will not be available for every

Table 19.2 Considerations when documenting baseline burden of illness

- Who has the condition (men, women, children, elderly, Blacks, Asians, Caucasians, etc.)?
- How long does the condition last?
- What is the impact of the condition and current treatment on the patient's functional status or quality of life?
- How satisfied are patients with current treatment options?
- Does the disease impact productivity?
- What health care and other resources are currently used to manage the condition?
- What percentage of patients with the disease are seeking treatment?
- What is the economic and humanistic impact if treatment is not received?
- What treatments or interventions are currently used to manage the condition?

question, neither will perfect data always be available for those answers that can be provided. The risk–benefit assessment of taking the time to answer each question thoroughly vs. applying some 'quick and dirty' estimates to the questions should be considered. Not every program requires a large-scale major prospective study to answer each question, for many of the reasons discussed above. However, in the long run it is usually less costly in terms of time and money to research the unknown issues before committing to the pharmacoeconomic development plan. The *post hoc* piecemeal approach almost always fails.

Case Study: Data Sources

A study to document the outcomes of epilepsy treatment, conducted by Hirsch and Van Den Eeden (1997), illustrates some of the challenges associated with collecting burden of illness data. The traditional clinical measure of seizure frequency is no longer considered appropriate as the sole measure of outcome of treatment or surgical intervention. The additional variables to document the burden of illness that were found illustrates the gap between the type of data desired and what is available. Hitherto, quality of life had been assessed in epilepsy patients using no fewer than 12 different instruments (both disease-specific and general). The economic impact of epilepsy had previously been assessed at a national level and in a few small studies.

These authors wanted to describe the overall disease impact for patients with chronic epilepsy, using a retrospective cross-sectional design in a managed care organization. Multiple data sources were required, since no single data base served as a repository for the various types of data required, and included administrative databases, medical charts, pharmacy databases, outpatient databases, hospitals, laboratories, outside services, memberships, etc. They found that all the identified sociodemographic variables were available in at least one automated database, as were two of the clinical variables, and 26 of the economic variables. None of the humanistic variables were available in any database.

In this case, about half of the data desired was available electronically, most of which was related to health as heavily weighted toward economic information. To gather the remaining desired data the investigators needed to collect prospectively humanistic as well as some additional clinical variables (Hirsch and Van Den Eeden 1997). It is quite typical that clinical data available electronically is often not complete and therefore not very useful, and that humanistic data is missing completely from the databases held by Health Maintenance Organizations.

When setting out to document the burden of illness, it is critical to ensure that the patients in the databases really are patients with the disease. In come cases, the ICD-9 codes are known to be inaccurate regarding patient capture, and means other than electronic data bases must be used. One advantage of using clinical trial patients is the certainty of having patients with the condition of interest—the trade-off being a concern for the generalizability of information to the larger population.

Pharmacoeconomic baseline data should not be considered in isolation, but as one aspect of data that must be considered as a part of the whole. Once the burden of illness information is collected and analysed, the development team must move to plan for ways to measure and document the clinical, economic and humanistic impact of the new pharmaceutical entity or other intervention.

STUDIES WITHIN CLINICAL TRIALS: TECHNIQUES

The information generated from the burden of illness component of a pharmacoeconomic strategy will serve as a useful guide for the design of pharmacoeconomic components within clinical trials. Obviously, this must be factored against the prior judgment of whether or not disease-specific quality of life instruments are required at all. Healthcare resource use, measures of lost productivity, and indirect financial cost measures may be all that is required.

The process of incorporating pharmacoeconomic measures into clinical trials should begin before a draft protocol is ever created.

Both the quantity and the types of data able to be collected will be affected by the nature of the clinical study: patients may be inpatients or outpatients, and this in turn will govern the nature of pharmacoeconomic data that can be recorded. It is also important whether a clinical trial is intended as a pivotal trial for registration or not: if a study is pivotal, then a clinical efficacy measure will have to be the primary endpoint. Pharmacoeconomic parameters can still be incorporated into such a study as secondary end-points, and still provide valuable information. If, on the other hand, the clinical research addresses a health system delivery issue, then the pharmacoeconomic end-points may well be primary, and the study design need not be constrained by FDA-mandated requirements for the double-blind, placebo-controlled aspects of proof of efficacy.

As the development moves from early Phase II through to Phase IV, the rationale for incorporating pharmacoeconomic parameters into studies should evolve. Initially, measures may be used in studies with small sample sizes to gain experience with certain instruments, or to determine which instrument is preferred for use in larger studies. Early on, the project team may think that everything but the kitchen sink is being included in a study. In some cases, it would be feasible to make the instrument determination in a separate study, but the costs in terms of additional patients needed, and other resources required, need to be carefully considered before a decision to reject the inclusion of several pharmacoeconomic instruments in one early study.

As the product moves from Phase II into Phase III, the number of seemingly redundant instruments should decline as the obvious choice, or best guess rises to the top. If the goal of Phase III studies is to file an NDA or gain regulatory approval, the studies may not be appropriately designed to capture the additional information deemed necessary for the product's success. In some cases it may be that separate pharmacoeconomic studies are needed to be completed prior to marketing (and thus almost prior to NDA submission, in an era where 180 days is the target review period), and separate from the pivotal clinical trials. Good advice is to prioritize at this stage of development: which pharmacoeconomic components are and are not critical for product launch or shortly thereafter? Thus, there is usually a need to strike a balance between getting information in a timely fashion, meeting regulatory demands, and

meeting demands of the marketplace; that balance may often have to be struck pragmatically.

Confidence and Validity of Data

As in any other scientific endeavor, the validation of the database is as important as its interpretation; pharmacoeconomic variables require two degrees of confidence, i.e. in the accuracy and the validity of what has been measured.

Consider two opposite examples of pharmacoeconomic measurement. In one case, patients could describe their impression of the impact of an intervention on their quality of life (QOL) following completion of a 2 week, open-label course of treatment. At the other extreme, a randomized, controlled trial (RCT), using a double-blind, placebo-controlled protocol and a 12 month follow-up in several hundred patients, could use a statistically validated QOL instrument. The results of the latter would probably inspire more confidence than the 'informal' scenario, all other things being equal. However, it does not mean that the answers given using the informal method are wrong, it simply requires an appreciation of the trade-offs involved in how data is collected. Furthermore, the former method might be of more use than the latter in exploratory pharmaceconomic research condicted in the earliest stages of drug development.

The RCT design, while often held as the gold standard, also has other problems. It is more costly, more time consuming, and not always ethical (12 months of placebo?). Some types of outcomes, such as compliance, do not lend themselves to double-blind designs because such designs mask one of the effects being measured. RCTs generally strive to maintain high levels of internal validity at the risk of reducing external validity. Biases to internal validity affect the accuracy of the results of the study, as they apply to those who participated in the study (e.g. patient selection bias, cross-over bias, and errors in measurement of outcomes). Biases to external validity affect how well the results may be generalized to the public at large. Obviously, the choice of study design must take potential biases into account. These factors are somewhat analogous for pharmacoeconomic and traditional clinical research.

Selecting a Quality of Life Instrument

It is always important to select an instrument that has adequate reliability and validity. Although many instruments have been published, many of these have little supporting validation. Another sources of information include the Medical Outcomes Trust (2001), www.outcomes-trust.org. Some instruments, such as the MOS-SF-36, a generic QOC instrument, seem to be gaining popularity, and it is tempting to routinely incorporate them into clinical studies. Many experts in the field recommend that both a disease-specific and generic instrument should be used in each study, in order to capture the broadest QOL information. Yet, excess burden on patients can defeat the accuracy and completeness of what is collected. Generally, if resources or patient burden threatens, then most experts would argue for retention of a disease-specific instrument when it is only possible to use a single measure.

The handling and analysis of pharmacoeconomic data should be along the lines familiar to those observing good clinical practices (GCP) for other purposes. Data collection instruments need to be selected, or created and incorporated into case report forms, just as for any other end-point. Data analysis plans should be created prospectively. The statistical analysis plan should be prospective, and should help put the pharmacoeconomic measures in the context of other properties of the test medication (Table 19.3). Are they included to test a hypothesis or is this a hypothesis-generating study for the pharmacoeconomic measures? Is the goal to evaluate patients, discriminate between patients, or predict how patients might act? The type of data collected should drive the level of analysis (continuous vs. categorical data). If there is an investigators' meeting for the study, the pharmacoeconomic components should be presented at the meeting so the investigators and/or the study coordinators fully understand their role in data collection. As the study is ongoing, appropriate levels of monitoring should be conducted. Queries that arise during the study and reconciliation of the data afterwards should be handled in the same manner in which clinical queries and data reconciliation are handled. Standard operating procedures and quality analysis should be a part of every study in which the company invests money to collect end-points, be they traditional or pharmacoeconomic end-points.

REPORTING AND PUBLICATIONS

Most companies have some form of standard operating procedure by which they generate clinical study reports. Pharmacoeconomic data should be handled and reported in a similar manner. In some cases it may be appropriate to issue the pharmacoeconomic component of a study as an appendix to a larger clinical report. This will depend on the

---

Table 19.3 Points to consider: incorporating pharmacoeconomic measures in clinical trials

- Document the pharmacoeconomic objectives, methodology and analysis plan within the study protocol
- Measure outcomes in the most appropriate and most disaggregate units. Categories can always be collapsed at a future time, but is impossible to split out variables beyond their original units. The sources of process and outcomes data may vary
- Clinical data may be captured from providers, patients, and medical records
- Resource use data may be obtained from patient, administrative databases, providers or charts
- Quality of life data should come from the patient. In some cases (very young, very old, mentally unstable) patient proxies are used, but the patient should be considered the optimal choice
- The study design can affect the *types* of outcomes that can be reliably collected, and the *manner* in which the outcomes can be collected
- Study design affects several parts of the evaluation process:
  - Cost of evaluation
  - Time required to conduct the evaluation
  - Accuracy of the information gained
  - Complexity of administering the evaluation
  - Ease of defending subsequent decisions made, based upon the evaluation

level of pharmacoeconomic involvement in the study and how closely related the end-points may be to the pathological measures. If there were just a few pharmacoeconomic measures that were being tested, an appendix to a clinical report might be appropriate. In contrast, for example, where recovery from anesthesia is measured by 'street fitness' (the humanistic outcome) and neurological measures of balance and coordination (the physiological end-point), then it could be cogent to report these two types of data together, and to examine how well they correlate; this would not be suited for an Appendix for the humanistic data.

External reports are most likely going to be manuscripts submitted to peer-reviewed journals. Placement of pharmacoeconomic articles in non-specialty journals is important but difficult; some editors do not understand the intrinsic properties of pharmacoeconomic data, and some reviewers will blindly apply statistical constraints that are inappropriate or not valid to humanistic outcomes (e.g. power calculations to measures of the adverse effects of drugs on quality of life measures).

The basic principles of scientific writing and reporting apply to pharmacoeconomic research, and little need be said here. The structure of the paper is the same (Introduction, Methods, Results, Discussion, etc.). It is important to be consistent and appropriate in the use of terminology (e.g. 'costs' is not synonymous with 'charges', and cost-effectiveness is not a cost–benefit analysis; Sanchez and Lee 1994). New mediums such as the Internet offer new possibilities for publication, dissemination, and debate (Medical Outcomes Trust (2001) www.outcomes-trust.org; American College of Clinical Pharmacy 1996).

It must be said that how such information gets disseminated is controversial in the USA. A good recent example is an investigation of atovaquone vs. i.v. pentamidine in the treatment of mild to moderate *Pneumocystis carinii* pneumonia. This report included a decision tree to estimate the costs and cost-effectiveness of atovaquone vs. Pentamidine for cotrimoxazole-intolerant patients (Zarkin et al 1996). Clinical outcomes were based on data from a previous randomized controlled trial (RCT) (Phase III) comparing the two medications, while economic outcomes were based on treatment algorithms derived from discharge data, published reports and clinical judgments by the co-authors. The clinical data was from a randomized, double-blind study, a key issue with the agency. A sensitivity analysis was conducted. The major conclusion of the study was that there were significant cost savings to be had from treating *Pneumocystis carinii* pneumonia on an outpatient basis. An FDA representative, during a platform presentation of this paper, even indicated that this data could be used in promotion.

CURRENT AND FUTURE USES OF PHARMACOECONOMIC OUTCOMES

The future for pharmacoeconomics is promising in the current health care environment. However, like any discipline, pharmacoeconomics has its limitations (Jennings and Staggers 1997):

1. *Competing perspectives create tension*, e.g. pharmacoeconomics vs. clinical importance. Differences in perspective may be irreconcilable because they relate to a perceived encroachment: 'turf wars' can erupt between clinical, marketing, and pharmacoeconomics departments within the same company, in spite of all three professing the same goal, i.e. to successfully market a worthwhile drug in a proper fashion.
2. *Need for rapid response*. Protocol in 2 weeks vs. 6 weeks? Sometimes it takes longer to develop the pharmacoeconomic portion of a protocol. There may be fewer people to do it, there are more likely to be unknowns, and there may be a need to decide which instrument to use; worse yet, there may be no baseline data to validate any chosen instrument. Studies that examine efficiency are especially likely to require more planning.
3. *Lack of prototype*. Some groups want these studies to be pragmatic and relevant to everyday practice, yet there is no prototype to delineate the basic tenets of such studies, meaning that the data may be riddled with inaccuracies and misrepresentations. Additionally, the regulatory agencies may be more concerned with internal validity than the pragmatic approach would allow.

4. *Performance measure pitfalls.* What gets measured reflects system values. If clinical groups are measured on the ability to meet target filing dates, then peak sales potential will be ignored. Relevant clinical indicators of performance may not be known, neither is it the best mix of data.

5. *Dearth of patient-centered outcomes measures in traditional drug development.* Physicians are usually relied upon for clinical data. Data from the patient is sometimes perceived to be 'soft'. Patient perspectives may also be missed when the traditional clinical focus may be diseases or organs-dominated.

6. *Discrepancies in terminology.* A new lexicon is emerging. The lexicon must be carefully and precisely translated in its application to health-care to avoid miscommunication. Marketing may ask for a CHA and not know the difference between a CHA and a CEA. They may not understand the approaches, but will only latch on to the buzzwords.

7. *When to measure.* A major challenge for clinical studies is when to measure. At what point in the process is the end-point reached? The decision can significantly affect the cost and time of conducting a study. Unfortunately, there are no obvious guides, but there should be sufficient proximity between process and outcome measures to believe the linkage.

8. *Value.* To what extent is value related to quality? If there is no standard definition of quality, quality may be overridden by cost. It is difficult to quantify non-monetary value into a neat formula. The challenge is to propose quality indicators that allow calculating a balance of quality and cost.

9. *Absence of clearly delineated perspective(s).* Outcomes can be categorized in a variety of ways, including disease, patient, provider and organizational. There will likely be multiple perspectives, but it still needs to be orderly.

10. *Outcomes are not processes.* Patient care and quality dimensions of outcomes must be considered.

This applied discipline of pharmacoeconomics is slowly evolving into a more sound science. Despite its lack of maturity, many people and systems are embracing it as a savior. While pharmacoeconomics is an important advancement in the contribution of decision making, it does need to be put in appropritae context. It is a new and essential part of an older, larger, and previously less sophisticated process. Used appropriately, pharmacoeconomic research can assist in rational decision-making at every level of drug development and drug therapy.

REFERENCES

American College of Clinical Pharmacy (1996) *Pharmacoeconomics and Outcomes: Applications for Patient Care.* A series of three modules created to develop in-depth working knowledge of pharmacoeconomic and outcomes assessment. ACCP Kansas City Mo 816 531 2177 **http://www.accp.com**

Bootman JL, Townsend RJ, McGhan WF (eds) (1996) *Principles of Pharmacoeconomics*, 2nd edn. Harvey Whitney: Cincinnati, OH.

Feldstein PJ (1983) *Health Care Economics*, 2nd edn. Wiley: New York.

Foundation for Health Sciences Research (1993) *Health Outcomes Research: A Primer.* Foundation for Health Services Research: Washington, DC.

Hirsch JD, Van Den Eeden SK (1997) Epilepsy: searching for outcomes data beyond seizure frequency in a managed care organization. *J Outcomes Managem* 1997; 4(1): 9–11, 14–17, 23.

Jennings BM, Staggers N (1997) The hazards in outcomes management. *J Outcomes Managem* 4(1): 18–23.

Kozma CM, Reeder CE, Schulz RM (1993) Economic, Clinical and humanistic outcomes: a planning model for pharmacoeconomic research. *Clin Ther* 15: 1121–32.

Lawrence WF, Fryback DG, Martin PA et al (1996) Health status and hypertension: a population-based study. *J Clin Epidemiol* 49(11): 1239–45.

"Medical Outcomes Trust (2001), www.outcomes-trust.org" 617 426 4046 **MOTRUST@worldnet.att.net**

Sanchez LA, Lee JT (1994) Use and misuse of pharmacoeconomic terms: a definitions primer. *Top Hosp Pharm Managem* 13: 11–22.

Steinwachs DM, Wu AW, Skinner EA (1994) How will outcomes management work? *Health Affairs* 13: 153–62.

Zarkin GA, Bala MV, Wood LL et al (1996) Estimating the cost effectiveness of atovaquone versus intravenous pentamidine in the treatment of mild to moderate pneumocystis pneumonia. *Pharmacoeconomics* 6: 525–34.

FURTHER READING

Bowling A (1995) *Measuring Health: A Review of Disease-specific Quality of Life Measurement Scales.* Open University Press: Buckingham, UK, and Bristol, PA.

Bowling A (1997) *Measuring Health: A Review of Quality of Life Measurement Scales*, 2nd edn. Open University Press: Buckingham, UK, and Bristol, PA.

Drummond MF, Stoddart GL, Torrance GW (1986) *Methods for the Economic Evaluation of Health Care Programmes*. Oxford: Oxford University Press.

Drummond MF, O'Brien B (1993) Clinical importance, statistical significance and the assessment of economic and quality of life outcomes. *Health Econ* 2: 205.

Eddy DM (1990) Should we change the rules for evaluating medical technologies? In Gelljns AC (ed.), *Modern Methods of Clinical Investigation*. National Academy Press: Washington, DC.

Freund DA, Dittus RS (1992) Principles of pharmacoeconomics analysis of drug therapy. *PharmacoEconomics* 1: 20–32.

Jolicoeur LM, Jones-Grizzle AJ, Boyer JG (1992) Guidelines for performing a pharmacoeconomic analysis. *Am J Hosp Pharm* 49: 1741–7.

Lee JT, Sanchez LA (1992) Interpretation of 'cost-effective' and soundness of economic evaluations in pharmacy literature. *Am J Hosp Pharm* 1992;48: 2622–7.

McDowell I, Newell C (1996) *Measuring Health: A Guide to Rating Scales and Questionnaires*, 2nd edn. Oxford University Press: New York.

Patrick DL, Deyo RA (1989) Generic and disease-specific measures in assessing health status and quality of life. *Med Care* 27(suppl): S217–32.

Sederer L, Dickey B (eds) (1996) *Outcomes Assessment in Clinical Practice*. Williams and Wilkins: Baltimore, MD.

Spilker B (ed.) (1990) *Quality of Life Assessments in Clinical Trials*. Raven: New York.

Ware JE Jr (1995) The status of health assessment 1994. *Ann Rev Public Health* 16: 327–54.

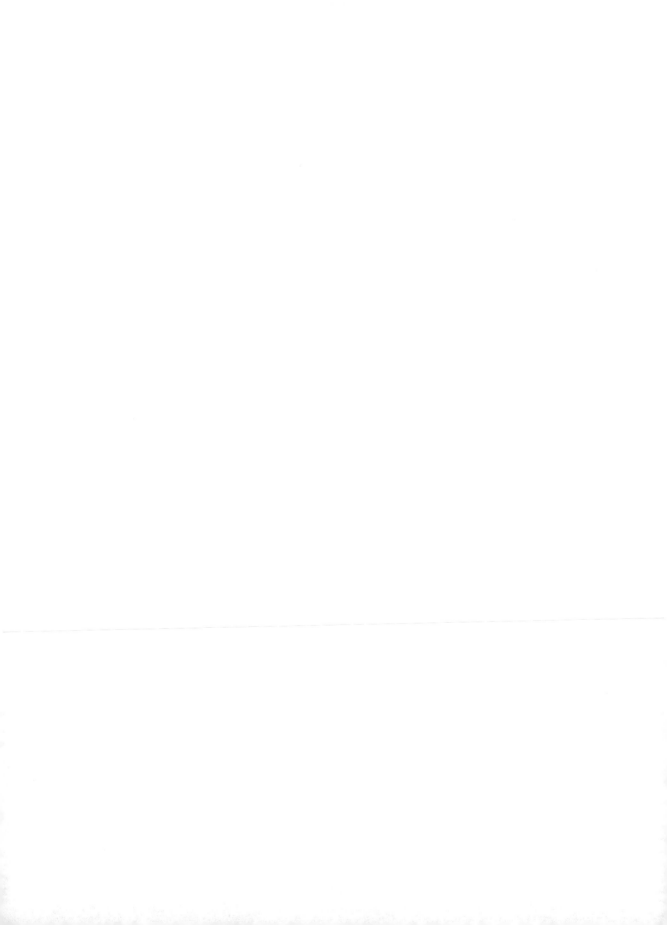

20

Pharmacoepidemiology and the Pharmaceutical Physician

Hugh H. Tilson

Department of Public Health, University of North Carolina, USA

The specialty practice of preventive medicine extends into the realm of pharmaceutical medicine just as deeply as better-recognized disciplines such as clinical pharmacology or toxicology. Pharmaceutical physicians may often be found practicing preventive medicine under the guise of clinical research or regulatory affairs, or in separate departments of pharmacoepidemiology, health economics or outcomes research, as well as the perhaps more predictable aegis of drug safety and pharmacovigilance.

Preventive Medicine/Public Health physicians, alias pharmacoeconomists and pharmacoepidemiologists, are trained in the core sciences of public health—epidemiology and statistics along with their non-physician pharmacoepidemiology colleagues. But, being physicians, they are also steeped in pathophysiology, diagnostics, therapeutics, and behavioral sciences. Additionally, specialization in preventive medicine requires detailed education in environmental health and general management and logistic skills. Many of these areas of expertise are shared with other types of pharmaceutical physicians, e.g. clinical trialists. It is not uncommon to find professionals moving (or oscillating) between pharmacoepidemiology and other departments within the same company.

Public health physicians use all these tools to identify, and control, public health hazards. In the pharmaceutical sector, these skills extend to such hazards associated with pharmacotherapy. Pharmacoepidemiologists have an additional dimension to their work, in that they may study drugs not only as a potential hazard to the public health (perhaps through drug surveillance programs) but also as a potential benefit to the public health (e.g. in large-scale interventional, clinical outcomes or economics studies). Identifying the types of patients who are most likely to benefit (or be harmed) by a therapeutic intervention is merely an extension of the orthodox world in which the public health physician practices. Thus, preventive medicine physicians may be found in pharmaceutical companies, CROs, academic, governmental, and international political environments.

EPIDEMIOLOGY

The word has three components, from the Greek *epi*, upon; *demos*, the people; and *logos*, the study. These elements describe the fundamentals of what epidemiology is all about, the application of scientific principles to the understanding of health issues which are 'upon the people'. *All* pharmaceutical physicians need an understanding of the fundamentals of this field, in order to understand and harness the value that epidemiology, and epidemiologists, can bring to drug development and product surveillance programs. Epidemiology is taught in all schools of public health and, in varying depth and quality, in schools of medicine. Epidemiological techniques are used by many people who would not describe themselves as epidemiologists. Board certification in preventive medicine requires a Master's degree with a large epidemiology component, and further tough examinations.

Such epidemiology training emphasizes the science of the observational research methodology as the core approach of the field. However, emphasis is also given on building expertise in clin-

Principles and Practice of Pharmaceutical Medicine. Edited by A. J. Fletcher, Lionel D. Edwards, Anthony W. Fox and Peter Stonier © 2002 John Wiley & Sons Ltd.

ical trials design and biostatistics. These disciplines require expertise and experience in the management of huge quantities of data and the attendant expertise in scientific computing/informatics. These are skills that find natural places in Phase III and Phase IV clinical study design and conduct within industry, and evaluation within the regulatory environment. However, it is in the understanding of the applications (and often more importantly the limitations) of the non-experimental/observational method that the epidemiologist brings special value-added to the pharmaceutical sector.

It is important to remember that epidemiology represents another set of tactics to address the same underlying motive as others working in and with the development enterprise. Just as much as a molecular biologist or clinical pharmacologist, the epidemiologist is trying to find out which set of conditions causes a particular disease or benefit or adverse event. The additional perspective of the impact upon actual populations (the actual effectiveness) complements the emphasis upon the experimental subject (the efficacy) of much of clinical research. The epidemiologist is faced with the substantial challenge of observational approaches. Without the benefits (comforts) of randomization and blinding afforded by the experimental method, only rarely can the epidemiologist imitate the pharmacologist, who can premeditate an intervention in a confined population, and then prospectively observe its effect. However, even when constrained by the observational approach, the epidemiologist is like other scientists in that findings are in the context of comparison among various structured observational groups, differing in their known exposures or outcomes.

EPIDEMIOLOGIC METHODOLOGIES

Prospective Cohort Studies

A prospective cohort epidemiologic study approximates to a parallel-group clinical trial in its scientific basis, and epidemiologists will be as aware as clinical trialists of the bias that can be introduced if the study groups do not contain comparable, well-balanced, and homogeneous groups of people. While the experimentalist uses exclusions, randomization and blinding as tools to control for unseen biases, the epidemiologist is, rather, required to measure and document attributes and control for those that may lead to skewed results, by selection in ascertainment and stratification in analysis. Furthermore, like others calling themselves drug surveillance specialists, the epidemiologist will be well aware that the size of the groups that must be studied increases with the rarity of the phenomenon that is sort. The latency of the effect (e.g. the duration between exposure to an unsuspected atheromatous stimulus and coronary artery disease) can define the desirable duration of follow-up, in a manner analogous to the study of the probability of adverse events arising only after prolonged multiple-dose drug exposure. Often, rather, the size of the available population and the duration for which it has already been followed (e.g. for other, administrative or clinical purposes) will dictate the extent to which an observational study is able to state the level of certainty of its observations.

Case-control Study Designs

These were developed to provide information more rapidly than when cohorts are followed for prolonged periods of time, using traditional hands-on methods; case-based research is, however, necessarily retrospective. Analysis begins with the characterization of a group of people that already have the disease of interest, the 'cases'. Control subjects are then drawn from a population with exactly the same attributes as that from which cases are selected (often a very difficult task!). The antecedent demographic, therapeutic and environmental factors of both groups are documented, often by a combination of record abstraction and interview. If differences are found in the proportion (rate) for some factor between the two groups, then this becomes suspected as an etiological agent for the disease of interest. This suspicion is strengthened when either the discovered factor corresponds with a predictive hypothesis at the start of the study, or when there is consistent evidence that would support its identification (perhaps a biochemical link between the factor and the disease).

DRUG RISK AS AN EPIDEMIOLOGIC PROBLEM

Drug-related epidemics have occurred, mercifully relatively infrequently. However, with each unfortunate episode, there is inevitably a variety of regulatory and clinical fallout. Indeed, the illnesses associated with ingestion of glycol-tainted linctus led to the Food, Drugs and Cosmetics Act in the USA, and the disastrous association of phocomelia with thalidomide propelled reforms of drug regulations worldwide. Other famous examples include, of course, practolol-induced oculomucocutaneous syndrome, and, more recently, fenfluramine-induced myocardial fibrosis, and isotretinoin-associated birth defects.

The major driver for the field of pharmacoepidemiology is the nature of the drug development process itself. Relatively small and often quite carefully selected clinical trials populations are followed for only limited periods, during and after exposure to the agent under study, in the populations that comprise typical product licence applications and NDA safety summaries. This leaves, for the post-approval scientific environment, the challenge to apply methods that can detect adverse events with relatively low frequency or relatively specific risk situations. Those who call for transfer of these burdens to the pre-approval environment would benefit from training in epidemiology, with the associated understanding that the only way to understand the real world is to study the real world!

Pharmacoepidemiology and pharmacovigilance do not pretend to be able to eliminate the occurrence of drug-associated epidemics. The challenge is to detect and quantitate problems as rapidly and accurately as possible, so that changes in the benefit–risk balance, as understood at the time of approval, can be quickly recognized and possible public health actions considered. Thus, pharmacovigilance may be understood as 'epidemiologic intelligence'. And thus, in turn, the physician pharmacoepidemiologist is a strong contributor to drug surveillance departments in industry and drug safety groups in regulatory groups. Typically, these epidemiologists will be supervising and/or providing expert counsel to groups of less special-ized or highly trained health scientists who implement the day-to-day running of these programs. Teamwork becomes an indispensable skill.

Consideration about the need for and technical considerations regarding one or more structured epidemiologic studies is a frequently recognized contribution of the epidemiologist in this enterprise. Less frequently extolled are the great contributions which epidemiologists make to consideration of approaches which, seductive because of their apparent simplicity, will *not* be likely to contribute, as options for reducing uncertainty around estimates of possible risk are considered. Observational science is very complicated, and the opportunities to failure of study are considerable! When epidemiologic studies are undertaken, and results are known, it falls to the physician epidemiologist to put on the public health hat and recommend whether an intervention in the interests of public health might be needed, and if so, then to suggest what its parameters might be.

THE 'WIRED' EPIDEMIOLOGIST

It probably goes without saying in the cybernetic environment of the twenty-first century that effective epidemiology of all types, including pharmacoepidemiology, can only be seriously conducted with the addition to the armamentarium of the epidemiologist, of the skillful use of large, automated, multipurpose, population-based systems (the LAMPS)—known by shorthand as 'the databases'. Often these databases have been developed with a primary intent of creating economic efficiency, quality assurance, or management controls within organized systems of healthcare. Hence, in the USA, the organizations that construct these databases include insurance companies, hospitals, health maintenance organizations, and other companies in the healthcare business. In Canada, and increasingly in Europe, such databases are emerging from provincial/regional or national reimbursement programs. If the database is equipped with patient identifiers (e.g. a unique membership number), then hospitalizations, prescriptions and combinations of healthcare transactions can be linked to a single individual across components of the system and over time: a so-called 'record-linkage' system. More recently, the evolution of a powerful clinical management tool, the electronic medical record, further powers the availability of linked data for entire populations under care. Such databases render it feasible to assemble cohorts of drug-exposed individuals and computer-matched comparator populations from historical (extant) data and observe them (using cohort analyses) forward over the time in the database (often decades) for evidence of excesses of events under study. Similarly, case-control methods may assemble cases and comparators, and use the powerful databases as the source of the antecedent information, so elusive in hands-on methods.

Recent regulatory efforts on behalf of the needs to protect patient privacy are no strangers to this field, which has established a long and successful record of systems that protect patient privacy while assuring access to necessary population-level, individual-linked data. The recent, excellent policy positions on data privacy protections of the American College of Epidemiology (ACE) and the International Society for Pharmacoepidemiology (ISPE) stand as evidence of this competence. The reader is referred to the websites of these organizations.

It is to be emphasized that such database work is often complicated, and requires a team of professionals comprising physician and non-physician pharmacoepidemiologists, statisticians, and specialists in information technology. Perhaps one of the greatest contributions that a clinician can make to such a team is to provide relevance to the hypotheses that are tested and as a reality check on the results that the computers generate, and which those less close to the field tend to regard automatically as 'fact'.

Despite the deserved enthusiasm for the contribution of the LAMPS to epidemiology, more traditional hands-on, structured observational studies, with enrollment of cohorts of persons exposed to an agent under study and proper comparator populations, and selection of cases (e.g. from medical records) and appropriate controls, still have specific applications in pharmaceutical medicine, thus characterizing part of the activity of pharmacoepidemiologists.

DEFINITIONS

The pharmaceutical physician, epidemiologist or not, must understand the concepts of prevalence and incidence *sine qua non. Prevalence* is the frequency of disease in a defined population, at any one moment. *Incidence* is the frequency of new cases of a disease in a defined population during a defined time interval.

Thus, influenza may have an incidence of 15% for the months December–April 1999 in the UK, whereas the prevalence of influenza in the UK probably ranges between 0% and 10% on any given day. Perinatal (and maternal) mortality rates are usually stated annually and for specified country or region. These are thus measures of incidence. The proportion of a population that will experience at least one seizure or one migraine attack in their lives is a measure of incidence and would likely be expressed as a number per thousand (or per hundred thousand) person-years, whereas the proportion of a population suffering from epilepsy or migraine during the year 2000 is an expression of prevalence.

In pharmacovigilance terms, the 'true frequency' in a treated population in a specified period, if it were known, of an adverse event (AE) observed in a marketed product, would be considered an incidence. All too often, the frequency of reported AEs (definitely not the complete or even estimated numerator), perhaps weighed against known sales (scarcely a true denominator), is mistakenly used to calculate a rate and called an 'incidence'. At best, such spontaneous reports data should be termed 'reports rates'.

Other, more complex terms are defined and described in standard textbooks of epidemiology and statistics (q.v.) and included in two excellent lexicons, the Dictionary of Epidemiology (Last) and, more recently, a very useful Lexicon from the International Society for Pharmacoeconomics and Outcomes Research (ISPOR).

EPIDEMIOLOGY IN DRUG DEVELOPMENT

The complexities of drug development include a decision web that is inevitably informed by incomplete information. While past, focused research may comprise some of the information for the next step, epidemiologic information can be of valuable assistance. The capturing and extension of population-based studies, often concerning the natural history of disease rather than the pharmacological properties of the test agent itself, can guide the choice of indication, market strategy, and even the viability of an entire project. Furthermore, the place of existing therapies, in the context of the natural history of disease, can also be investigated epidemiologically. 'If they don't need it, we can't sell it; then let's not pursue it' is an aphorism: but whether they need it is, of course, an epidemiologic challenge.

Population-based measures of burden of disease involve a formal quantitation of the opportunity for a new drug. These measures vary among organ systems, but typically involve the integral of lifestyle interference, duration of disease, prevalence, incidence, effectiveness and adverse effects associated with existing therapies, and reduction in lifespan. Such objective measures can be ascertained from population-based studies and existing national databases, e.g. from major ongoing population health surveys, and can often allow the pharmacoepidemiologist to contribute a substantial and useful evidence base to inform the difficult and emotion-laden decisions which must be made by senior executives in drug development.

During Phases II and III, an additional capability can be offered to the development team that might hitherto be comprised purely of clinical department staff—Are infrequently observed but highly dangerous adverse events being seen in a clinical trials program within the expected range for that study population? If so, then entire development programs in jeopardy could be saved; if not, appropriate actions may be undertaken more rapidly and decisively.

Under some circumstances, in the USA, widespread distribution of an investigational agent prior to NDA approval, involving large-scale populations, is permitted (the treatment IND is an extension of the old compassionate use notion). Under these conditions it is, of course, necessary to monitor safety in such broader use, and usually with greater scrutiny that might ordinary apply

after product approval. Adverse events are bound to occur; thus providing an ideal opportunity for early detection of infrequent but important adverse reactions; conversely, trouble-shooting these, in the context of a sound epidemiologic and clinical understanding of adverse events associated with the disease itself, and with alternative therapies, is also often needed to protect against false conclusions. Such interpretations also eventually are translated into labeling, either by exclusion or inclusion.

EPIDEMIOLOGY IN DRUG REGISTRATION AND LICENSING

During the registration process, there is typically repeated interaction between an NDA/PLA sponsor and the regulatory authority. Often these interactions revolve around whether the tolerability of the new drug is sufficiently well-characterized, and the criteria for the inclusion and exclusion of particular observed intolerabilities in labeling, as well as the weight that should be applied to each (e.g. adverse event list, warning, contraindication or, rarely, precluding drug approval). Often the question 'What level of risk is acceptable?' becomes quickly answered with 'Acceptable, compared to what?' These considerations are clearly based upon an insight into public health decision-making and are often well-served by inclusion of epidemiologists working with and/or consulting with regulators and sponsors.

Furthermore, the scientific proof of a negative is virtually impossible when fewer than an infinite number of patients have been studied. The more elusive problem, then, is to define acceptable uncertainty. Some of these decisions are based upon precedent rather than observation. Pharmacoepidemiology is often a useful source of precedents, as well as available for further, future study in the post-approval period to clarify residual questions and/or reduce the remaining uncertainty. While many of the activities described can then be orientated towards support of registration with fair and balanced labeling or education that is useful to the prescriber, recently regulators have requested and sponsors have proposed programs of 'risk management', in which provider and/or consumer interventions accompany the marketplace activities with a drug with a residual safety concern. These programs likewise include documentation of the effectiveness of the intervention, once again a challenge for the public health researcher, i.e. the pharmacoepidemiologist.

Post-marketing Surveillance Studies

Approval (especially in the USA) is now often contingent upon the agreement of the sponsor to conduct one or more postmarketing surveillance studies. Typically conducted on a scale of 5000 or more patients, the design of such studies poses classic epidemiologic challenges: the choice of control cohorts (if any), appropriateness of historical controls, power calculations, the nature and range of confounding variables, among others. Many of these may be addressed using the databases described above. It should be noted that postmarketing surveillance studies are often implemented by companies without any imposed regulatory requirement, simply due to the value that they bring in understanding a new product that may formerly only have been tested in several hundred patients.

General Pharmacovigilance

Whether or not a postmarketing surveillance study is used, all drugs undergo pharmacovigilance when in the market place. This can be especially challenging but vital during the early period after launch. The assessment of pharmacovigilance findings, inevitably adverse events with low incidence, has obligatorily to include an epidemiologic component. Recent product withdrawals provide a litany that need not be repeated here, but averages one or two major products and several minor ones each year. Product withdrawals are often misunderstood, particularly by the lay press hungry for a scandal. It is neither feasible nor desirable to 'know everything about a product' at the time of approval. But judicious product withdrawal, based upon substantial evidence properly collected and analyzed in the postmarketing environment, is a classic example of a robust and balanced system, with each component functioning as it should.

Pharmacoepidemiology contributes to the pursuit of the best-informed decision making, with the shared goal of optimization of the balance between patient benefit and the inevitable patient adversity.

Prescription-event Monitoring (PEM)

This is essentially an extension of traditional, hands-on epidemiology, which assembles all patients that are prescribed a drug into a cohort which is then followed. In the UK, for example, through the Drug Safety Research Trust, all or a sample of this cohort is assembled from the records of the prescription pricing authority, generally within the first year or two of initial marketing of the product. Each patient can be followed-up with a confidential enquiry for serious adverse events using a form that, in the UK, is popularly called by its appearance: the 'Green card' (this term has an entirely different meaning in the USA, and, curiously, describes a pink document!). It is a classic example of an observational as opposed to an experimental method, in which all uses and all outcomes (events) are observed, generally without a simultaneously collected comparison population. Thus, data stemming from these sorts of activities are fraught with analytical and methodological traps. However, PEM is a good method for generating hypotheses for further testing, usually after reconciliation with the known pharmacology of the drug of interest, other drugs in the same class, and the natural history of the disease and kindred disorders. These, of course, shed further light on these data, and may be gathered, e.g. from the spontaneous reports system. Indeed, sometimes this is also the first evidence of an unsuspected drug intolerability, perhaps in a previously unsuspected subset of the treated patient population. The ability in certain European areas and New Zealand to aggregate prescriptions from entire countries or regions, often as part of the reimbursement system, is obviously strategic to this approach.

Pregnancy Registries

Pregnancy registries (or, more properly, pregnancy follow-up studies) are being recommended with increasing frequencies for products that are likely to be used in women with child-bearing potential. Inevitably, all new drugs have not been studied in women who are, or become, pregnant, and equally inevitably, labeled warnings to that effect do not prevent exposures of embryos and fetuses to new drugs. The anticipated, spontaneous incidence of anomalies detectable *post partum* is in the range 3–7%, depending upon criteria such as severity (e.g. is a minor birthmark a 'birth anomaly'?), degree of scrutiny (follow-up until the age of 4 years or beyond is needed to detect some anomalies; some types of inguinal hernia presenting in adulthood are even thought to be congenital), geography, concomitant disease or toxin exposures (including tobacco, illicit drugs, and alcohol), and socioeconomic status. The key to a successful pregnancy registry is that pregnancies should be registered before their outcome is known: the diagnosed birth anomaly can cause bias in reporting frequency, and converts a prospective approach into a retrospective one. The choice of comparison population is highly complex. In general, the assumption of such registry studies is that the appropriate comparison is the general population, effectively a prospective cohort-controlled approach, i.e. the objective of such studies is to detect increases of specific defects over the expected rates in the general population. However, the detected occurrence of defects is a function of follow-up method and definition, and may be influenced by many (undocumented or even unknown) factors. Therefore, the conduct of registries and development of such comparisons must be done with great caution.

TRAINING TO BE A PHARMACOEPIDEMIOLOGIST

No parent has ever heard the statement: 'Mummy (or Daddy), I want to be a pharmaceutical physician pharmacoepidemiologist when I grow up'! Few physicians and very few pharmaceutical physicians choose this route. But what is along that route? The 'high road', in the USA at least, is graduation from medical school, obtaining at least 1 year of intense clinical postgraduate training (often leading to internal medicine or other primary care boards, the equivalent of MRCP in the UK), and then to undertake a further formal residency training program that leads to certification by the American Board of Preventive Medicine. Residencies are inspected and approved by the Board, and may be in one of four areas: public health, general preventive medicine, occupational medicine, or aerospace medicine. Various concentrations in medical management are also becoming recognized. In the UK, registrar positions in most of these specialties are advertised, and the Diplomas in Occupational or Public Health, membership of the Faculties of Occupational or Public Health, and the Diploma in Aviation Medicine would provide equivalent experience and certification.

In the USA, the academic equivalent of these, which can often be pursued in parallel, is to obtain the additional degree of Master of Public Health (MPH). Board certification through a preventive medicine residency requires such formal academic training and an MPH degree. Again, European equivalents exist. A 4–5 year program can accomplish all of these. Additionally, those interested in pharmaceutical matters which involve epidemiology, but do not aspire to board certification, can often attend specialized courses, and use case studies in this area to fulfill their academic requirements, or, of course, at least to enroll in a MPH degree program. Many of these now exist as 'off-campus' (so-called executive) degree programs, particularly for physicians.

More commonly, if not the 'high road', a pharmaceutical physician will stumble into this area by lateral transfer within a company, or due to the chance happening of being assigned a development project that requires extensive pharmacoepidemiologic support. Such physicians can supplement their training with *ad hoc* programs in statistics and epidemiology that are commonly offered on a short-term or part-time non-degree basis by many universities and training groups, or an executive MPH.

THE FUTURE

Pharmacoepidemiology has proved itself over the last 20 years, and will only grow during this new century. It is unlikely that society as a whole will understand the subtle but vital nuances of the concepts of risk and uncertainty any better in 50 years time than it does now. Governments and the

general public will require the pharmacoepidemiologist to protect their interests, and to accurately
assess the hazards that today's powerful drugs will
also bring. And tomorrow's drugs, driven by the
genomics revolution, will only further underscore
the need for epidemiology, to help us map the
genome to the 'phenome', i.e. the population manifestations of our genomic make-up. While it is
by no means clear where our earliest experiences
with genetic alteration will lead, it is clear that
any efforts in this arena will require long-term
population-based follow-up. Cost containment
will become increasingly a constraint on pharmaceutical medicine, and we must ensure that it
does not bring its own hazard. And risk management, with its accompanying accountability, is
emerging as a classic epidemiologic challenge. The
future for the pharmacoepidemiologist trained in

both epidemiology and medicine is bright indeed.
The lucky men and women who choose pharma-
ceopidemiology will be highly fulfilled in this subspecialty of pharmaceutical medicine.

REFERENCES

American College of Epidemiology (ACE). Data Privacy
    Protections. www.aceepidemiology.org <http://www.aceepi
    demiology.org>.
International Society for Pharmacoepidemiology (ISPE).
    Data Privacy Protections. www.pharmacoepi.org <http://
    www.pharmacoepi.org>.
Last JM. (2001). *Dictionary of Epidemiology*. Oxford University
    Press, Inc., New York.
Pashos C and Heissel A. (eds). International Society for Phar-
    macoeconomics and Outcomes Research, New Jersey.
    www.ispor.org <http://www.ispor.org>.

21

Statistical Principles and Their Application in Biopharmaceutical Research

Dan Anbar

Millennium Biostatistics Inc., Bound Brook, NJ, USA

THE SCIENTIFIC METHOD AND THE ROLE OF THE SCIENTIFIC EXPERIMENT

The purpose of science is to explain natural phenomena by uncovering the natural laws that give rise to them. The scientific method is a three-step process: (a) formulating theories as explanations of phenomena; (b) making predictions based on these theories; and (c) testing the theories through experimentation. Most people engage daily in the first two activities. Explaining the environment in which we live is an innate human characteristic. However, people rarely subject their theories to testing by experimentation.

What makes the scientific method unique is that it does not accept an explanation as valid until it has been validated through testing. However, a scientific experiment can never *prove* a theory. At best, it can provide evidence for the usefulness of the theory in predicting events under given experimental conditions, and help to define more precisely the relationship between these conditions and the implied events. The greatest value of a scientific experiment is in its ability to *disprove* a theory or identify limits of its applicability, either of which can lead to scientific advances. An experimental finding inconsistent with a theory suggests that a theory should be revised or rejected. Popper (1959) states that a necessary condition for a valid theory is the condition of *falsifiability*, i.e. it should generate predictions that can be tested experimentally. Experimental outcomes contradicting the theoretical predictions would lead to a reassessment of the theory requiring a revision or rejection. In other words, a scientific theory is always tentative and entirely dependent on experimental verification. Theories that are not falsifiable may be the subject of religious or philosophical discussions but not of scientific investigation, according to Popper.

Experiments designed to confirm a theory (or to falsify it) are called *confirmatory* and those designed to merely accumulate information are termed *exploratory*. Exploratory experiments are a useful first step in the process of formulating scientific theories. Either type must follow strict methodological procedures and adhere to a detailed experimental protocol describing the conditions of experimentation, the methods of measurement, and all other aspects that might affect the results. The experimenter must record the raw data prior to any analysis and document any protocol deviations, documenting all aspects of the experiment such that another scientist can precisely repeat it.

THE STATISTICAL METHOD: MAKING DECISIONS UNDER CONDITIONS OF UNCERTAINTY

The scientific method runs into difficulties when applied to random phenomena. A *random phenomenon* is one where the outcome cannot be predicted with certainty from the experimental conditions. One cannot guarantee the repeat of a coin toss, no matter how hard one tries to keep the conditions constant. Neither can one expect a drug to produce an identical effect in the same patient under identical conditions on separate occasions. Such phenomena can be described probabilistically. That is, one can assign numerical values describing the likelihood, *or probability*, of the possible outcomes.

Principles and Practice of Pharmaceutical Medicine. Edited by A. J. Fletcher, Lionel D. Edwards, Anthony W. Fox and Peter Stonier © 2002 John Wiley & Sons Ltd.

Because of the uncertainty, an isolated failure of a drug to produce a desired therapeutic effect does not prove that a drug is unefficacious. Similarly, an isolated successful drug treatment outcome does not prove that the drug is efficacious.

Unfortunately, it is impossible to design an experiment that will totally disprove a theory based on random phenomena. Various outcomes may occur, some of which may be unlikely but not impossible. Thus, Popper's falsifiability condition does not hold. The statistical method advocated by Fisher (1973) attempts to overcome this problem by substituting 'unlikely' for 'impossible', but otherwise follows the scientific process described above. This substitution raises a host of conceptual issues beyond the scope of this discussion, except to say that this approach has its opponents and is not accepted by all statisticians.

Let us illustrate the statistical method with an example:

A pharmaceutical company has developed an antihypertensive drug that is theorized to lower diastolic blood when given to subjects with moderate to severe hypertension. If the diastolic blood pressure were constant under given conditions, then failure to lower diastolic pressure by any amount in any patient treated with this drug under a constant set of conditions would disprove the theory. In reality, the subject's blood pressure is a random phenomenon. It varies with or without treatment. Thus, the simple experiment described above cannot be used to disprove the hypothesis (or the converse theory, that the drug has no efficacy). Since blood pressure is naturally variable, how do we know whether the difference in blood pressure before and after treatment is due to the drug or to the natural randomness of blood pressure? The experiment must: (a) measure the natural variability of diastolic blood pressure; and (b) determine whether the change in blood pressure is likely to result from natural variability.

A typical experiment might be as follows: Subjects are divided into two groups, A and B. Group A receives no treatment or a placebo. Group B receives the test drug. Diastolic blood pressure is measured in all subjects before treatment and at some time point when the drug effect should be measurable if the drug is efficacious. Mean change in blood pressure is compared between the groups.

Table 21.1 Type I and II errors in statistical decision making

True state	Decision	
	Accept hypothesis	Reject hypothesis
Hypothesis is true		Type I error
Hypothesis is false	Type II error	

If the difference appears random, the drug is probably ineffective. If the difference appears non-random, the drug is probably influencing diastolic blood pressure. If the starting point of the experimenter is the hypothesis that the drug is ineffective, then the smaller the probability that the observed difference is random, the higher the probability that rejecting the hypothesis of no efficacy is correct.

The key difference between the statistical method and the scientific method is that statistically, no matter how unlikely a result may be, it is not impossible. Therefore, any decision to confirm or reject a hypothesis is liable to error. Two types of error are possible, as summarized in Table 21.1.

THE STATISTICAL TEST: THE NULL HYPOTHESIS, ERROR PROBABILITIES, STATISTICAL POWER

Seemingly, therefore, whether a drug is efficacious or not is a dichotomy. In reality, however, it is a continuum. If we consider the effect (E) of our drug in lowering diastolic blood pressure, then lack of efficacy corresponds to $E = 0$. Positive efficacy corresponds to $E > 0$, which contains a continuum of possibilities depending on the strength of the effect. Thus, the hypothesis of no efficacy is very specific in terms of the size of the effect and is called a *simple hypothesis*, while a hypothesis corresponding to a range of values is called a *composite hypothesis*.

As we have seen, both the scientific method and the statistical method are designed to prove a claim false rather than prove it to be true. In drug testing, the statistical experiment is designed to reject the *null hypothesis*—the hypothesis that there is no difference between the treatments being tested.

Applying Table 21.1 above to the null hypothesis:

Type I error rejection of the null hypothesis when it is true (an ineffective drug is judged effective).

Type II error acceptance of the null hypothesis when it is false (an effective drug is judged ineffective).

Type I error is often also called 'false positive' and type II error 'false negative'. Because rejection of the null hypothesis enables one to make the scientific claim that the study was performed to prove, statisticians label such a rejection as *significant*. When the result of a test is declared significant, the only error that could occur is type I error. Clearly, the smaller the probability of type I error, the more secure one is in rejecting the null hypothesis. The probability of a type I error is called the *significance level* of the test and is denoted by α. The probability of a type II error is denoted by β; $1 - \beta$ is called the *power* of the test, often expressed as a percentage. The null hypothesis is usually a simple hypothesis. Therefore α is usually a single number. The alternative to the null hypothesis, on the other hand, is typically a composite hypothesis. In our antihypertensive drug testing example, this alternative was the whole region $E > 0$. In this case the value of β and the power $1 - \beta$ depends on the specific value of E. Thus, it is meaningless to talk about the power of a statistical test without specifying the alternative for which it applies. In our example, the power of the test at $E = 10$ is the probability that the statistical test would be significant if the effect of the drug is 10 mmHg.

An effective statistical test must have small α and β (i.e. high power) with regard to alternatives of interest. So if, in our example, the clinician estimates that the drug should lower diastolic blood pressure by an average of about 10 mmHg, the statistician would want α to be small, say ≤ 0.05, and $1 - \beta$ to be large, say ≥ 0.90, for the alternative $E = 10$. Can the statistician design a study such that the test would have any desirable α and β? Generally, yes, by selecting an appropriate sample size; that is, by including a sufficient number of subjects in the study. Once the sample size is fixed, the relationship between α and β is determined. A reduction in α increases β, and vice versa. For a given study design, the only way to decrease α and β simultaneously is by increasing the sample size. We will discuss this topic in greater detail later.

CAUSALITY

The ultimate goal of clinical research, is to establish causality—to determine efficacy outcomes that are due to the drug and to measure their magnitude, and to determine adverse effects related to the drug.

How does one know whether an effect A (e.g. giving a particular drug at a particular dose) causes an event B? A number of conditions must be satisfied. First, A must precede B. Second, whenever A occurs, B must occur too. These, of course, are not sufficient, since both A and B could be caused by an effect C. In addition, therefore, a theory is required that links A to B. This requirement is the Achilles heel of 'causality', since all theories are necessarily tentative. In an experimental science such as pharmaceutical research, the second condition can be established by conducting an experiment both when effect A is absent and when effect A is present, while all other conditions remain unchanged. If B requires the presence of A, then B is caused by A. However, if B is present regardless of A, then no causality is proven because B may be caused by an effect C that is present in both parts of the experiment.

In studying drug effects in humans, the controlled clinical trial is the preferred method to establish causality. In its simplest form, a controlled clinical trial is an experiment in human subjects in which some subjects are treated with an investigational drug and some are not, while all other conditions remain the same for the two treatment groups. In this way, any differences in clinical outcome should be due only to the investigational drug (controlled clinical trials will be discussed in greater detail in the section on The Controlled Clinical Trial, below).

VARIABILITY—THE SOURCE OF UNCERTAINTY

Virtually no drug has an identical response in all patients. For example, an effective antibiotic will, almost certainly, be ineffective in some patients, possibly because such patients are infected with a resistant strain or have a deficient immune response. Variability in response introduces uncertainty in establishing cause and effect. The fact that administering a drug to a given subject has not resulted with the desired therapeutic effect does not necessarily imply that the drug in ineffective. Causality, in the strict sense discussed in the previous section, can no longer be established when outcome of an experiment is subject to variability. However, one can still talk about causality in a probabilistic sense by modifying the requirement that 'whenever A is present B *must* be present, too' necessary for the establishment of causality, to 'the *probability* that B will occur is *greater* in the presence of A than when A is not present'.

Another issue is that when the measurement of efficacy is variable, it is impossible to determine what part of the measured outcome is due to the effect of the drug and what part is due to variability unrelated to the drug effect. The size of a drug effect is called the 'signal' while the variability associated with it is called the 'noise'. Clearly, the larger the 'signal-to-noise *ratio*', the easiest it is to establish a causal relationship. Thus, in a clinical drug trial, it is equally important to measure both noise and signal. How are these measured? The nature of variability is that it is random. When we measure the blood pressure of an individual subject repeatedly, the measurements will be dispersed around some central value in a random fashion; some will be larger and some smaller. The effect, on the other hand, is systematic. If, for example, we measure the blood pressure of an individual repeatedly before and just after administering an antihypertensive drug, the pre- and post-treatment measurements will be dispersed around different central values, the post-treatment lower than the pretreatment value. The magnitude of the effect

(signal) is usually calculated as the mean of the individual effects in a population of subjects. The variability (noise) is usually calculated as the standard deviation.

Example

Suppose 10 hypertensive subjects are treated with a novel antihypertensive drug. The subjects' blood pressure is measured at 8:00 a.m., just prior to the administration of the drug, and then again 1 hour later: the data are shown in Table 21.2.

The first and second rows of Table 21.2 give the diastolic blood pressure of subjects before and after treatment, respectively. The third row gives the change (Δ) in diastolic pressure (row 1 minus row 2). The mean of Δ given in the last column, is 12.8 mmHg. On the face of it, 12.8 mmHg looks like an impressive effect. However, as we have discussed before, we cannot assess its significance without considering the inherent variability, the noise. Indeed, the values of Δ range from -4 to 33, a substantial range. To assess Δ's variability, we calculated the deviations of the values of Δ about their mean, 12.8. These values are given in the next row. Naturally, since the mean is a value somewhere in the middle, some deviations are positive and others are negative. One property of the mean is that the sum of these deviations is always zero. Thus, the average (mean) of the deviations around the mean is always zero, and therefore is not useful as a measure of the variability. Instead, we calculate the mean of the squares of the deviations about the mean as a measure of variability. This measure is called the *variance*. The variance is an average of non-negative numbers and it is, therefore, always a non-negative number. It is equal to 0 if and only if all the deviates are equal to zero, meaning that all

Table 21.2 Diastolic blood pressure before and after treatment (mmHg) (hypothetical data)

Subject	1	2	3	4	5	6	7	8	9	10	Mean
Before treatment	102	78	95	86	109	107	100	86	96	92	95.1
After treatment	75	82	80	81	76	93	92	80	90	74	82.3
Difference (Δ)	27	-4	15	5	33	14	8	6	6	18	12.8
$[(\Delta - \text{mean}(\Delta)]$	14.2	-16.8	2.2	-7.8	20.2	1.2	-4.8	-6.8	-6.8	5.2	0
$[\Delta - \text{Mean}(\Delta)]^2$	201.64	282.24	4.84	60.84	408.04	1.44	23.04	46.24	46.24	27.04	110.16

the measurements are the same and thus equal to their mean, i.e. there is no variability at all. The *standard deviation* (SD), the most commonly used measure of variability, is the square root of the variance. In our case, SD = $\sqrt{110.16} = 10.50$. The advantage of using SD over the variance is that it is measured with the same units as the mean. The mean does not represent the response to treatment of any particular individual. It does, though, give us an idea of the magnitude of the response to treatment produced by the drug. Can we conclude, then, that the drug is efficacious? If the drug is ineffective, the mean change of 12.8 mmHg is due entirely to chance. Statistical theory shows that the likelihood that of a set 10 numbers generated at random with standard deviation of 10.5 would have a mean of 12.8 or larger in either a positive or a negative direction is less than 0.15%. Although this outcome is not impossible, it is highly unlikely. Thus, it is more prudent to conclude that the results of the experiment are due to the drug's effect rather than to chance.

The above example encapsulates many of the ideas and concepts behind the theory of statistical inference. The SD quantifies how widely a measurement is expected to deviate from theoretical typical value of the variable being measured. In our example, the variable being measured is the change between pre- and post-treatment in a patient's diastolic blood pressure. So, if the drug is ineffective, any change is due entirely to chance and therefore one would expect the change to be zero. This expected typical value is theoretical. In reality, blood pressure is affected by a variety of factors independent of the treatment and therefore actual measurements will not necessarily be zero. The SD enables us to calculate the probability that the measurements will fall close to, or far away from, zero, e.g. the probability is 95% that a measurement will fall within ± 2 SD. That is, assuming the drug is ineffective and the SD is 10.5, 95% of patients treated with the drug should have a change in their pre- and post-treatment diastolic blood pressure between -21 and $+21$. This is a fairly large range and indeed, all but two of the measurements in our example are within this range. This observation does not contradict our previous conclusion that the drug is effective. This is because our conclusion that the drug is effective was based on the mean of 10 measurements rather than on a single measure-

ment. The mean change is associated with experimental error. If we calculate the mean change for another set of 10 measurements obtained from different patients, it is unlikely that the result will be 12.8. The variability associated with a mean is smaller than that of a single measurement. The SD associated with the mean [also called the *standard error of the mean* (SEM)] is smaller than the SD by a factor equal to the square root of the number of measurements used to calculate the mean. In our example, SEM $= 10.5/\sqrt{10} = 10.5/3.16 = 3.32$. Thus, in our experiment the probability is 95% that the mean change will fall between -6.64 and $+6.64$. The mean of 12.8 is well outside that range. In fact, 12.8/SEM $= 3.85$. The probability of obtaining a ratio of 3.85 or larger is now approximately 0.15%.

To summarize, statistical methods are not intended to establish a cause-and-effect relationship between treatment and the response of any *individual* subject; rather, it is to establish a cause-and-effect relationship in the aggregate response (e.g. the mean) of a *population* of subjects. The key to this is the fact that, by considering aggregates, one can control the variability of a measured quantity. By increasing the sample size, one can reduce the SEM to a level that would make it possible to determine whether a signal is likely or unlikely to be due to chance, and thus decide whether a causal relationship is likely or unlikely to exist.

THE CONTROLLED CLINICAL TRIAL: BASIC DESIGN ELEMENTS

Randomization

The controlled clinical trial (CCT) is the scientific tool for demonstrating causality. Two essential elements characterize the CCT: (a) it contains a control group and an experimental group; (b) with the exception of treatment, all other conditions and procedures to which the subjects are exposed during the trial are constant. These two characteristics of the CCT enable the researcher to establish a causal relationship between treatment and the outcome of the trial. The tool for standardizing the trial is the study protocol, the document defining the subjects eligible for inclusion in the study, the study procedures and schedules.

A key element is the method of allocating subjects to the treatment groups. Subjects may possess a variety of characteristics that could influence their response to treatment. These could be related to the subjects' demographic background, such as age, sex and ethnic origin, genetic disposition or other prognostic variables. The method of allocating subjects to treatment must make sure that the resulting treatment groups are balanced with respect to such factors. The most effective way to achieve this is by randomization, i.e. assign each subject to a treatment group using a chance mechanism. Of course, one could achieve the desired balance by using a systematic, non-random allocation scheme that will force the balance. Randomization, however, has some important advantages. Any non-random method inevitably involves a decision by the individual making the allocation. This potentially could result with the preference of a certain type of subject for one of the treatments that may not be reflected as an imbalance in any of the identified prognostic variables. Furthermore, there might be some other variables which affect the response to treatment, which are either unrecognized as such at the time the study is planned, or are impossible to balance for logistical reasons. A random allocation, at least in large trials, can typically protect the investigator against such problems.

The most common method of randomization is by using *randomized blocks*. Let us illustrate this for a trial with three treatment Groups: A, B and C. Blocks containing the letters A, B, and C in a random order, with each letter repeated the same number of times, are generated. Such a block of length 6 might look like B, B, A, C, C, A. The requirement that each letter appears in the block as frequently as any of the other two letters implies that the length of the block must be a multiple of 3. Thus, for the case of three treatment groups, the block size must be either 3, 6, 9, etc. The number of such random blocks generated must be such that the number of letters in the resulting string equals or exceeds the number of subjects to be enrolled in the trial. Subjects are then assigned sequentially to the treatment group corresponding to the next unassigned letter in the randomization string. Because each individual block contains the same number of each of the letters, the treatment assignment sequence obtained from the randomized blocks

method is not exactly a sequence of random numbers. However, the method has the advantage that it guarantees a maximum balance in the resulting sizes of the treatment groups. This is a desirable feature because it increases the efficiency of the statistical analysis tools.

Bias and Blinding

An imbalance among the treatment groups might introduce a *bias*. In statistics, 'bias' has a specific technical meaning. Statisticians routinely use data obtained from a sample to estimate a parameter of interest. The estimate is subject to variability inherited from the data. Thus, using different and independent samples would result in different values of the estimate that are distributed around a mean value. Bias is the difference between that mean value and the quantity it intends to estimate. Thus, if this difference is positive, the method used tends to overestimate the quantity of interest, and when it is negative, it tends to underestimate it. We refer to this type of bias as *statistical bias*. For the purpose of our discussion, we will sometimes use the term 'bias' in a broader, although less precise, fashion. We would refer to bias as *the effect of any factor, or combination of factors, resulting in inferences which lead systematically to incorrect decisions about the treatment effect*. Because of its imprecision, this usage cannot be quantified. It is, however, useful in discussing problems that could result from a faulty design or inadequate conduct of a trial.

The most common source of bias is one resulting from subjects being selected to the different treatment groups in a way that creates an imbalance in one or more prognostic variables. This type of bias, known as *selection bias*, is usually the result of conscious or unconscious action on the part of the investigator or other people who can influence the enrollment of subjects into the trial, or a faulty treatment allocation method. Randomization is designed to take the treatment assignment decision away from the enrolling investigator and place it in the hands of chance. Unfortunately, it is not foolproof. An investigator who has a personal preference for one treatment over another for a particular type of subject may decide to postpone enrolling a subject until the 'right' treatment comes up on the randomization schedule. Also, there are many other ways that are not affected by randomization in which the investigator can influence the trial outcome. A simple talk with a subject reinforcing the subject's confidence in the efficacy of treatment can often have a real or transient effect on the subject's response to treatment.

Another potential source of bias is the subject him/herself. Often the mere expectation that the drug will have a therapeutic effect produces the effect. This effect is known as the *placebo effect*, and in some cases it could be considerable.

To counteract these types of bias, CCTs are generally *blinded*. That is, the identity of the treatment is concealed from anybody who can influence the treatment assignments and any procedure that could impact the trial outcome. When the treatments are masked from both the investigator and the subject, the trial is called *double-blind*. In drug trials, blinding is accomplished by using placebo, an inert substance, as a non-active control, and identical-looking packaging for the different treatments with labels that do not reveal the identity of the drug.

The use of double-blind randomized clinical trials has become the gold standard for good clinical research. However, it is not always possible to mask the treatments. A trial designed to compare the effectiveness of two surgical procedures is an example for a trial that cannot be blinded. Another example is a trial comparing an intravenous drug to an oral drug. In principle, one could blind such a trial by delivering an inert substance (e.g. saline) intravenously to the oral drug group and an oral placebo to the intravenous group. However, this procedure may be rejected as being unethical. When the comparators have distinct characteristics that would identify them, blinding can be achieved by using the so-called 'double-dummy' method, unless it is ethically unacceptable. The 'double-dummy' method means that all subjects receive identical-looking treatments, only one of which is active, while the others are placebos, e.g. in a com-

parison of two oral drugs, one of which is a tablet and the other a capsule, each subject receive a tablet and a capsule, one of which contains the treatment assigned to that subject and the other placebo. Sometimes even the 'double-dummy' method is not helpful. The drug might have a characteristic profile, such as identifiable smell, taste, or a specific adverse event or other biological effect that would reveal the identity of the treatment, either to the investigator or to the subject, or both, no matter how the drug is packaged or labeled. When blinding is not possible, special efforts must be made to minimize the possibility of introducing bias. The only effective way to handle it is by prevention; i.e. by incorporating appropriate bias prevention methods in the study design. Once bias is introduced, it is very difficult and sometimes impossible to adjust for it at the analysis stage.

Stratification

An efficient study design is one that maximizes the 'signal-to-noise ratio'. Thus, controlling the 'noise', or variability, is an important aspect of a good design. Consider the following example.

A graduate student in public health is conducting a research project on the health-related habits of the students at her university. As part of the project, she measures the resting heartbeat of 20 student-subjects. The results are listed in Table 21.3.

The mean is 56.8 and the SD is 3.57. The student then divides the subjects into two groups: group A consists of subjects who do aerobic exercises regularly, and group B of those who do not. The results are presented in Table 21.4

We notice that the two groups of subjects have different means and different SDs. Both SDs are smaller than obtained before separating the subjects into subgroups, i.e. the two groups are more homogeneous than the original group. When

Table 21.3 Heartbeat measurements of 20 students

Student	1	2	3	4	5	6	7	8	9	10	11	12	13	14	15	16	17	18	19	20
Heartbeat	60	53	56	56	56	57	56	52	63	51	59	63	55	58	56	53	64	56	58	55

Table 21.4 Heartbeat measurements of 20 students by exercise status

Group A	Subject	2	8	7	13	20	5	4	18	10	16	Mean	SD
	Heartbeat	53	52	56	55	55	56	55	56	51	53	54.2	1.81
Group B	Subject	12	15	14	1	11	6	9	3	17	19	Mean	SD
	Heartbeat	63	56	58	60	59	57	63	56	64	58	59.4	2.99

one combines the SDs into so-called 'pooled standard deviation', the result is $SD_{pooled} = 2.47$, which is substantially lower than the SD of the original combined group. The reason for this is that, when we calculated the mean of the combined group, we ignored the fact that the group consisted of two subgroups with different means. Thus, the calculated mean was, in fact, a mean of the two subgroups' means. Indeed, the overall mean, 56.8, equals the average of the means of the two subgroups $[(54.2 + 59.4)/2]$. The SD, therefore, represented the sum of two sources of variation: the intragroup variability, represented by the two subgroups' standard deviations; and the intergroup variability, represented by the difference between the two subgroup means.

The above example illustrates well the idea behind stratification. The study population is usually quite heterogeneous. If one measures the effect of treatment by calculating the overall mean effect in the population, although this mean represents an estimate of the treatment effect in this population, it might be associated with a large measurement error which could make it difficult to distinguish the signal from the background noise. In other words, the overall mean may be *an* estimate of the treatment effect but an *inefficient* one. If one can identify *a priori* certain subgroups, or *strata*, in the study population that are more homogeneous with respect to the efficacy variable of interest in the trial, then by estimating the effect within each of these strata, and combining these estimates, one may increase substantially the power of the analysis because the noise masking the effect of interest is reduced. It is well known, for example, that in multicenter trials the measured effect often differs between investigators. This could be a result of the physician's procedures, his/her instruments, the method of evaluating the subject's response, or a myriad of other reasons, especially when the measurement has a great degree of subjectivity. Sometimes the difference is due to the characteristics of

subject populations from which the different investigators draw their subjects. Whatever the reason might be, it is often common practice to stratify the subjects by investigators. It is also wise to identify important prognostic variables and design the trial so as to stratify according to them. Examples of some common stratification variables are sex, race, age, disease severity, Karnofsky status score (in cancer studies), disease staging, and so forth. When strata are identified, it is recommended that the randomization process will be done within the strata. This helps to equalize the number of subjects in the various treatment groups within each of the strata and to balance them with respect to the stratification variables. The drawback is that as the number of important prognostic variables increases, the number of strata increases multiplicably, thus complicating the trial's logistics. For example, if one wants to stratify by sex and race, when sex has two categories (male and female) and race four (White, Black, Hispanic and other), the number of strata is eight. Adding another variable with three categories, such as disease severity (mild, moderate, severe), will bring the number of strata to 24. If, in addition, 'investigator' is a stratification variable, then this would mean that each of the data centers performing the randomization would have to manage 24 randomization tables for each investigator, one for each stratum, which is utterly impractical. For a study of moderate size of 100–500 subjects, a large number of strata may mean that some strata may contain very small number of subjects, which complicates the statistical analysis and its interpretation.

In summary, stratification is a very useful tool for noise reduction, but it has its limitations. Usually, the one stratification variable used in a multicenter trial is the investigator. More than one additional variable can introduce serious logistical and methodological difficulties. If one is not concerned about the investigator's effect, then central randomization procedures can be very useful in situations of complex stratification requirements. Computerized central randomization procedures are now available that make complex stratification schemes possible.

Blocking

Another common method employed to decrease the background variability is *blocking*. Like stratification, blocking involves the subdivision of the subject population into homogeneous subgroups. The experimenter defines blocks of subjects and randomizes the subjects within each block to the study treatments, such that the same number of subjects are assigned to each treatment within each block. The blocks are defined so that the intrablock variability is minimal, e.g. to determine whether a drug is carcinogenic, rats of the same litter are randomized to received several doses of the drug or placebo. In this way, the variability due to genetic variation is minimized.

To take advantage of the block design, the treatments are compared within each block and then the information is pooled across blocks. When the 'within-block' or 'intrablock' variability is substantially smaller than the 'between-block' or 'interblock' variability, blocked designs could be very efficient in the use of subject resources. One disadvantage of blocked designs is that they do not allow for missing data. If data from one subject in the block are missing, the entire block may be disqualified.

A variation on the idea of blocking is the *cross-over* design. Here, each block consists of one subject, who receives the study treatments in a random order. Cross-over experiments are frequently used in bioavailability and pharmacokinetic studies. The reason is that the pharmacokinetic parameters that determine the absorption, distribution, and metabolism of the drug in the body and its elimination from the body depend on the biological make-up of the subject and vary, often considerably, from subject to subject. Thus, the intersubject variability is typically much higher than the intrasubject variability. In cross-over studies the treatments are compared within each subject and then summarized across subjects. The cross-over design is different from the blocked design described above, in that each block consists of a single subject, which

means that measurements within each block are not independent of each other. Furthermore, it is possible that a residual effect of one drug carries over to impact the effect of another drug administered subsequently. Statistical analytical methods are limited in their ability to adjust and correct for such effects. This is why the use of cross-over designs in clinical research is limited.

In summary, the design of a clinical trial incorporates methods of minimizing noise and the prevention of bias. This is done through the use of appropriate subject allocation procedures, such as randomization and blinding, or through the use of stratification and blocking.

THE STUDY POPULATION: INCLUSION AND EXCLUSION CRITERIA

Representation

The study of the pharmaceutical effect of a drug is always done in reference to a population of prospective patients, e.g. the clinical dose to be recommended for an older patient is often different from that for a younger patient. Thus, the target population for the study must be well defined in advance. Obviously, it is impractical to study the entire patient population of interest. Fortunately, this is also not necessary. Statistical sampling methodology enables us to draw conclusions from a sample to the population from which the sample had been drawn, to any desirable degree of accuracy and confidence. However, there is one important caveat to this ability: the sample must be 'representative' of the population of interest; meaning that it must preserve all the relevant characteristics of the population. That is, it must have the same proportion of females and males, the same racial distribution, the same percentage of hypertensives, and so on. Clearly, the creation of an exact replica of the population on a small scale is an impossible task. However, statistical sampling methods can produce very close to representative samples with very high probability. These are the methods utilized by pollsters to make highly reliable predictions and inferences on the population from relatively small samples.

In clinical research, the random selection of subjects to be included in the trial from the target population is not practical. Subjects are usually selected from the patient pools available to the investigators participating in the trial. This, in and of itself, is problematic. The patient pool available to a particular center usually reflects the population in the geographical area where the center is located, which may not represent the general potential patient population. To complicate things even further, some of the patients available at a given center may not be suitable for enrollment in a trial with an experimental drug. The investigator may wish to exclude certain patients because of certain known or unknown risks. The possible effects of drugs on the unborn fetus are often unknown, and thus pregnant or lactating women are usually excluded. Patients may be excluded if they are taking another medication which can potentially interact with the study drug. Also, some patients may refuse to participate in the trial for one reason or another. Finally, for the purpose of studying the efficacy of a drug, it is desirable to enroll only patients who are most likely to have a measurable response to treatment. Thus, every trial protocol contains a list of inclusion and exclusion criteria defining the subject population to be studied. Obviously, such a population is hardly ever fully representative of the target population. This raises a question regarding the generalizability of the trial's conclusions.

When defining a set of inclusion and exclusion criteria for a trial, the issue of generalizability must be kept in mind. The rule is that the more restrictive the criteria, the less generalizable the results. On the other hand, setting criteria for eligibility to participate in the trial provides the investigator with an important tool for controlling the variability. Thus, the choice of eligibility criteria must guided so as to balance the efficiency of the trial design against the need to ensure that the result are generalizable. Some of the guiding principles for defining subjects' eligibility are listed below.

Homogeneity

Homogeneity of the subject population is an important factor in controlling variability. The more homogeneous the subject population generating the data, the more informative it is. Thus, fewer subjects are required to achieve the desired control

of the statistical errors when a study is conducted in a homogeneous subject population, as compared to when the subjects are drawn from a heterogeneous population. The problem is that the more homogeneous the group of subjects, the less representative of the general potential patient population it is. In the early stages of drug development, where the goal is to establish the general perimeters for the drug safety and efficacy, and provide information for the design of future studies, studies are usually carried out on a limited number of subjects. In these early trials it is the subjects' safety that is of primary concern and the question of efficacy is secondary. The scope of the efficacy-related questions is limited to the 'proof of principle', i.e. a demonstration of clinical activity, the identification of a safe dose-range and information leading to the choice of dose and regimen for further studies. Subjects are selected who are most likely to respond to treatment, who present no obvious potential safety risks, and are as similar as possible. Later stage studies, such as confirmative Phase III trials, those providing pivotal information for the proof of the drug's efficacy and safety, are generally less restrictive.

Safety

The safety of the subjects enrolled in the trial is always the primary concern of the researcher. Individuals at high or unknown risk to treatment with the drug are excluded from the study. For example, women of child-bearing potential are usually excluded or required to be using an acceptable method of birth control. Similarly, patients taking medications that might interact with the experimental drug, or who have medical conditions that place them at increased risk, are also excluded from participation.

Selection of Subjects—Maximizing the Signal-to-noise Ratio

Clinical trials are very expensive undertakings. Also, because they involve human subjects, there is always an ethical imperative to use the subject resources judiciously. Often, the researcher has only one chance to conduct a trial designed to answer a given question. Thus, the efficiency of the trial design is critical. In other words, the design must be such that the signal-to-noise ratio is maximized. The selection of subjects by specifying certain inclusion and exclusion criteria may go a long way in this direction. The exclusion of patients with poor prognosis who are unlikely to respond to treatment, the inclusion of only patients with more than minimal severity of their condition, and similar measures, are often used to achieve this goal. Again, one must be careful not to narrow the subject population to the extent that the results could not be generalized to a broader patient population.

The Placebo Effect

Placebo is the preferred control in the double-blind randomized controlled clinical trial (RCCT). Although placebo is not supposed to have any relevant biological activity, it is well known that it often produces remarkable therapeutic responses. This phenomenon occurs across the therapeutic board. It seems that mere knowledge that is the subject is being treated for his/her condition often produces a measurable favorable response (see e.g. Gribbin 1981: Bok 1974). A high placebo response will tend to mask the response of the experimental drug. Since placebo is rarely used outside the clinical research setting, some people argue that the comparison with placebo tends to show lower response rates for the drug than would later be observed in general use. Thus, goes the argument, the placebo-controlled trial puts the test drug at a disadvantage. The counter-argument is that what one sees in the clinic is perhaps the combination of the placebo effect plus the drug's biological effect, and therefore, establishing the residual effect of the drug over its inherent placebo effect should be the true objective of the trial. Whatever the case might be, the placebo effect invariably results in decreasing the signal-to-noise ratio. Therefore, measures are often taken to select subjects whose placebo response is low or nil. One way of accomplishing this is by treating prospective subjects with placebo for some time prior to randomization. Patients whose response during this screening phase is high or very variable are then disqualified from participating in the trial.

In summary, the selection of subjects to be enrolled in the trial, using a list of entrance criteria, is an important tool in helping to sharpen the signal-to-noise ratio thus making the study more powerful. It also helps in understanding the extent to which the study conclusions can be generalized to a broader population of patients than those studied under the clinical trial's artificial conditions.

THE STATISTICAL MODEL

The statistical model is the mathematical framework in which the statistician operates. It provides the statistician with the tools to quantify the various information obtained during the trial and defines relationships among the various measurements. It provides a framework for evaluating the properties of the statistical methods used to analyze the data and answer the questions the study is designed to address.

What is a Statistical Model?

A statistical model consists of a set of assumptions about the nature of the data to be collected in the trial and about the interrelationships among various variables. These assumptions must be specific enough that they could be expressed by a set of mathematical expressions and equations.

As an example, in a placebo-controlled clinical trial for testing a new analgesic for treatment of migraine headaches, the key efficacy variable is the number of subjects whose headache is eliminated within 1 hour of treatment. A statistical model appropriate for this situation is as follows. Let p denote the probability that a subject treated with a drug will have his/her headache disappear 1 h after treatment following an episode of migraine headache. If the responses of different subjects are independent of each other, this probability can be expressed as:

$$\text{Probability (No. of responses} = k)$$
$$= cp^k(1 - p)^{N-k}(0 \leq k \leq N)$$

where N is the number of subjects treated and c is a constant representing the number of possible combinations of k elements out of N. This is known as the *binomial model*.

The trial objective is to determine if the new drug is more efficacious than placebo. Within the context of this model, one could declare the drug as 'more efficacious' if $p_d > p_p$, where p_d is probability of response for a subject treated with the new drug, and p_p the probability of response of a placebo-treated subject.

The data collected during the trial will provide information about p_d and p_p, enabling the statistician to test the null hypothesis, $H_0: \Delta = p_d - p_p = 0$ against the alternative hypothesis, $H_1: \Delta = p_d - p_p > 0$.

This very simple model provides sufficient structure for the statistician to design a statistical test to test these hypotheses. As was discussed in the section on The Statistical Test, above, the statistical test is a device providing a rule for decision-making associated with possible errors. The study design must be such that the error probabilities are properly controlled. In other words, the researcher must decide on acceptable levels of α and β, the probabilities of type I and type II errors. Typically, α is chosen to be 0.05, or 5%, and β between 0.05 and 0.20, depending on how serious the consequences are of committing a type II error ('false positive'). Since the type II error probability is calculated under the assumption that the alternative hypothesis is true, it depends on the value of Δ. The investigator must specify a value of Δ for which the type II error should be calculated. This value is the smallest clinically important Δ. In our example, the clinician might consider an increase in the probability of response of less than 50% not clinically meaningful. So, if it is known that 15% of patients treated with placebo report the disappearance of their headache, $\Delta = 0.075$, or 7.5%. Using the model and this information, the statistician can calculate the number of subjects required in the trial to guarantee that the statistical test will have the desired power, say 90%, to detect this increase if it is true, while maintaining the type I error below a desired low level, say 5%.

Another commonly used statistical model is the linear model, which represents a family of models of a similar structure, among which is the often referred-to-analysis of variance model (ANOVA). We shall illustrate this model with the simplest one-way ANOVA model.

The model is used to describe continuous data, such as blood pressure. The model assumes that the observed variable of interest Y (e.g. diastolic blood pressure) can be expressed as a sum of a number of factors:

$$Y = \mu + t + \varepsilon \qquad (1)$$

where μ represents the overall mean diastolic blood pressure in the population under study, t represents the increase (or decrease) of the blood pressure due to treatment, and ε represents a random error. The model makes two additional assumptions: (a) that ε behaves like a Normal (Gaussian) variable with mean zero and some (unknown) standard deviation (SD); and (b) that the measurements obtained from different subjects are independent of each other. The quantities μ and t are called the *model parameters*. There is one additional parameter in this model, which is the *standard deviation of the random error*, ε. It is not an explicit part of equation (1) above, but is it implicit in assumption (a). The model parameters are unknown quantities that must be estimated from the data. The data here are represented by Y. The relationship between the data and the model parameters is expressed by the linear equation (1), hence the name, the linear model.

Linear models can be quite complicated when additional structure, parameters, and assumptions are introduced. For example, one may include another term, c, in the model to account for the effect of the investigator (center) on the measurements, or another parameter, $t*c$ to account for the interaction between the treatment and the investigator effect. We will discuss this important parameter in some detail in the section on Issues in Data Analysis, below.

There are two common features to all linear models: the relationship between the data and the model parameters is always assumed to be linear, and the errors are assumed to be Normal.

It is important to remember that all the statistician's quantitative work and calculations are model-dependent. That is, their application to real life depends on the extent to which the model assumptions are satisfied in reality. Much of the work the statistician does in planning the trial, in discussing the nature of the efficacy and safety variables, randomization, blinding, and so forth, is expressed in the model. Obviously, the more complex the model and the more specific the model assumptions, the more the final results of the analysis will depend on it. Statisticians are advised to always start the statistical analysis by performing certain diagnostic procedures on the data to check to what extent the model assumptions are supported by the data. This process involves a certain level of subjective judgment, and different statisticians may reach different conclusions looking at the same data. Statisticians have at their disposal certain tools by which they can manipulate the data so as to conform better to the model's assumptions. For example, the distributions of measured pharmacokinetic (PK) parameters is typically skewed. The assumption of Normality of the distribution implies that it is symmetric. It turns out that if one calculates the PK parameters using the natural logarithms of the blood concentrations, rather than the raw measured concentrations, the distribution of the estimated parameters is less skewed. The choice of model is part of the study design, therefore, it is done before any data is available. It is not uncommon that at the analysis stage, it becomes evident that the model assumptions are grossly violated. It may become necessary to use different methods that are not as dependent on the model assumptions to analyze the data. This should be done with great care, so that spurious patterns in the data would not lead the researcher to reach wrong conclusions. Additionally, changing the analysis methods after an inspection of the data could result in an introduction of bias if the statistician is aware of the treatment assignments. For this reason it is prudent to perform these diagnostic examination of the data without revealing the treatment assignments. In blinded studies this means that these procedures are executed prior to the breaking of the blind. The statistical guidelines issued by the International Conference on Harmonization (ICH), which were adopted by the Food and Drug Administration (FDA) and the European regulatory authorities, address this issue as follows:

The [statistical] plan should be reviewed and possibly updated as a result of the blind review of the data...and should be finalized before breaking the blind. Formal records should be kept of when the statistical analysis plan was finalized, as well as when the blind was subsequently broken. If the blind review suggests changes to the principal features stated in the protocol, these should be documented in a protocol amendment (ICH, E9, 4.1).

It is important to remember that the question is not whether the statistical model is true or false. The statistical model is a theoretical construct and thus it is *always false*. The question is how well it approximates the situation under study. Or, in the words of a famous statistician, 'All models are wrong, but some are useful'.

STATISTICAL INFERENCE

Hypothesis Testing Revisited: The *p* Value; Power

Earlier in the chapter we discussed the concept of the statistical test and defined some basic terms. In this section we take a closer look at this idea and see, through an example, how this is actually done.

Let us look at the data presented in Table 21.4 above. The graduate student who generated the data did not, in fact, study 20 randomly selected students. The purpose of her study was to demonstrate that engaging in aerobic workout on a regular basis has a beneficial effect on the cardiovascular system, including slowing down the heart rate. To do this, the researcher set out to test the null hypothesis (H_0), that the mean heart rate of exercising students, μ_A, is the same as the mean of the non-exercising students, μ_B. The alternative hypothesis (H_1) is that $\mu_A < \mu_B$. In order to test H_0 against H_1, one would need to identify a variable (or a *statistic*), the distribution of which is sensitive to the difference between the heart rates of the different groups. Such a statistic is the signal-to-noise ratio, where the signal is the difference between the sample mean of Group B, $\overline{X}_B$ and the sample mean of Group A, $\overline{X}_A$, and the noise is the standard error (SE) of the difference $\overline{X}_B - \overline{X}_A$. Thus, the test statistic, T is defined as:

$$T = \frac{\overline{X}_B - \overline{X}_A}{SE(\overline{X}_B - \overline{X}_A)}$$

We have seen in the section on variability, above, that the standard error of the mean is $1/\sqrt{N}$ times the sample SD. The variance of the difference

$\overline{X}_B - \overline{X}_A$ is the sum of the variances of $\overline{X}_B$ and of $\overline{X}_A$. Therefore, from Table 21.4 we obtain:

$$\overline{X}_B - \overline{X}_A = 59.4 - 54.2 = 5.2$$

$$SE(\overline{X}_B - \overline{X}_A) = \sqrt{(1.81^2 + 2.99^2)} \div \sqrt{10}$$
$$= 1.105$$

Therefore $T = 5.2/1.105 = 4.7$.

Statistical theory teaches that the distribution of the variable T under the assumption that the population means of the two groups are the same, that is, if H_0, is true. This is the so-called Student's t-distribution. Using tables of the t-distribution, we can calculate the probability that a variable T, calculated as above, assumes a value greater or equal to 4.7, the value obtained in our example, given that H_0 is true. This probability is < 0.0001. Thus, the result obtained in our experiment is extremely unlikely, although not impossible. We are forced to choose between two possible explanations to this. One is that an unlikely event occurred. The second is that the result of our experiment is not a fluke, but rather that the difference $\mu_B - \mu_A$ is a positive number, sufficiently large to make the probability of this outcome a likely event. We elect the latter explanation and reject H_0 in favor of the alternative hypothesis, H_1.

The steps we have taken in the above example are quite generic. They could be summarized as follows:

Step 1   Describe a statistical model and identify the variable measuring the effect of interest.

Step 2   Define the statistical hypothesis to be tested.

Step 3   Define the test statistic to be used for testing H_0. This test statistic is always the signal-to-noise ratio.

Step 4   Perform the experiment and collect data.

Step 5   Calculate the value of the test statistic based on the data.

Step 6   Calculate the probability, under the assumption that H_0 is true, that the test statistic will assume a value equal or greater than the value obtained in the experiment. If this probability is small enough for you to decide that the value obtained in the experiment is highly unlikely, declare the test as statistically significant and reject H_0.

Step 6 reflects the logic driving statistical inference. It is based on the assumption that, if an event occurs in an experiment, it is not an unlikely event. Therefore, if a particular assumption leads to the conclusion that the event is highly unlikely, one should declare the assumption as false, rather than assume that the unexpected actually occurred.

The probability that the test statistics will assume a value as large or larger than the value obtained in the experiment is called the *significance probability* of the test, or the *p*-value. In our example, the *p*-value was less than 0.0001. Most people would consider such a value extremely unlikely and declare the test statistically significant. The question of what values should be considered small enough to declare statistical significance is a matter of judgment. Over the years of statistical practice, the number 0.05 became the standard cutoff point. Any *p*-value smaller than 0.05 is considered significant and any *p*-value greater than 0.05 is considered not significant. It should be emphasized, though, that this is an arbitrary value, and that there is no real difference between a *p*-value of 0.049 and a *p*-value of 0.051, although, if one follows the cutoff rule of 0.05 to the letter, one will declare statistical significance in the former but not in the latter case. This is, of course, absurd. These two *p*-values should not lead the researcher to conclusions with such diametrically opposed consequences. A choice of any other cutoff value will lead to a similar situation if followed blindly. A good measure of commonsense is always useful. There is, of course, no reason why anyone should not use a cutoff point other than the customary 0.05 if he/she feels it is more appropriate, But, as in any other situation when one deviates from a standard, one must explain one's reasons *before* the experiment is performed and before the data are known.

The statistical testing setup, as we have already seen, is geared toward the declaration of statistical significance. When a test is significant, we draw a conclusion about the cause of the effect of interest. If we decide to reject the null hypothesis, the *p*-value is the type I error associated with this decision. Therefore, the level of confidence in the correctness of the decision depends on the *p*-value; the smaller the *p*-value, the more confident one is that the decision is correct.

What if the statistical test is not statistically significant? If one accepts the null hypothesis, in this case the error to be concerned about is the type II error (see Table 21.1 above). At the design stage of the trial, the statistician usually ascertains that the test to be employed at the end has high power at clinically important alternatives. Since the power is 1 minus the probability of type II error, a well-designed study has built-in protection against making a type II error when one of these alternatives is true, but generally does not have this protection at other alternatives. In fact, for most statistical models used in practice, for alternatives close to the null hypothesis, the probability of type II error is near $1 - \alpha$, where α is the significance level of the test. Since the alternative hypothesis is usually composite, not all alternatives can be protected. Thus, accepting the null hypothesis when the test fails to achieve statistical significance is a decision associated with uncontrolled probability of type II error. For this reason, statisticians prefer to declare the test as inconclusive when it fails to achieve statistical significance.

Confidence Intervals: Precision and Confidence

Testing statistical hypotheses is a decision-making tool. The outcome of the test is a dichotomy, either the test is declared 'statistically significant' or it is not. The test provides directly very little information on the magnitude of the effect of interest. In the example of the heart rate data of Table 21.4, we have declared the test statistically significant and rejected the null hypothesis that the effect is zero. But we have not identified how large the effect is. It is often important to take the next step and estimate the magnitude of the effect. The obvious starting point is the 'signal' $D = \overline{X}_B - \overline{X}_A = 5.2$. This value is an estimate of the difference between the two population means, $\Delta = \mu_B - \mu_A$, and, as we have already seen, it is associated with a certain amount of variability measured by its standard error. This means is that if the experiment were to be repeated under exactly the same conditions, it is most likely that a value different than 5.2 is obtained. But how different? How much should

one expect the values obtained from repetitions of the experiment to spread about Δ? This information is provided by the standard error.

A method of simultaneously providing information on the magnitude of the estimated parameter and the range of likely values of the estimate is the *confidence interval*. The key idea rests on a fundamental mathematical fact that if $\overline{X}_n$ is a sample mean of a variable calculated from n independent samples of a variable, whose population mean and standard error are μ and σ, respectively, then the quantity:

$$Z = \frac{\overline{X}_n - \mu}{\sigma/\sqrt{n}} \qquad (2)$$

has approximately Standard Normal distribution (Gaussian distribution). The Normal distribution has the familiar bell-shaped curve and is tabulated in almost any elementary statistics textbook. The word 'approximately' here means that the actual distribution of Z may be different from the Normal distribution, but it becomes closer and closer to it as the sample size n increases. For all practical purposes, when the sample size is greater than 30, performing probability calculations on Z using the Standard Normal Distribution tables, will result in only minor errors.

Using the Standard Normal distribution tables, one can find for every number $0 < \gamma < 1$, a pair of numbers $Z_1(\gamma)$ and $Z_2(\gamma)$, such that:

$$\text{Probability } \{Z_1(\gamma) \leq Z \leq Z_2(\gamma)\} \\ = 1 - \gamma. \qquad (3)$$

For example, for $\gamma = 0.05$, then $Z_1(0.05) = -1.96$ and $Z_2(0.05) = 1.96$.

Now, by substituting the definition of Z in equation (2) and rearranging terms, the inequality $Z_1(\gamma) \leq Z \leq Z_2(\gamma)$ can be rewritten as:

$$L_\gamma = \overline{X}_n - Z_1(\gamma) \cdot \sigma/\sqrt{n} \leq \mu \leq \overline{X}_n + \\ Z_2(\gamma) \cdot \sigma/\sqrt{n} = U_\gamma \qquad (4)$$

Now, let us take a closer look at equation (4). The value at the center, μ, is the population mean, which is the unknown quantity we are estimating. The two expressions on the right and on the left-hand sides of (4) are variables calculated from the data. Thus, equation (4) represents a random interval containing the population mean, μ. Equation (3) assigns a probability of $1 - \gamma$ that (4) holds. The interpretation of this is that if we conduct an experiment and calculate the lower and upper limits of the interval, L_γ and U_γ, respectively, then the interval (L_γ, U_γ) will contain the true (and unknown!) population mean with probability $1 - \gamma$. The interval (4) is called a *confidence interval* for the population mean, and $1 - \gamma$ is called the *confidence level* of the interval.

Let us illustrate these ideas using the data of Table 21.4. Suppose we wish to estimate the difference Δ between the population means of the non-exercising and the exercising students by constructing a confidence interval with confidence level 95%. Then, substituting D for $\overline{X}_n$ and SE_D for $\sigma/\sqrt{n}$ in (4), and recalling that $Z_1(0.95) = -1.96$ and $Z_2(0.95) = 1.96$, we obtain the confidence limits:

$$L_{0.05} = D - SE_D \cdot Z_2(0.95) = 5.2 - 1.105 \cdot 1.96$$
$$= 3.03; \text{ and}$$

$$U_{0.05} = D - SE_D \cdot Z_1(0.95)$$
$$= 5.2 + 1.105 \cdot 1.96 = 7.26.$$

Thus, the interval (3.03, 7.26) is a 0.95 (or 95%) confidence interval for the effect Δ. It should be emphasized that the probability statement about the confidence level of 0.95 does not relate to the specific interval (3.03, 7.26) since this specific interval is an outcome of the specific sample used for the calculation, and it either contains the parameter Δ or it does not. It is a theoretical probability relating to a generic interval calculated from a sample following the steps we described above. Thus, if we could repeat the experiment many times, each time calculating a confidence interval in the way we have just done, we should expect 95% of these intervals to contain the true mean effect Δ. Of course, when calculating a confidence interval from a sample, there is no way to tell whether the interval contains the parameter it is estimating or not. The confidence level provides us with a certain level of assurance that it is so, in the sense we have just described.

Confidence intervals are often calculated after performing a statistical test. When the test is statistically significant, we have reason to believe that the effect is real. The confidence interval gives us additional information as to the size of the effect. Confidence intervals are also calculated during exploratory analyses. The purpose of such analyses is to explore the data, identify possible effects and generate hypotheses for future studies, rather than make specific inferences. Confidence intervals are extremely useful tools toward this goal.

Confidence intervals are often used in the establishment of equivalence between two treatments. Here 'equivalence' is not synonymous with 'equality'. It means that the difference between the effects of the two treatments, if any, is not considered of material importance. Let us illustrate this with the following example: suppose one is interested in determining whether two antihypertensive drugs are equivalent in their effect on diastolic blood pressure after 4 weeks of treatment. Let μ_A and μ_B denote the mean change from the pretreatment baseline for patients treated with drug A and drug B, respectively. Let $\Delta = \mu_A - \mu_B$. Furthermore, assuming that as long as the two means are within ± 3 mmHg, the two drugs are considered as having equivalent effectiveness. A trial to establish whether the two drugs are equivalent must be then designed so that a confidence interval for Δ with confidence level of 0.90 or higher (or another level considered by the researcher to be adequate) will have width not exceeding 6 mmHg. When the trial is concluded, the confidence interval is constructed. If it is entirely contained within the interval $(-3, +3)$ the two drugs are considered equivalent. Otherwise, they are not. It is possible to design a trial so that a desired confidence interval of a given confidence level will have a desired width. The width of a confidence interval for a parameter is the estimate's *precision*. It depends on: (a) the confidence level; (b) the inherent variability of the data; and (c) the sample size. The inherent variability of the data can be controlled only to a limited degree. For a fixed sample size, the width of the confidence interval is determined by the confidence level. The researcher can increase the precision of his/her estimate only by lowering the confidence level associated with the confidence interval. The only way to guarantee an acceptable level of confidence and precision is to include sufficiently large number of subjects in the trial. In our example, if the trial is poorly designed and the interval's width is larger that 6 mmHg, the trial could never establish equivalence because the criterion for this cannot be met.

To summarize, when estimating the magnitude of a parameter is an important objective of a trial, thought must be given at the design stage to what levels of confidence and precision are considered acceptable, and to make sure that the trial is designed to enroll a sufficient number of subjects to accommodate these requirements. There are no hard and fast rules about what levels of confidence are considered acceptable. However, rarely do researchers go below 80%, and more typically they require a confidence level of 90% or higher. The desired level of precision is depends entirely on the particular situation.

STUDY DESIGN: DETERMINING THE SAMPLE SIZE

We have already seen, through a number of examples, the interplay between sample size, variability, and the performance of the statistical procedures employed to analyze the data. The sample size determines the amount of information that will be available at the end of the trial. Therefore, the determination of an adequate sample size is one of the most important aspects of the trial design. A trial accumulating an inadequate amount of information is hopelessly flawed, as it will not enable the researcher to answer the questions the trial is intended to answer.

The determination of the sample size is intimately related to the trial objectives, the inferences the researcher wants to be able to make, and the maximal error probabilities in the case of hypotheses testing, or the minimal confidence and precision in the case of estimation, that the researcher is willing to accept. The following example illustrates the process of determining the required sample size for a clinical trial.

Suppose one wishes to conduct a trial to test the efficacy of a new antihypertensive drug. The clinical research physician plans to enroll a certain number of subjects with mild to moderate hypertension and randomize them to receive either drug or placebo. The primary efficacy variable is the decrease in the diastolic blood pressure as compared to a pre-treatment baseline. The subject's diastolic blood pressure is measured twice: once

prior to treatment, when the subject is free of any antihypertensive medication, and once following the administration of treatment (drug or placebo). The change in diastolic blood pressure between the two measurements is the primary efficacy variable. The researcher knows that, for the drug to be sufficiently efficacious to justify its development, it must reduce the subject's diastolic blood pressure by at least 10 points. So, if we denote by μ_D the mean decrease in diastolic blood pressure for the drug group, and by μ_P the corresponding decrease for the placebo group, then the null hypothesis the researcher is set to test is:

$$H_0: \mu_D = \mu_P$$

vs. the alternative hypothesis:

$$H_A: \mu_D > \mu_P, \text{ or } H_A: \mu_D - \mu_P > 0.$$

One particular alternative of interest is:

$$H_{10}: \mu_D = \mu_P + 10, \text{ or } H_{10}: \mu_D - \mu_P = 10.$$

In order to guarantee that the statistical test of H_0 will have a significance level α and power not less than $1 - \beta$ at the alternative $H_\Delta: \mu_D = \mu_P + \Delta$, each of the two treatment groups must have at least N subjects, where N is given by the equation:

$$N = 2(Z_{1-\alpha/2} + Z_{1-\beta})^2 \cdot (\sigma/\Delta)^2 \qquad (5)$$

where σ is the SD of the raw measurements (i.e. the decrease in diastolic blood pressure). For simplicity we assume that it is the same for both treatment groups. $Z_{1-\alpha/2}$ and $Z_{1-\beta}$ are two constants depending on α and β, that can be obtained from tables of the Standard Normal distribution. If in our case we assume that $\sigma = 12$, $\Delta = 10$, $\alpha = 0.05$ and $\beta = 0.10$, then $Z_{1-\alpha/2} = 1.96$, $Z_{1-\beta} = 1.28$, and (5) yields $N = 30.23$. That is, a sample size of at least 31 subjects per group is required. Equation (5) is specific to situations similar to our example. However, in general, the sample size required is calculated by a formula that looks like equation (6):

$$N = C_{\alpha,\beta}(\sigma/\Delta)^2 \qquad (6)$$

where $C_{\alpha,\beta}$ is some constant depending on α and β.

There are a number of important observations implied by equation (6):

(a) The sample size is proportional to σ^2. That is, the larger the noise, the larger must the sample size be to enable one to distinguish the effect of interest from the noise.

(b) The sample size is inversely proportional to Δ^2. That is, the smaller the effect of interest, the larger must the sample size be to enable us to separate it from the background noise.

(c) The sample size depends on the squares of the parameters σ and Δ; meaning that if we are able to reduce the noise in the experiment by one-half, the payoff is that the clinical trial will require one-quarter of the number of subjects. Similarly, if we wish to build in sufficient power to detect one-half of the effect, the clinical trial would have to enroll four times as many subjects.

During the design phase of the trial, the statistician will typically ask the clinical researcher questions leading to the determination of σ and Δ. The anticipated SD is often very difficult to estimate, and the best way of arriving at a useful number is either to look for such an estimate in the published scientific literature, or to estimate it from data obtained in similar studies performed by the pharmaceutical company. Underestimating σ can result in an underpowered study, resulting with unacceptable error rates, leading to ambiguities and an inability to make reliable inferences. For this reason it is always preferable to overestimate σ rather than underestimate it when information on σ is scanty. The value of Δ, the minimal clinically important effect, is usually arrived at by the clinician based on past clinical experience.

The Abuse of Power: Pitfalls of Overdesign

Equation (6) is expressing N in terms of σ and Δ. It is very easy to rewrite this equation and express any of the three parameters, N, σ, and Δ, in terms of the other two. If we express Δ in terms of N and σ, we could see that by increasing N, the statistical test could have high power to detect very small differences. Thus, it is often very tempting to 'overde-

sign' the study; that is, to enroll more subjects than are really needed, so that if the drug is not quite as efficacious as one hopes, the statistical test would still be significant at the end. By enrolling a large number of subjects, one can assure that the statistical test is so powerful that it would declare very small and possibly meaningless differences as statistically significant. This approach is not only wasteful, but it may lead to false inferences, and is outright unethical in the drug development arena. Clinical trials are very expensive enterprises and it is usually not feasible to repeat a trial to demonstrate that the results are reproducible. The variables studied in clinical trials are random, thus there will always be differences between the treatment groups that are due to chance. An overpowered study could find such differences statistically significant and lead the researcher to a false conclusion that a drug is efficacious when it is not, or that it is harmful, when it is not. In the absence of a second chance, these findings may never be repudiated.

An underpowered trial is wasteful and unethical for a different reason. Such a trial may not have enough power to detect clinically meaningful differences, resulting in missing clinically important medical advances. The subjects enrolled into such a trial are exposed to the risks involved in all clinical trials using experimental drugs, without the anticipated benefit to themselves and to society.

For these reasons it is important that the size of the trial is just right: not too small and not too large. The discussions taking place among the project research team leading to the appropriate choice of the sample size are therefore very important, and, although at the end it is the statistician who performs the calculations, the input from the other team members is critical.

ISSUES IN STATISTICAL TRIAL DESIGN

Multicenter Trials

Most Phase III clinical trials are multicenter trials; i.e. they are conducted in more than one clinical center. The number of centers participating in a clinical trial can vary greatly.

There are a number of good reasons to conduct Phase III trials as multicenter trials. The most obvious reason is an administrative and logistical one. Spreading the burden of subject recruitment among many centers will reduce the duration of the subject enrollment phase of the trial. This is an important reason considering that often the commercial success or failure of a new drug is the timing of its introduction to the market. There are also important scientific reasons to conduct the trial as a multicenter trial.

Noise Reduction

Different centers often draw subjects from different types of patient populations. Also, different centers may utilize different procedures and medical practices that are not controlled by the study protocol. It is, therefore, reasonable to expect that the within-center variability is smaller than the overall variability. In a multicenter trial, the center often serves as a stratification variable, thereby reducing the variability and increasing the efficiency of the trial design. In order to take advantage of this aspect of the multicenter trial, the number of subjects per center cannot be too small, so that the estimate of the intracenter variability is stable. A rule-of-thumb is that the number of subjects per treatment group within each center will be at least five.

Generalizability

A multicenter trial may be viewed as a number of identical small trials, each conducted at a different center. From this perspective, each center can be viewed as repeating the study conducted in other centers. In addition, different centers draw their subjects from different geographic areas, and thus a multicenter trial is more likely to enroll subjects who are representative of a cross-section of the general population. Consistency of the results among the different centers adds to the level of confidence that the results could be replicated anywhere. It is possible that the results across centers are inconsistent. There are two types of inconsistencies:

1. *The magnitude of the effect is different across centers.* When the magnitude of the response to treatment is different across centers, the relative effect between the two treatments is approximately constant treatment, referred to

by statisticians as the 'center effect'. The existence of a center effect means that the different centers contribute differently to the measured effect of treatment, but this contribution is the same for both the experimental treatment and the comparator. This situation is illustrated in Figure 21.1, which shows schematically the effects of two treatments across six centers. The magnitude of the treatment differs from center to center, but the difference between the effect of treatment A and treatment B is the same. Such a situation does not present a problem in comparing the treatments. It makes it impossible, though, to talk about the absolute magnitude of the treatment effect, since it is not constant. Observing a center effect is not unusual in clinical trials. The reasons for this may be many; it could be the result of a difference in the type of patients seen at the different centers, the center procedures and general nursing care, subjects' compliance in taking their medication, the equipment used in the different centers, and so on.

2. *Treatment-by-center interaction.* This is the type of inconsistency that may cause an invalidation of the entire study. Here, the relative response to the different study treatments is different across centers. There are two situations that present qualitatively different levels of difficulties:

   (i) *Quantitative interaction.* We say that the interaction is quantitative if the relative effect of the different treatments is in the same direction across centers, although the magnitude may be different. Figure 21.2 illustrates this type of interaction. This type of interaction means that the relative efficacy of the treatments is different in different centers, but the direction is always the same, i.e. treatment A is more efficacious than treatment B at all centers, but the magnitude of the difference between the treatment effects is different in the different centers. When this type of interaction occurs, one can say that one treatment is more efficacious than the other, but not by how much, because the relative efficacy of the two treatments is not constant.

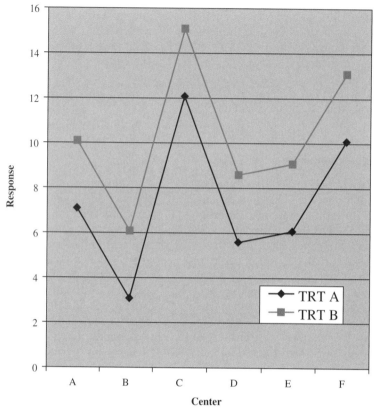

Figure 21.1   Center effect

(ii) *Qualitative interaction.* This type of interaction is the one that could invalidate the entire study. It occurs when the relative efficacy of the two treatment is different across the different centers in both magnitude and direction. This is illustrated in Figure 21.3. Here, treatment A produces a larger effect than treatment B in some centers and a smaller effect in other centers. If the researcher cannot find the cause of this interaction and correct for it, the study will be inconclusive. This type of interaction would occur if, for example, the data center mislabeled the treatments for some centers. This would be easy to rectify. However, often there is no reasonable and acceptable explanation for this and the entire study has to be invalidated.

The ICH guidelines address this issue as follows:

If heterogeneity of treatment effects is found, this should be interpreted with care, and vigorous attempts should be made to find an explanation in terms of other features of trial management or subject characteristics. Such an explanation will usually suggest appropriate further analysis and interpretation. In the absence of an explanation, heterogeneity of treatment effect, as evidenced, for example, by marked quantitative interactions implies that alternative estimates of the treatment effect, giving different weights to the centers, may be needed to substantiate the robustness of the estimates of treatment effect. It is even more important to understand the basis of any heterogeneity characterized by marked qualitative interactions, and failure to find an explanation may necessitate further clinical trials before the treatment effect can be reliably predicted (ICH, E9, 3.2).

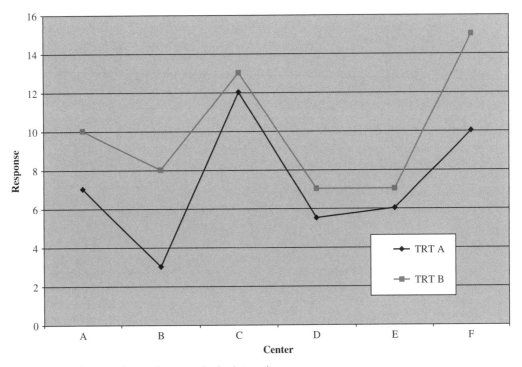

Figure 21.2 Treatment by center interaction: quantitative interaction

Multiplicity

Clinical trials always include multiple end-points and/or multiple comparisons between treatments. For example, in a clinical trial of a new drug for asthma, one may want to analyze the change in the forced expiratory volume in 1s (FEV_1), as well as the change in the total asthma symptoms score, the subject's morning and evening symptoms severity scores, the investigator's global improvement score, and perhaps other end-points. In a dose–response trial with placebo, low dose, middle dose, and high dose, the investigator may want to compare the three dose groups to the control and perhaps the different dose groups with each other.

The issue of multiplicity is that when performing multiple statistical tests, the error probability associated with the inferences made is inflated. To see this, let us consider a simple situation where one is interested in performing two statistical tests on independent sets of data, each at a significance level of 0.05. Thus, the probability that each of the two tests will be declared significant erroneously (type I error) is 0.05. However, the probability that at least one of the two tests will be declared significant erroneously is 0.0975. The probability that at least one of the tests of interest will be declared significant erroneously is called the *experimentwise error rate*. If we perform three 0.05 level tests, the experimentwise error rate increases to 0.143. In practical terms, this means that if we perform multiple tests and make multiple inferences, each one at a reasonably low error probability, the likelihood that some of these inferences will be erroneous could be appreciable. To correct for this, one must conduct each individual test at a decreased significance level, with the result that either the power of the tests will be reduced as well, or the sample size must be increased to accommodate the desired power. This could make the trial prohibitively expensive. Statisticians sometimes refer to the need to adjust the significance level so that the experimentwise error rate is controlled, as the statistical penalty for multiplicity.

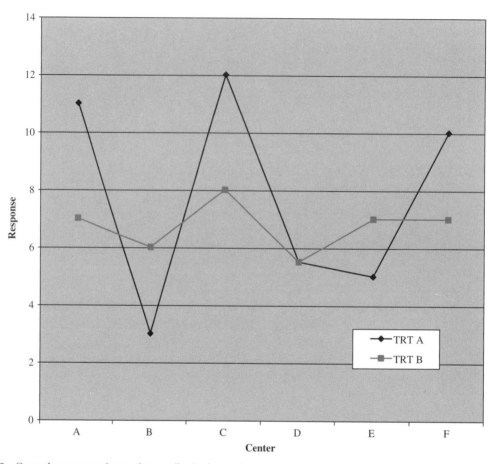

Figure 21.3 Center by treatment interaction: qualitative interaction

The need to control the experimentwise error rate may not apply to exploratory analyses. Statisticians often perform formal statistical tests for exploratory purposes, so no formal hypotheses are stated and no inferences are made based on them. Even though the act of performing an exploratory test formally involves the same steps as inferential testing, it is conceptually different because of the absence of a null hypothesis. The *p*-value obtained in such a test should be viewed as a measure of the level of inconsistency of the data with the underlying assumptions of the test, rather than error probabilities involved in making causal inferences.

In summary, one should limit the number of inferential tests to be performed to the minimum necessary for making the desired causal inferences.

They must be specified in the study protocol and the appropriate adjustments to the error probabilities must be made. Similarly, one should remember that when multiple tests are performed without adjustment, as would be the case in an exploratory testing situation, one should expect to see spurious statistically significant results that may or may not be meaningful. This last comment applies particularly to statistical tests performed on adverse events and laboratory data. Adverse events reported in a study are often summarized by reporting their incidences, summarized by body system. Often, dozens of categories are listed. When formal statistical tests are applied to these data, some of these tests will result in *p* values less than the customary 0.05. The researcher should be cognizant of this issue and not jump to conclusions. It is strongly advisable to specify in advance the particular safety tests to be performed inferentially if there is a known or suspected safety concern with the drug or the class of drugs tested.

Interim Analysis

In long-term clinical trials in life-threatening disease areas, or in diseases involving serious morbidities, or in the study of drugs with possible serious toxicities, it is imperative to monitor the data on an ongoing basis and to perform periodic interim analyses.

Interim analyses are performed for a variety of reasons. Some of the main reasons are:

1. To stop the development of an ineffective treatment.
2. To stop the development of a toxic treatment.
3. To terminate a trial in a life-threatening disease as soon as enough evidence has accumulated to conclude that one treatment is significantly more efficacious than the other.
4. To verify protocol assumptions (e.g. variability and sample size, assumptions on control group response rate).
5. To plan additional trials.
6. To plan for capital expenditures and product launch.
7. To make a regulatory submission for a short-term portion of a long-term trial.
8. For other regulatory reasons (e.g. opening the trial to previously excluded high-risk subjects).

The first three reasons in the list include the possibility of terminating the trial based on an interim inferential analysis. The fourth reason can potentially alter the trial's conduct. The other reasons should not, in principle, impact the trial.

Essentially, there are two separate issues involved in performing an interim analysis: a statistical issue, and an administrative or trial management issue. The statistical issue is very similar to the multiplicity issue discussed in the previous paragraph, and it applies to the reasons (1), (2) and (3) above. If we perform an interim inferential test, the overall error probability is inflated. Therefore, if one contemplates performing an interim analysis, with the option of making inferences early and possibly terminating the trial before its planned end, the procedure used for making this determination must be planned in advance and documented in the study protocol, just as any other inferential procedure. As we discussed above, there will be a statistical penalty in the sense that each of the interim analyses and the final analysis will have to be performed at a lower level of significance than the desired overall type I error rate. The statistical penalty depends on the decision-making procedure to be used.

The administrative issue involves the potential for the introduction of bias. Any interim analysis, regardless of whether or not it is done with the intention of affecting the ongoing trial, involves the possibility of introducing bias if the analysis requires the breaking of the blind. The FDA is particularly wary about these types of analyses, because even if every step and decision is well documented, it is impossible to anticipate the impact on the trial that a partial, even preliminary, knowledge of the efficacy results might have. For this reason, it is imperative that such analyses, regardless of their declared purpose, will be performed with strict guidelines as to who will be unblinded, and how the results will be disseminated. It is important to make sure that individuals directly involved in the trial conduct and management, such as investigators, monitors, and other project personnel, should remain blinded to the data and the results of the interim analysis. For this reason it has become standard practice in the pharmaceutical industry to appoint a Data Monitoring Board consisting entirely of people uninvolved in the trial conduct to review the interim data and analyses and make recommendations. The Pharmaceutical Manufacturers' Association (PMA) published a position paper discussing in details the various aspects of the issue as it relates to the specific circumstances of new drug development (PMA Biostatistics and Medical *Ad Hoc* Committee on Interim Analysis 1993). The ICH guidelines address this issue as well:

> The execution of an interim analysis should be a completely confidential process because unblinded data and results are potentially involved. All staff involved in the conduct of the trial should remain

blind to the results of such analyses, because of the possibility that their attitudes to the trial will be modified and cause changes in the characteristics of patients to be recruited or biases in treatment comparisons. This principle may be applied to all investigator staff and to staff employed by the sponsor, except for those who are directly involved in the execution of the interim analysis. Investigators should be informed only about the decision to continue or to discontinue the trial, or to implement modifications to trial procedures.

Also:

> Any interim analysis that is not planned appropriately (with or without the consequences of stopping the trial early) may flaw the results of a trial and possibly weaken confidence in the conclusions drawn. Therefore, such analyses should be avoided. If unplanned interim analysis is conducted, the clinical study report should explain why it was necessary and the degree to which blindness had to be broken, and provide an assessment of the potential magnitude of bias introduced and the impact on the interpretation of the results (ICH, E9, 4.5).

ISSUES IN DATA ANALYSIS

Clinical trials present unique problems during the analysis phase that other experiments do not. The inherent complexity of the clinical trial is compounded by the fact that it uses human subjects, and therefore is governed by a set of ethical rules, paramount of which is the voluntary and informed participation of the subjects in the study. Subjects are required to sign an informed consent form prior to their enrollment in the study in which they confirm their understanding of the trial procedures and the potential risks and benefits, and state their voluntary agreement to participate. Notwithstanding the informed consent form, subjects can at all times exercise their free will and choose to terminate their participation, refuse to undergo a procedure, skip a visit, or violate any of the study protocol procedures without penalty. The result is that clinical trials are rarely conducted exactly as planned. Some of the issues resulting from this are discussed below.

Non-compliance, Drop-outs and Missing Data

Non-compliance

In testing the efficacy of a new drug or studying a dose–response relationship, it is of critical importance that subjects take their medication as prescribed in the protocol. Most drugs exhibit a direct dose–response relationship in terms of the drug's efficacy and safety. Non-compliance with respect to the schedule and dose of the study medication may have serious impact on the researcher's ability to determine the recommended dose or even to show efficacy. When subjects underdose themselves, the drug efficacy may be missed and the true adverse event pattern of the drug may be underestimated. Clinical researchers always try to build in mechanisms into the trial's procedures designed to maximize compliance. However, it is not uncommon that, despite such efforts, some subjects will miss some doses.

It is impossible to adjust for non-compliance at the analysis phase without making assumptions about the dose–response relationship, which is often not well understood and might vary greatly from one subject to another. It is always important to assess the level of compliance at the end of the trial so that one might gain some appreciation, qualitative and incomplete as it may be, of what one should expect when the drug is taken as prescribed.

Another type of non-compliance is the subjects' adherence to the protocol procedures and schedules. It is the role of the investigator to make sure that the protocol is adhered to. Lack of adherence to the protocol complicates the analysis and may make the result difficult to interpret.

Drop-outs

Subjects may drop out of the trial for a variety of reasons. Some could be unrelated to the trial, such as relocation, but others, such as experiencing adverse events, the perception of no efficacy, or perception of well-being, could be strongly correlated with the study drug effect. The result is that some subjects will have no data to evaluate from some time point onward. When the reason for dropping out are treatment-related, the patterns of dropouts will be typically different between the different treatments and ignoring the missing data will introduce bias into the analysis. There are a number of methods for handling dropouts, none of which is entirely satisfactory. One common way is to use the last-observation-carried-forward (LOCF) method. In this method, the last available value is substituted for all missed measurements. The problem with this approach is that it assumes that, had the subject not dropped out, he/she would continue to respond in exactly the same way as on his/her last visit before dropping out. This assumption is never verifiable and often unreasonable. Another approach is to substitute the worse possible value for the missing data. The rationale for this approach is that the results of the analysis will show 'worst-case scenario' and if the drug passes this test and can be labeled safe and effective, it would still be so had subjects not dropped out. This rationale is certainly plausible. The trouble is that the efficacy of important and moderately efficacious drugs may be missed or mildly toxic drugs may end up with unnecessarily serious safety warnings on their labels. There are other methods of statistical 'imputation' where a value is calculated using some algorithm and is substituted for the missing value. The reasonableness of these procedures must be judged on a case-by-case basis by examining the underlying assumptions and judging their appropriateness in the given situation.

Missing Data

Dropouts present one type of missing data; namely, data are not available from a certain time point on. Data could be missing in many other ways. A subject may miss a visit, a sample could be invalid, or a subject may fail to fill out a form or a questionnaire. When data are missing at random, the effect is generally some loss in the power of the statistical analysis. When data are missing according to some pattern, bias can be introduced in addition. Some statistical study designs are particularly sensitive to missing data. Cross-over designs are such designs. The loss of one value in a cross-over study will result in a loss of the entire

sequence. Some designs require certain balances among the treatments and schedules of treatment. Missing data can destroy such balances, seriously handicapping the statistician's ability to analyze the data. Here too, imputation, with all the caveats going along with it, is the method of 'correcting' for missing data. When many data are missing, say 20% or more, one should seriously question the validity of the conclusions drawn from the study, since they might be driven more by the assumptions made about how to handle the missing data than by the data themselves.

Intent-to-treat Analysis

One possible way of handling protocol violations, non-compliance, missing data, dropouts, etc., is to remove from the analysis all subjects whose violations are considered to be serious, and analyze only the data obtained from the subjects who reasonably complied with all the requirements stated in the protocol. Such analysis is sometimes referred to as *per-protocol analysis* (PP). The problem with this approach is that the effectiveness of the randomization process as a mechanism to bestow balances among latent on non-latent prognostic factors, and set the stage for making causal relationship inferences, is disturbed. Also, if the reasons for these violations are not independent of treatment or the subject's condition, the removal of these subjects for the analysis may introduce a bias the analysis. Therefore, it is customary to always perform an *intent-to-treat-analysis* (ITT), in which all subjects randomized, or all subjects randomized who received at least one dose of study medication, are included. The proponents of this approach argue that, in addition to the preservation of the randomization process, the ITT reflects 'real-life' results. They argue that in 'real-life', as opposed to the artificial set-up of the clinical study, neither patients nor their physicians follow a specific rigorous protocol. So, if the outcome of non-compliance, for example, is reduced efficacy, this is what one should expect to see when the drug is used in clinical practice. The use of the ITT is required by the FDA as one of the analyses to always be presented to them. The problems we highlighted earlier in this section present challenges to the data analyst that can be addressed at the analysis phase only to a limited extent. It is impossible to design a trial so that these problems will be prevented entirely. However, a careful design and diligent execution and monitoring of the trial can minimize them.

SUMMARY: THE STATISTICIAN'S ROLE

Information derived from data collected in a clinical trial is the ultimate product of the trial. Every aspect of the trial, from its conception to its execution, impacts the quality of the data and the information they contain. The final step in the process, the analysis, is nothing but the application of statistical methods for organizing the data, summarizing them and extracting relevant information; i.e. separating the signal from the noise. The statistician's ability to make up for design deficiencies and for noisy data is very limited, and the same rule defining good practice of medicine applies here as well: the best treatment of a disease is to prevent it. The statistician's greatest impact could, therefore, be at the front end, i.e. during the trial planning, rather than the back end, i.e. at the analysis phase.

The Study Protocol and Case Report Forms

A clinical trial is a complex scientific undertaking that requires the collaboration of many people: clinical investigators, subjects, study coordinators, data managers, statisticians, programmers, and many more. It is therefore of critical importance that a study plan, procedures, and conventions will be laid out clearly in advance in a document, so that all the participants in this journey will follow the same road map, i.e. the study protocol. Like any good road map, the study protocol must be very clear about the ultimate goal and direction of the journey, i.e. the study objectives. Often, the clarity of the study objectives in the protocol determines the coherence of the rest of the protocol. Clearly and specifically stated objectives will help to identify when the primary measures of efficacy, for example, are inadequate, or when the design is flawed, or when superfluous data, which will not contribute anything to answer the questions posed in the objectives, are going to be collected.

The creation of the study protocol is a multidisciplinary and collaborative effort. Every aspect of the protocol impacts all other aspects. A medical procedure may impact the response of subjects to treatment, their compliance, or some other important aspect that ultimately will impact the data and the conclusions that can be drawn from them. For this reason, every member of the study design team must assume responsibility for the entire protocol. The statistician may be responsible directly for writing the statistical design considerations and the analysis plan, yet his/her involvement in all other aspects of the design that feed into it are equally important.

The case report form (CRF) is the data collection tool for the clinical trial. Often, the design of the CRF is viewed as a technical task auxiliary to the trial, and the statistician may not see it until the trial is ongoing and the data start coming in for processing. The CRF design is an important activity that can make a difference in the quality of the data obtained in the trial. It should be viewed as an integral part of the protocol development process, and input from the clinician, the clinical monitor, and the statistician must be obtained. The CRF is a multipurpose instrument: it serves the investigator as the tool for recording the data obtained in the trial; it must facilitate the review of the data by the clinical monitor; and it is the document used by the data manager to build the database for statistical analysis. The organization and structure of the CRF, the way the questions are phrased, and the use of codes all impact the quality of the data.

Analysis and Reporting

The analysis of the data at the end of the trial is, of course, the statistician's domain. A successful analysis is one that reaches unambiguous conclusions, not necessarily the ones the clinical researcher is hoping for. As we emphasized earlier, the success of the analysis depends entirely on the way the trial was conducted and monitored, and the way the data were generated and collected. The statistician's role is to utilize the appropriate tools, designed to most effectively extract the information from the data. The analysis tools do not create information. We emphasized the need to prepare for the analysis at the design stage. It is also important to think one step ahead and consider the need to analyze data obtained from a number of different studies. A new drug application usually consists of many different studies. The approval of the application is not based on any single study. Rather, it is based on the synthesis of the information obtained from all the studies. Data from some studies will have to be combined and analyzed. Such an analysis, called *meta-analysis*, must be planned for in advance, too. Two examples of meta-analysis are the integrated summary of safety (ISS) and the integrated summary of efficacy (ISE). These analyses must be planned for just as if the combined database represented data from a new study. It is recommended that plans for meta-analyses will be made at the time the individual studies are planned. This is not always possible, but it is the best way to ensure that the meta-database used for the analysis is coherent. For example, if the adverse events information is collected in two studies using different data collection forms, the combination of the individual databases may be difficult and some information may be lost.

An anonymous cynic once said that there are three types of liars: liars, damn liars, and statisticians. This statement reflects the discomfort many researchers feel when working with statisticians. The image of the statistician taking the data to his/her dark room, performing incomprehensible manipulations behind closed doors, and coming back with results, charts and magic numbers, throwing around vaguely understood terms, is unfortunate. It is our hope that this article helps to disperse the haze and clarify the statistician's role and mode of thinking. He/she is neither a liar nor a magician; rather, the statistician is a professional, trained in scientific methods that are devised to establish causal relationships under conditions of uncertainty. Our goal in writing this article was not to turn the reader into a statistician. Instead, it was to bring the statistician out of the dark room into the open and, by reviewing the issues he/she is concerned about, and clarifying the terminology he/she is using, facilitate communication between his/her and the rest of the study team. If the reader feels that he/she is better equipped to communicate with their statistical colleagues after reading this review, then our effort was successful.

REFERENCES AND ADDITIONAL READING

Armitage P (1971) *Statistical Methods in Medical Research.* Wiley: New York.

Bok S (1974) The ethics of giving placebos. *Sci Amer,* 231(17).

Fisher RA (1973) *Statistical Methods and Scientific Inference, 3rd Ed.* Hafner: New York.

Freedman D, Pisani R, Purves R. (1978) *Statistics.* W.W. Norton: New York.

Friedman LM, Furberg CD, DeMets DL (1981) *Fundamentals of Clinical Trials.* John Wright: Boston, MA.

Gribbin M (1981) Placebos: cheapest medicine in the world. *New Sci* 89: 64–5.

International Conference on Harmonization (ICH)(1998) E9: Statistical Principles for Clinical Trials, 1. *Fed Reg* 63(179): 49583–98, September 16.

PMA Biostatistics and Medical Ad Hoc Committee on Interim Analysis (1993) Interim analysis in the pharmaceutical industry. *Contr Clin Trials* 14: 160–73.

Pocock SJ (1983) *Clinical Trials: A Practical Approach.* Wiley: Chichester.

Popper K (1959) *The Logic of Scientific Discovery.* Basic Books: New York.

22

Data Management

T.Y. Lee and Michael Minor

ACER/EXCEL Inc., USA

Pharmaceutical research and development is a lengthy (8–12 years) and costly process (approximately US$500 millions in 2001 dollars). It starts from discovery of the compound, biological screening, animal toxicological studies, formulation, assay development/validation, clinical pharmacology, stability testing, clinical trials, data management, statistical and clinical evaluation, new drug application and promotional marketing. At each stage of the research and development, data are generated, processed and validated before being subject to statistical analysis. Data management plays a significant role in assuring the government agency and consumers that the database represents a pool of information that was accurately collected and processed and logically presented. With the advancement of pharmaceutical technology in identifying new compounds, and improved efficiency in software support and information processing, the duration of exclusivity enjoyed by a new drug has been drastically reduced before a competitive drug of the same or a similar class reaches the market. For example, the duration of exclusivity (PhRMA 1997) for several major drugs is summarized in Table 22.1.

Because of the accelerated shortening of the duration of the exclusivity, the pharmaceutical companies tend to initiate clinical trials in several countries simultaneously to obtain worldwide clinical data. This strategy will give the pharmaceutical companies a chance to market the drug in many countries simultaneously and recover as much cost as possible before the competitors join in. To collect worldwide data and pool them together presents a special challenge to data management professionals. It is necessary to consider differences in culture, medical practice, laboratory standards/units, classifications of disease and medication, drug reactions, religion, self-medication, drug interactions, etc. Therefore, a detailed and coordinated data management plan, standard operation procedures, quality control, and quality assurance are essential to produce a reliable database.

OBTAINING THE PROJECT MATERIAL

To develop a data management plan pertinent to the project, a checklist of the project material is necessary to enhance the planning. The items to be collected include: the protocol, annotated case report forms (CRFs), literature, log-in and tracking forms, file structures, coding rules, CRF review conventions, query handling procedure, required edit checklist, central laboratory address/file format, laboratory normal ranges, clinically significant ranges, timelines, quality control (QC) rules, quality assurance (QA) sampling, error analysis, criteria to release the database, disaster recovery plan, etc. Most of these rules and conventions are preliminary and are collected from earlier studies. These rules and conventions will be discussed by the project team from time to time to make them pertinent to the current studies.

Table 22.1 Duration of exclusivity for some major drugs

Drug name	Year approved	Exclusivity (years)
Inderal	1968	10
Tagmet	1977	7
Capoten	1980	5
Prozac	1988	4
Diflucan	1990	2
Recombinate	1992	1
Invirase	1995	0.25

Principles and Practice of Pharmaceutical Medicine. Edited by A. J. Fletcher, Lionel D. Edwards, Anthony W. Fox and Peter Stonier © 2002 John Wiley & Sons Ltd.

Table 22.2   Project team personnel list

Protocol #:	Project team coordinator:

Name of drug:
Directory location:

1. Regulatory associate:
2. Clinician/medical writer:
3. Primary statistician:
4. Secondary statistician:
5. Scanner
6. Primary CDC
7. Secondary CDC
8. Data entry screen designer
9. Edit check programmer
10. Quality assurance
11. Data entry
12. Data verifier

FORMATION OF THE PROJECT TEAM

Pharmaceutical companies usually assign a project manager to coordinate the formation of the project team (Table 22.2). The project manager works closely with the functional department heads to select the team members. The team usually includes representatives from the departments of regulatory affairs, clinical research, medical writing, biostatistics, data management, programming and document supports. The project manager should coordinate the activities to make sure that: the team has adequate resources; the project information is distributed in a timely fashion; the status is issued; milestones are reached at each stage; and the team members have a clear and detailed instruction of the priorities of the various protocols. For multinational projects, the quality of CRFs varies from country to country. It requires a great deal of management skill on the part of the project manager to balance national pride and quality requirements without sacrificing the quality of the final database.

PROJECT SETUP

From the data management perspective, the clinical data coordinator (CDC) is the central team member receiving and to distributing data-related information to the project team members. The CDC meets with the project team members to review the project material collected and to elicit the rules and special requirements from the statistician, clinician, safety officer, medical writer, and regulatory associates. These project materials, rules, and special requirements will be considered in conjunction with data management requirements to develop the data management plan. The CDC should prepare the following documents before the clinical trials are initiated:

Data creation flow chart (Figure 22.1).
Project team personnel list (Table 22.2).
CRFs log-in sheet (Table 22.3).
CRFs cover sheet (Table 22.4).
Data query sheet (Table 22.5).
Data processing status (Table 22.6).
Preliminary edit check document (Table 22.7).
Audit sheet (Table 22.8).
Audit document (Table 22.9).
Summary of audit results (Table 22.10).
Sample memo of notifying formal closure of database (Table 22.11).

DATA PROCESSING

Log-in and Scan Process

To prepare the CRFs to be scanned into the computer:

1. Verify the shipment of CRFs from clinical research department to the inventory of data management department (Table 22.3).
2. Check the CRFs to assure that the header information is accurate and complete.
3. Prepare the CRF file folder with the cover page (Table 22.4), which carries the following information: batch number, site, patient ID, visit number, log-in date, and the initials of the

Table 22.3   CRFs Login Sheet

Protocol #:
Name of drug:
Data Clerk name:

1. Log-in date:
2. Investigator number and name:
3. Patient number/initial:
4. Book/visit number:
5. Batch name:
6. Comments:

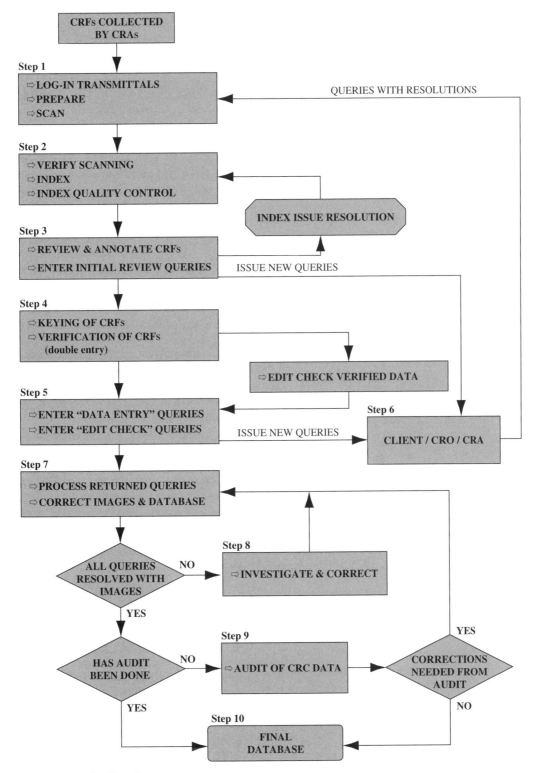

Figure 22.1 Data creation flow chart

Table 22.4   CRFs cover sheet

Protocol #:		Site/investigator:
Name of drug:		Patient # / visit #:
Data clerk name:		Batch number:

Process	Date	Initial
Log-in		
Review		
Key		
Verify		
Query		
Audit		

person who logged the CRFs. This will ensure that the scanner will assign the patient information to the correct fields of the electronic image files.

4. Scan CRFs into the computer image files.

CRFs Image Review Process

This process is to ensure that unexpected data problems or unusual interdata relations in various data fields are identified. It is a very important step in the data process: many companies have encountered data quality problems because of the lack of this step, which is not included to replace the computer edit check but rather to enhance it. The basic principles for the image review are checking the 'accuracy', 'completeness', and 'consistency' of the data within a subject and across subjects. This review and timely computer edit checks will provide feedback to the monitoring staff concerning a problematic investigator or CRF page, so that corrective action of monitoring practice or enhancement of the computer edit checks can be implemented promptly. The review should include:

1. Are there missing header information, missing pages, and visits.
2. Are randomization numbers allocated sequentially?
3. Are blanks are properly answered?
4. Check adverse events and prematurely discontinued subjects, with special attention to the comments for hidden information.
5. Has clinically significant laboratory abnormality has been followed by the investigator?
6. Does the drug inventory match the number consumed?

7. Clarify all text items, e.g. adverse events, concomitant medications, physical examinations, ECG, progress notes, etc.

Data Entry and Double Entry using CRF Images

-   Autocode the data using structured glossaries, including drug class, body system, preferred term and verbatim term.
-   Manual code the 'no-hit' terms and update the glossary.
-   Run computer edit checks (Table 22.5) and generate queries. Reconcile the discrepancies between the queries generated by manual review and computer edit check. Issue the queries (Table 22.6) to the investigators.

Query Resolution and Database Update

When the answers to the queries are returned, the CDC updates the database and CRF images. This is a continuous process during the course of the clinical trials.

Table 22.5   Preliminary edit check document

Protocol #:	Edit check programmer:
Name of drug:	Version date:
CDC name:	Revision date:

General checks:
   D-1) Subject initials should be consistent throughout casebook
   D-2) All dates should be within valid ranges
Inclusion criteria:
   D-1) Inclusion # 1 should be yes or no
   D-2) Inclusion # 2 should be yes or no
   D-3) Inclusion # 3 should be yes or no
   D-4) Consent date should be equal to visit date
Exclusion criteria:
   D-1) Exclusion # 1 should be yes or no
   D-2) Exclusion # 2 should be yes or no
   D-3) Exclusion # 3 should be yes or no
   D-4) Exclusion # 4 should be yes or no
   D-5) Exclusion # 5 should be yes or no or na
   D-4) Exclusion # 6 should be yes or no or na
Demographics:
Efficacy:
Safety:
(etc.)

Table 22.6 Data query sheet

Protocol #:	Data submitted:
Name of drug:	Date returned:
CDC name:	

Site/pat. no. Page Visit   Problem   Resolution

Investigator signature: Date:
CRA signature: Date:

Create Test Datasets for Various Analysis population

To make the adequate inferences of the efficacy and safety of the study drug, *Federal Reg* (1996) should be followed: in Section 11.1, 'Data Sets Analyzed', it states:

> Exactly which patients were included in each efficacy analysis should be precisely defined, e.g. all patients receiving any test drugs/investigational products; all patients with any efficacy observations or with a certain minimum number of observations; only patients completing the trial; all patients with an observation during a particular time window; or only patients with a specified degree of compliance. It should be clear, if not defined in the study protocol, when (relative to unblinding of the study) and how inclusion/exclusion criteria for the datasets analyzed were developed. Generally, even if the applicant's proposed primary analysis is based on a reduced subset of the patients with data, there should also be, for any trial intended to establish the efficacy, an additional analysis using all randomized (or otherwise entered) patients with any on-treatment data ... A diagram showing the relationship between the entire sample and any other analysis groups should be provided.

Therefore, an algorithm has to be developed to precisely define how each analysis population of the dataset is defined. For example, there are at least four analysis population datasets, e.g. the intent-to-treat (ITT) population, the per-protocol (PP) population, the safety population, and the microbiological population, as indicated in the diagram (Figure 22.2). During the derivation of various analysis populations, it may be necessary to issue new

queries and update the database, based on the resolution of the queries.

Status Reporting (Table 22.7):

1. From the image files and the database, a weekly production report is generated.
2. A cross-check of milestones and progress achieved should be made, and the status be reported to the department heads for review and action.
3. The department heads may adjust the resources, depending on the progress report.

Create Audit Sheet for Audit

The computer-generated audit sheet (Table 22.8) should be formated in the same sequence as the fields in the CRFs. This will enhance the speed of the audit task. The QA auditor will check the audit sheet against the CRF images.

Issue Interim Audit Document and Audit Summary

When 10% of the CRFs have been scanned and entered into the computer, the interim audit should be conducted in order to tune up the CDC review manual and edit-check programs. Findings regarding the quality of the database should be given to the head of the data management group for possible action. The audit document (Table 22.9) should include: patient ID; the initials of the keyer and verifier; CDC; editing programmer; type of audit; number of errors; description of errors. It

Table 22.7 Data process status

Protocol #:					
Name of drug:					
CDC name:					
Site/inv.	Logged (no.) (%)	Reviewed (no.) (%)	Keyed (no.) (%)	Verified (no.) (%)	Audited (no.) (%)
Total:					

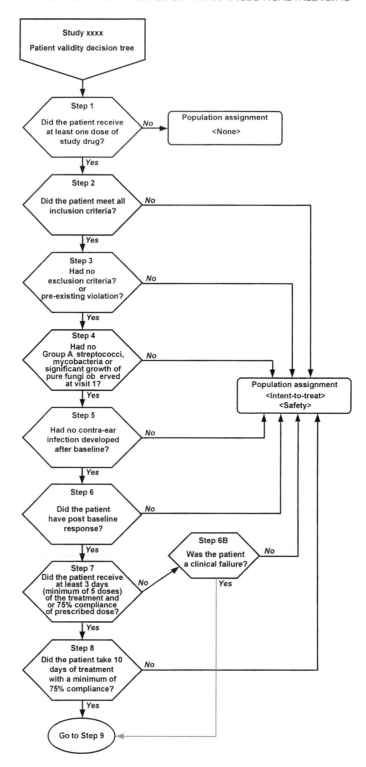

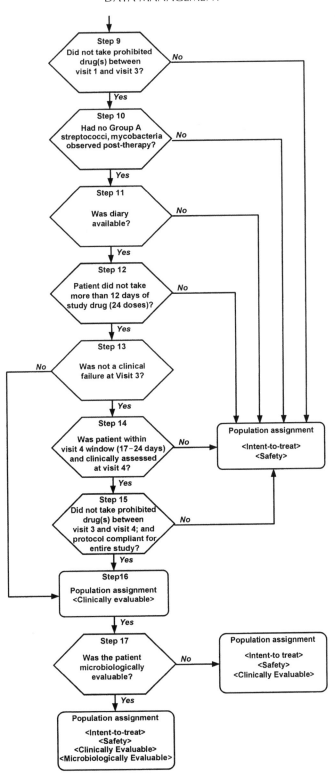

Figure 22.2 Derivation of study population

Table 22.8 Audit sheet

Protocol #:	Audit sheet programmer:
Name of drug:	Version date:
Name of CDC:	Revision date:

CRF Page 1:
Eligibility criteria:
        Initial: RLD   Visit date: 02/10/97

                Inclusion Criteria

1	2	3	4	5	6	7
1	1	1	1	1	1	1

                Exclusion Criteria

1	2	3	4	5	6	7	8	9	10	11
2	2	2	2	2	2	2	2	2	2	2

CRF Page 2:
Infection history:
Initial: RLD Visit date: 02/10/97

Number of infections in past year: 3
Therapy for infection in past year: 2

Medication: Drug aaa   Effective: 1   Complete med.: 1
(etc.)

is a tool to find out which records tend to produce more errors and who tends to make most of the mistakes. Is CDC review adequate? Are the programs written for the computer edit checks sufficient? Did the data entry verifier find the problems of the keyer and fixed them? Once the CDC review manual and computer edit checks have been improved, a second interim audit should be repeated when 50–60% of the CRFs have been scanned and entered. Final audit should be performed when all the CRFs are scanned and entered. In addition to the audit memo issued during the interim audits, an audit summary report (Table 22.10) should be issued to summarize the quality of the final database. This will also give management an index of the error rate, which measures the confidence level of releasing the database.

Database Release Memo

Once all the queries have been resolved and updated to the image files and database, the database is officially locked. A database release memo (Table 22.11) should be issued to the project statistician, all other team members and management. The project statistician will then merge the file of the randomization codes to the database to generate the analysis data sets.

DISASTER RECOVERY PLAN

The data files and the completed CRFs generated from the clinical trials are more precious than the hardware. In addition to daily and monthly backup, pharmaceutical companies should have a detailed recovery plan in case of unexpected disaster. The disaster recovery plan should include:

1. *Key personnel contact list*, with home telephone and pager numbers listed.

Table 22.9 Audit document

Protocol #:	Date audit start:						
Name of drug:	Date audit stop:						
Auditor name:							
Pat. no.	Keyer	Verifier	CDC	Auditor	Type of audit	No. of errors	Description of errors
01/002	ka	jp	sr	et	Full	0	
01/005	ka	jp	sr	et	Full	0	
01/009	ka	jp	sr	et	Full	1	Med. His—'Pnemonia' should be 'Pneumonia'
01/014	ka	jp	sr	et	Full	0	
01/018	ev	cc	jf	wa	Full	0	
02/005	js	cc	jf	wa	Full	1	Diary—3/24/98 bedtime 11:10 pm should be at 11:00 pm
.							
.							
.							
(etc.)							

Table 22.10 Format of summary of audit result

Protocol #: Name of drug: Auditor names:	Date audit start: Date audit stop:						
Page description	Dataset #	Variables/ pat #	Pat audited #	Records checked #	Values checked #	Errors found	Error rate (%)
Adv. Exper	Adverse	26	497	558	14508	0	0.0000
Study Complete	Complete	7	497	497	3479	2	0.0575
Conc. Med.	Conmed	18	497	602	10836	4	0.0369
Eligibility Criteria	Criteria	29	497	497	14413	1	0.0069
Diary	Diary	160	497	497	79520	17	0.0214
Drug Accountab	Drugacct	6	497	497	2982	1	0.0335
Overall					270771	51	0.0188

Table 22.11 Database release memorandum

Date:
To: Project statistician
From: CDC
Subject: Database Release

The master files of the following study have been audited by the QA department and passed. The database is therefore signed off and released by Data Management.

Drug:
Protocol number:
Investigator number and name:
Date master files signed off:
Time master files signed off:

Please verify that you have received the master files. Via this memo, QA department is requested to release the randomization codes to the project statistician. Thanks.

Clinical Data coordinator
cc: Project team members

2. *List of critical applications and operations*. It should be a company's policy to set up an off-site processing center with the same hardware–software set-up. This should be able to be made operational within 2 hour should it become necessary if a disaster strikes the data center. Critical applications and operations include upcoming NDA studies, safety database, NDA summaries.

3. *Off-site storage*. In order to be operational at the off-site process center for critical applications, the files that need to be updated to the off-site center are master files for all completed projects, daily back-ups for ongoing studies, monthly system files, monthly glossary up-dates, monthly safety monitoring, NDA files, and production job streams. The protocols, CRFs, regulatory documents, rules, and manuals should also be stored off-site. A drill of the disaster recovery plan should be put to test at least every 6 months to reveal any un-anticipated problem.

REFERENCES

ICH (1996) International Conference on Harmonization: Guideline on Structure, Content and Clinical Study Reports; availability; notice. *Fed Reg* 61(138): 37326.
PhRMA (1997) *Facts and Figures*.

23

Patient Compliance

Jean-Michel Métry

AARAEX Ltd, Zug, Switzerland

Patient non-compliance with prescribed drug regimens is a long-recognized aspect of ambulatory health care that has only recently been analyzed. It was only in 1987 that objective, satisfactory methods became available for measuring compliance. Since then, much new information has been gained. Studies with low-dose chemical markers have shown that subjective methods grossly overestimate patient compliance in clinical trials and medical practice. Reliable measurements of drug exposure in ambulatory patients require methods that make it difficult for patients to misreport delayed or omitted doses. Electronic monitoring now has a decade of research experience and a strong consensus has developed for considering this to be the 'gold standard' for measuring drug exposure in ambulatory patients. Recent advances in electronics and manufacturing technology have brought the cost of electronic monitoring down substantially.

A major reason for poor compliance is simple negligence. Neither good intention nor a professional level of understanding of medicine and pharmacology competes well for priority in busy lives: 35–40% of well-informed, cooperative patients frequently delay or omit scheduled doses (Pullar et al 1989; Van der Stichele 1991; Kruse 1992; Urquhart 1994; Kass et al 1987; Wakerhouse et al 1993; De Klerk and van der Linden in press). The resulting range and patterns of drug intake are remarkably similar for a wide range of drugs, diseases, prognoses, and even symptoms (Kass et al 1987; Wakerhouse et al 1993; De Klerk and van der Linden in press; Steiner et al 1994). Yet, while compliance patterns may be similar, the medical and economic consequences vary widely, and are dependent on drug, disease type, disease severity, and co-morbidity (Urquhart 1995). The need for intervention thus varies, and considerations of cost-effectiveness require proper targeting of those patients who may incur bigger problems and higher costs if their poor compliance is not improved.

Two basic issues are (a) reliable detection of poor compliance, and (b) reliable measurement of the consequences of the steps taken to improve it. Given that traditional clinical assessments of compliance (e.g. the taking of treatment histories) leads to such gross underestimates (Pullar et al 1989; Van der Stichele 1991; Kruse 1992; Urquhart 1994; Kass et al 1987; Wakerhouse et al 1993; De Klerk and van der Linden in press; Steiner et al 1994; Urquhart 1995; Kass et al 1986; Cramer et al 1989), real-time electronic monitoring is now the accepted standard (Bond and Hussar 1991).

Several levels of feedback to the patient will probably have importance in the future. These may range from audible or visual status alerts for the patients themselves to more intensive approaches, using modems or pagers, which can also communicate with the professionals willing to assume responsibility for pharmaceutical care. The latter must focus on well-defined, high-risk situations, in which the consequences of delayed or omitted doses are severe and costly, and where remedial actions can be shown to be cost-effective.

WHAT DOES 'COMPLIANCE' MEAN?

Prior to the technical advances described below, patient compliance was vaguely defined. A typical definition might have been, 'following the instructions of the health care provider' (Cramer 1991). With the advent of electronic monitoring methods, it has become practical to use a definition of compliance with pharmacologic and quantitative meaning

Principles and Practice of Pharmaceutical Medicine. Edited by A. J. Fletcher, Lionel D. Edwards, Anthony W. Fox and Peter Stonier © 2002 John Wiley & Sons Ltd.

in terms of drug exposure. Today, we can define compliance as: 'The degree of correspondence between the actual time history of dosing and the prescribed regimen' (Temple 1969). The time history of dosing describes drug exposure, not only in quantity but also in respect to the timing of individual doses. Full therapeutic benefit, and fewest adverse events, can only be achieved by meeting certain standards with respect to the quantity of drug taken and the accurate timing of doses. Every drug, depending upon its pharmacokinetics and pharmacodynamics, has its own scientifically definable standard, and these are found from properly conducted dose–response and dose–frequency studies (Feely et al 1987).

METHODS OF EVALUATING COMPLIANCE

There are two general classes of compliance evaluation, termed 'direct' and 'indirect'.

Direct Compliance Evaluation

Direct methods rely simply on the measurement of plasma drug concentration. Unfortunately, this method is biased because sporadic venesection can usually reflect only the dosing history of the previous day or two. Most drugs are eliminated quite quickly from the bloodstream and measurement of a drug level in plasma reflects dosing only during a small fraction of the duration of dosing (Crawer 1991; Feely et al 1987). Furthermore, when they know that a blood sample will be taken, patients commonly improve their dosing behavior for a day or two before (Feinstein 1990), and for most drugs, these samples indicate atypically good compliance and overestimate total compliance. For those few drugs that have exceptionally slow turnover (amiodarone is an important example), periodic measurements of drug concentration in plasma may suffice, and give comparable results to the use of low-dose, slow-turnover markers, described below. Random, unannounced sampling of blood can help, but is often inefficient, costly, impractical, and intrusive during clinical trials and ordinary medical practice.

Another useful method of direct compliance evaluation uses slow-turnover chemical marker-substancs incorporated into the drug formulation (Feely et al 1987; Mäenpää et al 1987). One example is phenobarbital, where a single measurement of its concentration in plasma can indicate the most recent 4–7 days of dosing history (Feely et al 1987).

Low-dose marker methods cannot, however, indicate the actual timing of doses. Blood samples can only indicate aggregate dosing during the time window that is defined by the marker's pharmacokinetics. A large number and high frequency of blood samples are usually needed to develop a longitudinal record of dosing over an extended period of time.

Indirect Compliance Evaluation

Prior to 1987, all indirect methods of compliance evaluation failed to prevent patients censoring the data that was collected. History taking, diaries, and counts of returned dosage forms can all be manipulated to conceal evidence of delayed or omitted doses, and have repeatedly been shown to be unreliable (Cramer et al 1989; Cramer 1991; Kruse et al 1993; Guerrero et al 1993) and to grossly overestimate compliance in both clinical trials and ordinary practice.

However, in 1987, the first solid dosage form monitor was introduced. This device records the opening of the drug package, and has time-keeping microcircuitry. The opening and closing of the package can be recorded separately. Intervals between each pair of opening/closing events can be calculated, and become part (for example) of a clinical trial record.

The disadvantage of solid dosage form monitors is that the patient's actual ingestion (and absence of regurgitation) of the drug cannot be confirmed. However, research experience suggests that patients rarely go to the length of opening the drug package at the scheduled times but not actually taking the medicine. To do this consistently, day in and day out, throughout the whole course of prescribed treatment, has never been reported.

COMPLIANCE DURING CLINICAL TRIALS

A growing consensus supports the reliable measurement of compliance with the protocol-specified treatment regimen; this consensus obtains within both the clinical and statistical communities (Meier 1991; Efron 1991, 1998; Rubin 1991, 1998; Cox 1998). The 'gold-standard' method for evaluating patient compliance is now electronic monitoring (Crawer 1995; Urquhart 1997; Kastrissos and Blaschke 1997) and standard methods to present this type of data are well known (Urquhart and de Klert 1998). Less reliable methods, e.g. counting returned, unused tablets, cannot now be justified because of well-documented, high incidences of tablet dumping by poorly compliant patients (Pullar et al 1989; Rudd et al 1989; Wakerhouse et al 1993), although some researchers are still oblivious to this well-documented fact (Pocock and Abdalla 1998). But what, precisely, are the advantages of measuring compliance in the different phases of development of a drug?

Phase I Clinical Studies

Typically, the aim of Phase I is to evaluate tolerability, some pharmacodynamic properties, and the human pharmacokinetics of a new drug. When witnessed administration of a single dose is all that the protocol requires, then compliance evaluation is not an issue. However, subsequent normal volunteer studies may examine the tolerability of repeat doses, even outside of a research facility, and the problems outlined above then apply. Furthermore, in studies of drug interactions, it is essential to know whether and when the subjects took the test drugs.

Phase II Clinical Studies

Limited numbers of patients take part in these studies, and the requirement that as little harm as possible should be created is therefore much greater than in normal volunteers. Identification of effective doses, and dose–effect and concentration–effect relationships must be efficiently demonstrated, as well as tolerability, in an automatically more complicated setting. Differences between pharmacokinetics in healthy subjects and patients are common and the evolution of the drug formulation during the development program adds another complexity. Controlling the intake of the

drug is thus of utmost importance: the future of the product depends inherently upon it, because the study results are governed by the degree of drug exposure that takes place.

Whether it is a Phase II study of efficacy or tolerance, one tactic is to use a run-in or preselection period, with the aim of choosing only 'good compliance' patients for the definitive assessment of the study end-points. The criteria for the measurement of compliance with electronic monitors in this case are: (a) the ratio of the number of administrations observed to the number of intended doses; and (b) the mean intervals between the administrations (e.g. a patient in a trial requiring a dose of a single tablet daily might be considered a 'good complier' if he she took 90% of the total doses with a mean interval between doses of 26 ± 2 hours (h)).

Using such a run-in period adds complexity to the trial. The study takes longer and is hard to manage, with relatively quick decision making about whether or not to allow patients to continue in the study. A larger number of patients are also needed, and all these factors cost money. However, by including only 'good compliers', precise knowledge of the dose for Phase III studies becomes more reliable, and the tolerability of the test-substance has been tested more rigorously.

The other method is to enroll the patients into the study from the beginning and to follow their compliance during the whole trial. Patients can be prospectively stratified in the statistical analysis, using compliance as an independent variable (e.g. examination of an efficacy end-point for two subgroups of patients who took more than or less than 80% of the prescribed drug doses). Initial assessment of product assessment is also possible with this approach, although this must be in the context of whether or not the proposed market formulation has been used in the Phase II study; this assessment might even drive the development of better dosage forms.

Phase III Clinical Studies

The object of Phase III is to evaluate the efficacy and tolerance of the product over a long period of time and in a large number of patients. Ideally, conditions should be close to the anticipated ordinary clinical practice. It is known from a great number of Phase III clinical studies that compliance is only partial and evaluations of effect–risk often differ from those observed during Phase II. Whatever design of trial is used (e.g. controlled against placebo or active comparator, with or without measurements of compliance of the alternative treatments), an analysis of the results with respect to treatment is inevitable.

Again, run-in periods which would preselect patients with good compliance could be used, but this moves away from the ordinary clinical situation. If a separate compliance study is performed, it is more rational to include the subjects from the onset and to follow their compliance over the whole course of the trial. The results may be factored against the intent-to-treat philosophy being employed. Later, in a secondary analysis, the results can be stratified according to the level of compliance, either according to prospective definitions or on an *ad hoc* basis. From these different analyses it should, for example, be possible to conclude whether, in a large number of patients, good compliance improves the efficacy of the product. The study of compliance again, of course, entails additional costs (the higher the number of patients, the longer the duration of the trial), but will improve the quality and reliability of the results with a view to the compilation of the product dossier.

Marketing may also benefit from Phase III clinical trials where compliance has been evaluated. It may become possible to estimate whether or not a patient will take his/her medicine regularly. Education of clinicians about the stages of treatment when the patient is most likely to either forget his/her tablets or deliberately discontinue treatment (e.g. the 'weekend effect') can permit relevant intervention and superior therapeutic results.

Phase IV Clinical Studies

Specific Phase IV studies of compliance can: (a) understand the different profiles of compliance; (b) test systems created to improve compliance; and (c) experiment, among other things, with conditioning, memory aids, sensitization of the doctor and the patient. Often more than one of these goals can be accomplished during a single study. The economic justification, and financial resources needed for such maneuvers, will vary from drug to drug, and even between different indications for a single drug.

COMPLIANCE STANDARDS FOR ANALYZING REAL-TIME COMPLIANCE DATA

Data saved in electronic monitors may be transferred and collated in larger computers; the data transfer may be hard (cable) or soft (telephonic). Patients' medication histories can then easily be charted using software that is not sophisticated by today's standards, and hard copy compliance reports can become part of the patient's clinical chart or case report form.

Compliance Reports

The central part of the compliance report is a quantitative and qualitative evaluation of the compliance data that was collected real-time. *Calendar displays* should show the number of daily dose units taken by the patient on ordinary monthly calendars. This form of illustration makes patterns of drug intake easy to see, e.g. an increase in compliance during the last days before the consultation (so-called 'white-coat compliance') or the 'weekend effect' (see above). Compliance with prescribed drug holidays, or accuracy of 'tailing off' of therapies, can also be assessed. Understanding these often subtle regimen behaviors may also help the evaluation of reported effects (wanted and unwanted).

Chronology diagrams show dose units on a graph according to a system of coordinates. The abscissa might show the observation period in days, and the ordinate the hours of the day from 0.00 to 24.00 h. Every plotted point then represents when the dose unit was opened. The distance between clusters of points corresponds to the accuracy of dose frequency, and the relative density or spaciousness of each cluster gives an impression of accuracy of dose timing.

Therapeutic coverage is defined as the percentage of time during which the patient had a therapeutically adequate effect of the drug during the observation period. The assumed optimum duration of action of the preparation (e.g. for a once-daily application 24 h, or for a prescribed twice-daily application 12 h) is balanced against the typical interval between the times that the patient actually takes the drug. The difference of this percentage to 100% is termed 'uncovered hours' and represents the times with an insufficient drug effect due to missed applications. If desired, the distribution of uncovered hours can also be charted, and characteristic patterns of inadequate therapeutic coverage (e.g. specific hours of the day) become evident.

Neither therapeutic coverage nor 'uncovered hours' will be scientifically exact, and may vary from day to day. As rating parameters they are inexact, but they may form useful tools for feedback to the patient, illustrating his drug-taking behavior within the observation period, and allowing comparisons between observation periods that can motivate an improvement in compliance. For the patient, this heightens the understanding of the complex problem of compliance, and the doctor and the pharmacist can instruct the patient in specific and individualized ways.

Calculation of the shortest and longest interval between two doses, the percentage of days with correct number of doses taken, and the distribution of intervals between doses are other aspects of compliance reports. These can be related to the known pharmacology of the drug, as discussed above.

HOW IS COMPLIANCE CLASSIFIED? COMMON PATTERNS

Full Compliance

This is the patient who respects the doctor's instructions to a high degree. Approximately 80–100% of the prescribed doses (e.g. tablets, capsules) are taken according to instructions. Depending on the medication and the aim of treatment, the rating of this type of compliance varies: e.g. in the treatment of hyperlipidaemia, a long-acting lipid-lowering agent may be effective with a compliance of 80%. In the case of a contraceptive, a compliance as good as 80% can still have unfortunate consequences. The general maxim is: the more regular the dosing frequency, the better.

Partial Compliance

This describes a situation in which the patient frequently 'forgets' to take his/her medication. Perhaps 50–80% of the prescribed doses (e.g. tablets, capsules) are taken according to instructions. The medication cannot provide its full action, and the patient does not profit fully from treatment. For example, antihypertensives may appear to work when blood pressures are satisfactory at the consultation (a common 'white coat compliance'), but at other times the patient still has uncontrolled hypertension. These patients may unconsciously or consciously be responding to adverse events, too; in some cultures they may be reticent to tell their doctors about this, and in other situations patients may want to avoid being withdrawn from clinical trials. Close treatment history taking is mandatory when such a patient is identified.

Non-compliance

This patient takes the prescribed medication very irregularly. Approximately 0–50% of the prescribed dose units (e.g. tablets, capsules) are taken according to instructions. The patient is quite insufficiently treated and the disease progresses. 'White coat compliance' may still exist.

Over-compliance

This term is used when there is evidence that the patient has taken more than the prescribed amounts of medication. More than 100% of the prescribed dose units (e.g. tablets, capsules) are taken. As a consequence, the treatment results are not better but the adverse effects increase in severity and frequency. Drugs with abuse liability are perhaps the commonest cause of this compliance pattern.

Drug Holidays

This term includes both prescribed drug withdrawal, and the patient who him/herself decides to discontinue medication for, say, 3 or more consecutive days. These so-called 'drug holidays' may tend to occur on days on which the patient changes his/her usual daily activities, i.e. chiefly at weekends, holidays and vacations. Usually, 50% of patients can be expected to have at least one such treatment-free phase within a 4 week treatment period, and 'drug holidays' may typically occupy 15% of outpatient observation periods (Kruse and Weber 1990).

Skewed Dosing

This uncommon type of patient continually changes his dosage. Overdosage and underdosage are about equally frequent. The result is a high fluctuation of the plasma levels and an inadequate therapeutic effect. This is especially true for the induction phase of preparations with a protracted onset of effect, but also for substances with a short half-life.

Skipped Dosing

The patient frequently omits a dose unit, e.g. if the prescription is 'twice daily', the patient often takes the medication once a day; if the recommended dosage is 1 tablet daily he/she often takes one tablet every second day. The most frequent consequence is therapeutic deficits occurring at intervals, which can lead to a considerable reduction of the overall therapeutic success.

Timing Non-compliance

The daily intake of the medication is not at a regular, set time but with large temporal deviations or completely unstructured. This type of non-compliance often fails to ensure adequate therapeutic coverage.

ACTIONS TO ENHANCE COMPIANCE

The prevalence of suboptimal compliance in all fields of chronic, ambulatory pharmacotherapy is well-established. This begs the question: how to ensure good therapeutic outcomes in a world of imperfect compliers?

Drugs can only exert their full benefit if they are taken within certain limits of full compliance with the recommended regimen. These limits are, for most drugs, undefined, although progress is being made with studies that define these limits.

In this effort, the patient should be the focus. His/her ability to cope with the prescribed regimen is crucial for good compliance, and if this is understood by the patient then a good outcome becomes more likely. Health professionals have an important role to play in helping patients comply properly and thus get the fullest possible benefit from their prescribed medicines. When compliance is insufficient, the outcome of the treatment is put in jeopardy and the costs of care rise, due to the needless addition of second or third agents, unnecessary dose escalations, or repeated diagnostic tests to ascertain the nature of a clinical problem that has been created simply by persistent, clinically unrecognized, poor compliance.

Many studies have shown that patients undergoing long-term treatment in particular do not succeed in taking their medication correctly over a long period of time, and the scale of this problem can only be described as epidemic! For example, 15% of all general practitioners' prescriptions fail to result in a pharmacy dispensing (Beardon et al 1993); half of all patients who have their prescriptions filled then do not take the prescribed medication at all or do not take it correctly; 30% of all prescriptions are used incorrectly and cause harm to health; and about 7–8% of all hospitalizations could be avoided with earlier detection of non-compliance or reduction of excessive drug intake.

Overall, it appears that there are four times as many errors of dose omission than errors of excess dosing. Both can result in clinical complications that mimic worsening disease (Urquhart 1997).

Two groups have now independently presented evidence that future compliance can be modeled and faithfully simulated during future months, after 30–60 days of electronic monitoring of dosing history. Many patients fail to realize that it is important to take medication regularly and that they can make hazardous mistakes in the application of their medication. This may be because of prejudice against the prescribed treatments, incomprehensible or disturbing package leaflets, or the misguided advice of lay friends and relatives. The compliance of the patient is not only influenced by this array of different factors, but these factors are also under dynamic change.

IMPROVE COMPLIANCE: BUT HOW?

The crucial step is to use the objective record of the patient's dosing history as a management tool, in a non-pejorative manner. These tools can allow the patient to see that errors were made, to identify difficulties with therapy, and to discuss options for how to avoid such errors in the future. This step is wholly new, for prior efforts to improve compliance have relied on patients (self-reported compliance), which is subject to errors due to imperfect memory, mixed feelings about the treatment program, and a desire to please the physician.

If the results of treatment are unsatisfactory, the following basic questions must be answered:

1. Is the cause pharmacological, due to failure of correctly taken drug to work as hoped, or is the cause due to inadequate compliance?
2. Is the compliance problem a static phenomenon or a dynamic process?

Many studies have clearly shown that the compliance of most patients deteriorates as treatment duration progresses. Diseases without major symptoms also are associated with high rates of partial compliance or non-compliance after a few months of treatment. If the treatment results are inadequate, the doctor must judge whether the disease is taking a progressive course, whether the drug is losing in effect with prolonged treatment (phenomenon of tachyphylaxis), or whether the cause must be thought in inadequate compliance.

Studies have shown that even experienced doctors often fail to recognize partial compliance or non-compliance in their patients. There is no proven relationship between compliance behavior and parameters such as age, sex, educational background and social status, specific drugs, adverse effects of medication, and nature or severity of the disease.

Compliance Monitoring with Feedback of the Results to the Patient Enhances Compliance

Reviewing the recorded dosing history with the patient is a powerful tool to help patients recognize when they have made errors in dosing likely to undermine efficacy or cause safety problems. This review may usefully be done by physicians, pharmacists, and nurse-educators, depending on the local circumstances. These reviews should not be isolated events, but part of an ongoing process. The patient should understand that, at the next visit, the dosing history will again be reviewed, and that the only way to compile a correct record is to pay careful attention to the prescribed regimen and link it closely to established routines in daily life. Children may even respond to rewards, based upon how satisfactory the reviews become.

Despite the disciplinary aspect of the review, the vast majority of patients regard the review as a logical extension of the interest of the prescribing physician in their care. Furthermore, knowledge of the compliance behavior of the patient can facilitate communication between pharmacist and doctor, increasing the attention to the patient with compliance problems, identifying misunderstood aims of treatment, clarifying details of the treatment regimen, and uncovering prejudices against treatment. Individualization of the treatment, adapting dose timings to the habits of the patient, and thus enhancing his compliance, can only become possible using this approach.

WHO ARE THE POTENTIAL PLAYERS INVOLVED IN THE FIELD OF REAL-TIME COMPLIANCE?

Every health care professional who has, directly or indirectly, contact with the patient is a potential player. In the forefront is the treating physician, who has to make sound decisions about the prescription, basing such judgment in part on average values coming out of clinical trials, but tempering judgment with understanding of the patient's individual characteristics. During the past two decades, much has been learned about many of the various influences on drug absorption and metabolism that arise from dietary factors, concomitantly prescribed drugs, and changes in renal or hepatic function. Yet, a major but hitherto inaccessible component of this dynamic process is the patient's actual dosing history, which has the potential to influence the clinical manifestations of drug response over its full range. The physician who has a reliable measure of the patient's dosing history can interpret the patient's response to the drug in far more realistic manner than the physician who can only guess at the patient's actual drug intake, and who will usually substantially overestimate the patient's true drug intake (Kass et al 1986; Cramer et al 1989; Bond and Hussar 1991; Kruse and Weber 1990; Matsui et al 1992; Matsuyama et al 1993; Cramer 1995; Feinstein 1990).

The pharmaceutical company also stands to benefit. Accurate understanding of compliance by physicians can reduce the probability that they will hold fallacious opinions of product ineffectiveness. The prescriber's perception of the drug's reliability and overall value will be falsely diminished by patients who appear to be unresponsive to the drug, but who actually have taken too little drug to produce a clinically useful response.

Needless to say, the economic consequences of poor compliance will sooner or later attract serious attention from insurers and other payers for health care. Prescription drugs, after all, are a principal interventional arm of modern medicine, and their actions are invariably dose-dependent. Ineffective or suboptimal dosing represents an inefficiency in medical care that is potentially remediable. Stefan Norell, a pioneer in this field, wrote in 1980:

> ...the aim of 'improving' compliance is not to achieve perfect agreement between behavior and prescription, but to increase compliance only to the level where the satisfactory outcome of treatment is assured. In practice, however, this level is often unknown.. (Norell et al 1980).

Several large pharmaceutical firms are now making promotional claims for products, based on evidence of therapeutic 'forgiveness' for the more common errors in compliance. Delayed doses, skipping a single dose, and skipping two sequential doses have been studied systematically (Urquhart 1994; Meredith and Elliott 1994; Detry et al 1994, 1995; Mallion 1995; Boutelant et al 1995). The 'therapeutic coverage' variable (see above) has become an end-point in itself (Urquhart 1991; Rubio et al 1992).

WHAT SHOULD INTERACTIVE PACKAGING OFFER TO IMPROVE PATIENT COMPLIANCE?

It is clear that patients have individual preferences and needs, and so will decide what fits them best: audible alerts, visible alerts, integrated or not with the phone system. Technology is available to meet foreseeable preferences. It seems highly unlikely that a single type of electronically monitored packaging will accommodate the whole range of patient needs. Instead, one can expect a variety of electronically monitored packages to emerge as the recognized need for such information grows.

Consider the following scenario: a 60 year-old patient is diagnosed as having high cholesterol levels, and is prescribed a once-daily cholesterol synthesis inhibitor, essentially a life-long therapy. The patient has a certain tendency to forget doses, which can be minimized by use of a simple reminder device. Perhaps, with practice, the patient develops a strong routine of drug intake, linked to some regular routine in his/her life. If that occurs, the reminder device becomes superfluous, although it has served its purpose during the start-up phase of treatment, to make the patient aware of the frequency of missed doses. Meanwhile, the consequences of missing an occasional dose of cholesterol-lowering drug are, as far as anyone knows, negligible. After a decade of treatment, however, the patient develops coronary heart disease with congestive heart failure, and now is in a situation where the punctual maintenance of a strict regimen is essential to prevent hazardous retention of fluid. In this setting, the types of errors that had little or no consequence for cholesterol regulation can create major problems: omission of the daily diuretic dose for as few as three days in sequence can trigger acute pulmonary congestion, requiring hospitalization that costs on the order of US$ 10,000 (Lasagna and Hutt 1991). If the patient's condition is additionally complicated by chronic obstructive pulmonary disease, the impact of fluid retention is all the more severe, with even less latitude for error.

In this rather common scenario of disease progression, one sees how the changing nature of drugs, diseases, severity of diseases, and co-morbidity can radically change the medical and economic implications of compliance errors.

The type of devices needed to accommodate this particular patient can be as follows:

1. *A device with an acoustic or visual reminder* for the patient and a memory capability, so that the treating physician will get that patient's actual history of dosing. When a strong routine exists, this device may be used then only sporadically to check whether the patient is continuing to dose satisfactorily.
2. *An electronic dose organizer* will help the elderly patients with multiple diseases and multiple medications, and may help them cope with the more complex regimens.
3. *An effective program of medication management* may prevent the patient having to abandon home-based care—an obvious issue in both the economics of care and the quality of life.

We should not forget, in this world of technology, that the patient should still come before, not after, the technology. Technology by itself will not solve all the problems created by erratic compliance. Technology is a tool than can help healthcare professionals to identify, track, and potentially solve many of the issues created by partial and poor compliance. The patient will decide which type of intervention or what level of monitoring he/she wants to have. It will not be helpful to have the patient forced into a world that he/she does not understand. When all is said and done, the patient will have to perceive the value of available services, and adopt one of them.

WHAT WILL BE THE REACTION OF THIRD-PARTY PAYERS ?

Studies will be needed to provide data on the cost-effectiveness of such approaches (Urquhart 1995). Studies done prematurely, before the 'learning curve' has been substantially traversed, will only confuse and delay matters. A key step (see above) is

targeting of high-risk patients, whose well-being depends very directly on maintenance of the dosing schedule. Moderate–severe congestive heart failure appears to be one such situation (Kruse and Weber 1990), and chronic hormonal receptor blockade in hormonally-dependent tumors is probably another.

The field of therapeutics is vast and complex, with many areas in which special problems arise due to seemingly inadequate response to the prescribed drug regimens. If there is one lesson taught by the past decade of research on patient compliance, it is to put uppermost the question: non-responder or non-complier? The economic opportunities for value-added packaging are to be found in our growing understanding of the medical and economic advantages of correctly answering this basic question in situations where the wrong answer is very costly in both medical and economic terms.

CONCLUSION

A decade ago the problem was how to measure drug intake in ambulatory patients. That problem has been solved by a variety of approaches, which integrate time-stamping, recording microcircuitry into a variety of drug packages, to record times when the package is used in the manner needed to provide a dose of drug for the patient. Electronic monitoring is an indirect method of measuring drug intake in ambulatory patients (Bond and Hussar 1991), and does not show actual ingestion of the dose. But it has the virtue of continuity over long periods of time, and has proved itself in a variety of settings to be the superior method of measurement (Bond and Hussar 1991; Matsui et al 1992; Cramer 1995). The key question facing us today is how best to target the methods now in hand, so that they improve care and reduce costs.

REFERENCES

Beardon FHG *et al* (1993) Primary non-compliance with prescribed medication in primary care. *Br Med J* 307: 846–8.
Bond WS, Hussar DA (1991) Detection methods and strategies for improving medication compliance. *Am J Hosp Pharm* 48: 1978–88.

Boutelant S, Dutrey-Dupagne C, Vaur L et al (1995) Electronic compliance monitoring and antihypertensive coverage evaluation. Abstracts of the Seventh European Meeting on Hypertension, Milano, Universita degli Studi di Milano. *Ricerca Scientifica ed Educazione Permanente* Suppl 103, 25(103).

Cox, D (1998) Discussion—The Limburg Compliance Symposium. *Stat Med* 17: 387–90.

Cramer J (1991) Overview of methods to measure and enhance patient compliance. In Cramer JA, Spilker B (eds), *Compliance in Medical Practice and Clinical Trials*. Raven: New York; 3–10.

Cramer JA (1995) Microelectronic systems for monitoring and enhancing patient compliance with medication regimens. *Drugs* 49: 321–7.

Cramer JA, Mattson RH, Prevey ML et al (1989) How often is medication taken as prescribed? A novel assessment technique. *J Am Med Assoc* 261: 3273–7.

De Klerk E, van der Linden SJ. Compliance monitoring of NSAID drug therapy in ankylosing spondylitis, experiences with an electronic monitoring device. *Br J Rheumatol* (in press).

Detry J-MR, Block P, De Backer G et al (1994) Patient compliance and therapeutic coverage: amlodipine vs. nifedipine (slow-release) in the treatment of angina pectoris. *J Int Med Res* 22: 278–86.

Detry J-MR, Block P, De Backer G et al (1995) Patient compliance and therapeutic coverage: amlodipine vs. nifedipine (slow-release) in the treatment of hypertension. *Eur J Clin Pharmacol* 47: 477–81.

Efron B (1991) Rejoinder. *J Am Stat Assoc* 86(413): 25.

Efron B (1998) Foreword—The Limburg Compliance Symposium. *Stat Med* 17: 249–50.

Efron B, Feldman D (1991) Compliance as an explanatory variable in clinical trials. *J Am Stat Assoc* 86(413): 9–17.

Eisen SA, Woodward RS, Miller D et al (1987) The effect of medication compliance on the control of hypertension. *J Gen Intern Med* 2: 298–305.

Feely M, Cooke J, Price D et al (1987) Low-dose phenobarbitone as an indicator of compliance with drug therapy. *Br J Clin Pharmacol* 24: 77–83.

Feinstein AR (1990) On white-coat effects and the electronic monitoring of compliance. *Arch Intern Med* 150: 1377–8.

Goetghebeur EJT, Pocock SJ (1993) Statistical issues in allowing for non-compliance and withdrawal. *Drug Inf J* 27: 837–45.

Guerrero D, Rudd P, Bryant-Kosling C, Middleton BF (1993) Antihypertensive medication-taking. Investigation of a simple regimen. *Am J Hypertens* 6: 586–92.

Hasford J (1994) Compliance bei Klinischen Pruefungen. In Hasford J, Staib AH (eds), *Arznei-Mittelpruefungen und Good Clinical Practice*. MMV Medizin Verlag: Munich; 166–78.

Kass MA, Gordon M, Meltzer DW (1986) Can ophthalmologists correctly identify patients defaulting from pilocarpine therapy? *Am J Ophthalmol* 101: 524–30.

Kass MA, Gordon M, Morley RE et al (1987) Compliance with topical timolol treatment. *Am J Ophthalmol* 103: 188–93.

Kastrissios H, Blaschke TF (1997) Medication compliance as a feature in drug development. *Ann Rev Pharmacol Toxicol* 37: 451–75.

Kruse W (1992) Patient compliance with drug treatment—new perspectives on an old problem. *Clin Invest* 70:163–6.

Kruse W, Nikolaus T, Rampmaier J et al (1993) Actual vs. prescribed timing of lovastatin doses assessed by electronic compliance monitoring. *Eur J Clin Pharmacol* 44: 211–15.

Kruse W, Weber E (1990) Dynamics of drug regimen compliance—its assessment by microprocessor-based monitoring. *Eur J Clin Pharmacol* 38: 561–5.

Lasagna L, Hutt PB (1991) Health care, research, and regulatory impact of non-compliance. In Cramer JA, Spilker B (eds), *Compliance in Medical Practice and Clinical Trials*. New Raven: York; 393–403.

Levy G (1993) A pharmacokinetic perspective on medicament noncompliance. *Clin Pharmacol Ther* 54: 242–4.

Mäenpää H, Manninen V, Heinonen OP (1987) Comparison of the digoxin marker with capsule counting and compliance questionnaire methods for measuring compliance to medication in a clinical trial. *Eur Heart J* 8 (suppl I): 39–43.

Mallion JM (1995) Le pilulier electronique: une nouvelle approche du suivi therapeutique des patients. Seminaire Roussel Cardiovasculaire No. 3: *Observance des Traitements en Pathologie Cardiovasculaire*. Siege Roussel–UCLAF. Paris, 10 February.

Matsui D, Hermann C, Braudo M et al (1992) Clinical use of the Medication Event Monitoring System: a new window into pediatric compliance. *Clin Pharmacol Ther* 52: 102–3.

Matsuyama JR, Mason BJ, Jue SG (1993) Pharmacists' interventions using an electronic medication-event monitoring device's adherence data vs. pill counts. *Ann Pharmacother* 27: 851–5.

Meier P (1991) Discussion. *J Am Stat Assoc* 86(413): 19–22.

Meredith PA, Elliott HL (1994) Therapeutic coverage: reducing the risks of partial compliance. *Br J Clin Pract* 73(suppl): 13–17.

Norell SE, Granstrom PA, Wassen R (1980) A medication monitor and fluorescein technique designed to study medication behaviour. *Acta Ophthalmol* 58: 459.

Pocock SJ, Abdalla M (1998) The hope and the hazard of using compliance data in randomized controlled trials. *Stat Med* 17: 303–18.

Pullar T, Kumar S, Tindall H, Feely M (1989) Time to stop counting the tablets? *Clin Pharmacol Ther* 46: 163–8.

Reichard P, Nilsson B-Y, Rosenqvist U (1993) The effect of long-term intensified insulin treatment on the development of microvascular complications of diabetes mellitus. *N Engl J Med* 329: 304–9.

Rubin D (1991) Comment: dose–response estimands. *J Am Stat Assoc* 86(413): 22–4.

Rubin DS (1998) More powerful randomizationn-based *p*-values in double-blind trials with non-compliance. *Stat Med* 17: 371–86.

Rubio A, Cox C, Weintraub M (1992) Prediction of diltiazem plasma concentration curves from limited measurements using compliance data. *Clin Pharmacokinet* 22: 238–46.

Rudd P, Byyny RL, Zachary V et al (1989) The natural history of medication compliance in a drug trial: limitations of pill counts. *Clin Pharmacol Ther* 46: 169–76.

Salsburg D (1994) Intent to treat: the reductio ad absurdum that became gospel. *Pharmacoepidemiol Drug Safety* 3: 329–35.

Sheiner LB (1991) The intellectual health of clinical drug evaluation. *Clin Pharmacol Ther* 50: 4–9.

Sheiner LB, Rubin DB (1995) Intention to treat analysis and the goals of clinical trials. *Clin Pharmacol Ther* 57: 6–15.

Steiner TJ, Catarci T, Hering R et al (1994) If migraine prophylaxis does not work, think about compliance. *Cephalgia* 14: 463–4.

Tashkin DP, R and C, Nides M et al (1991) A nebulizer chronolog to monitor compliance with inhaler use. *Am J Med* 91(suppl 4A): 33–6S.

Temple R (1969) Rose-response and registration of new drugs. In Lasagna L, Erill S, Maranjo CA (eds), *Dose–response Relationships in Clinical Pharmacology*. Elsevier: Amsterdam; 145–67.

Urquhart J (1991) Therapeutic coverage: a parameter for analyzing the pharmacodynamic impact of partial patient compliance. Program and Abstracts, Society for Clinical Trials/International Society for Clinical Biostatistics, Joint Meeting, Brussels; p 12.

Urquhart J (1992) Time to take our medicines, seriously. *Pharm Weekbl* 127: 769–76.

Urquhart J (1994) Partial compliance in cardiovascular disease: risk implications. *Br J Clin Pract* 73(suppl): 2–12.

Urquhart J (1994) Role of patient compliance in clinical pharmacokinetics: review of recent research. *Clin Pharmacokinet* 27: 202–15.

Urquhart J (1995) Correlates of variable patient compliance in drug trials: relevance in the new health care environment. In Testa B, Meyer UA *Advances in Drug Research*, vol 26. Academic Press: London (in press).

Urquhart J (1997) The electronic medication event monitor lessons for pharmacotherapy. *Clin Pharmacokinet* 32: 345–56.

Urquhart J (1997) The electronic medication event monitor—lessons for pharmacotherapy. *Clin Pharmacokinet* 32: 345–56.

Urquhart J, de Klerk E (1998) Contending paradigms for the interpretation of data on patient compliance with therapeutic drug regimens. *Stat Med* 17: 251–67.

Van der Stichele R (1991) Measurement of patient compliance and the interpretation of randomized clinical trials. *Eur J Clin Pharmacol* 41: 27–35.

Wang PH, Lau J, Chalmers TC (1993) Meta-analysis of effects of intensive blood-glucose control on late complications of type I diabetes. *Lancet* 341: 1306–9.

Waterhouse DM, Calzone KA, Mele C, Brenner DE (1993) Adherence to oral tamoxifen: a comparison of patient self-report, pill counts, and microelectronic monitoring. *J Clin Oncol* 11: 1189–97.

24

Complementary Medicines

Anthony W. Fox

EBD Group Inc., Carlsbad, CA, USA

Complementary medicines are very widely used. Their relevance to pharmaceutical medicine is that:

- Many patients in clinical trials will be using complementary therapies (and we often omit to ask on the case report form).
- Many are pharmacologically active.
- Some risk well-described drug interactions or other adverse events.
- People uncritically pay for worthless therapies (e.g. the laetrile scandal).
- Pharmaceutical physicians are rarely trained in this area.

Geographical and cultural factors are as important as in any aspect of medicine; e.g. there are especially strong complementary therapy traditions in places as different as Germany and Utah. Furthermore, the popularity of drugs varies between places: e.g. the UK apparently has the greatest faith in garlic. The market for complementary therapies is huge: the *Nutrition Business Journal* reported in 1999 that, in the USA alone, about $14.7 billion (i.e. $14.7 thousands of millions) of complementary therapies are sold each year, and that it is a growing market.

Historically, complementary therapies were the only therapies available. Some orthodox drugs have their origin in complementary medicine: Withering's discovery of digoxin came long after the gypsy had been prescribing it for dropsy, and the Revd. Edmund Brown's willow-bark extracts were the result of his belief in the doctrine of similarities. Much of the Third World has little allopathic medicine available to it, and complementary therapies continue to be offered for a wide variety of diseases. Even in the developed world, most good hospices will have complementary therapists on staff.

The ethical aspects of this area of medicine are as varied as the therapies themselves, and could be debated almost *ad infinitum*. Thus, the purpose of this short chapter is to alert pharmaceutical physicians to this topic, discuss the most commonly encountered therapies (recognizing that this changes with time), and describe their regulatory status (which is generally quite simple).

TERMINOLOGY

The Cochrane Collaboration defines 'complementary medicine' as:

> Complementary and alternative medicine (CAM) is a broad domain of healing resources that encompass all health systems, practices, accompanying theories and beliefs, other than those intrinsic to the politically dominant health system of a particular society or culture, within a defined historical period. CAM includes all such practices and ideas self-defined by their users for prevention or treatment of disease, or promotion of health and well-being. Boundaries within CAM and between the CAM domain and that of the dominant system are not always sharp or fixed.

The term 'alternative medicine' is often now avoided in Western, developed countries, because it (often erroneously) suggested a mutual exclusivity between these therapies and conventional or 'allopathic' approaches. However, most of the diverse disciplines now prefer 'complementary medicine', so as to emphasize that the patient can benefit from a combination of orthodox and alternative approaches. There is no reason why complementary therapies may not be subject to evidence-based analysis, although there are very few such

Principles and Practice of Pharmaceutical Medicine. Edited by A. J. Fletcher, Lionel D. Edwards, Anthony W. Fox and Peter Stonier © 2002 John Wiley & Sons Ltd.

published examples, in comparison to orthodox medicine (see Critchley et al 2000).

The factor in common to all complementary therapies is that they are prescribed or recommended by practitioners that approach the patient as a whole (*holistic practitioners*). It might be said that so does any good general practitioner. However, the clinical variables used by complementary therapists are often unquantitated, may lack an orthodox clinical correlate or, occasionally, even defy translation into English, e.g. the clinical variable 'slipperiness' that is used in oriental medicine). Zollman and Vickers (1999) have pointed out that the same patient may be described as having deficient liver Qi by an acupuncturist, as having a pulsatilla constitution by a homeopath, or having a peptic ulcer by a Western physician.

Complementary therapists may or may not be graduates of orthodox medical schools. Other complementary therapists are organized professionally, if separate from orthodox medicine (the UK operates a General Chiropractic Council that regulates chiropracters in a manner exactly analogous to the General Medical Council). Other complementary therapists are trained privately, or in more informal ways, such as by experienced older relatives. Chinese traditional medicine is codified and relies on the accumulated experience of both ancient and modern practitioners (Cheng 2000).

The complementary therapies themselves also vary in their degree of characterization. Less well-characterized therapies include some forms of over-the-counter products (especially in the USA), aromatherapies, crystal therapies, and various forms of psychotherapy. This is a book about drugs, and non-pharmacological therapies (e.g. the well-regulated areas of acupuncture and physiotherapy) are beyond the scope here. 'Herbal medicines' (a term widely used in the USA) are basically unregulated pharmaceuticals; confusingly, materials that are not of vegetable origin (e.g. shark cartilage, oyster calcium, or selenates) are often included under the category of herbal medicines. 'Alkaloid' is an older term referring to any drug with a plant origin (e.g. digoxin, aspirin, and warfarin), including both orthodox and complementary therapies. Incidentally, *opiates* are alkaloids (e.g. morphine, codeine) and *opioids* are semi-synthetic or synthetic drugs, such as diacetyl-

morphine or pentazocine. '*Pharmacognosy*' is the science of plant-related, pharmacologically-active materials.

Homeopathy is the art and science of the treatment of disease using microscopical drug doses. *Homeopaths* believe that the most potent homeopathic products are those that have been most extremely diluted: in many cases, calculations based on Avagadro's number and the number of sequential dilutions suggests there may not be a single alkaloid molecule left in the administered dose. However, it is believed that the pharmaceutical method, which is at least as rigourous as for the manufacture of allopathic drugs, creates an emergent property in the administered vehicle that still has the therapeutic effect. Homeopathic medicines are available with and without prescriptions. Homeopathic prescribing resembles orthodox, if historical, prescribing. Homeopathic drugs are identified using the Latin terms for the (usually alkaloid) starting materials, and a set of apothecaries' symbols for dose size, dose frequency, and the number of dilutions required before dispensing. In the UK, homeopaths are regulated by law, and there is a *Faculty of Homeopathy* within the Royal Colleges in an analogous manner to the Faculty for Pharmaceutical Medicine. Associate members of the Faculty of Homeopathy may include any clinician with statutorily registered qualifications; the *Licence* of the Faculty is available by examination, again to all clinicians, usually after study at any of five nationally-recognized homeopathic colleges. *Membership* of the Faculty is by examination and restricted to medical practitioners, and dental and veterinary surgeons; *Fellows* are selected from among the more prominent members. The Royal Household includes one or more homeopathic practitioners.

COMMON COMPLEMENTARY MEDICINES

The nine most commonly used complementary medicines in Europe and North America are derived from St John's wort, saw palmetto, *Gingko biloba*, black cohosh, glucosamine/chondroitin, SAM-e, ephedra, ginseng, and kava. While there is a certain amount of contemporary fashion that seems to govern which products sell best, all have a long tradition in complementary therapy. These complementary medicines are not without adverse effects (Tomlinson et al 2000).

Extracts of St John's Wort (*Hypericum perforatum*)

These are used for the prevention of migraine, depression, and anxiety. The clustering of indications for neurological purposes suggests that it contains an active alkaloid or alkaloid mixture. The remittent, relapsing nature of these diseases make assessment of the limited reports of its efficacy difficult, but there are one or two fairly sound papers concerning migraine and depression. Most formulations of St John's Wort can reduce rates of absorption of antiviral drugs. Serotoninergic drugs (antimigraine agents, antidepressants, whether serotonin-specific uptake blockers or not) ought to be most likely to interact with St John's Wort, while, on its own, St John's Wort can cause photosensitivity. Pharmaceutical physicians should investigate herbal drug use whenever this unusual adverse event arises (see also Kava, below).

Saw Palmetto (*Palmito caroliniensis*)

This is the State tree of South Carolina, being the only palm indigenous to the east coast of North America. Its seeds (which are used to derive the pharmaceutical) are rich in fatty acids, their esters, and sterols. The extract of these seeds is recommended for mild symptoms referable to the prostate, without pharmacological rationale, and with the danger that patients will use the product to temporize for symptoms that could lead to the early diagnosis of malignancy. The doses administered are usually insufficient to reduce the absorption of oral fat-soluble drugs, but it would seem wise to separate the administration of vitamin D, warfarin, etc. and this complementary therapy.

Gingko biloba

A robust tree that has remained essentially unevolved for far longer than almost all other tree species, hence this is also known as the 'fossil tree' in the far east, where most of its fossils are found. A specimen of *Gingko biloba* was the only living thing to survive at ground zero, Hiroshima, recovering its stature from the surviving root within about 10 years. The product is used for memory loss and mental alertness, without good clinical trial evidence, but it has enjoyed this reputation for centuries in Asia, and now worldwide. Ginkaloids are antioxidant, but how this mechanism relates to its proposed neurological and cardiovascular effects is unclear. Some *G. biloba* extracts increase both the antiplatelet properties of aspirin and the anticoagulant properties of warfarin, perhaps suggesting that the interaction takes place at the level of plasma protein binding; which flavanoid or terpene lactone is responsible for this is unknown, and perhaps it is due to some other, unidentified component of these particular formulations. Hydrolysed amino acids from cow brain is recommended for the same purpose in Central Europe (e.g. Cerebrolyticu® in Romania).

Black Cohosh (*Cimicifuga racemosa* or 'Bugbane')

This is native to the eastern USA and was first identified by the Algonquin tribes as an aid to inducing labour, and treating peri- and postmenopausal symptoms. Separation scientists have found no factors with known oestragenic activity. It would be therefore be illogical to impute beneficial effects of this material on prevention of coronary heart disease or osteoporosis.

Glucosamine/Chondroitin combinations

These are promoted as 'optimal support for joint health', and to 'repair joint cartilage' in the USA. Both materials may be prepared from either bovine or ovine sources, which reputable manufacturers usually obtain from herds that are free from scrapie or bovine spongiform encephalopathy prions. Glucosamines are also found in chitin (the material giving strength to insect exoskeletons and the shells of marine arthropods) and some plant cell walls. Patients with allergies to crabs and lobsters are also liable to be allergic to glucosamine formulations derived from these sources. Chondroitin is a sulphated mucopolysaccharide found in mammalian cartilage or tendons. Glucosamine, in large doses, can increase insulin requirements in diabetics. Chondroitin increases the likelihood of relative overdose with warfarin, probably by competition for plasma protein binding sites and increase in free warfarin concentrations.

SAM-e

Recently this became popular in North America, although it has been used for much longer in Europe. It is recommended for the kindred syndromes of fibromyalgia and chronic fatigue syndrome, as well as unrelated diseases such as osteoarthritis and Parkinson's disease. SAM-e is also recommended for depression and anxiety, which can obviously be either primary or secondary to the other indications. Pure SAM-e is (usually) the *S*-isomer of adenosyl (L-) methionine, but it is often formulated with B vitamins; endogenous adenosyl methionine is found in the mammalian liver, and thus swallowing 200 mg/day (a typical dose) may not be able to materially change the biological economy of this substance. Perhaps by extrapolation from the known detoxicating properties of sulphydryl-containing amino acids, it proposed that SAM-e removes 'harmful metabolites' and that these in turn are responsible for the diseases for which the drug is indicated. It is also proposed that SAM-e can 'optimize the synthesis of neurotransmitters, glutathione, and cartilage'; since glutathione is synthesized in many mammalian tissues at high concentration, always from glutamate, cysteine and glycine, this claim cannot be entirely correct. One manufacturer's trade mark for SAM-e is 'Nature's Wonder®' and sells SAM-e formulated with unidentified 'methylation factors' as a 'complete methylation support formula'.

Ephedra spp.

Known as 'ma huang' in Chinese medicine, this is a large genus of woody, jointed, desert shrubs. These shrubs appear to be leafless from a distance, but on close inspection possess scale-like leaf structures at the nodes. Ephedrine, pseudoephedrine, and related alkaloids are the active principles. *Ephedra* is marketed for many logical purposes, e.g. as decon-

gestants, bronchodilation, etc. Less appropriate uses are to heighten awareness, remain awake when studying for examinations, and a street-sold alternative to illegal amphetamines. The predictable adverse events are hypertensive episodes, stroke, cardiac arrhythmias and seizures, many in young people, and after doses as low as 1–5 mg, reported at a rate of about 100/year to the US Food and Drug Administration (FDA). During general anaesthesia, unexpected hypertensive problems occur due to supra-additive interactions. Renal stones have been reported to be associated with *Ephedra* use in one or two case reports, although a causal relationship must be viewed, at present, as uncertain. It would be illogical to recommend *Ephedra* to patients with glaucoma, diabetes, hyperthyroidism, and any other condition that would usually cause contraindication of sympathomimetic agonists.

Ginseng

This is an extract of *Panax schinseng* (China) or *P. quinquefolius* (North America). It is a five-leaved herb with red berries. The part used for making complementary therapies is the aromatic root. Ginseng is recommended for holistic measures of good health, usually stated, at their most specific, as enhancing resistance to stress and improving sexual function. There are one or two case reports that ginseng can antagonize the effects of warfarin, but otherwise this herbal medicine appears to cause almost no adverse events. Ginseng is more widely used in North America and the Far East than in Europe.

Kava

This is an Australasian shrubby pepper (*Piper methysticum*). Amidst much ceremony, its crushed roots are made into an intoxicating beverage by the peoples of the Molucca Islands and the Northern coast of Australia. Kava is usually recommended for anxiety. Kava has sedative and extrapyramidal effects, in common with some anticholinergic and antidopaminergic drugs, and probably has synergistic sedative effects when administered with benzodiazepines, barbiturates (barbitals), alcohol, and some antiepileptic and antipsychotic drugs. Kava makes parkinsonism worse, and can cause drug rash, photosensitivity, and itching.

Other Complementary Medicines

There are many thousands of other complementary medicines. These range from large doses of vitamins or minerals to extracts of many other plants and animals. Most are not characterized toxicologically or pharmacologically; the properties of the simplest may be anticipated with a good clinical biochemistry textbook at hand.

In Hong Kong, limited regulatory control of many traditional medicines has been found to be necessary, due to their toxic nature. These regulations extend over root extracts from several *Aconitum* spp. (containing C_{19} terpinoid sodium channel-blocking drugs), various herbs containing anticholinergic substances, toad venoms (which containg Na–K ATPase-inhibiting bufotoxins), and even preparations from the more familiar geneta *Impatiens*, *Rhododendron*, and *Euphorbia* (Tomlinson et al 2000). The view through the window of a Chinese pharmacy, in the Chinatown of any city in Asia, Europe or the Americas, may cause different emotions in the pharmaceutical physician and pharmacologist. While both may feel daunted, the true pharmacologist also beholds an almost inexhaustible new supply of drug development leads!

ADVERSE EFFECTS DUE TO COMPLEMENTARY THERAPIES

It should be noted that almost all types of adverse event have been described. These include agonist–antagonist interaction, protein binding competition, metabolic adaptation, and pharmacodynamic synergy.

The general public seems to have a preconceived notion that drugs with 'natural' origins, or those which may be bought without prescription, are automatically safe (perhaps this notion complements the uncritical assumption that there is no need to rigorously prove efficacy). It is curious and illogical to assume that a complementary therapy has sufficient pharmacological activity to make an improvement in health (however imprecisely that may be defined) and yet insufficient properties to cause harm. Perhaps only the homeopathic medicines are safe in overdose.

Part of the problem is that adverse reactions to 'natural' therapies are not reported in the same way as for orthodox drugs (Barnes et al 1998). Reporting bias also tends towards the association of adverse effects with the condition being treated, rather than from the 'harmless' over-the-counter or herbal remedy that has been administered.

REGULATORY ASPECTS

Homeopathic drugs are regulated in much the same way as allopathic drugs; there are some over-the-counter formulations, but most are prescribed and can only be dispensed by a pharmacist in the UK. Chinese medicines are essentially unregulated; as in mediaeval Europe, these can be prescribed by both a Chinese medical practitioner and a Chinese pharmacist (using the term 'Chinese' to describe their disciplines, not their nationality), and much responsibility rests on the pharmacist for identification of the correct plants, resisting the purchase of cheap materials from unreliable suppliers, and knowing what to look for in quality control. Other forms of herbal remedy (including all nine examples discussed above) are freely available in supermarkets and pharmacies in most jurisdictions. Mail order, using the Web for advertising, is increasing, and will doubtless cause legal issues with cross-border commerce and transportation in the future.

In the USA, most herbal manufacturers simply write a letter to the US FDA notifying when a new product is being introduced, and sometimes with an example of the labels and tablets for identification purposes. It is unclear whether the Food, Drug and Cosmetic Act applies in this situation, but if so, then it is certainly not enforced. FDA does maintain adverse event registers for all forms of drug through the usual Medwatch forms.

REFERENCES AND FURTHER READING

Barnes J, Mills SY, Abbot NC et al (1998) Different standards for reporting ADRs to herbal remedies. *Br J Clin Pharmacol* 45: 496–500.

Cheng JT (2000) Review: drug therapy in Chinese traditional medicine. *J Clin Pharmacol* 40: 445–50.

Critchley JAJH, Zhang Y, Suthisisang CC et al (2000) Alternative therapies and medical science: designing clinical trials of alternative/complementary medicines—is evidence-based traditional Chinese medicine attainable? *J Clin Pharmacol* 40: 462–7.

Eisenberg DM, Kessler RC, Foster C et al (1993) Unconventional medicine in the United States. Prevalence, costs, and patterns of use. *N Engl J Med* 328: 246–52.

Ernst E (1996) *Complementary Medicine: A Critical Appraisal.* Butterworth-Heinemann: Oxford, UK.

Tomlinson B, Chan TYK, Chan JCN et al (2000) Toxicity of complementary therapies: an Eastern perspective. *J Clin Pharmacol* 40: 451–6.

Zollman C, Vickers A (1999) What is complementary medicine? *Br Med J* 319: 693–6.

Section V

Drug Registration

Introduction

Anthony W. Fox

EBD Group Inc., Carlsbad, CA, USA

Regulatory affairs is the art of making drug development and marketing comply with the requirements of governments. This section starts with the Food and Drug Administration (FDA) in the USA because its requirements are the most comprehensive in the world. Furthermore, much of the lore and history of drug regulation has developed from historical events in that jurisdiction. We then consider the European Community (EC) and Japan separately.

Of all industries in the world, pharmaceutical companies are, by far, the most closely regulated. This is one aspect of governmental care for the public health, which is quite proper: motor car manufacturers do not have the benefit of domestic and foreign government departments overseeing the design of their next year's model! The costs of this regulation are immense, and comprise a major fraction of drug development budgets. However, given the diversity of approaches that have been taken by different national governments, there is scope for debate about their relative merits. The International Conference in Harmonization (ICH) is now making major contributions in this area, and drug development will become more efficient as a result, thus commanding a chapter of its own.

The impact of regulatory compliance on preclinical and clinical drug development is almost limitless. At the strategic (clinical development plan) level, the target, right from the start, should be draft labeling that is compliant with the various jurisdictions in which the drug is to be marketed. At the tactical level, the need for permission to study investigational drugs, and its reporting, are part of the daily life of the pharmaceutical physician. Some regulatory authorities involve themselves in broader areas. For example, the FDA scrutinizes promotional materials, imposes restrictions on trademarks that exceed those associated with their national registration, and awards favorable proprietary protections for the study of rare diseases or to encourage research in pediatrics. All regulatory authorities are interested in drug tolerability, both before and after marketing.

It behooves the pharmaceutical physician, in any subspecialty, to have a firm grasp of the principles of regulation.

25

United States Regulations

William Kennedy

Consultant, Delaware, USA former V.P. Regulation Affairs

THE FOOD AND DRUG ADMINISTRATION: HOW WE GOT TO WHERE WE ARE

Once upon a time... there was no FDA. However, the history of food and drug regulation began well before any modern government administration, anywhere in the World. Drugs and foods have only become distinguished from each other in the relatively recent past, and, it can be argued, as yet incompletely in the USA.

The ancient Greeks, Romans and Arabs all regulated food and drugs. Principally, their concern was with product *purity*, one of the three pivotal concepts that still form the basis for drug approval today. The typical penalty in ancient times for violating the standards was the loss of the dominant hand that had made the adulterated product. The Arabs were probably the most conscientious of regulators, with standards for about 2000 drug products, and, like today's FDA, they were the first to establish a professional staff of food and drug inspectors. Their penalty for a baker of underweight loaves exceeded that of the drug adulterer: the bakers went summarily into their own ovens.

In 1202, the first English regulation is identified, traditionally, as the Assize of Bread. In fact, this assize had been held by manorial lords for a lot longer than this, and the lords were often also the exclusive owners of the ovens. To remedy this small aspect of local despotism, presumably with skepticism about self-regulation, the new national law forbade the incorporation of ground peas or beans in the flour meal. Meanwhile, the London grocers had organized, and formed their own Guild, again with self-regulation of a wider range of foodstuffs. In the seventeenth century, the London apothecaries (makers of medicines and also licensed medical practitioners in their own right) devolved from the Grocers. The Worshipful Society of Apothecaries of London still exists, can still award a medical license (although this is quite rare among British physicians), and is now the largest of all the London Guilds.

What with 1776 and all that, the British jurisdiction of food and drug regulation ceased to obtain in what were to become the USA. The apothecaries were still people who had trained mostly in London or Germany, or had graduated to professional status by apprenticeship. However, there was a void in national regulation of food and drugs. British patents, which had already been awarded to American drug recipes, also became null and void.

Over-the-counter (OTC) medicines (or 'patent' medicines) thrived in this void. The American patent process was also undeveloped, so these became what we would perhaps view as trade secrets, held by named apothecaries and their apprentices. There were also no inspectors. Moreover, the British were not quickly mollified by the new political reality: European medicines were included in the embargo, and yankee ingenuity began to be expressed to the full. The problem quickly evolved: who was to say that the 'eye of newt' in the Scottish witches' potion was not actually a bit of chicken?

It has been said that the drug law in the USA developed in the eighteenth and nineteenth centuries with all the red, white and blue of the aniline dyes that quickly became available. Regulations in this country rapidly developed in a characteristically idiosyncratic manner.

Sewers and food do not mix. This was the era of rapid expansion of Boston, Philadelphia, New York, Baltimore, and eventually Washington DC itself. Massachusetts regulated food for the first time in 1784, but this again was a feeble attempt

Principles and Practice of Pharmaceutical Medicine. Edited by A. J. Fletcher, Lionel D. Edwards, Anthony W. Fox and Peter Stonier © 2002 John Wiley & Sons Ltd.

to control purity. No attempt was made to address the potions used to treat ineffectively the infectious diseases that were rampant.

'Dr. Feelgood' potions, typically named after the apothecary who compounded them, had eponymous effects. These potions usually contained alcohol and morphine, were used indiscriminately, and at least made people feel good. One of these survives, ironically enough in England, and is called 'Dr. John Collis-Brown's Compound'.

The American geography constrained the regulatory environment. First, there was a lot of pioneer activity in the West: trained professionals were not the first to climb on the covered wagons. Second, new religions were being spawned at a rate far faster than had ever occurred in any European country. Third, worthless medicines were being distributed and used over millions of square miles with, at best, only rudimentary communications. The promotion of medicines became a form of entertainment, by bogus professors, showmen, fakers, and embezellers in Desert Gulch! Meanwhile, little opportunity was taken to learn from the Native Americans, whose herbals were often quite well developed, with active pharmacognosy. But the national government was not stirred into action until its own interests were directly affected: soldiers in the Mexican–American War were poisoned by ineffective antimalarials south of the Rio Grande.

And so it was, in 1848, that the first drug regulation was established in the USA. It simply banned the import of impure drugs. The medicine man shows were left to local regulation (a legislative omission that is still with us today). And so it was that in 1850, the State of California became the first to enact anything resembling a comprehensive drug regulation.

By 1900, it is estimated that about $40 million per annum was being spent on drug advertising. This was mostly in newspapers, who were thus only too happy to ally with potion makers in stirring up public opinion against the national regulation of their products. Medicines (some up to 50% alcoholic tinctures) became the only source of alcohol in some communities where religion forbade wine and whisky. For the more adventurous, morphine, opium, cannabinoids, and cocaine were available, even in some of the earliest formulations of Coca-Cola, although not, of course, today.

Harvey Wiley was a hero among the villains. He headed the Federal Bureau of Chemistry, and began calling for national regulation in 1890. His 'poison squad', the forerunners of the Inspectorate Branch of FDA today, began documenting and, on occasion, prosecuting the makers of fake and poisonous drugs. The convictions were usually for things that were very egregious, probably because Dr. Wiley could only prosecute under the general laws. Unlike today's FDA Inspectors, the members of this squad were expected to sample the questionable product themselves, and then give first-hand evidence of the adverse effects that they experienced!

Specific regulation began in 1902, and concerned the purity of serums and vaccines to be used in humans: the Center for Biologics Evaluations and Research (CBER) thus has a longer history than its colleague center for drugs (CDER).

Part of US food and drug regulatory lore includes, at this point, an unlikely convergence of two famous characters. One was President Theodore Roosevelt, nationalist ex-'rough-rider', soldier in Cuba, and hero of San Juan Hill. The other was Upton Sinclair, America's first published communist, and author of *The Jungle*, intended as an éxposé of North American capitalism at its worst. Sinclair's book was being serialized in the DC newspapers, which the President habitually read during his high-cholesterol breakfast, which always included sausages. In one daily episode of the book, Sinclair described the use of offal, floor-waste, and other abominations at the end of the daily sausage run, in the attempt to maximize profits. Dr. Wiley had his political ally, and the Pure Food and Drug Act (PFDA) and Meat Inspection Act were the result (1906).

The PFDA banned adulterated or misbranded drugs from interstate commerce, and this remains the legal basis for FDA actions to this day. Today's definitions of 'adulterated' and 'misbranded' are also those of nearly a century ago. The philosophy, however, has long been forgotten: if you made bad drugs, then you had to sell them within your own community, and the local law enforcement people should have found you out fairly easily for themselves. This is, arguably, a survival of the Anglo-Saxon principle of frankpledge within the twentieth century US laws.

From among the wide variety of dyestuffs available in the north-eastern factories before the First World War, just seven were authorized for human consumption by the Certified Color Regulations (1907). This brought dyestuffs within the canon of interstate commerce law. This is not as incongruent as it might seem, because among these dyestuffs were the first primitive antibiotics.

But, then as now, the US Supreme court was not averse to getting involved in unprecedented situations. In 1911, the Court held that the 1906 Act did not prohibit false or misleading therapeutic claims, but was strictly to be interpreted in terms of purity and composition. PFDA was thus amended in 1912, to include specifically false therapeutic claims. However, the Act now required proof of intent to be fraudulent: it was essentially a criminal matter. This need for proof of intent made the Act hard to enforce, and few could be punished or made to change their ways. In 1914, a further amendment defined that the presence of poisonous or adulterous substances was specifically a violation of the Act, although the definitions of precisely what was a poisonous or adulterous substance would have to be developed on precedent.

It was not until 1924 that a further PFDA amendment that made mere statements potentially a violation under the Act. For the first time, exaggerated claims of therapeutic effectiveness could be proscribed. This amendment went further to specify that even true statements that nonetheless deceive or misinform would henceforth fall foul of the Act (malt vinegar, without any written claim to be apple cider vinegar, but with an apple depicted on the label, was cited as an example of how this situation could arise).

Ever since 1906, there had been many challenges to the Act and its amendments, and this consumed much administrative time and money. The innovation of 1930, expansion of the Bureau of Chemistry into a renamed Food and Drug Administration, was designed to relieve this administrative burden. The new Agency introduced a Bill into Congress, that was designed to invigorate and modernize the, by now patchwork and creaking, amended PDFA.

Once again, there was resistance to the Bill. However, communications were modernized, and public opinion was moulded not only by newspapers but also by radio—and radio could be heard hundreds of miles away. One small fly in the proverbial ointment, however, was that Teddy Roosevelt's nephew, Franklin Roosevelt, was now President; the President was wheelchair-bound due to polio, and believed in the therapeutic value of hot springs and other complementary therapies.

At about this time (1931), an OTC potion called 'Jake' poisoned hundreds of people. It was probably a peripheral neurotoxin, due to an adulterant in an extract of Jamaican ginger: 'Jake-leg' became a recognized syndrome. While Jake 'the Peg', with an extra leg (i.e. an axillary crutch), became famous, it needed a much bigger disaster to move legislative and public opinion.

Domagk demonstrated in 1935 that sulphonamide-containing dyes could protect mice from infection; he became a Nobel laureate in 1938. The nostrum artists could hardly believe their luck: now they could peddle a drug that actually worked! The favoured formulation at the time was an elixir, probably a holdover from evasion of alcohol restrictions due to religion, or the earlier flirt with prohibition. In any case, one company, supposedly laudibly, searched for a non-alcoholic solution for their sulphonamide. They chose diethylene glycol. In four weeks of marketing, the product was not a success: only 353 patients drank it, and of these, 107 died. They were mostly children, and there was no renal dialysis in 1936. Thousands could have been killed had the company's market analysis been accurate.

But finally, there was sufficient groundswell, and FDA obtained passage of the Food, Drug and Cosmetic Act (FD&C Act) in 1938. Thus, the FD&C Act added *safety* as the second pivotal leg of drug approval. There was still no requirement to prove product efficacy. But in 1941, with most of the world at war, an often overlooked piece of US legislation was passed. The FD&C Act was amended, to reflect an FDA proposal. Henceforth, FDA was empowered to certify the potency of insulin. This required a bioassay, and for the first time FDA was able to regulate pharmacodynamics. It was short step to therapeutic efficacy.

In 1943, the Supreme Court again got involved. In an otherwise obscure case, it held that FDA was empowered to establish standards for products labeling. The four principal arms of drug approval were finally concentrated in the hands of a single Agency: purity, safety, efficacy, and labeling. To this day, much of the power of FDA is exercised by its control of what a label says, and not by the pharmacological characteristics of the particular drug in question. To Europeans this is sometimes a surprising concept, but in fact the principal extends to other areas of American commerce: e.g. cars may be imported into California, depending upon not whether the vehicle meets the emissions standards, but rather whether it is labeled as meeting those standards.

In the 1950s, the Delancy Amendment to the FD&C Act authorized an investigation into the new dyes, flavorings, and preservatives that were becoming available in an era of unprecedented chemical innovation. There was already a clear need to update the FD&C Act, and the Food Additive Amendment of 1958 was one result, which, among other things, prohibited carcinogenic materials from foods and drugs. This required a method to establish carcinogenicity, which is now an important element in the toxicology package for an overwhelming majority of approved drugs. There are now exceptions. Antineoplastic drugs are often themselves carcinogenic, and the absolute restriction on such materials is somewhat tempered. Furthermore, we now understand the dose relationships for chemical carcinogenesis, and how to measure it, very well; high school exercises now routinely exceed limits of detection available in the 1950s. But the princip had been established in law. November 1958 saw FDA recalling the entire cranberry crop, just before the Thanksgiving holiday, because there was a fear of weedkiller contamination which they had established was a carcinogen in animals!

The other major piece of legislation in the 1950s was the Durham-Humphrey Amendment to the FD&C Act. Humphrey (unsuccessful Presidential candidate and later Vice-President) had been a pharmacist; he wanted to clarify what should and should not be an OTC drug. Hitherto, the only reason to get a prescription from a physician, and have it filled by a pharmacist, was because the patient did not know of an OTC drug to meet his/her need, and the prescription was one which needed to be compounded by a professional. The Amendment provided, perhaps artificially, that when a disease or a drug side effect needed a physician's attention, then any treatment required a prescription, and that only a licensed pharmacist

could fill a prescription. Some view this as the genesis of general diagnostic education by the pharmaceutical industry, and, in turn, the origins of direct-to-consumer advertizing designed to drive patients into their doctors' offices.

In the late 1950s, there were also many other reasons to seek reform. FDA's ability to regulate efficacy assessments was still restricted to a small number of highly specialized products, and modern advertising techniques were getting under way. As usual, there was public resistance, and it required a big disaster to get things done—to be precise, thalidomide.

Dr. Frances Kelsey had the thalidomide application on her desk. She was busy and had simply not got around to it. Then from Europe she heard about a question of peripheral neuropathy, and possibly thyrotoxicity; at that point she made an active decision to hold up the approval. It was an Australian dermatologist who identified drug-induced phocomelia, and the rest is well known. Only nine cases of phocomelia were reported in the USA, from an exposure of about 4000 women of child-bearing potential, most of whom were pregnant. Kelsey received a medal from President Kennedy.

Amazingly enough, the 1962 amendments would still not have kept thalidomide off the market in the USA. The precise strain of rodent that would have been required to identify the lesion was not in common use, and the adverse event frequency in neonates, in the average-sized new drug application (NDA) of the day, might not detect adverse events of such low frequency. However, the 1962 amendments required, in the general case, that drugs should be demonstrated to be effective prior to approval, for the first time.

The 1962 Kefauver–Harris amendments provided further capability to the FDA. They set forth the requirements of the investigational new drug application (IND) process. The FDA was empowered, for the first time, to seize a drug and cause it to be withdrawn. Adverse event reporting to FDA became mandatory. Labeling and advertizing requirements were clarified, and transferred that responsibility to FDA from the Federal Trade Commission. Inspections of manufacturing sites were also facilitated by these far-reaching amendments.

In 1966, it was estimated that there were about 4000 drugs available that had been approved on pre-1962 criteria. FDA commissioned the National Academy of Sciences/National Research Council (NAS/NRC) to review these 'grandfathered drugs' against the modern standards. Some of the reviews lasted 15 years, and were contentious, while other drugs felt to be important had to be transferred to new manufacturing sites. The abbreviated NDA (ANDA; mostly thought of today in connexion with generic drug approvals) was invented in 1970 for the latter purpose. The NAS review was extended to OTC drugs in 1972. Meanwhile, devices came under the FDA aegis in 1972, and biologics and vaccines were subsumed under the FDA umbrella in 1972.

As regulations increased, then so did the risks of drug development. Complaints were loud that rare diseases, offering small potential markets, were increasingly ignored because the costs of drug development to address those markets had become so high as to deter research and development by the pharmaceutical manufacturers. After much debate, a compromise was reached in the Orphan Drug Act (1983). If it could be demonstrated that the incidence of the disease in question was fewer than 200 000 persons year in the USA, then Orphan Drug designation would be allowed. This provided tax credits and exclusivity guarantees, should an eventual NDA succeed. Currently, there is criticism that this absolute number of 200 000 patients has not been raised with time, since the US population is now greatly increased since 1983, and, unless amended, this legislation will eventually become moot. Meanwhile, there is also often debate with FDA on borderline cases of calculation of incidence. Several drugs that are on the market in Europe are denied to Americans by reason of FDA not granting Orphan Drug designation, and there being no other method for gaining exclusivity for at least the 7 years that the Orphan Drug Act provides.

The Waxman–Hatch Amendment (1984) traded off patent term restoration for innovative drug development with generic drug ANDA approval. The contents of the ANDA were clearly stated for the first time. Furthermore, FDA review times could be added to the patent-awarded period of exclusivity. Currently FDA compares these review periods in a highly conservative manner: the review period is compared to the period that the drug company has been conducting IND research, and

the public is led to the view that FDA review is a trivial component of total development time. Furthermore, FDA stops this artificial clock every time they send a question about the NDA back to the Sponsor, even though review activities at the Agency continue. In one case, in the 1990s, when these procedures had been well-established, 30 months elapsed between NDA submission and approval, but the patent term restoration was only 9 months; no new clinical trials or toxicology studies were needed during this review.

The generic scandal of the 1980s involved pharmaceutical companies making, and FDA staff accepting, bribes in the interests of rapid generic drug approval. No new legislation resulted, even though two Vice-presidential commissions (one Republican, the other Democratic) inquired into the matter. Similarly, there was no new legislation following the massive Clinton initiative; drug pricing was probably the principal missed target on that occasion. It is arguable whether or not these vents triggered the subsequent spate of mergers and acquisitions within the pharmaceutical industry.

The Prescription Drug Users Fee Act (PDUFA; 1992) traded off fees paid upon NDA submission for performance standards on the part of FDA. This was the first time that any effective accountability had been applied to FDA, somewhat reversing the orientation of the Agency. PDUFA is due for reauthorization in 2002, and an analysis of its effect is being conducted by several industry and government organizations.

The last major revision of food and drug law took place in 1997, coincident with the first reauthorization of PDUFA. The Food and Drug Administration Modernization Act (FDAMA) of 1997 was only the third major overhaul of the original 1906 Act. It was the first to occur without the impetus of a disaster or perceived disaster. After a troubled start in 1996, FDAMA received overwhelmingly positive support in both houses of the US Congress, getting 98 of 100 votes in the Senate, and a unanimous vote in the House.

The perceived need for FDAMA by Congress, the industry and ultimately the FDA was the recognition that while the law and the regulations had changed little from the 1962 Amendments, the requirements made by the FDA of the industry had increased dramatically. Part was due to advances in technology and medicine, but part was due to FDA reviewer preferences. Both of these contributed to the phenomenon known as 'regulatory creep', which was demonstrated by wide variances across the FDA in requirements. While there were some significant breakthroughs that advanced health care and the regulatory process, a major portion of the legislation focused on the formalization of 'best practices' that existed within the FDA and making these the standard throughout the FDA.

Some of the major breakthroughs of FDAMA included:

- Formalized the evidence needed from pharmacoeconomic studies.
- Authorized and regulated the dissemination of information on unapproved uses of approved products to health care providers by pharmaceutical companies.
- Enhanced the availability of labeling information for use in pediatric patients, by recognizing the difficulties of developing drugs for this group and providing an incentive to undertake this work.

Examples of modernization which were the result of identifying 'best practices' within FDA and making them the standard include:

- Improving access to unapproved drugs.
- Clarifying the definition of 'substantial evidence of efficacy' to include only one pivotal study, provided there is adequate confirmatory evidence. This had long been used for the approval of oncology drugs, but was now able to be applied more widely.
- Formalization of various administrative aspects of the IND and NDA process.

While PDUFA and FDAMA offered significant opportunities to improve the drug development process and make more drugs available to more people, more quickly, for the most part, the promise has yet to be fully realized. There are two reasons for this, both acknowledged before the legislative changes were initiated. The first reason is that the 'regulatory creep' that was being corrected was something that took place over the period 1962–1997. It would be unrealistic, not to

mention unsound, to expect 35 years of change to be corrected overnight, and at the same time maintain a productive regulatory agency. Congress allowed for an implementation period. The second reason flows from the first. The drug development process is long and resource-intense. It is difficult to turn midstream. Once the FDA starts changing, the industry will have to respond with changes in the development process. This takes even more time. Simply stated, many of the changes have just not had sufficient time to get into the process.

ECONOMIC CONSIDERATIONS

FDA has jurisdiction over about 20–25% of the gross national product (GNP) of the USA. In 1996, the FDA-regulated industries comprised about $1750 billion (i.e. 1.75×10^{12}), thus dwarfing the US Department of Defense budget by about a six-fold difference. This is about 150% of the entire GNP of the UK. These regulated industries include all medical devices, all drugs, many other OTC or *in vitro* diagnostic materials, and almost all food (meat is still the responsibility of the Department of Agriculture, under Teddy Roosevelt's 1906 Act). These activities are all mandated by the FD&C Act, and its various amendments.

In addition, FDA engages in various cooperative projects with organizations such as the National Institutes of Health, the Centers for Disease Control, the Drug Enforcement Agency, and the US Public Health Service (many of whose officers serve attachments to FDA). A certain amount of independent research is supported in the FDA budget, as well as international liaisons. FDA, too, conducts lobbying and legislative functions.

ORGANIZATIONAL ASPECTS

FDA is part of the Department of Health and Human Services, which is represented at Secretary level within each president's cabinet. The secretary appoints a commissioner to head the FDA, and this is usually a political appointment (i.e. not held by a career civil servant). The commissioner appoints assistants or deputies to head the following centers or offices:

- CDER
- CBER
- Center for Food Safety and Applied Nutrition
- Center for Devices and Radiological Health
- Center for Veterinary Medicine
- Office of Regulatory Affairs
- Office of Orphan Product Development
- National Center for Toxicological Research

The assistant and deputy commissioners might be either political appointees or career civil servants. Each of these sub-divisions is typically further subdivided. For example, CBER has offices of Management, Compliance, Therapeutic Research and Review, Vaccines Research and Review, Establishment Licensing and Product Surveillance, Blood Products, and Communications and Training. Each are typically led by career civil servant Office Directors, although, currently, the Office of Orphan Product Development is headed by an Admiral from the US Public Health Service.

CDER has a larger product development responsibility than CBER, and thus has five Therapeutic Review Divisions, each led by a career civil servant Division Director. But the other divisions are similar to the CBER model, with divisions for Epidemiology and Statistics, Compliance, Pharmaceutical Sciences (including a specialized office of New Drug Chemistry), Biopharmaceutics, and Generic Drugs. It seems likely that an Office for Toxicology will soon be established.

Most centers or offices have access to a wide network of inspectors. These inspectors operate worldwide, and audit both animal and clinical studies, as well as manufacturing processes and premises. Such audits can be 'for cause', e.g. a complaint from the public or an emergent safety issue, or 'routine'. Pivotal clinical trials in a submitted NDA or BLA will usually garner an inspection of the clinical trials sites and statutory documentation.

This inspection process has recently been augmented with the establishment of an Office of the Inspector General (OIG), which reports at the level of the Secretary, not the FDA Commissioner. One of the first announced targets of the OIG, selected from the entire realm of foods and drugs that FDA regulates, is clinical trials. In particular, the OIG is actively investigating informed consent documents, and also has notified Institutional Review Boards

(the US equivalent of the Ethics Committee) that they are in for close scrutiny.

Make no mistake. One big difference between the EMEA and FDA is that the FDA are also the police (and often the judge and jury, as well). Do not take lightly the appearance of your name on Form 1571.

INVESTIGATIONAL NEW DRUGS (INDS)

The student is urged to read the Code of Federal Regulations with this title, beginning at 21CFR310. The legal basis for an IND was set up in the 1962 amendments. It is unlawful to transport an unapproved drug across state lines unless FDA has issued an exemption. The IND is technically an exemption from the requirements of an NDA. Drugs labeled 'Not for human use' are also exempt from the NDA requirements before being transported, but carry regulatory restrictions. Note that, technically and legally, these regulations apply just as much to non-commercial research physicians, for example, in universities, as to pharmaceutical companies.

The structure of an IND the application is contained in the regulation and is quite easily followed. Almost all pharmaceutical companies, contract research organizations, and universities have templates for the writing of these documents. All the animal data, the proposed clinical study protocol, a clinical investigators' brochure, and the chemistry and manufacturing controls must be described. Once an IND is active, then it can be amended with further clinical protocols, additional toxicology data, etc., as the development program proceeds.

The IND differs in a number of ways from its European counterparts. First, it is much longer; a typical IND is at least 1000 pages, and for drugs with foreign human experience often many multiples of this number. The UK Clinical Trials Certificate, used very rarely for this reason, and not the Clinical Trials Exemption (CTX), would be the nearer comparison. Second, an IND is required for all human exposure to investigational new drugs, and this includes normal volunteer studies. Third, all being well, there is only a 30-day wait between filing and commencement of the clinical study; no news from FDA after this time period has elapsed is presumptive evidence that the study may proceed (most FDA divisions will, in fact, issue affirmative letters that this is the case, within 30 days). Fourth, once an IND has become active, there is no subsequent 30 day wait when further clinical protocols are submitted.

FDA is at liberty to impose partial or total clinical holds on any protocols that it receives. Partial holds might limit, for example, the maximum dose that can be employed, prevent commencement until additional safety monitoring measures have been instituted, or restrict dose frequency.

It is no longer the case that an IND is needed merely for the export of an investigational agent to another jurisdiction, provided that the regulations that obtain in that jurisdiction are adhered to. This was one former peculiarity of the restriction on transportation of unapproved drugs across state lines.

There are variants of the IND process.

MEETINGS WITH FDA

Many Europeans are surprised at the access that pharmaceutical companies have to the reviewing divisions of FDA. The typical investigational drug will be the subject of a pre-IND meeting, which FDA will provide at its discretion, and for which the agenda may be set by the prospective applicant. These meetings can be also held by telephone conference, and FDA is getting quite good at accepting electronic files of data. An IND is, however, only allotted a number upon its submission.

It is fair to say that US companies differ on their approach to pre-IND meetings. Most companies probably view pre-IND meetings as desirable. However, under the law, proprietary information is only required to be kept confidential by FDA when it is the subject of an IND. No known major disclosure has happened, but companies would have little recourse if FDA leaked information following a pre-IND meeting. The other problem is that without an IND in place, FDA has no obligation to meet with clinical trials sponsors: reviewers up against a PDUFA deadline on another project are unlikely to prepare thoroughly for a pre-IND meeting, and may entirely change their views after the IND, when they become

obligated to adopt a position. Some companies file the IND first, with a simultaneous request for a meeting.

Typically, during Phase I and II development there will be sporadic communications between the developers of investigational drugs and FDA. These might be to clarify issues over post-IND clinical protocols, reach agreement on compatibility of toxicology data with clinical study design, carcinogenicity testing requirements (typically starting at this time due to their long duration and the necessity for their completion before filing the NDA), and the many technical matters associated with the scale-up of the chemistry and production processes.

It is typical to hold an end-of-Phase II meeting (EOP2). At this meeting, the FDA will review the current Phase I and Phase II clinical data, and the state of the toxicology program. The objective is to reach agreement on the design of the Phase III studies that will support NDA approval, as well as to identify any further problems that may be ameliorated without delaying the NDA. FDA can also begin planning for the resources needed when the NDA arrives.

A pre-NDA meeting is typically held as the Phase III clinical trials are concluding. The principal objective is to check how the issues identified at the EOP2 meeting have been resolved. At this meeting, the entire structure of the forthcoming NDA can be agreed, and technicalities surrounding electronic submissions can also be arranged.

THE NEW DRUG APPLICATION (NDA)

The best NDAs have a table of contents before the EOP2 meeting, and are built as the various component non-clinical and clinical study reports become available. Most companies do this both electronically and as paper hard copy. At present, FDA requires the submission of both, although PDUFA requires FDA to be able to accept just an electronic version by 2002. The structure is well-described in the regulation, which the student is again urged to read.

Two sections of the NDA are markedly different from a European submission. These are the Integrated Efficacy and Safety. In some respects, these are the biggest intellectual exercises that are encountered during the NDA process. These documents require the pharmaceutical physician to have thoroughly reviewed and understood the other sections of the NDA. But further than this, these summaries risk–benefit assessment, crystal clear arguments that arrive at the choice of dose size, and a full justification of how the NDA data place the new drug into the current understanding of the pathology and indication. The new drug must also be reviewed in comparison with the pharmacology and toxicology of kindred drugs. Justification for every statement in proposed labeling must also be provided. These Integrated Summaries, in contrast with a European expert report, are often 300–400 pages long.

Assembling an NDA is a long process. Usually there is a cutoff date for data that by then may be accruing from all over the world, but which is not pivotal for NDA approval.

The Integrated Safety Summary is then supplemented 4 months after NDA submission. This usually provides a significant increase to the safety database, either from ongoing studies that are rapidly accumulating patients in Phase IIIB, or from marketing data from foreign countries where the drug may be already approved. The FDA requires updating on all safety information that has been gathered subsequent to the filing of the NDA.

Federal law requires that FDA issue a notice of action within 180 days of filing the NDA. There are three forms of action: Approval, Approvable, or Non-approvable. Approvable letters must indicate all the deficiencies that FDA has identified that can, upon rectification, lead to approval. If such deficiencies require the submission of additional data, however slight, then FDA has another 180 days to review the application. If the deficiencies are administrative (e.g. debate over the precise wording in labeling), then the FDA must act within 90 days of a resubmission. Lack of agreement on labeling is the major reason for issuance of an Approvable letter rather than an Approval letter. While most FDA reviewing divisions will only negotiate the proposed label, word for word, after the issuance of an Approvable letter, some companies have been able to go directly to an Approval letter as the first action by a combination of good communication with the FDA and the submission of a realistic package insert. The labeling negotiation itself will often be done by fax and counter-fax, possibly culminating in a face-to-face meeting at FDA premises.

NDA approval is sometimes contingent on the sponsor making various commitments. Most recently, the company is being asked to conduct post-marketing surveillance studies for safety issues that may be more or less well defined. Post-NDA safety report frequency will also be agreed prior to approval. Occasionally, there may be a toxicology study that FDA regards as outstanding but not crucial to drug launch. There may also be stated requirements for additional indications that have been refused the company at the initial NDA approval.

SOURCES OF GUIDANCE

Both CDER and CBER have published a large number of guidance documents that are now also available at the www.fda.gov website. Some of these are simply ICH documents in English. However FDA has gone far beyond this, in supplying a large amount of valuable information. Guidances are not binding (on either sponsor or FDA), but it would be fair to say that clear reasons would have to be enunciated by FDA when requiring the guideline to be exceeded, and by the sponsor when suggesting a variance from them.

One of the difficulties in dealing with FDA is that reviewing divisions interpret these guidances differently. These differences can be profound. The term 'adequate and well-controlled studies' is used to describe the requirement for complying with the need to demonstrate drug efficacy. Most reviewing divisions in CDER still tend to interpret this to mean two, independent, large-scale Phase III clinical trials, despite the clarification in FDAMA. Yet CBER will approve drugs with a single Phase III study and some consistent Phase II data. Similarly, while the ICH guideline states that drugs used for intermittent, acute therapy do not need to have lifespan carcinogenicity tests, there can still be different interpretations within FDA regarding the definition of 'intermittent'. Anesthetic drugs are usually exempt from these long and resource-intense animal studies; but should this apply to acute treatments for disease, labeled for a maximum of three doses per week, and with relatively short half-times of elimination, or not?

Another example was the computer-assisted NDA (CANDA). The cardiorenal division within CDER embraced this technology rapidly and developed its own guidelines as to the technical parameters for this innovation. When the rest of CDER caught up (several years later), it was clear that consistency with an established and successful CANDA format was not on the agenda.

A further example relates to the pre-IND meeting. Some FDA divisions don't like them, and if reviewers attend, they have a tendency to provide less valuable information than they would for an EOP2 meeting or a pre-NDA meeting, the so-called 'entitled meetings'. But, within the industry, there are a number of companies who have similar attitudes about the value of pre-IND meetings. The notable difference is that the FDA has to go to the pre-IND meeting if scheduled. The companies who see little value merely don't schedule them.

The bottom line is that guidances are merely that—guidances. Individual reviewers at FDA are unlikely always to agree with what are essentially consensus documents.

CBER has innovated further with documents entitled *Points to Consider*. These rank below guidances in terms of their gravity. These are designed to accommodate rapidly developing technologies, which, to be fair, is probably a greater challenge for CBER than CDER. These *Points to Consider* are almost completely outside the ICH process, and have been very well received by the regulated industries.

FDA has also been keeping its eye on the public. Advisory committee hearings are typically held by the reviewing divisions prior to any significant NDA approval. These hearings are open to the public, and specifically include an agenda item that provides for public commentary, quite apart from the dialog that goes on between FDA staff, their recruited outside experts, and the NDA Sponsor (again, all in public). FDA has also begun to publish its policy statements. The AIDS community, in particular, has been especially effective in deflecting FDA from its otherwise default-mode course in the review of investigational and new drugs.

INFLUENCES ON FDA ACTIVITIES

The FDA, like any other branch of the US government, is subject to the oversight of Congress. It is Congress that writes the laws that FDA must implement as regulations. FDA must understand the congressional intent in any law, or will find itself called before them to justify their actions. FDA is also dependent upon Congress for its budget, which it must get approved yearly. The court of public opinion has had more of an influence on the FDA in the past 20 years than any other time in its history. This influence is directly focused at the FDA, or indirectly through interaction with Congress or the media. The AIDS community broke the ground in this arena in the 1980s, when they demanded access to more drugs for this dreadful disease more quickly. Fueled by the success of their actions, other patients groups have challenged FDA authority since then. Groups such as the American Association of Retired People have voiced their concern on a wide range of activities. The American Academy of Pediatrics continues to fight for more drugs for children. A number of cancer patient groups seek the ear of the FDA on a regular basis. Pharmaceutical trade associations are also active voices.

SUMMARY

No apology is made for the extensive historical narrative that opened this chapter. Dealing successfully with the FDA requires an understanding of how the institution thinks, and how the individuals within it are constrained. The way the FDA thinks is predicated on its legislation, and how and why that legislation has evolved, mostly in reaction to crisis, but recently, at last, in progressive negotiations with the industry and patient groups to bring about change that is of mutual benefit. The FDA has a complicated structure, and remains the most stringent regulatory authority in the World. We are likely to see further changes in the years to come.

26

Emergency and Compassionate-use INDs and Accelerated NDA or ANDA Approvals—Procedures, Benefits and Pitfalls

Anthony W. Fox

EBD Group Inc., Carlsbad, CA, USA

The special types of investigational new drug application (IND) and new drug application (NDA) probably represent the greatest differences in regulatory practice between Europe and the USA. These differences reside not only in the particular procedures themselves, but also in the differences of philosophy between regulatory authorities, including differences in the nature of, for example, IND, clinical trials exemption (CTX), NDA and Product Licence Application (PLA) documents. Emergency INDs, Treatment INDs, and accelerated approvals are essentially of USA interest, and the Code of Federal Regulations, Title 21, Chapter I (21CFR) is where most of these rules are published (the Orphan Drug regulations may, perhaps, also be seen as a special type of IND or NDA, and are described in detail in Chapter 18). It is probably fair to say that these procedures are have created a quiet revolution in the US drug approval process and have increased the likelihood of timely drug development. Their careful and gradual introduction has not damaged the public health. This chapter covers:

- Emergency INDs.
- Compassionate Use: the treatment IND.
- Accelerated approvals: serious and life-threatening diseases.
- Accelerated approvals: ANDAs and generic drugs.

It should be noted that an 'investigator's IND', or 'physician's IND', is not a specific practice defined by regulation, and that these are orthodox INDs. It is true, however, that these INDs are usually abbreviated in comparison to those from pharmaceutical companies (see the 'treatment IND' section below).

EMERGENCY INDS

All INDs in the USA are legally based on the need for Food and Drug Administration (FDA) permission to convey investigational (i.e. unapproved) drugs across state or international boundaries. This defines the jurisdiction of the federal government in comparison to the state governments in all matters of commerce, not just drug development. The FDA imposes control over this process by requiring information of appropriate quantity and quality before granting its permission. Much of the documentation is judged by how well it supports a clinical protocol, and thus the latter is one of the most important pieces of information that FDA quite properly demands. Normally, a 30-day waiting period applies to the first submitted clinical protocol; provided FDA is notified by IND amendment of succeeding protocols, there is no mandatory waiting period when new sites or whole new studies are proposed after an initial review of the IND. Of course, at any time thereafter, FDA may impose clinical holds on particular dosing regimes, patient populations, protocols or entire projects, should safety issues present themselves. For a detailed discussion of the typical IND, see Chapter 25 and Fox (1996).

The Emergency IND (21CFR para 312.36) is designed to permit a physician to treat a particular

Principles and Practice of Pharmaceutical Medicine. Edited by A. J. Fletcher, Lionel D. Edwards, Anthony W. Fox and Peter Stonier © 2002 John Wiley & Sons Ltd.

patient with an investigational drug with an urgency that precludes the writing and filing of a protocol, or indeed of an entire orthodox IND. An emergency IND does not require the 30-day waiting period. Part of the philosophy behind the perceived need for this regulation is that the federal government does not wish to interfere directly in the relationship between an individual physician and an individual patient. The emergency procurement of materials that are unapproved for human use would be illegal, without this regulation.

It should be noted that the experimental (or 'off-label') use of approved (i.e. 'lawfully marketed') drugs is exempt from the need for an Emergency IND, under 21CFR paras 312.2(b)(i)–(v), provided that the intended use:

1. Is not designed to support of an NDA or NDA supplement for a new indication to FDA.
2. Is not designed to support promotional materials.
3. Does not involve a significantly greater risk than the usual use of the agent (whilst not defined more precisely, large increments in dose, strange routes of administration or special patient populations would all violate this provision).
4. The ethical provisions of the Declaration of Helsinki still apply, and informed consent (which need not necessarily be in writing) have been obtained, i.e. the patient is fully informed of the unusual drug usage.
5. No representations of safety or efficacy, and no monetary charges (ordinarily) are made (21CFR para 312.7).
6. The usage is not prolonged beyond the time period needed to reasonably ascertain its failure.

It may be noted that in anesthetics, pediatrics and intensive care medicine in particular, drugs are used 'off-label' almost routinely, and in practice it is doubtful that physicians in these specialties are even aware of these nuances in the IND regulations. Reimbursement systems in the USA will, however, often refuse to pay for drugs used 'off-label', and use this part of the regulations as their justification.

When the need for an investigational drug is too urgent for the filing of an IND, then the procedure is for a physician to identify a source of his desired compound, and then telephone the FDA for Emergency IND permission. For biologics, the telephone number is (301) 443 4864 (the Center for Biologics Evaluation and Research, HFB-230), and for all other drugs (301) 443 1240 (the Center for Drug Evaluation and Research, HFD-53; *note that the telephone number published in the 1995 Edition of 21CFR is out of date*). Out of ordinary office hours (0800–1600 Eastern Standard Time), FDA's Division of Emergency and Epidemiological Operations maintains a 24 h availability on (202) 857 8400. A confirmation will be provided to the requesting physician, either with a number or by a named FDA officer. The physician may then notify those details to the pharmacy or pharmaceutical company holding the investigational agent, and who may then ship the drug. This information is also available by Internet. It should be noted that this permission can only be obtained by the treating physician him/herself; the pharmaceutical company cannot obtain an Emergency IND on behalf of a treating physician. It should be noted that a paper IND must follow within reasonable time after the event.

The contrast in philosophy between these arrangements in the USA and the emergency use of unapproved drugs in Europe was succinctly put by one German pharmaceutical physician recently: 'We don't need any of that; I can prescribe cyanide if I want to!'. Although an exaggeration, this comment is nonetheless telling. Compared to the USA, there has always been a general tendency for European regulatory authorities to place more discretion and responsibility on pharmaceutical companies and individual physicians when using investigational materials. For example, the previous absence of the need for a CTX for normal volunteer studies in the UK, and indeed the CTX procedure itself (in comparison to Clinical Trials Certification), as well as the limited review of investigational packages after filing in Germany, are all examples of this consistent difference in philosophy between regulatory authorities, and expectations of pharmaceutical companies and physicians to maintain appropriate self-discipline in clinical trials, even when $n = 1$. In the USA, the regulatory process, like much else in other areas of government, is conceived in terms of full disclosure of data in their final form, enforcement, and affirmative acts of the granting of permission by the government.

'COMPASSIONATE USE': THE TREATMENT IND

Although the term is still in common usage, 'Compassionate Use INDs' no longer exist. The intention was to make an investigational new drug available to patients with a defined disease state that is serious (usually life-threatening), and for whom there is no alternative therapy. Furthermore, for the investigational drug, there must be information that is already available that indicates that the new drug is promising; the judgment of what is and what is not 'promising' lies with the relevant reviewing division of FDA, and in practice it is usually the reviewers that have been responsible for an antecedent, ordinary IND that makes this recommendation.

Frequently, circumstances arise during the interval between NDA submission and approval which make it desirable for the (still) investigational drug to be made more widely available. This need is accommodated by the Treatment IND (21CFR paras 312.34 and 312.35), or the Emergency Use IND (21CFR para 312.36, see above).

The stated objective of this section of the regulation, under 21CFR paras 312.34(a) and (b) can, however, often be achieved using an intelligently designed ordinary IND. A seriously interested physician can pursue this in his/her own name, and pharmaceutical companies can cooperate by notifying the FDA that the physician may refer to the chemistry and toxicology sections of the company's IND own IND, and by quoting these cross-references. In this way, the physician's IND usually becomes rather abbreviated.

The clinical protocol needs only be an open-label, tolerability study in patients for whom inclusion and exclusion criteria are kept broad and to a bare minimum for safety. These abbreviated INDs are of orthodox composition (21CFR para 312.23), but have the advantage that the complexities of the Treatment IND can be avoided. Furthermore, even with a rudimentary case report form, the pharmaceutical company can gather tolerability information by this means, even for products approved for other purposes, because the exemptions

of 21CFR paras 312.2(b)(i)–(iv) have not been exploited (see above). One pharmaceutical physician maintains a skeleton word processing file for these physician's INDs, can complete the details for the particular physician over the phone, and mail it to him/her for signature and forwarding to FDA; however, the disease state in question, whilst life-threatening, is rare and congenital, and diagnosed by a simple clinical chemistry test. Such patients tend to congregate in the practices of the few physicians who are experts in the disease; once the FDA reviewer grasps and understands one such submission, and the pharmaceutical company or physician provides sufficient required information, then subsequent similar applications draw clinical holds very rarely. The administrative burden, once this is set up, can be relatively light, and is often very much quicker and easier than navigating the complexities of a *de novo* Treatment IND.

The Treatment IND takes these concepts one step further. This type of IND provides for the use of an unapproved, investigative drug in patients who are not taking part in clinical trials at all, and may not require a protocol.

There are several criteria which must be met for a Treatment IND to be acceptable to FDA, under 21CFR paras 312.34(b)(i)–(iv). Within these criteria are several terms that further require definition or justification to the reviewers:

- The disease process must be serious or life-threatening.
- There must be no feasible alternative therapy.
- The drug is already under investigation in an orthodox IND.
- The sponsor of the drug must be actively pursuing marketing approval of the drug with all due diligence.

Treatment INDs are thus for pharmaceutical companies, not for individual physicians.

FDA considers Treatment IND proposals on the basis of a preponderance of evidence of effectiveness, such as may be available at the time of submission, but which has, obviously, not been definitively decided in an NDA review. There will be close attention paid to all tolerability data that can be marshaled in favour of the Treatment IND, but taken in context of the serious nature of the natural history of the disease process. All the usual clinical hold provisions apply.

ACCELERATED APPROVALS: SERIOUS AND LIFE-THREATENING DISEASES

In the USA there are very active, non-medical communities that are interested in the treatment of human immunodeficiency viruses (HIV), age-associated or Alzheimer's dementias, and, to a lesser extent, emergency medicine and various rare genetic diseases. Another community has formed to support the availability of generic drugs, because of concern about healthcare costs (with drug prices as a small but highly visible part of this). These communities have accomplished a very rare thing: using various parts of the political process, they have brought about a change in the practice of a government administration. Specifically, they have caused the FDA to alter, accelerate, and amend its drug approval process.

The accelerated approval of new drugs for serious or life-threatening illnesses is provided for in 21CFR314.500–560 ('Subpart H'). This new practice dates from 1992, and applies to all types of drug, including antibiotics. In concept, the structure of NDAs that may be submitted under these regulations are the same as the structure of all ordinary NDAs (see Chapter 25 for a full discussion). But the *reviewing practice* and the composition of the NDA within the ordinary structure is very different for these types of accelerated approvals. For example, azathioprine was approved under these regulations with a single well-controlled trial in its support, as well as various *in vitro* and uncontrolled human data as confirmatory; CD4 lymphocyte counts were accepted as a surrogate end-point. Sub-part H also carries requirements for pre-approval of promotional materials, and specifies how FDA may withdraw approval.

In contrast, 21CFR312.80–88 ('Subpart E'), also provides for expedited approvals; reviews can be accelerated for 'drugs intended to treat life-threatening and severely debilitating illnesses'. This is generally understood to be disease states where there is no effective, alternative therapy. Subpart E anticipates flexibility, but continued observance of the statute, as for all drugs. However, Subpart E is also clearly compatible with the 1997

'Modernization Act' [21 USC 351, section 506 (a) (1)], where FDA is required:

> ... at the request of the sponsor of a new drug, [to] facilitate the development and review of such a drug if it is intended for the treatment of a serious or life-threatening condition and it demonstrates the potential to address unmet medical needs for such a condition.

Such products are officially termed 'Fast Track Products'.

Within Subpart E, there is no specific anticipation of a relaxation of the requirement for two adequate and well-controlled studies. These regulations prescribe meetings and schedules, and simply suggest that there ought to be more flexibility in the application of the existing regulations to this type of drug. In contrast, the 'Modernization Act' specifically amends the previous Statute [Section 505 (d) of 21 USC 355 (d)] stating that:

> If the Secretary determines, based on relevant science, that data from one adequate and well-controlled clinical investigation and confirmatory evidence (obtained prior to or after such investigation) are sufficient to establish effectiveness, the Secretary may consider such data and evidence to constitute substantial evidence ....

In other words, the definition of substantial evidence of efficacy has been loosened.

The differences in reviewing practice for accelerated approvals, in comparison to more typical NDAs, are that the regulations specifically permit FDA: (a) to judge efficacy on the basis of surrogate end-points; (b) to grant marketing permission on condition of greater degrees of monitoring for safety than the norm; and (c) to control promotional practices more stringently than usual.

The definitions for illnesses that are serious or life-threatening are not repeated in the accelerated approvals regulations. Thus, the assumption is that these definitions are similar to those provided elsewhere in the IND regulations (21CFR para 312.32(a), 21CFR para 312.34, and see Chapter 25). One problem that arises is in the interpretation of regulations couched specifically in terms of adverse events or justification of a Treatment IND, and how these apply to NDA approvability or the clinical definitions of a disease process. 'Life-threatening' usually is taken to mean that the patient's life is actually under threat by the currently observed disease process (or adverse event), and not that the same *type* of disease or adverse event, but in worse *degree* than that actually observed in the patient, could be life-threatening. Clearly, the burden of proof for demonstration that a disease is serious or life-threatening, and thus an NDA may be considered for accelerated approval, falls squarely with the pharmaceutical company, and FDA will certainly need to be convinced of this as part of its judgment whether to accept the NDA application under these regulations.

Surrogate end-points are those which may be accepted as being predictive of clinical deterioration, but which are not themselves measures of increasing morbidity or mortality. Lymphocyte counts, differentiation, and vitality in patients with AIDS is a good example. However, this is not as radical as it may first appear: antihypertensive drugs are approved using blood pressure as the surrogate end-point, and, until recent huge studies, no approved antihypertensive had been demonstrated to actually reduce strokes or myocardial infarctions. This concept of surrogate end-point should not be too unfamiliar to those involved in drug development: the selection of development candidates at the IND stage, and assessing their worth during Phase I or II clinical investigation, often requires development decisions based upon surrogate end-points, again because these are usually quicker to obtain than (for example) mortality data in support of the proposed indication for the drug (see Chapter 25).

Safety monitoring, after NDA approval, is required for almost all drugs in the USA (21CFR para 314.98). The difference in practice with accelerated approvals is that almost always, *specific* postmarketing safety studies (and sometimes efficacy studies) will be required as a condition of approval. These postmarketing safety studies range from agreement on drug surveillance procedures in detail, through the maintenance of patient registries, to specific studies with protocols.

Postmarketing safety studies are considered in depth in Chapter 33. However, it should be noted here that patient registries have been associated with grave jeopardy of litigation in the USA, and not necessarily on a sound scientific basis. On more than one occasion, pharmaceutical companies have been deterred from marketing new drugs when FDA has required a patient registry as a condition of NDA approval.

The greater control over promotional practice, under the accelerated approval process, usually places less burden on an ethical company than the postmarketing safety requirements. Promotional materials must be submitted for review before NDA approval; the obviously desirable intention is that promotion should not be any broader than the approved indication, which under these special circumstances is likely to be narrower than usual. Furthermore, the package insert should usually quantitate how narrow or broad the tolerability experience with the drug might be, and this will then necessitate fairly frequent updates, as NDA supplements, as the post-marketing data become available.

These special arrangements create two unusual situations where withdrawal of an NDA approved on an accelerated basis is more likely than for an ordinary NDA. First, the approval may be conditional on further clinical studies; FDA can withdraw NDA approval if unconvinced that these studies are being conducted with due diligence. Usually, the interim reporting frequency for these studies will be agreed as part of the NDA pre-approval meeting. Since regulators often have no experience of clinical study management, and since also the difficulties of the disease under study may be substantial, there can be controversy on what does and does not constitute due diligence under these conditions. Secondly, it is possible that the postmarketing studies either fail to confirm efficacy of the drug, or uncover a serious tolerability issue that was not evident in the limited clinical experience in the original NDA. This, again, increases the likelihood that an NDA should be withdrawn. Thirdly, failure to adhere to agreements over promotion can also lead to NDA withdrawal, although this is under the pharmaceutical company's control, and is far more predictable than the results of postmarketing studies. All the usual reviewing and appeals processes are available to both FDA and pharmaceutical companies when NDA withdrawal becomes a possibility (see Chapter 25).

It should be noted that postmarketing study results more often lead to package insert changes than withdrawal of the entire NDA in practice, and that, so far, the accelerated approval process has not led to any serious threat to the public health. This is a new reviewing practice that appears to be working well.

ACCELERATED APPROVALS: ANDAS AND GENERIC DRUGS

The abbreviated new drug application (ANDA) is another form of accelerated approval. In this case, the submission document is not of the same structure as an ordinary NDA, and this is quite unlike the accelerated approval for serious and life-threatening diseases (described above). In this case, the acceleration is accomplished, as the name suggests, by a massive reduction in the documentation needed for FDA review and approval. For all practical purposes, this can only be accomplished when introducing a generically equivalent challenger to a previously approved, innovative drug. The process is described in 21CFR paras 314.3 and 314.92–314.99.

For all practical purposes, the generic equivalent will challenge a trademark drug, probably by price competition, in the marketplace. However, there are rare situations where a trademark drug may have been withdrawn from marketing for purely commercial reasons. Although absent from the market, such a drug could still be followed by an ANDA from another company. The commonest case is where a large company withdraws an innovative but off-patent drug due to insufficient market size. For strategic reasons, the innovator company may not wish to license the product to some other company, nor to continue its manufacture. The niche thus created can be filled by a small generic company for whom that small market size can still comprise a large fraction of its financial revenues.

The FDA publishes a current list of drugs which it considers suitable for ANDA applications. This may be obtained from the Superintendant of Documents, US Government Printing Office, Washington, DC 20402, USA; telephone +1 (202) 783 3238, and will shortly be available on the World Wide Web. This includes both antibiotics and orthodox drugs within the Center for Drugs Evaluation and Research, although there are very few biological therapeutics on the list.

An unusual aspect of the ANDA is that there are two ways to apply. The first way is to file a straight-forward ANDA, which describes a copy of an approved drug. The second way is to file a petition for a drug that is not identical but which may be sufficiently similar for the ANDA process to apply.

The straightforward ANDA demonstrates that the generic drug is identical in its route of administration, active components, dosage form, strength, and stability. The previously approved drug must be identified specifically [21CFR para 314.93(d)], or, exceptionally, the applicant can identify more than one previously approved product and demonstrate that the new product falls within the ranges of previously approved specifications. The Freedom of Information Act, which provides free access to the Summary Basis of Approval documents for all approved drugs in the USA, facilitates this exercise.

If one has a close, but not identical, copy of a drug, then the second way to an ANDA is to file a petition under 21CFR para 314.93(b), identifying what the differences may be from the approved product, and making a case why the new drug should be the subject of a forthcoming ANDA. Successful examples have included differences in excipients, minor differences in *ex vivo* dissolution studies, and other matters which can be argued not to have much clinical impact. FDA will rule on this petition, and there are various appeals procedures if the ruling is unfavourable. The checklist of matters to cover in the petition is:

- Identity of active ingredients.
- Expectation of the same therapeutic effect.
- Failure of the new product to meet the definition of a 'new drug' under 21CFR para 314.1 and Section 201 (b) of the Federal Food, Drug and Cosmetic Act (21USC, 301–392).

It should be noted that the therapeutic equivalence expectation is precisely that: no comparative clinical studies are required. A phase I pharmacokinetic study, in support of the therapeutic equivalence, may be helpful, but need not contribute any pharmacodynamic data. With a favourable ruling on this petition, the ANDA may then follow.

The structure of the ANDA is described in 21CFR para 314.94. Its component parts are:

- Application form.
- Table of contents.

- Basis of the ANDA, covering either the question of identity, or the results of a petition, as described above.
- description of the conditions of use, and showing its similarity to the previously approved drug (usually best done simply by plagiarizing large sections of the previous package insert).
- Description of the active ingredients.
- Route of administration, dosage and strength.
- Bioequivalence data.
- Previous drug's label and proposed labeling.
- Chemistry, manufacture and controls.
- Samples for testing in FDA's own laboratories.
- Other information.
- Patent certification.

In practice, in comparison to an NDA, the Chemistry, Manufacturing and Controls section of an ANDA is just as long, but all the other sections are much abbreviated from an ordinary NDA. The issue of patents is covered in Chapter 37, but prescribed wording for the certificates is provided, according to the various types of patent, in 21CFR paras 314.94–314.95.

The post-marketing requirements for an ANDA are similar to those for an orthodox NDA, and not as stringent as for an accelerated approval for a serious or life-threatening disease (see above). The usual processes are available for amending ANDAs, either before or after approval. The FDA is committed to reviewing complete ANDAs within 6 months.

The ANDA process has permitted large numbers of generic drugs to be provided to the general public at lower cost. The process was created at the same time as the Orphan Drug procedures (Chapter 18), and the Waxman–Hatch Act in the US Congress. Many view the ANDA and the Orphan Drug initiatives as *quid pro quo*, and certainly both were the subject of negotiation with the US pharmaceutical industry.

It should be noted that regulatory practices with FDA are evolving all the time. Pharmaceutical physicians should check each annual re-issue of the 21 CFR for any changes that may have occurred since this chapter went to press.

The intent of this chapter has been to provide the context and philosophy behind these special procedures. All these special IND and NDA procedures are now widely used by pharmaceutical companies, and they have all been developed with a lot of industry input. By these measures, they can be judged to have been successful.

REFERENCES

Code of Federal Regulations (1997) Title 21, Chapter 1, various paras as mentioned above.

Federal Food, Drug and Cosmetic Act (1938) Title 21, sections 201–901.

Fox AW (1996) The US IND: practical aspects. *Reg Aff J* 7: 371–7.

27

Japanese Regulations

Etienne Labbé

Sanofi-Synthelabo, Paris, France

Japan is a country of 125 million inhabitants, 200 000 medical practitioners, and the second-largest drug market in the world. Economically very attractive, it remains for Westerners a country difficult to understand and to communicate with. A strong Dutch, then German, influence during the eighteenth and nineteenth centuries, respectively, opened Japan to Western medicine; it then developed its own techniques to become internationally recognized as one of the most advanced countries in the world of biological and medical sciences. However, Japan, land of contrast, also preserved its traditional therapies of Chinese origin: herbal medicine ('kampo') is still popular and commonly co-prescribed with ethical drugs. Such co-prescription seeks to add different pharmacological effects at low doses without inducing adverse drug reactions. It is unethical for a physician to be responsible for iatrogenic incidents and drug safety has long been a priority to the detriment of efficacy. Japanese regulators developed the most severe guidelines regarding drug safety studies in animals and, paradoxically, clinical development remained, until recently, a pragmatic approach totally in the hands of medical doctors, not prepared (or educated) for clinical drug investigation. Nowadays the rules regulating clinical trials recommend the use of international standards, and Japan became the leader of several topics at the International Conference on Harmonization. This chapter will present the main preclinical and clinical regulations governing drug development on Japanese territory.

ORGANIZATION OF JAPANESE HEALTH AUTHORITIES

General Organization

Under the authority of the Minister and the Vice-Minister, the Ministry of Health and Welfare (MHW) is responsible for social security, public health and the promotion of social welfare. For such purposes, the organization includes (Figure 27.1):

- A main body (central offices).
- An external bureau: the Social Insurance Agency.
- An advisory body: the central Pharmaceutical Affairs Council, involved in drug evaluation.

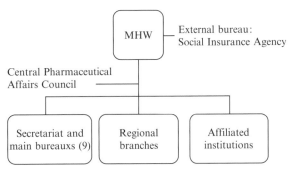

Figure 27.1 General organization of the Ministry of Health and Welfare

Principles and Practice of Pharmaceutical Medicine. Edited by A. J. Fletcher, Lionel D. Edwards, Anthony W. Fox and Peter Stonier © 2002 John Wiley & Sons Ltd.

The main body of the MHW is divided into three branches:

1. *The core administration*, which consists of: the Secretariat (including the Statistics and Information Department); and nine bureaux, as follows: Health Policy Bureau; Health Service Bureau; Environmental Health Bureau; Social Welfare and War Relief Bureau; Health and Welfare for Elderly Bureau; Children and Families Bureau; Health Insurance Bureau; Pension Bureau; and the Pharmaceutical Affairs Bureau; which plays a major part in drug regulation. Around 2000 officials work full-time in the central offices.
2. *Regional branches.* Each prefectural government (47 prefectures) offers a local branch of the Health Authorities: the Regional Medical and Pharmaceutical Affairs offices, and the District Narcotics Control offices. New drug applications are made through the regional office of the prefecture where the company is settled.
3. *Affiliated institutions.* In the present organization, three affiliated institutions operate under MHW supervision:
   (a) The National Institute of Hygienic Sciences, performing tests and research on drugs, food and chemical substances.
   (b) The National Institute of Health, conducting research on pathogenicity, etiology, prevention of certain diseases, and tests and research on vaccines and blood products.
   (c) The National Institute of Public Health, training public health technicians and conducting surveys related to public health.

More than 58 000 officials are working for the MHW general organization.

Pharmaceutical Administration

The Pharmaceutical Affairs Bureau, with the assistance of the Central Pharmaceutical Affairs Council (CPAC) and the Organization for Adverse Reaction Drug (ADR) Relief, Research and Devel-opment Promotion and Product Review (the 'Drug Organization'), represent the managing authorities of Japanese pharmaceutical administration, in charge of reviewing drug application for approval, re-examination, or re-evaluation.

The Pharmaceutical Affairs Bureau (PAB)

Headed by the General Director, 180 officers work for the eight divisions of the PAB (Figure 27.2):

Planning Division. This division coordinates all activities of the PAB, enforces the Pharmaceutical Affairs Law, manages questions related to the Central Pharmaceutical Affairs Council, and provides guidance and supervision to the Drug Organization. Two offices are attached to the Planning Division:

1. The Office of Blood Products Management, which defines the basic policy regarding blood products business in relation to the Japanese Red Cross Society.
2. The Office of Drug-induced Damages, which supervises the organization of the Drug ADR Relief, R&D Promotion, and Product Review Law.

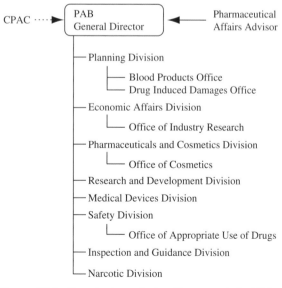

Figure 27.2 Organization of the Pharmaceutical Affairs Bureau (PAB)

Economic Affairs Division. This division surveys and coordinates regulation of production, research, and trade of drugs, quasi-drugs, and medical devices. The Office of Industry Research, attached to this division, collects information related to the pharmaceutical industry and favors consultations between the industry and the Authorities.

Research and Development Division. Many services are provided by this division: surveys and coordination related to drug research and development; designation of orphan drugs and medical devices; guidance to the 'Drug Organization'; supervision of standards and specifications for drugs, quasi-drugs, and cosmetics; guidance for the Japanese Pharmacopoeia, etc. This division also promotes basic research on health sciences through the Japan Health Sciences Foundation, a joint public and private foundation.

Pharmaceutical and Cosmetics Division. This division provides technical guidance and supervision of the production of drugs, quasi-drugs, and cosmetics, as well as services for drug approvals or licences for manufacture or import. The Office of Cosmetics, attached to this division, supervises the production of quasi-drugs and cosmetics and deals with matters related to their approval for import or manufacture.

Medical Devices Division. As in the former division, this supervises and provides guidance for the production of medical devices, promotes research in this field, and deals with matters related to their approvals and licences for import or manufacture.

Safety Division. The responsibility of this division is to provide services related to re-examination and re-evaluation (cf. section or Postapproval Activities, below), postmarketing surveillance regarding safety and efficacy of drugs, quasi-drugs, medical devices and cosmetics. The Office of Appropriate Use of Drugs, attached to this division, collects and evaluates information related to ADRs and promotes the appropriate use of drugs.

Inspection and Guidance Division. The role of the division is 'control and inspection', looking for quality issues, faulty labeling, unlicensed drugs, quasi-drugs, medical devices, and cosmetics. It gives guidance for advertising, testing, official certification, and good manufacturing practice (GMP).

Narcotic Division. The division provides services for the enforcement of laws and investigations regarding the control of narcotics, psychotropics, cannabis, opium, and stimulants.

The Central Pharmaceutical Affairs Council (CPAC)

CPAC is an advisory organ of the MHW, established under the provisions of Article 3 of the Pharmaceutical Affairs Law. Upon request of the minister, the CPAC will investigate and discuss important matters related to pharmaceutical affairs. CPAC members are experienced specialists in the field of medicine, pharmacy, dentistry, and veterinary medicine, coming from universities, public hospitals and research institutes; there are 55 permanent members and 480 temporary members (this last number may vary according to the issues to be discussed). Major subjects treated by the CPAC include:

- Revision of the *Japanese Pharmacopoeia.*
- Determination of standards for drugs.
- Evaluation of the relevance of allowing import or manufacturing of drugs.
- Designation of drugs to be submitted for re-examination and re-evaluation.
- Judgments concerning the payment of relief funds under the provisions of the Adverse Drug Reaction Relief and Research Promotion Fund Law.

For such purpose the CPAC is organized into 17 committees and 54 subcommittees, of which 23 committees and subcommittees are involved in drug review and evaluation.

The Drug Organization

In 1979, the Law concerning the Drug Fund for ADR Relief was enacted in order to facilitate rapid relief for damages caused by ADRs, provided that the drug had been approved and used properly.

This law was revised in 1987 and in 1994, when its name was changed to the Organization for Drug ADR Relief, R&D Promotion, and Product Review, also called the 'Drug Organization'.

This organization, under the supervision of the MHW, evaluates medical costs and pensions for disabilities related to ADRs, under particular conditions as assessed by the CPAC. Nowadays, the Drug Organization also provides other services, including:

- Guidance for the development of orphan drugs.
- Investigation on the equivalence of generic drugs.
- GLP inspection.
- Communication with drug consumers.
- Guidance on the necessity of different types of certificates.
- Finance for joint research projects involving several companies.

From April 1 1997, the Drug Organization started clinical trial consultation services which are of four types:

- Consultation on initial plans for clinical trials (Phase I).
- Consultation at the end of Phase II.
- Consultation before filing (dealing with long-term trials).
- Consultation on protocols.

Fees of ¥1–2.3 million are charged for consultation services; records of the guidance and advices are kept and can be used as attached data for a new drug application.

JAPANESE PHARMACEUTICAL LAWS

Japanese pharmaceutical administration has a long story; it started during the reign of Emperor Meiji, a period during which Japan reopened its frontiers to Western countries. The first law, enacted in 1874, dealt with pharmaceutical sales and handling, but it was limited to three areas (Tokyo, Osaka, and Kyoto). Fifteen years later, the law covered the whole country and was merged with another law, the Patent Medicine Law, in 1925; it

was then renamed the 'Pharmaceutical Affairs Law' in 1943.

Pharmaceutical Affairs Law

The first 'modern' law was born in August 1960, when it was split into the Pharmaceutical Affairs Law and the Pharmacists' Law. The original goal of the Law is to ensure the quality and safety of drugs. Following the evolution of medicines, technique, quality standards, etc., the Law was revised and amended several times in order to incorporate new regulations, such as the GCP. Nowadays, the Pharmaceutical Affairs Law and the Enforcement Regulations of the Pharmaceutical Affairs Law regulate drugs from production and development to marketing and distribution, its scope covering new drugs, quasi-drugs, cosmetics and medical devices.

The Law contains 11 chapters and 89 articles. Surveying this Law in brief, we find:

Chapter 1   *General provisions.* Purpose of the Law and definitions of drug, quasi-drug, cosmetic, medical device and pharmacy.

Chapter 2   *Pharmaceutical Affairs Council.* The CPAC is established, as well as local prefectural councils.

Chapter 3   *Pharmacies.* Defines license standards and supervision of the pharmacies.

Chapter 4   *Manufacture and import of drugs, etc.* Here it is specified that import or manufacture of a drug needs official approval and that the drug should be re-examined and then re-evaluated after a certain period of marketing.

Chapter 5   *Selling drugs and medical devices.* deals with licenses for sales and restrictions.

Chapter 6   *Standards and tests for drugs, etc.* Establishes the Japanese Pharmacopoeia and other standards.

Chapter 7   *Handling of drugs, etc.* Specifies the handling of poisonous and powerful drugs, drugs requiring prescription, package inserts, containers, labeling, sales, and manufacturing restrictions.

Chapter 8   *Advertising of drugs, etc.* Regulates drug advertising.

Chapter 9   *Supervision.* Defines on-site inspection and potential sanctions, orders for improvement, cancellation of approvals and licenses, etc.

Chapter 9.2   *Designation of orphan drugs and orphan medical devices.*

Chapter 10   *Miscellaneous provisions.* Deals with data submission and the handling of clinical trials, etc.

Chapter 11   *Penal provisions.* Defines and fixes the penalties for violation of different articles of the Law.

The Law generally describes the frame of the regulations; for most of the articles, more details and complementary information are provided by the Enforcement Regulations of the Pharmaceutical Affairs Law, which regulates most of the drug development. These regulations will be reviewed in the next chapters.

Other Pharmaceutical Laws

Separated from the main Law in 1960, the Pharmacists' Law deals with the activities of pharmacists, examination, licensing, and duties. As we have seen in the previous section, the Drug Organization is also governed by the Drug ADR Relief, R&D Promotion and Product Review Organization Law. Several other laws are involved in pharmaceutical administration. Their scope are restricted to limited areas and most of them aim at preventing drug abuse and health damages. They are: the Poisonous and Deleterious Substances Control Law, the Narcotics and Psychotropics Control Law, the Cannabis Control Law, the Opium Law, the Stimulants Control Law, and the Blood Collection and Blood Donation Services Control Law.

DRUG DEVELOPMENT REGULATIONS OVERVIEW

In order to clarify the following sections, we have artificially separated some regulations, guidelines and standards described in this chapter. For Western people not familiar with Japanese regulations, these rules, delivered through hundreds of notifications from the Pharmaceutical Affairs Bureau, are a huge maze. We have tried to simplify this review and we apologize for the lack of precision consequently induced.

Generalities

Approval, Manufacturing and Import Licenses

To be authorized to market a new drug in Japan, it is necessary to obtain a drug approval and a license to manufacture or import the drug. Drug Approval ('shonin' in Japanese) is an official confirmation, based on scientific data, that the drug is effective and safe. The Approval is granted for a drug to a person or a juridical person. The License ('kyoka' in Japanese) for manufacturing or importing a drug is granted after ensuring that the applicant is healthy and sane, legally competent, and that the personnel, facilities and equipments comply with the Pharmaceutical Law requirements and quality standards, in order to be able to manufacture or import the approved drug properly. The License is granted for a specific drug to the facilities where the drug will be manufactured. Manufacturing approval can be transferred to legally authorized manufacturers, e.g. through contracts or mergers.

In-country Caretaker System

Approval might be obtained by either a domestic company or directly by a foreign company settled abroad, since the revision of the Pharmaceutical Affairs Law in May 1983. However, clinical data establishing efficacy and safety should be generated in Japanese patients, on Japanese territory; therefore, if the foreign company has no means of conducting these clinical trials on its own, it should appoint an in-country caretaker, domiciled in Japan. A clinical research organization (CRO) is allowed to perform such clinical development in respect to the Pharmaceutical Affairs Law; the CRO may be subject to spot inspections or other specific requests from the MHW, such as report submission regarding ADRs. The CRO should be able to take necessary measures to prevent the occurrence or spread of health damages induced by the drug under investigation (for more information about CROs in Japan, please refer to Bentley 1997).

Substances and Devices Regulated by the Pharmaceutical Affairs Law

Main Groups Defined by the Law

Four groups are defined, which usually need an Approval and a License to be marketed in Japan, unless specifically designated by the MHW:

1. Drugs, including substances listed in the *Japanese Pharmacopoeia*, substances for diagnosis, treatment or prevention of human and animal diseases, and substances affecting any structure or function of the human or animal body. Apparatus or instruments are, of course, excluded. This group can be divided in prescription drugs (or ethical drugs) and non-prescription drugs.
2. Quasi-drugs are substances that exert a mild action on the body, such as drugs used to prevent nausea, bad breath, body odour, hair loss, heat rash, etc.
3. Cosmetics are substances also having a mild action or no action on the body but for external use, applied by rubbing or spraying on the skin or hair and used for cleaning or beautifying.

4. Medical devices are instruments or equipment used for the diagnosis, treatment, or prevention of human or animal diseases. They are designated by ministerial ordinance.

Drug Classification

The four groups outhead above include numerous subclasses, which vary according to the function of different parameters: e.g. approval procedures, approval authorities, handling of standards, list of data to be submitted. Regarding drugs and data to be submitted for approval, Figure 27.3 gives a good example of a possible classification.

Orphan Drugs

Within the ethical drug class, a particular group should be distinguished: orphan drugs. Orphan drugs status was defined in 1993 as follows: a drug is designated as orphan by the MHW after recommendation by the Central Pharmaceutical Affairs Council, when efficacy is scientifically established and when it can benefit less than 50 000 patients. Orphan drugs are subject to financial aid, priority review, and extension of the re-examination period for 6–10 years.

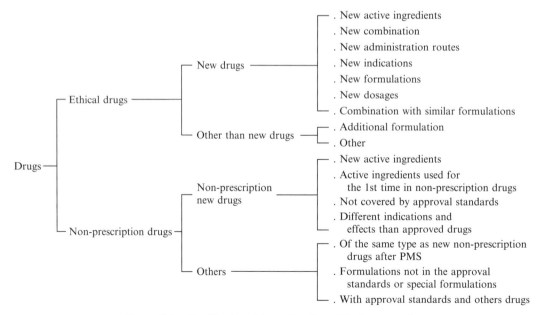

Figure 27.3 Classification of drugs, function of the data to apply

Data Required for a New Drug Application (NDA)

According to Notification 698 from the PAB, dated May 1980, the whole original list of data required for a NDA includes:

1. Data on origin, details of discovery, use in foreign country, etc:
   (a) Data on origin and details of discovery.
   (b) Data on use in foreign countries.
   (c) Data on characteristics and comparison with other drugs.
2. Data on physical and chemical properties, specifications, testing methods, etc:
   (a) Data on determination of structure.
   (b) Data on physical and chemical properties, etc.
   (c) Data on specifications and testing methods.
3. Data on stability:
   (a) Data on long-term storage test.
   (b) Data on severe test.
   (c) Data on acceleration test.
4. Data on acute toxicity, subacute toxicity, chronic toxicity, teratogenicity, and other toxicity:
   (a) Data on acute toxicity.
   (b) Data on subacute toxicity.
   (c) Data on chronic toxicity.
   (d) Data on reproductive effects.
   (e) Data on dependence.
   (f) Data on antigenicity.
   (g) Data on mutagenicity.
   (h) Data on carcinogenicity.
   (i) Data on local irritation.
5. Data on pharmacological action:
   (a) Data on effectiveness.
   (b) Data on general pharmacology.
6. Data on absorption, distribution, metabolism, and excretion.
7. Data on the results of clinical trials.

Some of these requirements are omitted when applying for a new dosage, a new indication or a new route of administration with regard to a drug already approved.

Quality Standards

Quality Standards for Substances and Devices Regarding Properties, Technical Specifications and Test Methods

1. The Japanese Pharmacopoeia (JP). The main and oldest document specifying standards for drugs is the Japanese Pharmacopoeia, first published in 1886. The JP is established by law (Article 41). It aims at regulating quality for important drugs used in healthcare and specific standard test methods. The JP is revised by law every 10 years, but in practice the revision is carried out every 5 years. The Thirteenth Edition was published in 1996 and already contains some monographs harmonized with the US and European Pharmacopoeias.
2. For drugs not mentioned in the JP, Article 42 of the Pharmaceutical Affairs Law indicates that the MHW can lay down necessary standards for drugs, etc., requiring particular cautions. The following standards for drugs have been gazetted through ministerial ordinance:

   (a) Requirements for antibiotic products of Japan.
   (b) Minimum requirements for biological products.
   (c) Minimum requirements for blood grouping antibodies.
   (d) Radiopharmaceutical standards.

   Other standards were published for quasi-drugs (e.g. sanitary products standards), cosmetics (e.g. standards for the quality of cosmetics), and medical devices (e.g. standards for blood donor sets, for cardiac pacemakers, for medical X-ray apparatus).
3. For substances not mentioned in the JP and not covered by Article 42 of the Law, additional standards were notified by the MHW, e.g. the Japanese standards for pharmaceutical ingredients, standards for crude drugs, standards of raw materials for clinical diagnostics, etc.
4. Finally, for drugs having particular manufacturing technology and test methods, such as

biotechnological products, a government certification based on 'batch tests' is necessary.

Quality Standards for Data, Facilities and Functional Organizations

These standards cover different fields describing 'good practices' ensuring the quality of the drug, the quality and reliability of the data generated with the drug and, finally, they warrant the efficacy and safety of a given drug for a given disease, with respect to scientific and ethical considerations for both humans and animals.

Good Manufacturing Practice (GMP). Enforced in 1976, GMP establishes the requirements ensuring drug production of a high and constant quality. It contains guidance on:

- Controls during the manufacturing process.
- The duties of the Control Manager (quality control, validation, self-inspection, etc.).
- The standards for buildings and facilities for manufacturing plants.

In 1988, GMPs for medical devices were also enforced. A group of inspectors attached to prefectorial government perform regular on-site inspections of manufacturers, importers, and distributors, in order to check their compliance to GMP.

GMP compliance certificates for Japanese drug plant have been issued since 1982, and bilateral agreements have been signed with the USA and European countries regarding GMP compliance recognition.

Quality Assurance of Imported Drugs and Medical Devices (GMPI). Also related to drug quality, the standards for quality assurance of imported drugs and medical devices were notified in 1993, establishing basic quality assurance requirements with which the drug importer should comply.

Good Laboratory Practice (GLP). In order to ensure the reliability of animal data, GLP standards were published by the PAB in March 1982, enforced 1 year later and revised in October 1988. GLP describes standards for personnel and organ-

ization (management, quality assurance unit, etc.) for animal care facilities and equipment, standard operating procedures for the operation of testing facilities, test and control articles, the conduct of a study, the study report, and the storage of the raw data.

These standards originally concerned animal safety studies; today they are applied to all animal studies, e.g. toxicology, pharmacology and animal pharmacokinetics. Testing facilities are inspected by MHW officers in order to certify their GLP compliance. Foreign data are acceptable if they meet specific study guidelines and GLP, as certified by a local inspection.

Mutual GLP agreements have been signed between Japan and the USA, Germany, France, The Netherlands, and Sweden.

Good Clinical Practice (GCP). Written in 1985, Japanese GCP standards were notified by the MHW in 1989 for a general application from October 1990. They laid down rules for conducting a clinical trial properly from an ethical and scientific standpoint:

- Definition of the respective role and responsibilities of the sponsor, the investigator and the medical institution.
- The contract for a clinical trial between the sponsor and the hospital conducting the study.
- The institutional review board (IRB) in each medical institute, its role and organization.
- The informed consent of patient to participate into the trial, which was not originally a 'written' consent.
- The storage of the study records (source data) during a certain period of time.

These rules, however, were to be applied to a clinical development organization specific to Japan, and were very different from our Western ones (cf. section on Clinical Development, below). Within the framework of the International Conference on Harmonization (ICH), GCP were rediscussed for several years and finally concluded in 1996. New harmonized GCP standards are now applicable to the USA, Europe, and Japan as well, but they require profound changes of the Japanese system to be fully applied; the Pharmaceutical Affairs Law had to be amended in order to permit the enforcement of the new GCP from April 1997.

The main changes for the Japanese clinic (Takahashi 1997) include:

- New obligations for the sponsor, such as the preparation of the clinical protocol and the writing of a clinical study report.
- The abolition of the 'chairman' of the investigator steering committee.
- The designation by the medical institution of an IRB which can be outside the hospital, such as an academic society, and which will compulsorily have a member from outside the institution.
- The sponsor must establish an independent monitoring system in order to conduct an adequate evaluation of progress of the clinical trial, safety information, and efficacy endpoints. This means that Japanese companies will now have to hire medical doctors to handle medical matters.
- The informed consent becomes a *written* consent and necessitates true and complete information for the patient, including risk and compensation for damage to the health of subjects.

The new GCP standards are, of course, similar to those of the US and European GCP, to which the reader should refer for detailed regulations.

The Good Post-marketing Surveillance Practice (GPMSP). The postmarketing surveillance (PMS) system is a well established system in Japan for collecting safety data in order to prepare the documentation requested for re-examination which will be described in the section on Post-approval Activities, below.

GPMSP standards were enforced in April 1994 after revision of the text published in May 1993.These standards specify the rules to be observed by the manufacturer in order to ensure the reliability of the postmarketing surveillance data, mainly:

- The manufacturer shall establish a PMS department independent of the marketing division and shall employ sufficient staff.
- PMS managers shall prepare standard operating procedures for PMS in order to collect information on drug use, assess this information and take appropriate measures, undertake surveys and special surveys when necessary, perform postmarketing clinical trials, conduct self-inspections, train and educate PMS personnel, contract-out PMS works, and store the information records properly.

Specific Guidelines for Drug Development

In addition to the Law and Quality Standards, specific guidelines have been notified for both preclinical and clinical studies. They regulate the preparation of the data to be submitted for approval by the Authorities and they should generally be strictly followed. These guidelines explain what kind of data have to be produced and indicate the methodology to generate these data; some of the guidelines are under discussion by Expert Working Groups at the International Conference on Harmonization, and some are already harmonized and implemented on Japanese territory.

Other guidelines or recommendations regulate the administrative procedures surrounding development works, such as the import or labeling of the study drug. The Pharmaceutical Affairs Law directly describes the procedures for notifying clinical trials in its section 'handling of clinical trials'. These regulations will be reviewed with the next section.

DRUG DEVELOPMENT PROCEDURES

After the chemical research and screening test periods, the development of a new chemical entity (NCE) follows preclinical and clinical steps similar to Western ones. It takes 8–10 years to establish the efficacy and safety for a new drug and to prepare the documentation required for a NDA.

Regarding the development in Japan of a new drug already approved in a foreign country, 6–8 years are necessary to conduct clinical development on Japanese territory, since Notification 660 of June 1985 requests the duplication of clinical studies in Japanese subjects and patients from Phase I to Phase III.

Preclinical Studies

Physicochemical Properties, Specifications and Test Methods

Basic chemical data, identification, purity and test methods should follow the Guidelines for the Establishment of the Specifications and Test Methods for New Drugs, notified by the MHW in September 1994. When available, standards published in the Japanese Pharmacopoeia or other quality standards (cf. section on Quality Standards) represent the references for specifications and test methods.

Stability Studies

Stability data on the active principle and on the formulation(s) are required on three batches, according to the Stability Test Guidelines issued in April 1994. These guidelines are now harmonized between the three ICH regions. Long-term data and tortured conditions test data should be submitted for new drug application; accelerated conditions tests only are necessary for applications regarding new dosages or new indications of a drug already registered.

Animal Safety Data

In May 1980, Notification 698 from the MHW specified the type of data required for the evaluation of safety in animals and Guidelines for Toxicity Studies were subsequently established in 1984. It is necessary to generate data on acute, subacute and chronic toxicity, effect on reproduction, dependence, antigenicity, mutagenicity, carcinogenicity, and local irritation.

After several revisions, including ICH agreements in 1993 and 1994, the present Guidelines for Toxicity Studies cover almost all these items, describing the tests methods to be conducted for:

- Single-dose toxicity study (ICH standard).
- Repeated-dose toxicity study, 1 or 3 months and 6 or 12 months administration (ICH standard).
- Reproductive and developmental toxicity studies (ICH standard).
- Drug dependence studies were notified in 1975 by the Narcotic Division (for drugs having a pharmacological effect on the central nervous system).

- Antigenicity studies were under drafting in 1997.
- Skin sensitization and skin photosensitization for dermatological preparations.
- Mutagenicity study (under discussion at the ICH).
- Carcinogenicity study (dose selection for carcinogenicity study has been harmonized).
- Local irritation tests are under review.

All toxicity studies supporting a new drug application should comply with GLP standards.

Pharmacology

Pharmacological data should include two different types of data:

- 'Specific pharmacology' data provide information regarding the main effects on the target disease in animal models and try to clarify the mechanism of action as far as possible. There are no guidelines for specific pharmacology.
- 'General pharmacology' studies are conducted to assess the overall pharmacological profile and to obtain information about the effects on the main physiological functions and potential adverse events. Three dose levels are studied (low, intermediate, and high or very high doses) in a battery of tests exploring the main body functions (category A). If some remarkable effect is observed, a second test battery (category B) is conducted. For certain substances, other tests should be performed (category C). General pharmacology studies are regulated by guidelines notified in January 1991.

All pharmacological studies should also comply with GLP standards.

Animal Pharmacokinetics

Data on absorption, distribution, metabolism, and excretion in animal are necessary to clarify the drug's biological fate in the body and to establish an appropriate dose regimen in animal studies, and ultimately in man.

The guidelines for non-clinical pharmacokinetic studies were notified in January 1991. They request those studies to be performed after single and repeated administration. Japan was traditionally the only country to systematically conduct a 2 or 3 week administration test in order to detect tissue accumulation.

Recently, the ICH-harmonized tripartite guideline, Guidance for Repeated Dose Tissue Distribution Studies, opened the door for such repeated-dose studies, but recognized that there was no consistent justification to conduct these tests systematically.

Clinical Development

Efficacy and safety data supporting a NDA approval does not differ fundamentally from the Western clinical data package. They are generated through similar phases, which are:

- The clinical pharmacology phase (Phase I)
- Dose determination studies (Phase II)
- Confirmation studies for safety and efficacy vs. a reference drug (Phase III).

However, Japanese clinical trials show some differences in their organization and methodological approaches, which are still in practice in spite of regulations requesting the application of internationally validated standards.

Clinical Trials Regulations

The Pharmaceutical Affairs Law and its Enforcement Regulations establishes some basic rules for clinical trials, i.e. in summary, it is necessary:

- To conduct preclinical tests (toxicity, pharmacology, etc.) before starting human administration.
- To request in writing to an adequate medical institution to conduct a clinical trial.
- To inform the patient before his/her enrollment into the trial.
- To submit to the MHW information regarding the clinical protocol for each study, with information regarding the study drug and a summary of the preclinical tests.

Each change in the study course should be notified to the authorities by filling specific administration forms (protocol modification, study suspension, study completion).

Notification 698 of May 1980 does not provide much more information regarding clinical trials, requesting to submit 'at least 150 cases in at least five institutions' for a new ethical drug application for approval.

Two guidelines notified in 1992 brought more detailed guidance on the purpose, methodology, and assessment of the three clinical development phases:

- General Considerations for the Clinical Evaluation of New Drugs (June 1992)
- Guidelines for the Statistical Analysis of Clinical Study Results (May 19992).

Phase I should estimate a range of safe dose levels up to a maximum tolerated dose, and characterize the pharmacokinetic profile of the study drug in humans. Generally a single dose study and a 1 week repeated-dose study are conducted in a small number (6–8) of healthy male volunteers. Food effects, drug interactions, and bioequivalence studies nowadays belong to this clinical pharmacology phase, as well as pharmacokinetics in the elderly and studies in subjects with poor kidney or hepatic function.

Phase II is divided in two sequences: Phase IIa or early Phase II; and Phase IIb or late Phase II. Phase IIa is generally an open study with three or four arms, performed to explore efficacy and safety of three or four doses in patients, and it should also bring supplementary information regarding pharmacokinetic parameters. Phase IIb is a double-blind study comparing the effects of two or three doses to placebo effects, aiming at the determination of the optimal dose and dose regimen for a specific indication. It should be noticed that placebo use is not mandatory, but is used 'if necessary'. The final galenic formulation and dosage forms of the study drug is required for the conduct of Phase IIb.

Phase III should confirm the efficacy and safety of the optimal dose and dose regimen in a large group of patients under the usual therapeutic conditions. A large randomized double-blind trial should be conducted vs. a reference drug (traditionally, a reference drug in Japan has been marketed for at least 6 years, and its efficacy and safety has been confirmed through the re-examination procedure).

Long-term trials have now to be conducted and meet international standards, the Extent of Population Exposure to Assess Clinical Safety (it was difficult in the past to obtain long-term data). Some open Phase III trials might be added to study particular patient subgroups, e.g. the elderly, or a specific subgroup of the disease.

The guidelines on statistics indicate how to analyse the study results properly and introduce international and validated standards for the statistical evaluation.

Specific guidelines. With regard to certain pharmacological or therapeutic classes, several specific guidelines have been published since 1980, describing the type of data necessary for a NDA and how to generate these data. Guidelines for clinical trials on urinary tract infections and on dysuria are to be announced soon; other therapeutic fields should be covered in the coming years.

ICH guidelines. In addition to these Japanese original guidances for clinical development, internationally harmonized guidelines are now implemented in Japan:

- Clinical Trials in Special Population (Geriatrics).
- Dose–Response Information to Support Drug Registration.
- The Extent of Population Exposure to Assess Clinical Safety.
- Clinical Safety Data Management (Definition and Standard for Expedited Reporting).
- Clinical Study Reports: Structure and Content.

International Good Clinical Practices. Finally, all clinical studies supporting a drug registration should comply with the harmonized *Good Clinical Practices*, which were enforced in April 1997.

Other Development Rules

1. Regarding the clinical development organization, some aspects are unique to Japan (Labbé 1995). Traditionally, an investigators' committee will take full charge of the clinical development from Phase I or Phase IIa through Phase III (Figure 27.4). The committee consists of a chairman, a senior leader in his speciality who is chosen by the pharmaceutical company. The chairman recommends key investigators and well-known experts to the sponsor.

    Each of the five or eight key investigators will recommend several medical institutions, public or private, where the investigators will performed the clinical trial. The investigators' committee is supposed to write the clinical protocol, to follow the study progress and to propose action when something wrong happen (serious adverse events for instance), to decide whether to keep or reject a case report form before statistical analysis, and to write the clinical study report. They meet and work under the supervision of a government controller (often a clinical pharmacologist). There is usually, for one indication, one study per phase from Phase IIa, and all trials are multicenter studies. Regulations require around 100 patients for Phase II and 200 for Phase III; however, 1000–1500 cases are commonly submitted to date in the NDA; since one investigator may

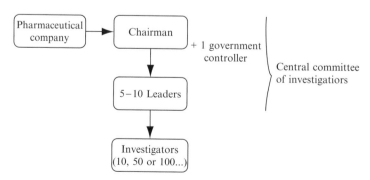

Figure 27.4 Clinical trial investigators organization

produce only one, two or three case reports, 30, 80 or 120 investigators may consequently be involved in a Phase II or III trial.

Clinical development has to progress step by step, according to the general guidelines; after each phase, the steering committee of investigators decides whether the study results justify whether or not to proceed to the next step. It is surprising to notice that the placebo is not considered as mandatory in dose determination studies (always mentioned in the protocols as 'placebo if necessary'), and it is never used in Phase III studies, for ethical reasons, unless no reference treatment is available.

These specificities and many others will change with the implementation of further ICH guidelines, e.g. the enforcement of the new GCP abolishes the traditional Steering Committee of Investigators. However, it generally takes a long time in Japan to modify such strong traditions, and they will probably still be in practice for some years more.

2. Foreign data could be helpful to reduce the 6–8 years necessary for clinical development in Japan. However, the clinical development of a foreign drug has to be duplicated in Japan from Phase I to Phase III, because of potential racial differences and diet differences (Notification 660 of June 1985). Key data are Japanese data; the foreign clinical data package is only considered as complementary information, only used when safety issues are raised during the approval process.

    Some clinical pharmacology studies only can be accepted as key data, such as drug interaction studies or kinetic studies in renal or hepatic insufficiency. The topic 'Ethnic factors in foreign data acceptability' is ending a 5 year discussion within the frame of ICH; it is now recognized that cultural factors are far more important than genetic differences (ICH 2 Proceedings 1993; ICH 3 Proceedings 1995). This allows hope for a regulated mutual recognition of clinical data within the next few years, which should significantly reduce the number of useless duplications of clinical studies and consequently save development resources.

3. The import of a foreign study drug is strictly regulated: imported amount of bulk and/or pharmaceutical form should be clearly justified and limited to the exact quantity necessary for the development. When a clinical trial protocol is available, a copy has to be submitted for approval by a customs officer with a Drug Import Report Slip (Form 12) and a copy of the invoice. When the protocol is not available, a certificate from the Inspection and Guidance Division must be obtained after submission of the following documentation: an Import Report Form (Form 1), a Drug Import Report Slip (Form 13), a Memorandum (Form 2), a protocol outline, a Memorandum stating that the protocol will be submitted within 3 months, and a copy of the Drug Import business license.

The labeling of the study drug should mention, on the drug packaging, container or wrapper, the fact that the drug is for study purposes, the name and address of the institution, the chemical name or symbol, the manufacturing code number, storage instructions and expiry date.

The anticipated brand name, indications or effects, and directions for use and doses of the trial drug should not be mentioned on the drug container or wrapper or on any document attached to the trial drug.

NEW DRUG APPROVAL PROCESS

Content of the New Drug Application (NDA)

Once the clinical development is completed, 4–6 months are necessary to prepare the presentation of the NDA, which should be as perfect as possible. The file consists of seven sections and additional documents:

- Section A. General information:
  - History of the discovery and development of the drug in the country of origin and in Japan.
  - Main characteristics of the drug and its conditions for use.
  - Patent situation in Japan and abroad.
  - List of countries where the drug is registered and samples of local data sheets.
  - International Non-proprietary Name (INN) and Japanese Accepted Name (JAN) publications.

- Comparison of the main characteristics of the drug with those of similar drugs already registered in Japan.
- Section B. Physical and chemical characteristics, specifications and test methods, for the bulk material and the pharmaceutical formulation(s).
- Section C. Stability data, for the bulk material and the pharmaceutical formulation(s).
- Section D. Toxicology.
- Section E. Pharmacology: general and specific pharmacology in animals.
- Section F. Pharmacokinetics in animals and humans, on absorption, distribution, metabolism, and excretion.
- Section G. Clinical data are organized phase-by-phase for each indication. For each study, the clinical report is integrated in section G with no specific analysis from the sponsor.

The main preclinical data and all clinical data should be published, or at least accepted for publication, in order to be accepted as key data. For each foreign study, three reprints are signed by the main author, certifying that he/she conducted the study and that the study results are reliable.

Additional documentation is required as follows:

- One original and two copies of the application form.
- A proposed summary of the product characteristics, clearly detailing contraindications, warnings, and precautions for use.
- A list and outline of the data included in the application.
- For preclinical data and clinical pharmacology studies, a description of the facilities and equipment, with photographs (if available) and an organigram of the personnel, in order to be able to position the main authors within the organization.
- The curriculum vitae of the main study authors.
- GLP and GCP compliance certificates and documentation.
- A brochure summarizing all data from chemistry to clinics: the 'GAIYO', in Japanese, for which the presentation and page number is regulated by Notification 21 of March 1992. It contains a small summary of all preclinical and

clinical data, and tables of all numerical data generated during development. Regarding clinical matters, a global summary of efficacy and safety is given, with a listing of all adverse events as functions of age, sex, doses, disease severity, in- or outpatients, concomitant treatment or not, etc., as well as a listing of all abnormal laboratory values.
- Reference data if available.

The final presentation should be almost perfect, with no copies 'difficult to read' for any reason; units and terms should be appropriate, and foreign data must be filed in the original language, with an English and Japanese translation. The official filing format is A4 (B5 until 1993). *Note* that there is no Expert Report in the Japanese dossier.

Review Process

Before submission of the NDA to the Authorities, the dossier is carefully checked because no other data, unless specifically required by the MHW, can be added after submission. No clinical trial with the study drug is allowed on Japanese territory once the review process has started.

The application for approval is submitted to the Health Authorities through the prefectural branch of the MHW (Figure 27.5). Application fees are ¥5 180 400 (around $ 44 000) for a new ethical drug, ¥534 900 ($4500) for a generic drug, ¥65 600 ($560) for a quasi-drug or a cosmetic and ¥34 500 ($300) for a non-prescription drug.

A first review is carried out by MHW officers regarding the format, contents and quality (source data should be provided upon request). A hearing can take place after this preliminary review and instructions are given to the pharmaceutical company to amend or complete the application. Samples of the active principle might also be requested, for analytical control by the National Institute of Hygienic Sciences. The application is then transferred to the Central Pharmaceutical Affairs Council.

The scientific assessment is carried out by the appropriate subcommittees of the New Drug Committee ('chosakai' in Japanese). After a few months, MHW officers meet with the industry during a hearing (a short meeting, usually) and a list of technical

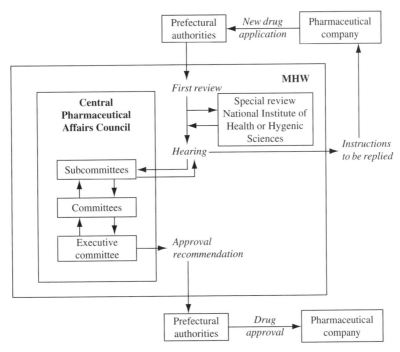

Figure 27.5 Approval process overview

questions is handed to the company; sometimes new preclinical or clinical studies are requested for complementary information, to be replied within a reasonable time frame.

When the subcommittees are satisfied with the answers, the dossier is reviewed by the committees ('tokubetsu bukaï') and a new hearing can take place with new questions. The approval recommendation is given to the MHW by the executive committee ('jioninbukaï') and then notified to the pharmaceutical company through the prefecture. Around 2 years are necessary to obtain a new drug approval if there are no special issues, 6 months for a quasi-drug, 3 months for cosmetics, and 12 months for a medical device.

Summary of the Product Characteristics

The data sheet is called the 'package insert' in Japan, since it can be found in the drug packaging. The data sheet is drafted by the company and checked and completed by the authorities after the NDA review and the recommendation for Approval. The content has been defined by the MHW

notification, and was revised in May 1997. Besides general information on the product, the most important entries are warnings, precautions and contraindications, and a list of adverse events quantitatively reported. These entries will be revised if necessary, with the safety data regularly analysed for the periodic safety update report; however, an *ad hoc* revision is made at any time in case of serious events.

NHI Price Fixing

Prescription drugs are listed on the National Health Insurance Drug Price List in order to be reimbursed under the National Health Insurance Program. The price is fixed by a commission, including medical doctors, consumers, Central Social Insurance Medical Council representatives ('chuikyo' in Japanese). Recent available treatments serve as price references and premiums of 3–10% are added to compensate for novelty and clinical advantages. The NHI price needs 2–3 months after the drug Approval to be listed on the drug tariff. The product can be launched the following day.

Summary Basis of Approval (SBA)

In order to ensure the transparency of the Approval process and to promote the appropriate use of new drugs, the MHW decided to publish the data on which the Approval was based. The SBA includes mainly clinical results and information regarding safety and precautions for use. The first SBA was published in April 1994 by the New Drugs Division: nine SBAs have been issued to date.

POSTAPPROVAL ACTIVITIES

From the first day of its launch, the drug enters the postmarketing surveillance (PMS) period until the end of its marketing life cycle. Besides Phase IV trials, the regulation of which are under reorganization and which should soon meet GCP standards, postapproval activities mainly aim at ensuring the new drug's safety and efficacy. For such purposes, a surveillance system has been settled by the Pharmaceutical Affairs Law. It consists of three different types of investigations: the adverse drug reaction collecting system; the re-examination; and the re-evaluation. Quality standards for those three activities are defined in by Good Postmarketing Surveillance Practice (cf. section earlier in this chapter).

Postmarketing Surveillance Organization

Several systems allow the collection of drug adverse events and their assessment by the MHW as shown in Figure 27.6:

- *Adverse Drug Reaction (ADR) Monitoring System.* Voluntary reports on ADRs are sent to the MHW from around 3000 facilities designated by the MHW, including national hospitals, and university and municipal hospitals; it is also called the 'hospital monitoring system'.
- *Pharmacy Monitoring System.* This is a similar system, collecting ADRs related to non-prescription drugs, by designated pharmacies. Around 2800 pharmacies report ADRs to the MHW.
- *Medical Device Monitoring System.* Another similar system reports to MHW the problems encountered with medical devices.
- *Manufacturers (and wholesalers)* should also report ADRs to the MHW, according to the Law.

The type of ADR to report and the time limits are defined by the international guidelines on Safety Data Management. In addition, periodic safety update reports are sent to the MHW with respect to these international standards. Traditionally in Japan, ADRs are classified according to severity criteria, in three grades (mild, moderate, severe), and in function of the body apparatus.

The MHW collects and exchanges ADR information through other sources:

- WHO International Drug Monitoring Program.
- Relations with foreign health authorities, such as the FDA in the USA and the European Union Health Commission.

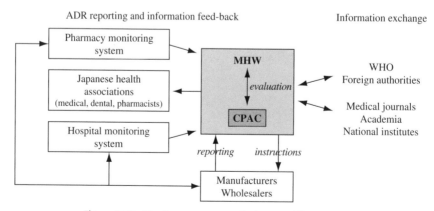

Figure 27.6   The Japanese postmarketing surveillance system

- Survey of medical journals.
- Relations with universities and national institutes, etc.

The safety information collected on a drug is assessed by the Central Pharmaceutical Affairs Council (the Adverse Reaction Committee) and when necessary the MHW instructs the manufacturer to take measures such as:

- The revision of the data sheet (warning, dose, etc.).
- To conduct new investigation in animal or in man.
- To discontinue import or manufacturing.
- To recall drugs from the market.

Re-examination

The re-examination system is part of, and complementary to, the PMS. After a certain period of marketing, safety and efficacy data are re-examined in the light of data collected during this period, which is:

- 6 years for new drugs, combined drugs and new administration route.
- 4 years for a new indication, or a new dosage.
- 10 years for orphan drugs.

Re-examination aims at confirming the conclusions from the drug Approval and particularly the daily recommended dose, treatment duration, safety in long-term use, etc. The manufacturer should apply a re-examination file 3 months before expiration of the 6 year period for a new drug.

The dossier contains data from case report forms collected from hospitals. The number of cases is around 3000–4000 observations, reporting pre-scriptions on a routine basis (survey of use). Safety information comes from this particular survey and from spontaneous ADR reporting (serious events reports and the synthesis of the periodic safety update reports). Of course, information on measures taken during the period should be added (modification of the data sheet, etc.) as well as updated information regarding approval of the drug in foreign countries.

The Safety Division is in charge of reviewing the application; subcommittees and committees of the CPAC will carry out the scientific assessment of the data and will either confirm the usefulness of the drug or ask for modification of the data sheet.

Re-evaluation

The spirit of the re-evaluation system is different from the that of re-examination. Here, the efficacy and safety are reconsidered in the light of the evolution of medical sciences and regulatory progress. The re-evaluation is nowadays periodical, i.e every 5 years after the re-examination (Figure 27.7); however, *ad hoc* re-evaluation can occur at any time upon request of the MHW, when efficacy or safety is questioned for some therapeutic groups. Re-evaluation is done for each drug designated by the MHW; drugs are usually grouped by therapeutic categories for re-evaluation; consequently, it may happen that for a given drug, re-evaluation is performed just before the re-examination, since re-evaluation is not directly dependent on the Approval date. Additional studies might be requested by the MHW to keep the drug on the market if the available data are not consistent with the present regulations and/or medical knowledge. If a drug designed by the MHW does not undergo re-evaluation or does not show evidence of usefulness, the drug Approval is cancelled.

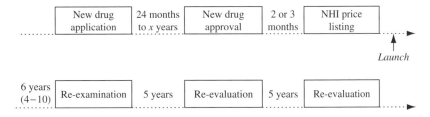

Figure 27.7 Flow-chart of the regulatory process after new drug application

So, from Approval to market withdrawal, the drug dossier is a 'living substance', regularly completed by the pharmaceutical company and periodically revised by the Health Authorities.

CONCLUSION

Japanese regulations regarding drug development and PMS were recently amended, because of the progress of the ICH program, and for other reasons, such as recent incidents related to contaminated blood infusion and a fatal interaction between an antiviral and an anticancer drug, which most probably prompted the changes. However, there is a strong will from the Japanese Authorities to apply international standards to drug development, particularly in the clinical field. The introduction of new GCP and GPMSP rules deeply modifies the background of the traditional Japanese R&D: the industry has to modify its structure and take over new responsibilities, hiring medical doctors in order to organize medical departments for clinical R&D and to assess ADRs. The predominant role of the investigators will decrease. The drug evaluation system by the authorities will have to be modified as well.

However, the move is not limited to drug research and development. Many other fields are involved in this general evolution of the Japanese healthcare system: e.g., the separation of prescription from dispensing ('bungyo') made recent progress; an important NHI price reform is under discussion, which could be a step toward a large change of the health insurance system.

In conclusion, the rapid evolution of the drug regulations may invalidate this chapter within a few years, but it is important for the pharmaceutical industry to understand that the whole drug environment moves toward international standards under the pressure of the scientific progress, quality requirements and economical issues. It represents a chance to integrate Japan in the conception of the global dossier, for which ICH has already laid the foundations.

BIBLIOGRAPHY

All information provided in this chapter comes from official information published by the MHW. More details can be found in good English translation of books published by Japanese editors. The following list is not exhaustive but covers all the items reviewed in this chapter.

Bentley S (1997) *Clinical Research and CROs in Japan. Appl Clin Trials* 8(4): 30–34.
Drug Approval and Licensing Procedures in Japan (1995) Yakugyo Jiho: Tokyo.
Drug Registration Requirements in Japan, 5th edn (1993) Yakuji Nippo: Tokyo.
Guidelines for Clinical Evaluation of New Drugs (1986) Yakugyo Jiho: Tokyo.
Guidelines for Clinical Evaluation of New Drugs (II) (1988) Yakugyo Jiho: Tokyo.
Japanese Guidelines for Non-clinical Studies of Drugs Manual (1995) Yakuji Nippo: Tokyo.
Japanese GMP Regulations 3rd edn (1988) Yakuji Nippo: Tokyo.
Japan Pharmaceutical Reference, 4th edn (1996) Japan Medical Products. International Trade Association: Tokyo.
Japanese Pharmacopoeia, 13th edn (1996) Yakuji Nippo: Tokyo.
Labbé E (1995) Clinical trials in Japan: overcoming obstacles. *Appl Clin Trials* 4(1): 22–32.
Pharmaceutical Administration in Japan, 7th edn (1996) Yakuji Nippo: Tokyo.
Pharmaceutical Affairs Law, Enforcement Ordinance and Enforcement Regulations (1996) Yakugyo Jiho: Tokyo.
D'Arcy PF, Harron DWG (eds) (1993) *Proceedings of the Second International Conference on Harmonization*, Orlando 1993, Queen's University: Belfast; 427–74.
D'Arcy PF, Harron DWG (eds) *Proceedings of the Third International Conference on Harmonization*, Yokohama 1995, Queen's University: Belfast: 421–58.
Takahashi Y, VandenBurg MJ (1997) Implementing the ICH GPC Guideline in Japan. *Appl Clin Trials* 8(4): 22–8.

28

The Development of Human Medicines Control in Europe from Classical Times to the Year 2000*

John P. Griffin

Quartermans, Welwyn, UK

THE EVOLUTION OF HUMAN MEDICINES CONTROL FROM A NATIONAL TO AN INTERNATIONAL PERSPECTIVE

'The past shapes the present'. It is this that justifies the study of history, since without it we cannot truly appreciate the present or shape the future.

From Classical Times to the end of the Eighteenth Century

To few belongs the privilege of being credited with the invention of a medicinal formulation that endured the test of time for 2000 years. Belong it does, however, to Mithridates VIth, King of Pontus, surnamed Eupator (Geddie and Geddie 1926). He succeeded to the throne about 120 BC as a boy of 13 years, had received a Greek education and it was claimed that he could speak 22 languages. He subdued the tribes who bordered on the Euxine as far as the Crimea and made incursions into Cappadocia and Bithynia, which were then in the Roman sphere of influence. In the First Mithridatic War he defeated the Romans and occupied Asia Minor, but in 85 BC he was defeated by Flavius Fimbria and compelled to make peace with Sulla, giving up all his conquests in Asia Minor, surrendering 70 war galleys and paying 2000 talents in reparations. In the Second Mithridatic War, which endured from 83 to 81 BC, Mithridates was wholly successful.

In the Third Mithridatic War, 74–64 BC, Mithridates VI was finally defeated on the banks of the Euphrates by Pompey the Great. New schemes of vengeance by Mithridates upon the Roman Republic were frustrated by his son's rebellion in 63 BC. When he found himself under siege by his own son, he killed his wives and his concubines and then committed suicide.

Pontus abounded in medicinal plants and Mithridates acquired considerable knowledge of them. Like every despot of that period, Mithridates lived in fear of being assassinated by poisoning, in consequence of which he sought the universal antidote to all poisons. Mithridates proceeded along a simple line of reasoning. Having investigated the powers of a number of single ingredients, which he found to be the antidote to various venoms and poisons individually, he evaluated them experimentally on condemned criminals. He then compounded all the effective substances into one antidote, hoping thereby to produce universal protection. A daily dose was taken prophylactically to give the immunity he sought.

After Mithridates VI's defeat by Pompey, a store of his writings containing detailed information on medicinal plants was captured. Pompey instructed a freed slave, Lenaeus, to translate these writings into Latin. It was said that by the value of these writings, Pompey did a greater service to the Roman Republic than by his military prowess. Our knowledge of these writings of Mithridates (Watson 1966) has come down to us in the writings

---

* This chapter is an adapted and expanded update of the chapter on drug regulation in Europe, published in Griffin JP, O'Grady J, D'Arcy PF (eds), *Textbook of Pharmaceutical Medicine*, 3rd edn. The Queen's University of Belfast Press: Belfast, 1998. The author retains sole copyrights on this chapter.

Principles and Practice of Pharmaceutical Medicine. Edited by A. J. Fletcher, Lionel D. Edwards, Anthony W. Fox and Peter Stonier © 2002 John Wiley & Sons Ltd.

of Pliny and Galen, since the translation by Lenaeus has been lost.

Pliny writes:

> By his unaided efforts Mithridates devised the plan of drinking poison daily after first taking remedies in order to achieve immunity by sheer habituation. He was the first to discover the various antidotes, one of which is even known by his name

So effective was Mithridates' formulation that he tried unsuccessfully to commit suicide by poisoning, and finally killed himself with a 'Celtic sword'.

Galen, writing in the second century A D at a time when he was physician to the Roman Emperor, Marcus Aurelius, refers to 'mithridatium' and a formulation derived from it by one Andromachus, Nero's physician. It is said that Andromachus removed some ingredients from Mithridates' formulation and added others, particularly viper's flesh. To this new product he gave the name 'galene', which means 'tranquillity'. Galene became known as theriac. Details of various theriacs, including mithridatium and galene, were given in Galen's 'Antidotes I' and 'Antidotes II'. In Galen's 'Antidotes I' he distinguishes three kinds of antidote, those that counter poisons, those that counter venoms, and those that counter ailments. Some will counter all three, and Galen claimed that to this class belong mithridatium and galene. According to Galen, mithridatium contained 41 ingredients and the galene of Andromachus 55 components.

The preparation of galene was simple, in that its ingredients were free of fractional measures. Four vipers, cut down small, were placed in a solution of sal ammoniac, about 1 gallon, to which were added nine specified herbs and Attic wine, together with five fresh squills, also cut down small. The pot was covered with clay and set upon a fire. When the vapor came out of the four small holes left in the clay seal, dark and turgid, the heat had reached the vipers and they were cooked. The pot was left to cool for a night and day. The roasted matter was taken out and pounded until all was reduced to powder. After 10 days the powder was ready for the next stage of manufacture.

At the final stage, the prescribed quantities of 55 herbs, previously prepared by various processes, along with the prescribed quantity of squill and viper flesh powder (48 drachms), were added to hedychium, long pepper and poppy juice (all at 24 drachms); eight herbs including cinnamon and opobalsam (all at 12 drachms); 18 herbs including myrrh, black and white pepper, and turpentine resin (at 6 drachms); 22 others and then Lemnian earth and roasted copper (at 4 drachms each); bitumen and castoreum (the secretion of beaver); 150 drachms of honey and 80 drachms of vetch meal. The concoction took some 40 days to prepare after which the process of maturation began. Twelve years was considered by Galen the proper period to keep it before use. Galen records that Marcus Aurelius consumed the preparation within 2 months of its being compounded without ill effect.

Mithridatium was similar, but contained fewer ingredients and no viper, although it did contain lizard! The other differences were that the opium content of Andromachus' theriac was higher than that of mithridatium, which also differed in containing no Lemnian earth, copper or bitumen and 14 fewer herbal ingredients.

Both mithridatium and galene were taken orally with water or wine, but were also used topically on the skin, or even in the eye. The theriac, galene, was also used by Galen to treat quartan fever (malaria), which was prevalent in the Pontine Marshes near Rome. Aetius (first century A D) stated that beyond question the best remedy for venomous bites is theriac of Andromachus, applied as a plaster– 'The patient should also drink this theriac or mithridatium or some similar compound'.

Paul of Aegina was the last of the physicians of the Byzantine culture to practice in Alexandria, which fell to the Arabs in his professional lifetime in 642 A D. He refers to both mithridatium and theriac. Paul of Aegina was a link between Greek medicine and Mohammedan medicine. His book was used by Rhazes (854–930 A D), one of the greatest of the Arab physicians. Avicenna (980–1037 A D) approved of mithridatium as an antidote to poisons, and Maimonides, a Jew born in Moslem Spain, was also familiar with mithridatium. Mithridatium re-entered Western medicine culture by two routes. A Saxon leechbook of the eleventh century records that Abel, the Patriarch of Jerusalem, sent mithridatium or theriac to King Alfred the Great, who died on 26 October 899 (Stenton 1947).

The *Leechbook of Bald* (Rubin 1975) is the most important piece of medical literature to have survived from the Saxon period. The document is in two parts or leechbooks; the first contains 88 chapters and the second 67 chapters. They were written circa 900–950 AD from an earlier ninth century Latin text. Following them is a third book, consisting of 73 sections, written in the same hand, but which is nevertheless a separate and additional work. It, too, is of similar age and likely to be a copy of earlier material. A verse at the end of the second leechbook suggests that these books belonged to a physician or leech called Bald, and were written down by a scribe called Cild. These three leechbooks were obviously intended as manuals of instruction for the treatment of a variety of illnesses, injuries, and mental states, together with instructions for the preparation of herbal mixtures. Interspersed with these remedies are sections dealing with rites, charms, and invocations. Christian and residual heathen practices are represented, the latter including Greek and Roman traditions in addition to Germanic and Celtic folklore, which the Saxons had either brought with them from their homeland or found persisting on their arrival in Britain. There can be no doubt that these leechbooks were intended to be consulted in the physician's everyday practice. Certain phrases and remedies can be traced to classical times, e.g. the sixth century Alexander of Tralles, and the fifth century Marcellus Empiricus. A most important passage is contained in the second leechbook and concerns King Alfred. It refers to his request that the Patriach Elias of Jerusalem send him remedies which the prelate had found to be effective. A theriac formulation appears in this leechbook.

The second route was when the works of the Greek and Roman medical writers again became available in Italy, possibly via Spain or through the university at Salerno. Theriac appears to have been more greatly favored than mithridatium as a remedy for poisons. In the twelfth century, theriac was being manufactured in Venice and widely exported. In England it became known as 'Venetian treacle' ('treacle' is a corruption of theriac). Theriac became an article of commerce, with Venice, Padua, Milan, Genoa, Bologna, Constantinople, and Cairo all competing. The manufacture of these theriacs took place in public, with much pomp and ceremony.

It was commonly thought by those in authority that if mithridatum or theriac did not produce the desired cure, this was due to incorrect preparation (perhaps with adulterated or poor quality materials) or to incorrect storage after use. Since the only cause for therapeutic failure therefore lay with the pharmacist who compounded the mixture, the remedy lay in careful scrutiny of manufacture, which should be in public. Any misdemeanour should then be detected and immediately punished.

The earliest written code of quality control in Britain seems to be the *Ordinances of Guild of Pepperers of Soper Lane* in 1316. The Pepperers in the twelfth century took over the distribution of imported drugs and spicery (which includes spices, sugar, confections, and fruit). They were not always easy to distinguish from the Spicers, who themselves became intermingled with or perhaps succeeded by the Grocers. The Ordinances of 1316 possibly included the Apothecaries and the Spicers and forbade the mixing of wares of different quality and price, the adulteration of bales of goods, or falsifying their weight by wetting.

For the next several hundred years the story is a confused one, containing the roots of the later separation of the Apothecaries as a craft guild and their emergence, first as compounders of medicine and then as a division into those who ultimately became general medical practitioners and those who, together with the emergent chemists and druggists, founded the Pharmaceutical Society and became the pharmacists as we know them today.

The Apothecaries were originally part of the Guild of Grocers and unsuccessfully petitioned Elizabeth I in 1588 for a monopoly of selling and compounding of drugs. It was not until 1607, however, that James I was to grant a Charter to the Grocers, who recognized the Apothecaries as a separate section. Ten years later, in 1617, James gave the Apothecaries a Charter to separate them from the Grocers as 'The Worshipful Society of the Art and Mistery of Apothecaries'.

The story over this period and for much later is that of a long fight with the physicians, and as early as 1423 the 'Commonalty of Physicians and Surgeons of London' appointed two apothecaries to inspect the shops and their colleagues and bring any who offended in the quality of their wares before the Mayor and Aldermen.

The College of Physicians was founded in 1518 by Henry VIII, and in 1540 one of the earliest British statutes on the control of drugs was passed (32 Henry VIII c.40 for Physicians and their Privileges), which empowered the Physicians to appoint four inspectors of 'apothecary wares, drugs and stuffs'. Section 2 of the Act gave the Physicians the right to search Apothecaries' shops for faulty wares, with the assistance of the 'Wardens of the said mysterie of Apothecaries within the said City'. If the search showed drugs that were 'defective, corrupted and not meet nor convenient to be ministered in any medicines for the health of man's body', the searchers were to call for the Warden of the Apothecaries and the defective wares were to be burnt or otherwise destroyed.

This Act of Henry VIII was obviously incorrect in defining the Apothecaries as a separate body, and was corrected later in the reign of Queen Mary by an Act of 1553 (1 Mary sess 2 c.9), in which it was enacted:

> for the better execution of the searche and view of Poticarye Wares, Drugges and Compositions according to the tenour of a Statue made in the Two and Thirtieth yeare of the Reigne of the said late King Henry Eighth That it shall be lawfull for the Wardeins of the Grocers or one of them to go with the say'd Physitions in their view and searche.

It is revealing that, whereas the penalty for refusing to have wares examined was 100 shillings in Henry's day (of which he took half), by Mary's day this had been raised to £10. The wording of the Act was also changed slightly, in that under Henry the Wardens were to be called for, but under Mary they had to go. Henry was also determined that the 1540 Statute would be obeyed and an errant apothecary punished and not allowed to make excuses:

> ...in the Kings Court...no wager of law, esoin (excuse) or protection shall be alloweth... apothecaries to sell or prescribe any poisonous substance or drug...to the body of any man, woman or child save on the written prescription of a physician or upon a note in writing from the purchaser.

The Apothecaries hotly disputed this Order and there is no record of any action being taken on it. They asked the Physicians to tell them of specific abuses and that they would then co-operate in reforming them. The Apothecaries said that others, such as druggists, grocers, and chandlers, could sell poisons quite freely and many craftsmen used them daily. The Apothecaries further said that to restrict them to providing poisons solely at the request of the physicians would take away their livelihood and interfere with the liberty of the subject to have free use of all medicines.

In England, after the founding of the Royal College of Physicians in 1518, the making of theriac and mithridatium was made subject to supervision under the Pharmacy Wares, Drugs and Stuffs Act of 1540. In the reign of Elizabeth I, the making of theriac was entrusted to William Besse, an apothecary in Poultry, London. He had to show the finished product to the Royal College of Physicians. In 1625, three apothecaries made respectively 160 lb, 50 lb and 40 lb of mithridatium when London was stricken with plague.

Another technique to control the quality of drugs is the issue of a pharmacopoeia (Greek 'pharmakon', a drug; 'poiia', making). The official and obligatory guide for the apothecaries of Florence was published in 1498 and is generally regarded as the first official pharmacopoeia in Europe in the modern sense, i.e. of a specific political unit. Other cities soon followed in the publication of obligatory formularies: Barcelona in 1535 (*Concordia Pharmacolorum Barcinonesium*); Nuremberg in 1546 (*Dispensatorium Valerii Cordis*). Similar compilations were also issued in Mantua in 1559; Augsburg, 1564; Cologne, 1565; Bologna, 1574; Bergamo, 1580; and Rome, 1583. Britain was somewhat slower, and it was not until Elizabethan times that it became obvious that there was a need for such a pharmacopoeia or formulary. This was first considered by the College of Physicians in 1585. However, work proceeded very slowly and the *Pharmacopoeia Londinensis* was not published until 1618. There were two issues: one on May 7, and the first 'official' edition on December 7. This latter was by no means a reprint of the earlier one and was substantially enlarged and changed. The publication of the *London Pharmacopoeia* in December 1618, setting out detailed formulations of theriac and mithridatium, had made supervision easier and the manufacture was clearly no longer entrusted to a single apothecary.

Nicholas Culpepper, in his *Dispensatory* (1649), refers to both mithridatium and 'Venetian treacle'. References in English literature to theriac always refer to it as treacle. Miles Coverdale translated balm as treacle in his *Bible* of 1538. This was repeated in the *Matthew Bible* and *Bishops' Bible* of 1568. Jeremiah 8 v 22 therefore read: 'Is there no treakle in Gilead? Is there no physician there?'.

In 1665 the Great Plague of London broke out and Charles II turned to the Royal College of Physicians for advice. It was eventually published as '*Advice set down by the College of Physicians (at the Kings Command) containing certain necessary directions for the cure of the Plague and preventing infection*'. The streets were to be kept clean and flushed with water, in order to purify the air, fires were to be lit in streets and houses and the burning of certain aromatic materials, such as resin, tar, turpentine, juniper, cedar, and brimstone, was enjoined. The use of perfumes on the person was recommended. Special physicians, attended by apothecaries and surgeons, were appointed to carry this out. The main internal remedies for the plague that were recommended were London treacle, mithridatium, galene and diascordium, a confection prepared from water germander. Victims of the plague who developed buboes were treated with a plaster of either mithridatium or galene, applied hot thrice daily.

Doubts as to whether theriac and mithridatium were the universal panacea had been voiced by Culpepper and other physicians such as Dr John Quincy, who died in 1722. The real attack on these two long-standing remedies came from Dr William Heberden (1745) in a 19 page pamphlet entitled *Antitherica: Essay on Mithridatium and Theriac*. Heberden concludes his attack on the lack of efficacy of these products with the words:

> Perhaps the glory of its [mithridatium's] first expulsion from a public dispensary was reserved to these times and to the English nation, in which all parts of philosophy have been so much assisted in asserting their freedom from ancient fable and superstition, and whose College of Physicians, in particular, hath deservedly had the first reputation in their profession. Among the many eminent services which the authority of this learned and judicious body hath done to the practice of Physic, it might not be the least that it had driven out this medley of discordant simples . . . made up of a dis-

sonant crowd collected from many countries, mighty in appearance, but in reality, an ineffective multitude that only hinder one another.

In William Heberden's entry in Munk's (1878) Roll it is stated that he was always ready to attack the 'idle inventions of ignorance and superstition'.

William Heberden was born in 1710, entered St John's College, Cambridge University, in 1724 at the age of 14, graduated BA in 1728, became an MA in 1732, and obtained his MD in 1739. Heberden published his *Essay on Mithridatium and Theriac* in the same year as he obtained his FRCP. William Heberden founded the *Medical Transactions of the Royal College of Physicians* in 1767 and in the first three volumes, 1768–1785, he published 16 papers. Heberden is known for his description of Heberden's asthma (cardiac asthma) and Heberden's nodes, which are calcipic spurs on the articular cartilage at the base of the terminal phalanges in osteoarthritis. He made the clear point that they had no connection with gout, which was the main and highly fashionable arthritic ailment of his time. Heberden died in 1801 and was buried in Windsor Parish Church, where there is a memorial plaque to him and his son William Heberden Junior, who was Physician to George III during his years of insanity, which we now believe was due to porphyria.

The 1746 *London Pharmacopoeia* was the last in which mithridatium and galene appear; they were absent from the 1788 edition. The *Edinburgh Pharmacopoeia*, first published in 1699, dropped mithridatium and galene from the 1756 edition. Not all Western European countries were so quick to expunge these formulations, for galene with its vipers appears in the *German Pharmacopoeia* of 1872 and in the *French Pharmacopoeia* of 1884. With the disappearance of mithridatium from the *French Pharmacopoeia*, the long-used complex remedy attributable to an experimental toxicologist from the first century BC came to an end.

Prior to the doubts on the efficacy of mithridatium raised by a number of English physicians, including Culpepper and Quincy, and culminating in William Heberden's attack and condemnation of these products, there had been occasions when these formulations had been noted to be ineffective. In all these circumstances, it was believed that the formulations had been inadequately compounded; or that the quality of the ingredients was suspect (the quality of cinnamon was frequently raised); or even the species of viper used in theriac was questioned. These concerns to maintain the quality of mithridatium and theriac led to the introduction of strict controls over the quality of ingredients and blending. For example, the manufacture had to be done in public in Venice and the ingredients had to be open to inspection. Pharmacopoeias were produced, which laid down standards, not only for mithridatium and theriac, but for other therapeutic substances. Perhaps, in the final analysis, the contribution of mithridatium and theriac to modern medicine was that concerns about their quality stimulated the earliest concepts of medicine regulations.

The *Medical and Physical Journal*, one of the earliest to supply regular information on new work in medicine, pharmacy, chemistry, and natural history, suggested in its first volume in 1799:

> ... we would submit to the legislature the propriety of erecting a public board composed of the most eminent physicians for the examination, analysation and approbation of every medicine before an advertisement should be admitted into any newspaper or any other periodical publication and before it should be vended in any manner whatsoever.

THE NINETEENTH AND TWENTIETH CENTURY TO THE MEDICINES ACT 1968

Compulsory vaccination against smallpox was established by the Vaccination Act of 1853 after the report compiled by the Epidemiological Society on the state of vaccination following the first Vaccination Act of 1840. The 1840 Act had provided free vaccination for the poor to be administered by the Poor Law Guardians.

Under the Vaccination Act of 1853, all infants had to be vaccinated within the first 3 years of life, default of which meant the parents were liable to fine or imprisonment. New legislation incorporated in the Vaccination Act of 1867 made it compulsory for children under the age of 14 years to be vaccinated, and encouraged the notification of default by doctors by providing financial inducements for compliance and penalties for failure.

The law was further tightened in 1871, when the appointment of vaccination officers was made compulsory for all local authorities. A House of Commons Select Committee, set up in 1871 to investigate the efficacy of the compulsory system, was concerned by a report by Dr Jonathan Hutchinson, who gave an account of the transmission of syphilis in two patients by arm-to-arm inoculation of the material from the pustule of one patient to the arm of another. The use of calf lymph vaccine did not become standard until 1893, when a commercially available preparation was introduced. Prior to this it had been impossible to standardize the material used for vaccination.

In 1858, the Medical Act created the General Medical Council, one of whose duties was to compile an official pharmacopoeia for the whole of the UK to supersede the three current ones for London, Edinburgh, and Dublin. The first *British Pharmacopoeia* was published in 1864 (the 1958 and 1993 editions were published by the Health Ministers on the recommendations of the Medicines Commission; *vide infra*).

It has to be acknowledged that there was little momentum during the nineteenth century concerning the general requirement for scrutiny of medicines for safety and efficacy, in addition to the quality requirements already in existence, before products were marketed in Britain. A few attempts were made to do this and, as far back as 1880, a British Medical Association (BMA) working party investigating sudden deaths occurring in chloroform anesthesia had suggested the establishment of an independent body to assess drug safety. Chloroform was first used as an anesthetic in 1847 and, as its use increased, it was found that occasionally people died unexpectedly during the induction of anesthesia. In 1877 the BMA appointed a committee to investigate this and the final report was published in 1880. They found that chloroform not only depressed respiration but had a deleterious effect upon the heart in very small doses and could cause cardiac arrest. This was the first major collaborative investigation of an adverse reaction to a drug ever carried out.

This study had very little impact on generating public or political concern to set up a regulatory authority. However, the appearance of two publications by the BMA concerning certain proprietary medicines, entitled *Secret Remedies* (1909) and

More Secret Remedies (1912), caused a Parliamentary Select Committee on Patent Medicines to be set up. This Select Committee reported in 1914, but World War I intervened and all the proposed legislation was shelved. It is worth listing several of the recommendations of this Committee, some of which had to wait until the Medicines Act (1968) controlled and kept standards under review, and many of these became internationally recognized.

Recommendations

- 56(1). That the administration of the law governing the advertisement and sale of patent, secret, and proprietary medicines and appliances be coordinated and combined under the authority of one Department of State.
- 56(5). That there be established at the Department concerned a register of manufacturers, proprietors, and importers of patent, secret, and proprietary remedies...
- 56(6). That an exact and complete statement of the ingredients...and a full statement of the therapeutic claims made...be furnished to this Department...
- 56(7). That a special Court or Commission be constituted with power to permit or prohibit...the sale and advertisement of any patent, secret, or proprietary remedy...
- 56(12). That inspectors be placed at the disposal of the Department...
- 58(2) That the advertisement and sale (except the sale by a doctor's order) of medicines purporting to cure the following diseases be prohibited: cancer, consumption, lupus, deafness, diabetes, paralysis, fits, epilepsy, locomotor ataxy, Bright's disease, rupture.
- 58(3 and 4) That all advertisements...[of] diseases arising from sexual intercourse or referring to sexual weakness...[or] abortifacient...be prohibited.

Still, little attention was paid to the efficacy of drugs and treatment. The Venereal Disease Act of 1917 and the Cancer Act of 1939 prevented the public advertisement and promotion of drugs for these conditions, to prevent sufferers from inadequate or unsuitable treatment and from fraudulent claims. It was necessary to wait until the Medicines Act was in force before further consideration was given to efficacy (but see Therapeutic Substances Act), but it may be noted here that this was a foretaste of control of advertisement and promotional literature for medicines.

The antisyphilitic drug arsphenamine (Salvarsan) had been discovered in Germany in 1907 and was imported into Britain until the outbreak of World War I, when the Board of Trade issued licences to certain British manufacturers to make it. Each batch had to be submitted to the MRC for approval before marketing. The problem was that, although synthetic, and hence the chemical identity of the product was known, highly toxic impurities could only be detected by biological testing.

It began to be realized also that the increasing use of potent biological substances and the extension of immunization were raising new questions of proper standardization of such preparations and of the competence of manufacturers. The only law at this time concerned with the purity or quality of drugs was the Food and Drugs Act of 1875, and this had a very limited application.

Control of biological substances was difficult to contain within a pharmacopocial monograph, for it demanded the use of biological standardization, as the purity and the potency of these substances could not be measured by chemical means. The Therapeutic Substances Act (TSA) aimed to regulate the manufacture and sale of such substances and to provide standards to which they must conform, to regulate their labeling and, to a certain extent, their sale. The principal substances to which the Act applied were vaccines, sera, toxins, antitoxins, antigens, arsephenamine and related substances, insulin, pituitary hormone, and surgical sutures. Certain suture material had been found to be contaminated with *Clostridium welchii*, and this was the reason for inclusion of sutures under the TSA. It provided for a licensing system, with the Minister of Health as the Licensing Authority for England and Wales, the Department of Health for Scotland, and the Minister of Home Affairs for Northern Ireland. The TSA also recognized that the competence of the employees of the manufacturer and the conditions under which they worked were equally as important as the tests applied to the end products. Factory inspections and in-process control therefore played a large part in supervision by the Licensing Authority. Records of sale also had to be kept by the manufacturer, and the container had to identify both the manufacturer and the batch.

This Act began modern concepts of safety. Further regulations issued between 1925 and 1956 brought more substances under control and kept standards under review, and many of these became internationally recognized. The whole TSA was revised and consolidated in 1956, but has now been superseded by the Medicines Act (1968).

The Biological Standards Act (1975) established the National Biological Standards Board. This Board, appointed by the UK health ministers and funded by the Health Department, is responsible for standards and control of biological substances, i.e. substances whose purity and potency cannot be adequately tested by chemical means, such as hormones, blood products, and vaccines. The Board operates through the executive arm, the National Institute for Biological Standards and Control.

THALIDOMIDE AND ITS AFTERMATH

The story of thalidomide is too well-known to bear much repetition here but, as it was the stimulus that laid the ground rules on which the Medicines Act in the UK and most other modern European states' legislation, including the European Community's Directive 65/65EC, was built, it is relevant to summarize these events.

Thalidomide first went on sale in 1956 in West Germany and enjoyed good sales, both there and in other countries, as a sleeping aid and as a treatment of vomiting in early pregnancy, because of its prompt action, lack of hangover, and apparent safety. Adverse reports of peripheral neuropathy and myxoedema appeared in the literature in late 1958 and 1959, associated with thalidomide. In 1961 reports began to be made of a remarkable rise, in West Germany since 1959, in the incidence of a peculiar malformation of the extremities of the newborn. This condition was characterized by the defective long bones of the limbs, which had normal to rudimentary hands or feet. Owing to its external resemblance to a seal's flipper, it was given the name 'phocomelia'. This condition had previously been very rare in West Germany but whereas no cases had been reported in the 10 years 1949–

1959, there were 477 cases in 1961 alone. In the UK, 400–500 cases were reported during 1959–1961. The public and government were not prepared for these unforeseen consequences of the therapeutic revolution that had been taking place for 30 years. This complacency was now shattered, public concern was vocal, and the government was galvanized into action.

The joint subcommittee of the English and Scottish Standing Medical Advisory Committees, under the chairmanship of Lord Cohen of Birkenhead, made recommendations regarding future legislation for the control of medicines, in addition to the immediate establishment of the Committee on Safety of Drugs, which came into operation in 1963 and whose function was to review the evidence on new drugs and offer advice on their safety. The Committee consisted of a panel of independent experts from various fields of pharmacy, pathology, etc. The Committee was serviced by a professional secretariat of pharmacists and medical officers, who undertook the assessment of the submissions and presented these to the committee and various subcommittees.

The Committee on Safety of Drugs was set up in June 1963 by the Health Minister, in consultation with the medical and pharmaceutical professions and the British pharmaceutical industry, with the following terms of reference:

1. To invite from the manufacturer or other person developing or proposing to market a drug in the United Kingdom any reports they may think fit on the toxicity tests carried out on it; to consider whether any further tests should be made and whether the drug should be submitted to clinical trials; and to convey their advice to those who submitted reports.
2. To obtain reports of clinical trials of drugs submitted thereto.
3. Taking into account the safety and efficacy of each drug, and the purposes for which it is to be used, to consider whether it may be released for marketing, with or without precautions or restrictions on its use; and to convey their advice to those who submitted reports.
4. To give to manufacturers and others concerned any general advice they may think fit.
5. To assemble and assess reports about adverse effects of drugs in use and prepare information

thereon which may be brought to the notice of doctors and others concerned.

6. To advise the appointing Ministers on any of the above matters.

The Committee had no legal powers, but worked with the voluntary agreement of the Association of British Pharmaceutical Industry and the Proprietary Association of Great Britain. They promised that none of their members would put on clinical trial or release for marketing a new drug against the advice of the Committee, whose advice they would always seek.

The joint English and Scottish Standing Medical Advisory Committee also recommended that there should be new legislation regarding many aspects of drug safety, and after a review and consultation, a White Paper, *Forthcoming Legislation on the Safety, Quality and Description of Drugs and Medicines* (Cmnd 3393), was published in September 1967, and the Medicines Act, based on these proposals, received the Royal Assent in October 1968. The Act is a comprehensive measure replacing most of the previous legislation on the control of medicines for human use and for veterinary use. The first provisions laid down in the Act, regarding licensing of medicinal products and other aspects of control, came into effect on September 1 1971. The Act was administered by the health and agriculture ministers of the UK, acting together or in some cases separately, as the health ministers or the agriculture ministers in respect of human and veterinary medicines, respectively.

The Medicines Commission was appointed by ministers to give them advice generally relating to the execution of the Act. A number of expert committees with specific advisory functions were appointed by ministers after considering the recommendations of the Commission, as proposed in Section 4 of the Medicines Act.

Under the Medicines Act (1968), the Licensing Authority consists of the Secretaries of State for Health and Social Services, the Secretary of State for Agriculture, and the Secretaries of State for Wales, Scotland and Northern Ireland. The Medicine Act (1968) was implemented to operate from September 1971. The day-to-day administration of the Act for human medicines was conducted by the Medicines Division of the Department of Health and Society Security (DHSS), and was

managed jointly by an under-secretary and the professional head of the Division, who held the rank of Senior Principal Medical Officer.

In 1988 the DHSS was split into two departments, the Department of Health (DoH) and the Department of Social Security (DSS). Following the Evans–Cunliffe report, from April 1989 the Medicines Division of the DoH became the Medicines Control Agency (MCA) under a director, and was expected to self-fund its operation from fees commensurate with the services provided. The UK MCA in 1997 had 458 staff, of whom 150 approximately worked in licensing, 130 in postlicensing, including pharmacovigilance, 75 in licensing inspection of manufacture and enforcement, and 28 on the *British Pharmacopoeia* and the UK contribution to the *European Pharmacopoeia*. This has now increased to 600 staff in 2002.

The Licensing Authority is advised by expert committees, appointed by ministers, as advised by the Medicines Commission under Section 4 of the Medicines Act. These advisory committees consist of independent experts, such as hospital clinicians, general practitioners, pharmacists and clinical pharmacologists, not the staff of the DoH, and are appointed by ministers on the advice of the Medicines Commission. The relevant advisory committees since 1971 have been the Committee on Safety of Medicines (CSM), the Committee on Review of Medicines (CRM), the Committee on Dental and Surgical Materials (CDSM), the *British Pharmacopoeia* Commission (BPC) and the Veterinary Products Committee, which is administered through the Ministry of Agriculture, Food and Fisheries (MAFF).

The Licensing of New Medicines

The UK joined the European Community (EC) in 1973, but the data requirements for granting marketing authorizations has, since the implementation of the Medicines Act (1968), been in accordance with *EC Directive 65/65* and the subsequent *Directive 75/318*, which elaborated on the requirements for preclinical testing, pharmaceutical quality and manufacture. Both these Directives and the Medicines Act (1968) envisaged that marketing authorizations issued on the basis of these requirements would be valid for 5 years and subject to review and/or renewal.

During the period 1971–1981, after the implementation of the Medicines Act (1968), the Licensing Authority granted 204 marketing authorizations for new chemical entities (NCEs), granted 3665 marketing approvals for new formulations, and 6898 variations of marketed formulations (Griffin and Diggle 1981). In the period 1971–1994, there were 525 NCEs approved for marketing, 30 new biological entities (NBEs) and 28 products of biotechnology (Jefferies et al 1998). Of these new active substances, 35 product licences were surrendered by the manufacturers and a further 22 were withdrawn for safety reasons.

National marketing authorizations were intended to be phased out after January 1 1998, but it is likely that national approvals for marketing will continue beyond that date. The future foresees that all marketing authorizations within the European Union (EU) will have been issued under the Rules governing medicinal products in the EC by virtue of the Centralized Procedure or the so-called 'mutual recognition' or 'decentralized procedure' (*vide infra*).

Controls on Conduct of Clinical Trials in the UK

In the UK, when the Medicines Act (1968) came into operation, all clinical trials in patients had to be covered by a clinical trial certificate (CTC). Under the Medicines Act, studies on normal healthy human volunteers (Phase I studies) were exempt.

A clinical trial in the terms of the Medicines Act (1968) is an investigation, or series of investigations, consisting of the administration of one or more medicinal products, where there is evidence that they may be beneficial, to a patient by one or more doctors or dentists for the purpose of ascertaining what effects, beneficial or harmful, the products have. The Licensing Authority does not lay down rigid requirements concerning the data, which must be provided before authorization can be given for the clinical trial of a new drug. It issues guidelines for applicants.

By the late 1970s it had become apparent that the need to apply for a CTC and the regulatory delay that this caused was driving clinical research out of the UK. The Secretary of State for Social Services approved the introduction of a new scheme in 1981, the details of which were announced by Griffin and Long (1981). The new procedures allowed for a clinical trials exemption (CTX) from the need to hold a CTC; the applicant company was required to produce a certified summary of data generated to support the proposed clinical studies, signed by a medically qualified advisor or consultant to the company. The regulatory authority has 35 days to respond to the notification, but can in exceptional circumstances require a further 28 days to consider the notification. If the CTX is refused, the applicant can apply for a CTC, in which circumstances complete data have to be filed. If the CTC application is refused, the statutory appeal procedures come into play if the applicant company wishes to avail itself of this provision. These appeal procedures are identical with those for marketing applications.

The basis of the CTX scheme is that, together with a detailed clinical trial protocol, summaries of chemical, pharmaceutical, pharmacological, pharmacokinetic, toxicological, and human volunteer studies may be permitted instead of the additional details normally required for a CTC or product licence application. This CTX scheme is based on the requirement that:

(a) a doctor must certify the accuracy of the data; (b) the supplier undertakes to inform the Licensing Authority of any refusal to permit the trial by an ethical committee; and (c) the supplier also undertakes to inform the Licensing Authority of any data or reports concerning the safety of the product.

Speirs and Griffin (1983) described the effect of the CTX scheme in attracting clinical studies on NCE in the first year of operation of the scheme. In 1980 there were 87 applications for CTC; in 1981, the first year of the CTX scheme, there were 210 applications for CTX, of which 79 were for NCEs. Speirs, Saunders and Griffin (1984) studied the effects of the CTX in encouraging inward investment into research in the UK; 23 companies had increased their research investment by 100%.

Clinical trial provisions vary greatly between EU member states and the EC, in accord with their prevailing philosophy of 'harmonization', wish to change this.

The Review of Products on the Market Pre-1971

At the start of product licensing in the UK in 1971, products already on the market were granted Product Licences of Right (PLRs), which were subject to review. Between 1971 and 1982, 22 376 lapsed or were revoked or suspended, and 598 had been converted to full product licences. The Committee of Review of Medicines was deemed to have completed its work in 1991 and was disestablished on 31 March 1992.

All member states of the EC were similarly required to review the quality, safety and efficacy data of products on their market. Various dates were set for the completion of such national reviews, and the time schedule had to be revised on a number of occasions due to slow progress of the exercise. The various national review processes have not led to harmonized marketing approvals for these older products within Europe.

Pharmacovigilance and the Adverse Reactions Voluntary Reporting System

One of the most important aspects of the UK regulatory system is the scheme provided by the voluntary reporting of adverse reactions to a marketed drug. Since most serious adverse drug reactions (ADRs) are rare events, they are unlikely to be detected in early clinical trials. The problem is essentially one of numbers, since relatively small numbers of patients are exposed to a new drug before it is released on to the market. Marketing may, therefore, be the first adequate safety trial. The main functions of the adverse reactions reporting system are:

1. To provide an alerting signal of a risk due to a particular drug.
2. To provide confirmation of an alert detected by some other method.
3. To provide data to assist in the evaluation of comparative risks of related drugs.

The spontaneous adverse reaction reporting system in the UK is based upon the submission of ADR reports by doctors and dentists by means of reply-paid 'yellow cards'. The system was intro-

duced in 1964 by Professor Witts, the first chairman of the Adverse Reactions Subcommittee of the original Committee on Safety of Drugs (CSD). The system has continued unchanged to the present time, and the number of reports and fatal reactions each year of the scheme's operation is shown in Table 28.1.

Membership of the EU and the establishment of the European Medicines Evaluation Agency (EMEA) has imposed a European dimension upon ADR monitoring and given it a new title—'pharmacovigilance'. The requirements of the

Table 28.1 Annual input of adverse reaction reports to CSM and total number of fatal reports

Year	Total ADR reports	Total deaths	Fatal reaction as a percentage of total ADR reports
1964	415	86	5.9
1965	3987	169	4.2
1966	2386	152	6.4
1967	3503	198	5.7
1968	3486	213	6.1
1969	4306	271	6.3
1970	3563	196	5.5
1971	2851	203	7.1
1972	3638	211	5.8
1973	3619	224	6.2
1974	4815	275	5.7
1975	5052	250	4.9
1976	6490	236	2.6
1977	11 255	352	3.1
1978	11 873	396	3.3
1979	10 881	286	2.6
1980	10 179	287	2.9
1981	12 357	303	2.5
1982	14 701	340	2.3
1983	12 689	409	3.2
1984	12 163	340	2.8
1985	12 652	348	2.8
1986	15 527	403	2.6
1987	16 431	390	2.4
1988	19 022	410	2.2
1989	19 246	475	2.5
1990	18 084	377	2.1
1991	20 272	541	2.7
1992	20 155	478	2.4
1993	18 066	480	2.7
1994	17 546	412	2.3
1995	17 668	467	2.6
1996	17 191	393	2.3
1997	16 637		
1998	18 062		
1999	18 505		
2000	33 094		

European dimension can be summarized as obligations for Regulatory Authorities and obligations for the pharmaceutical company holding a marketing authorization (MA):

Agency granted under the centralized procedure (the Agency referred to is the EMEA) and member state responsibilities:

- Receive all relevant information about suspected adverse reactions to medicinal products authorised by the centralized procedure.
- Marketing authorization holders and member states are required to provide such information to the Agency.
- Member states must record and report to the Agency within 15 days all suspected serious adverse reactions.
- The Agency is responsible for informing national pharmacovigilance systems and the establishment of a rapid network for communication.
- The Agency shall collaborate with WHO on international pharmacovigilance issues, and submit information on Community measures which are relevant to public health protection in Third World countries.

MA holder's responsibilities:

- To have a qualified person responsible for pharmacovigilance.
- Establishment and maintenance of a system for collection, evaluation and collation of all suspected adverse reaction information so that it may be accessed at a single point in the Community.
- Preparation of 6 monthly scientific reports and records of all suspected serious adverse reactions for the first 2 years after marketing, annual reports for the next 3 years and thereafter at renewal of the authorization.
- Reporting to the member state concerned within 15 days of receipt information on all suspected serious adverse reactions within the community.
- Reporting to member states and the Agency within 15 days of all suspected serious unexpected adverse reactions occurring in Third World countries.

Good Manufacturing Practice (GMP)

Manufacturers' licences were issued by the UK Licensing Authority from the inception of the Medicines Act to cover all manufacturing operations, including those previously embraced by the Therapeutic Substance Act (TSA). The Medicines Inspectorate laid down standards in its Guide to Good Manufacturing Practice, otherwise known as 'The Orange Guide'; the most recent edition was issued in 1997. Although the issue of manufacturers' licences remains a national regulatory function, it is governed by the standards set in EC Commission Directive 91/356 EEC, which can be summarized as follows.

The directive lays down the principles and guidelines of good manufacturing practice to be followed in the production of medicines, and requirements to ensure that manufacturers and member states adhere to its provisions. Manufacturers must ensure that production occurs in accordance with GMP and the manufacturing authorization. Imports from non-EC countries must have been produced to standards at least equivalent to those in the EC, and the importer must ensure this. All manufacturing processes should be consistent with information provided in the marketing authorization application, as accepted by the authorities. Methods shall be updated in the light of scientific advances, and modifications must be submitted for approval.

Principles and Guidelines for GMP

- Quality management—implementation of quality assurance system.
- Personnel—appropriately qualified, with specified duties, responsibilities, and management structures.
- Premises and equipment—appropriate to intended operations.
- Documentation.
- Production—according to pre-established operating procedures with appropriate in-process controls, regularly validated.
- Quality control—independent department or external laboratory, responsible for all aspects of quality control. Samples from each batch must be retained for 1 year, unless not practicable.

- Work contracted out—subject to contract, and under the same conditions, without subcontracting.
- Complaints and product recall—record keeping and arrangements for notification of competent authority.
- Self-inspection—by manufacturer of his own processes with appropriate record keeping.
- Good manufacturing standards are enforced by the Medicines Inspectorate of the Medicines Control Agency. The UK has been involved in the Pharmaceutical Inspection Convention since its inception and, through the Orange Guide, set standards which are now reflected in the EC Directives.

Wholesale Dealers' Licences

This activity, established under the Medicines Act 1968, still remains wholly within the remit of national regulatory authorities but in accordance with *Directive 92/25 EEC* on the wholesale distribution of medical products for human use (*Official Journal* L113/1–4 30 April 1992).

Routes of Sale and Supply

In the UK the Medicines Act 1968 assumes that all medicinal products will be sold through a pharmacy unless it is decided by the Licensing Authority that supply of the product should be limited to being dispensed only on a registered medical practitioner's prescription. Such products appear on the Prescription Only Medicines List and their packaging is marked 'POM'. Certain products are also available through outlets other than pharmacies and are designated as General Sales List (GSL) products and listed as such. Additional restrictions on supply are imposed by the Misuse of Drugs Act 1971, and the Misuse of Drugs Regulations substances that have a potential for abuse are scheduled under three categories, Classes A, B and C:

- *Class A* includes: alfentanil, cocaine, dextromoramide, diamorphine (heroin), dipipanone, lysergide (LSD), methadone, morphine, opium, pethidine, phencyclidine, and class B substances when prepared for injection.
- *Class B* includes: oral amphetamines, barbiturates, cannabis, cannabis resin, codeine, ethylmorphine, glutethimide, pentazocine, phenmetrazine, and pholcodine.
- *Class C* includes: certain drugs related to the amphetamines, such as benzphetamine and chlorphentermine, buprenorphine, diethylpropion, mazindol, meprobamate, pemoline, pipradol, and most benzodiazepines.

The Misuse of Drugs Regulations 1985 define the classes of person who are authorized to supply and possess controlled drugs while acting in their professional capacities, and lay down the conditions under which these activities may be carried out. In the regulations, drugs are divided into five schedules, each specifying the requirements governing such activities as import, export, production, supply possession, prescribing, and record keeping which apply to them:

- *Schedule 1* includes drugs such as cannabis and lysergide, which are not used medicinally. Possession and supply are prohibited, except in accordance with Home Office authority.
- *Schedule 2* includes drugs such as diamorphine (heroin), morphine, pethidine, quinalbarbitone, glutethimide, amphetamine, and cocaine, and are subject to the full controlled drug requirements relating to prescriptions, safe custody (except for quinalbarbitone), the need to keep registers, etc. (unless exempted in Schedule 5).
- *Schedule 3* includes the barbiturates (except quinalbarbitone, now Schedule 2), buprenorphine, diethylproprion, mazindol, meprobamate, pentazocine, phentermine and temazepam. They are subject to the special prescription requirements (except for phenobarbitone and temazepam) but not to the safe custody requirements (except for buprenorphine, diethylproprion and temazepam) nor to the need to keep registers (although there are requirements for the retention of invoices for 2 years).
- *Schedule 4* includes 33 benzodiazepines (temazepam is now in Schedule 3) and pemoline, which are subject to minimal control. In particular, controlled drug prescription

requirements do not apply and they are not subject to safe custody.

- *Schedule 5* includes those preparations which, because of their strength, are exempt from virtually all controlled drug requirements other than retention of invoices for 2 years.

There is no 'harmonized' comprehensive legislation to control drugs of abuse under an EU Directive.

THE EUROPEAN CONTROLS OF MEDICINAL PRODUCTS

Directive 75/319 laid down the legal basis for the establishment of the Committee on Proprietary Medicinal Products (CPMP). This met for the first time in November 1976, at which time there were nine member states in the EC. Each member state was represented at the CPMP by its named representative and specified alternate.

At this time a procedure was laid down in *Directive 75/318*, a scheme for 'mutual recognition' of marketing authorizations. Article 9 of this Directive envisaged that:

> The member state which has issued a marketing authorization for a proprietary medicinal product shall forward to the Committee a dossier containing a copy of the authorization, together with particulars and documents specified in Article 4

second paragraph of Directive 65/65, if the person responsible has requested the forwarding to at least five other Member States.

This was later changed to 'at least two other member states' in *Directive 83/570* to encourage the use of the procedure, which was initially very slow in taking off.

This 'Mutual Recognition procedure', initially called the 'CPMP procedure', has had several other names attached to it, e.g. the 'multistate procedure', and the 'decentralized procedure'. Manufacturers could choose the country that they would wish to be the initiating or reference country to forward their dossier into the multistate procedure. Some countries were more popular than others (see Table 28.2).

In December 1986, The Council Directive on the approximation of national measures relating to the placing on the market of high-technology medicinal products, particularly those derived from biotechnology (87/22/EEC), was published. This Directive introduced the concept of two classes of high technology medicinal product:

ANNEX A.   Medicinal products developed from the following biotechnologic processes:
- Recombinant DNA technology.
- Controlled expression of genes coding for biologically active proteins in prokaryotes and

Table 28.2 The distribution of work to the rapporteur countries under the former CPMP procedure (*Directive 75/319/EEC*) 1978–1986, and the multistate procedure (*Directive 83/570/EEC*) 1986–October 1992

Country	CPMP procedure		Multistate procedure	
	Country of origin	Recipient country	Country of origin	Recipient country
Belgium	5	33	14	147
Denmark	7	26	27	106
Germany	5	25	17	195
Greece	–	12	0	124
Spain	–	–	0	144
France	7	15	51	101
Ireland	–	24	32	87
Italy	–	38	16	142
Luxembourg	–	37	0	139
The Netherlands	–	35	20	131
Portugal	–	–	0	38
UK	16	18	75	82
Total dossiers/applications	41	263	252	1436

eukaryotates including transformed mammalian cells.
- Hybridoma and monoclonal antibody methods.

ANNEX B.
- Other biotechnological processes.
- Medicinal products administered by means of a new delivery system which, in the opinion of the competent authorities, constitutes a significant innovation.
- Medicinal products containing a new chemical entity.
- Medicinal products based upon radioisotopes.
- Medicinal products the manufacture of which employs a significantly novel process.

This directive required that products covered by the Annex classification had to be referred to the CPMP for an opinion before a marketing authorization (MA) could be granted in any member state. This process became known as the 'concertation procedure', or 'central procedure'. Products covered by Annex B could, at the request of the manufacturer, be dealt with by the concertation procedure or by an individual national authority, and then achieve entry into other EU member states markets if requested by means of the multistate procedure. In the concertation procedure, the opinion given by the CPMP was not binding upon member states.

Directive 2309/93 introduced further changes. It established a new body that is based in London, The European Medicines Evaluation Agency (EMEA), established January 1 1994, and two procedures for the obtaining entry to the markets of the member states, namely the 'multistate or decentralized or mutual recognition procedure' and the 'centralized procedure'; see Figures 28.1 and Figure 28.2, which show schematically the procedures which became operative on January 1 1995.

Under the mutual recognition procedure, the applicant company would receive a number of national marketing authorizations from national drug regulatory authorities. Under the centralized procedure, the applicant company would receive a single marketing approval from the EMEA, valid in all EU countries.

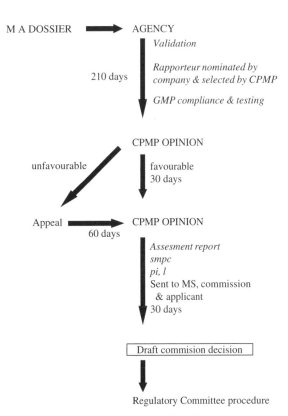

Figure 28.1 Centralized procedure for biotech (mandatory) and high-tech (optional) medicines (from January 1 1995)

Centralized Procedure

In the centralized procedure, products falling within Annex A have to be processed by this route, products in Annex B may be processed by this route at the discretion of the manufacturer. Applicants using the centralized procedure may nominate a member of the CPMP to act as rapporteur and co-rapporteur. However, the final choice of rapporteur and co-rapporteur remains within the remit of the CPMP. The membership of the CPMP has been made so that it is now a technically expert committee which advises the EMEA. The opinions of the CPMP are referred to member states, who have a period of time to comment back to the CPMP. Thereafter an opinion is issued which is binding upon member states.

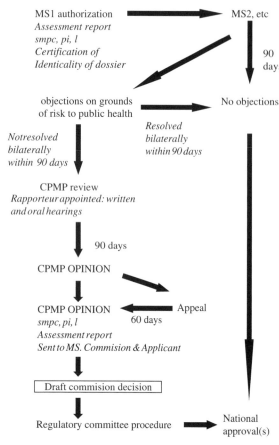

MS1 authorization → MS2, etc

Assessment report
smpc, pi, l
Certification of
Identicality of dossier

90 days

objections on grounds of risk to public health → No objections

Resolved bilaterally within 90 days

Not resolved bilaterally within 90 days

CPMP review
Rapporteur appointed: written and oral hearings

90 days

CPMP OPINION

CPMP OPINION ← Appeal
smpc, pi, l   60 days
Assessment report
Sent to MS. Commision & Applicant

Draft commision decision

Regulatory committee procedure → National approval(s)

Figure 28.2 Mutual recognition procedure for all products except those of biotechnology. MS1, 1st member state; MS2, 2nd member state; pi, 1, package insert and labelling

Table 28.3 Centralized marketing applications to EMEA

Centralized procedures	1997	1998	1999	Total 1995–1999
Applications received				
Part A	20	12	18	224
Part B	40	33	29	
Withdrawals				
Part A	3	8	1	38
Part B	4	12	7	
Opinions adopted by product				
Part A	6	11	9	133*
Part B	19	30	17	
Opinions adopted by substance				
Part A	6	11	8	105*
Part B	13	19	15	

* These figures include negative opinions given for seven products (representing four substances), and for two variations.

Table 28.4 Variations and line extensions to marketing applications processed by centralized procedures

Centralized procedures	1997	1998	1999	Total 1995–1999
Type I variations				
Part A	57	50	68	569
Part B	52	108	207	
Type II variations				
Part A	19	26	48	239*
Part B	28	40	61	
Extension and abridged applications				
Part A	32	11	6	73
Part B	2	4	13	

* These figures include negative opinions given for seven products (representing four substances), and for two variations.

Tables 28.3 and 28.4 show the work of the EMEA in terms of centralized procedure applications dealt with since the inception of the current scheme on January 1 1995 to December 19 1999. Table 28.3 shows the new applications submitted to the EMEA under the centralized procedure, and Table 28.4 shows the number of variations to marketing authorizations granted under the centralized procedure. It can be envisaged that variations are going to comprise the major part of EMEA's workload, in the same way as it does for national drug regulatory authorities.

The MCA has remained the dominant regulatory authority regarding the share of work conducted under the two revised community procedures, e.g. in March 1996, the Annual Report of the MCA for 1995/96 states: 'The MCA was responsible for eight of the 21 mutual recognition procedures that had been successfully completed (38%) and was the reference member state for 10 of the 23 procedures in progress at that date'. The UK was also the rapporteur or co-rapporteur for 19 of 81 applications made to the centralized procedure in 1997 (European Agency for the Evaluation of Medicinal Products, Third General Report 1997). The distribution of work on centralized applications is shown by member state in Table 28.5. The processing times for centralized applications is shown in Table 28.6.

Table 28.5 Distribution of work on centralized procedure applications among EC member states

Country	Number of times a country has been rapporteur or co-rapporteur
Belgium	17
Denmark	25
Germany	34
Greece	2
Spain	19
France	37
Ireland	25
Italy	18
Luxembourg	6
The Netherlands	33
Austria	12
Portugal	12
Finland	15
Sweden	36
UK*	36

* UK has been rapporteur for 21 applications.

Decentralized or Mutual Recognition Procedure

Table 28.7 shows the use of the 'decentralized' or 'multistate' or 'mutual recognition' procedure during 1997. In this procedure the initial or reference member state that granted marketing approval forwards the necessary documents for registration

Table 28.7 Total number of finalized mutual recognition procedures by type, August 1995–December 1997*

	Number	(%)
New active substance	77	31.5
Generics	45	18.4
Line extensions	29	11.9
Fixed combination	20	8.2
OTC	6	2.6
Herbal	2	0.8
Others	65	26.6

* The number includes multiple procedures (total = 244).

to the other member states where the manufacturer wishes to market his product, and a copy is also sent to the EMEA/CPMP. If one or more member states raise objections, the applicant had the right, until December 31 1997, to withdraw his request for a marketing authorization in that member state. Thereby the applicant avoided the application being forwarded to the CPMP for arbitration (Table 28.8).

Application for Marketing Approval

Application for marketing approval, using either the centralized or decentralized procedure, has to

Table 28.6 Processing times (days) of centralized applications to EMEA, 1995–1999

Year	Assessment phase	Decisions process	EMEA post opinion phase	Company clockstop	Total
1995	189	45	119	59	412
1997	169	40	79	119	407
1997	178	32	86	139	435
1998	185	42	83	109	419
1999	183	38	70	148	439

Table 28.8 Mutual recognition procedure and Arbitrations for 1999.

Mutual recognition procedure	Total submitted in 1999*	Under evaluation in 1999	Ended positively in 1999	Arbitrations in 1999
New applications	275	48	210	2
Type I variations	695	90	625	0
Type II variations	254	109	292	2

* The number includes multiple procedures

be accompanied by three expert reports, which cover: (a) chemistry, pharmacy, manufacturing route; (b) preclinical aspects, including pharmacology, safety pharmacology, pharmacokinetics, single and repeat-dose toxicological evaluation, reproduction studies, mutagenic potential, and carcinogenicity; (c) clinical studies covering Phase I–III studies; ADRs notified to the company during clinical studies. If the product has been marketed, then all postmarketing experience should be assessed. Expert reports are not a promotion platform for the product but an assessment of the data generated, an explanation of the results and an interpretation. An expert report should not normally exceed 25 pages of A4. The expert reports should also make clear whether or not the studies submitted have been conducted according to GLP standards and whether the clinical studies have been conducted to GCP principles and in accord with the Declaration of Helsinki. A statement of the enviromental effects of the product is also necessary.

SOME OUTSTANDING ISSUES IN EUROPEAN MEDICINES CONTROL

Future Clinical Trial Legislation in the EU

At present, the EU Directives covering medical products are all directed at the marketing of such products. There is currently a draft Directive aimed at harmonizing the requirements for clinical trials in the EU.

The various member states' level of control on clinical evaluations vary. These were surveyed by Griffin (1987); the UK, Eire, The Netherlands and Italy did not have legislation requiring regulatory approval affecting human volunteer (non-patient) studies; Germany, Denmark and Sweden did control such studies. This survey indicated that a clear definition of what was meant by a 'human volunteer' was also lacking between national regulatory authorities in Europe.

Various sectors of the pharmaceutical industry have lobbied hard against this proposed Directive, particularly the industry based in the UK, who object to Phase 1 studies being brought under legislation. These objections are largely based on the negative effects on research of the CTC scheme introduced by the 1968 Medicines Act, and the stimulus that the deregulation achieved by the CTX scheme had on UK clinical research.

While at present no European Directive has been agreed concerning the conduct of clinical trials in the EU, a draft Directive was submitted to the European Parliament by the Commission in September 1997 [*COM(97) 369*]. This draft directive consists of:

- *Preamble*.
- *Chapter I*: Scope and definition.
- *Chapter II*: protection of confidentiality of clinical trial subjects and Ethics Committees.
- *Chapter III*: commencement of clinical trials (timing of regulatory processes) and provision for exchange of detailed information between member states.
- *Chapter IV*: manufacture, import, labeling of investigational medicinal products.
- *Chapter V*: compliance and good clinical practice inspections, which, it is envisaged, will be coordinated by the European Agency for the Evaluation of Medicines (EMEA).
- *Chapter VI*: clinical safety deals with the reporting of adverse drug reactions and events by the investigator to the sponsor, who shall report to the regulatory authority of the member state where the trial is in progress. The member state has the obligation to ensure that all serious adverse reactions and events are reported immediately to the EMEA.
- *Chapter VII*: includes general provisions and the proposed implementation date of the Directive on January 1 1999.

The implementation date of January 1 1999 was not met and has not been met at the time of writing.

DG XXIV Scientific Committee on Medicinal Products and Medical Devices

In a communication to the Council and European Parliament on 'Consumer Health and Food Safety' [*COM(97) 183 Fund*], the European Commission emphasized that high quality scientific committees are an essential foundation for EC rules in this area.

It was decided in August 1997 that DG XXIV Consumer Policy and Consumer Health, now renamed the Health Directorate in 1999 Protection, should set up a number of eight new advisory committees, including a Scientific Committee on Medicinal Products and Medical Devices. These committees are expected to meet 10 times/year and the Committee on Medicinal Products and Medical Devices met for the first time on November 10–14 1997. The *European Drug and Device Report* stated: Feathers are understood to be ruffled in the EU's Committee for Proprietary Medicinal Products; however, up to now, the CPMP has largely held a monopoly on scientific opinion.

The Commission said the new Scientific Committee will not overlap CPMP and there does appear to be a role for both panels.

Unlike the CPMP its minutes would be public.

Drug companies have feared that the committee would lean more towards consumers than industry.

The interaction between CPMP (which reports to the Enterprise Directorate, formerly the Commissions DGIII Industry Affairs) and the new Medical Products and Medical Devices Committee, which reports to the Health Directorate, formerly DGXXIV Consumer Policy, is very uncertain. It has to be borne in mind that the objective of Directive 65/65 was to advance the free movement of goods within the EC, i.e. an industrial/commercial objective. In the future it might be more logical for the functions of EMEA to be the responsibility the Health Directorate rather than the Enterprise Directorate.

The CPMP and European Harmonization of Data Requirements and ICH

It might not be immediately apparent that the drive towards 'harmonization' of regulatory requirements had its birth at the first meeting of the CPMP in November 1976. The CPMP at that juncture had been established to operate a 'mutual recognition' procedure, laid out in Directive 75/318, but it had no work to do initially. It was, however, immediately clear to the CPMP that the data requirements laid down for registration were being interpreted differently by individual member states' regulatory authorities. For example, there was no agreement on requirements for reproduction studies, carcinogenicity, studies etc. At that first meeting two expert working groups on safety and efficacy were established to draw up guidelines (later, other expert working groups were established). A great deal of international harmonization of requirements and thought was achieved, and this could clearly be extended beyond the confines of the EC.

By June 1994, the EC Commission decided that a meeting with the Japanese authorities, attended by Mr Fernand Sauer and the Chairmen of the Safety and Efficacy Groups J.P. Griffin and J.M. Alexander should take place in Tokyo. As a result of this, a second meeting with the Japanese authorities (the JPMA), the EC Commission and EFPIA representatives took place. This was the stimulus for EFPIA, JPMA and the PMA, as it then was in the USA, to press for wider consultation. From such a start, the International Conference on Harmonization (ICH) was born. The ICH Steering Committee established expert working groups (EWG) to discuss areas where harmonization was possible and to produce universally acceptable guidelines. Thus, under the auspices of the ICH, a considerable number of guidelines have been issued in the areas of quality, safety, and efficacy, with the object achieving harmonization of requirements for registration between regulatory authorities, and thus reducing the need for duplicating studies. It must be made clear that these documents should be regarded as *guidelines*, not requirements. These guidelines are not at the cutting edge of science but represent acceptable compromises. Guidelines will need updating, and this must be coordinated, otherwise there will be 'regulatory drift' towards disharmony.

If harmonization can be achieved, as it has been, across sufficiently broad areas of quality, safety, and efficacy, there is no logical reason why a common technical document (CTD) or dossier cannot be prepared that would be acceptable to all drug regulatory authorities. Movement to a CTD would appear to be the next step towards further internationalization.

The ICH guidelines and details of their evolution can be obtained in the Proceedings of the First, Second, Third and Fourth International Conferences on Harmonization, held in Brussels (1991), Orlando, USA (1993), Yokohama, Japan (1995), and Brussels (1997), published by the Queen's University of Belfast and obtainable from the IFPMA Offices, 30 Rue du St Jean, PO Box 9, 1211 Geneva 18, Switzerland.

The clinical guidelines applicable to the EC may be obtained from the Medicines Control Agency (MCA), EuroDirect Guideline Service, Room 1615, Market Towers, 1 Nine Elms Lane, London SW8 5NQ, UK Tel: +44 (0) 171 273 0352/0228.

Mutual Recognition of Established Products and Line Extensions

The bulk of national licensing activities relates to new formulations of older products, generics and line extensions. However, over the years the indications, contraindications, warnings, dosages, etc. of even well-known products differ significantly from member state to member state. The national reviews required of older products that were conducted by each member state of the EC were not accompanied by any international concertation of effort and did not lead to harmonization within the EC. This has made it difficult for companies to use the mutual recognition procedure for the introduction of generic products, since the summary of product characteristics (SPC) differs between member states. The same problem can affect the originator of an established chemical entity when the company wishes to introduce a line extension, because even under the operation of the mutual recognition procedure, where the CPMP opinion was not binding, there were differences in dosages, indications, contraindications, and warnings between member states.

In 1996, the Swedish Government proposed a solution to the impasse affecting the use of the mutual recognition procedure for generic products. This would have allowed generic companies to apply for recognition only of the quality and bioequivalence data, the rest of authorization to market, i.e. indications, contraindications, and warnings, would be decided by the national authorities, bearing in mind these factors as they applied to the originator's product in each member state.

In April 1997 the EC Commission announced that, rather than change the Directives to allow the 'core SPC idea' as advanced by Sweden, it would 'reinterpret' them. In practice, this means that generic companies would, from January 1 1998, be able to use the mutual recognition procedure only when the originator's SPC was identical in all member states, i.e. the originator's product had mutual recognition status or a centralized licence. In practice, this means that generics will have to use national procedures 'which were due to be phased out on December 31 1997'. Line extensions of existing products, i.e. new dosage forms, etc., would logically be caught in the same net as generics if the initial product did not have an identical SPC in all member states. Currently, some companies are withdrawing products from the market and replacing them with a new salt of the same active substance in an attempt to thwart generic products entering the market.

Changes Ahead for European Regulation?

Possible Changes to the Centralized Procedure

In view of the increased membership of the EU, in future years, if standards of granting marketing authorizations for medicines are not to decline, measures will have to be taken to preserve the standards that operated in Northern Europe prior to 1994. It could be conceded that all NCEs should be handled through the centralized procedure. This could only be acceptable in terms of consumer safety if the competence of advice available to the EMEA was increased. EMEA staff themselves must be technically competent to do the assessment work currently done by those national drug regulatory authorities, appointed to act on behalf of the rapporteur and co-rapporteur. The use of national drug regulatory authorities to do the work of rapporteur and co-rapporteur would cease. The staff recruited to the EMEA to do this expert work should be recruited on the basis of quality, rather than having regard to the adherence of 'national quotas' of staff. The CPMP, currently composed of two members from each member state's regulatory authority, should be disbanded. The technical advisory committee serving the EMEA should be served by expert panels, covering chemistry and pharmacy, pharmacology, and toxicology, and multiple clinical panels of experts, covering e.g.

cardiovascular, respiratory, diabetic, and endocrine disorders, oncology, etc. on the pattern used by the US Food and Drug Administration (FDA). This would be a way forward, with synthesis of an overall view done by a standing expert committee. It would have to be recognized that not all EU member states would be involved in every committee or expert panel. Although attempts should be made to involve all member states at some level in the procedure, it must be accepted that, in the public interest, expertise should predominate over national representation. The role of selection of the experts to serve on this standing committee and expert panels should be the role of the EMEA Management Board, and nominations should be made by the Ministers of Health of the Member States of the EU, on a similar basis to the way the membership of the British Committee on Safety of Medicines is drawn together.

Possible Changes to the Decentralized or Mutual Recognition System

The current mutual recognition system is cumbersome and could be improved. A true mutual recognition system for marketing applications that did not involve a NCE could be devised, drawing on the system operating in the medical devices area, where authorization by one regulatory agency leads to an EU-wide approval, provided that marketing in all EU member states is identical with the approval granted in the reference member state. A single chemical entity marketing authorization number would be used to cover the authorization in all member states of the EU. Applicant companies would be wise to select a credible national drug regulatory authority to process such a mutual recognition. In fact, it might be better if the scheme were to designate competent national authorities to operate such a procedure, and laid down strict criteria for delegating such authority to competent national regulatory bodies (not all national authorities would necessarily qualify).

Single Assessment/Single Marketing Approval

Both systems, modified as outlined, would lead to a single EU-wide marketing approval, following a single assessment.

CONCLUSION

The European system for granting marketing authorization for medicinal products will continue to evolve and perhaps must change; however, like the advice given to the man seeking directions (I wouldn't start from here if I were you), we do not have an option. Finally, it has to be understood that the EU is not a country—it is a collection of member states, and there is much fertile ground for continuing dissent.

REFERENCES

Geddie WM, Geddie JL (1926) *Chambers Biographical Dictionary. The Great of All Nations and All Times*. WR Chambers: London; 662.

Griffin JP, Diggle GE (1981) A survey of products licenced in the United Kingdom, 1971–1981. *Br J Clin Pharmacol* 12: 453–63.

Griffin JP, Long JR (1981) New procedures affecting the conduct of clinical trials in the United Kingdom. *Br Med J* 283: 477–9.

Griffin JP (1987) An international comparison on legislation regarding human volunteer studies. *Int Pharm J* 1: 57–60.

Heberden W (1745) *Antitherica: Essay on Mithridatium and Theriac.*: London.

Jefferys DB, Leakey D, Lewis JA et al (1998) New active substances authorized in the United Kingdom between 1972 and 1994. *Br J Clin Pharmacol* 45: 151–6.

Munk W (1878) *The Roll of Royal College of Physicians of London*, vol II, 1701–1800. Royal College of Physicians: Pall Mall East, London; 159–64.

Rubin S (1975) *Medieval English Medicine*. David & Charles: Newton Abbot; 43–128.

Stenton FM (1947) Anglo Saxon England. *Oxford History of England*, 2nd edn. Oxford University Press: Oxford; 266.

Speirs CJ, Griffin JP (1983) A survey of the first year of operation of the new procedure affecting the conduct of clinical trials in the United Kingdom. *Br J Clin Pharmacol* 15: 649–55.

Speirs CJ, Saunders RM, Griffin JP (1984) The United Kingdom Clinical Trial Exemption Scheme—its effects on investment in research. *Pharm Int* 5: 254–6.

Watson G (1966) *Theriac and Mithridatium. A Study in Therapeutics*. The Wellcome Historical Library: London.

RECOMMENDED INFORMATION SOURCES

The European Agency for the Evaluation of Medicinal Products (1995, 1996, 1997) *First, Second and Third General Reports.*

EMEA: 7 West Ferry Circus, Canary Wharf, London E14 4HB, UK.

EC *The Rules Governing Medicinal Products in the European Community*, vols I–IV. Commission of the European Communities: Brussels.

Medicines Control Agency (1994/5, 1995/6, 1996/7) *Annual Report and Accounts*. HMSO: London.

29

Ethnic Issues in Drug Registration

[1]Lionel D. Edwards, [2]J.M. Husson, [3]E. Labbé, [4]C. Naito, [5]M. Papaluca Amati, [6]S. Walker, [7]R Williams and [4]H. Yasurhara

[1]Novartis, East Hanover, USA, [2]Paris, France, [3]Sanofi-Synthelabo, Paris, France, [4]Teikyo University, Japan, [5]EMEA, London, UK, [6]Centre of Medicine Research, Carlshalton, UK, [7]US Pharmacopia, Rockville, USA

BACKGROUND

The international need for quicker national approval of significant drugs offering improved therapy, less toxic effects, and even cure, had been delayed and restricted by differing mandatory regulatory requirements between nations. Thus, by 1980, the need for an international cohesive policy was apparent. Discussions between the regulatory authorities of Europe (EMEA) and the USA (FDA) were aimed at the harmonization of regulations governing the approval process of drugs and devices, and have been going on since the first International Conference of drug regulatory authorities, which met in October 1980 (Annapolis, USA), and latterly under the auspices of the International Conference on Harmonization (ICH). In their first meeting in Brussels (November 1991) the Japanese regulatory authorities (Ministry of Health and Welfare (MHW)) participated as a full member; these three major regional members were joined by representatives from the pharmaceutical industry of Japan (JPMA), Europe (IFHPA) and USA (PhRMA) and observers from the World Health Organization (WHO) Nordic countries, and Canada's HPB, thus covering about 92% of the current regulatory activity and global spending on pharmaceuticals.

The International Conference on Harmonization (ICH) continuing series of meetings has resulted in success in the areas of quality control, toxicology, pharmacology and clinical development, including good clinical practice (GCP) and the recent issue of guidances on the acceptability of foreign clinical data, the technical document and electronic submissions.

The clinical area has proved much harder to harmonize because of the lack of clear-cut regional or national concordance on many clinical issues. The very existence of some diseases is in dispute, e.g. the USA temporomandibular joint dysfunction and premenstrual syndromes, the European hypotension syndrome (Pemberton 1989), and the Swiss 'heavy leg' prevaricose vein syndrome. The emphasis on treatment, overprevention, and the real physical and genetic differences between national populations with variety of health care systems, can cause disparity of results, observations, and conclusions. Again, diversity within a national population, geographic influences, diet, varied measurement standards, religious and cultural effects, and patient–doctor relationships also play a part in making interpretation and agreement difficult.

To date, it is by no means clear that harmonization has reduced the overall burden of regulations for either the regulators or the regulated, but it has already eliminated some inconsistencies. To those ends, 'Ethnic Factors Influence on the Acceptability of Foreign Data' was proposed by Japan and Europe and accepted as an ICH II topic by the ICH Steering Committee, Washington (March 24 1992). This chapter will give an account of the ethnic issues faced by the working party, ending in the tripartite implementation of the 'Guidance' of 1998. A working party made up of representatives from each of three major regions was set up and met many times for 2-day working sessions. A major study of approved drug dosage and pharmacokinetics between the three regions was undertaken by Japan's MHW and JPMA. A further

Principles and Practice of Pharmaceutical Medicine. Edited by A. J. Fletcher, Lionel D. Edwards, Anthony W. Fox and Peter Stonier © 2002 John Wiley & Sons Ltd.

study, commissioned by IFFPA, was undertaken by the Centre of Medicines Research (CMR, UK). In addition, the type and incidence of spontaneous adverse events reports occurring with eight drugs marketed in the European community were examined for consistency by the EC representative, and concurrently, the data files of one pharmaceutical company of four drugs in different therapeutic areas was examined for any varaitions of pharmacokinetics, dosage, and adverse events between regions by the EFPIA member. Only their major findings are included in this chapter, more information can be found in the individual reports (Naito and Yasuhara, Walker and Harvey: Papaluca; Labbé Edward: Williams (Orlando 1993)).

REGULATORY PRACTICE

In the USA, initially, non-US studies, not under the investigational new drug applications (INDs), were considered primarily as a source of supportive safety data. By the early 1970s, it was appreciated that well-controlled non-US clinical data could be utilized to support US new drug applications. US regulations have allowed for the use of non-US data as the sole basis for approval, so long as certain conditions were met, including the stipulation that 'foreign data are applicable to US populations and US medical practice' (FDA 1975, 1985). No specifics were given regarding the definition of 'applicable'. Thus, clinical data from Phases I–III were allowed, but in practice such data could not be the sole source of safety and efficacy for new drug approvals. The reasons given for why Japanese data were not used more widely in the USA and Europe involve differences in medical practice, such as the use of different end-points, lower dosages, and differences in research methodology, such as the emphasis on a large number of physicians and their experience in Phase III, resulting in a large number of investigators with a low ratio of patients enrolled. In Europe, while there may be preference by individual countries to have local clinical data developed, it did not appear that actual regulations precluded the use of 'foreign' (usually US) data in most European countries (Safety Workshop—ICH 1 1992), although some nation (France, Italy, and Ger-

many) required some clinical experience in their countries prior to approval.

In Japan, there has been harmonization with the other regions in the area of toxicology (animal studies); the Japanese Ministry of Health and Welfare (MHW) accepts appropriate foreign animal data, and animal safety studies performed according to ICH guidelines. Indeed, Japan played a major role and Japan's current fertility and reproductive animal studies requirements have been adopted by the other two regions.

However, the acceptance of 'foreign' clinical data has been a major issue to the Japanese for a long time. Previously, all Phase II and III clinical studies needed to be performed on Japanese people. Phase I studies could be done outside Japan, *but only* if the drug was in wide use in that country (which had to be a developed country) and if the drug's performance was unaffected by racial differences in physiology. The Japanese position has been that diet, and perhaps genetics, can play a significant role in pharmacodynamics, and that because of subsequent metabolic differences, a drug's safety or efficacy may be different in the Japanese than in other races (MHW Notification 660 and Notification June 1987). Clearly there are a few drugs where this rationale is justified, but there are many others where metabolism may be largely irrelevant (e.g. ophthalmologicals, topicals). However, these differences appear to constitute a major reason why (without exception) Phase II and III trials had to be carried out on Japanese patients (Uchida 1988; Fairburn 1989; Homma 1991; for further discussion, see Apple, and Weintraub 1993).

OBJECTIVE DIFFERENCES

We must first examine those differences which can be quantified more readily.

Population Demographics between Tripartite Areas

The USA is a nation of many racial, ethnic and national origins and is the most heterogeneous population of the three areas. Given the successive waves of European, African and Asian immigrants, themselves imposed upon even earlier waves of Bering Straits immigrants (Native North and South American Indian, and Eskimo), this makes the US population the most diverse in the world. While intermarriage has occurred, many major racial groups remain regionally or locally clustered and still adhere to cultural aspects of their area of origin. However, many of the smaller distinct racial and ethnic groups may not be represented in US pharmaceutical databases, either due to the realities of setting up clinical studies or because only small numbers are present in that population. In general, only Caucasians, Blacks, Asians and Hispanics may have measurable populations in a database (Edwards 1992). As of 1990, American Indians comprise 0.8% of the population, with the other minorities larger or smaller percentages of the population: Hispanic (any race), 9.8%; Pacific Asian, 2.9%; Black, 12.1% (US Bureau of the Census 1991). Europe has a Caucasian 'heterogeneous' population made up of Anglo-Saxon/Celtic, Germanic, Gaelic, mid-European and 'Latin' races. There are sizeable populations of migrant foreign workers, as much as 10% in Germany, and many resident Asian and African citizens of Britain and in France (5%). In contrast, Japan is populated almost entirely by ethnic Japanese, truly homogeneous, although a sizable non-national immigrant population of other guest Asian workers exists.

The definitions of racial groups are not totally satisfactory (e.g. what is 'Black'?), and ethnicity and geography can wreak havoc on the meaning of 'representative' e.g. Pacific Islanders and Asians make up 9.8% of the Pacific states population and 61.8% of the US state of Hawaii (US Bureau of the Census 1991). What is Hispanic, other than a language group that contains a combination of genetic groups from Europe, Africa, and Native America? Diseases such as stroke are associated with high levels of Von Willebrand factor (Folsom et al 1999), found commonly in the Black population. Sickle cell anemia, thalassemia and glucose dehydrogenase deficiency are ethnically linked, but how do they effect drug metabolism?

The small genetic variation (DNA), only 0.5% of the 11% total variations between individuals of these groups among the three major divisions of humans (Caucasian, Negroid, and Mongoloid), makes up of the total variation between individuals of these groups (Vesell 1989). Thus, it would not be a surprise if race gives rise to fewer differences than does individual variation of drug metabolism and dynamics. That is, genes of race have less influence than an individual's genetic makeup.

Pharmacokinetics/Pharmacodynamics and Ethnic Differences

One of the earliest reports of differences was described by Chen and Poth (1929). They noted that the mydriatic response to cocaine was greatest in Caucasians, less in Chinese and least in Blacks. When pharmacokinetic differences were first reported in the literature, they usually involved the genetic polymorphisms of acetylation, the debrisoquine–sparteine and mephenytoin pathways, the second phase of metabolism or selective protein transport systems. Drugs such as clonazepam, hydralazine, sulphonamides, isoniazide, nitrazepam, and procainamide undergo acetylation in the liver. Most Asians, especially Japanese (88–93%), are fast acetylators compared to 50% of Caucasians and Blacks (Wood and Zhon 1991). Fast acetylators may be at greater risk of isoniazide hepatitis from toxic metabolites (Drayer and Reidenberg 1977), whereas slow acetylators may respond better to treatment (sustained levels) but be at greater risk of toxic reactions. Those drugs which extensively use both acetylatiy as to second phase of metabolism, and also we use either of two Cytochomes enzymes in the first phase, are more likely to induce Cupus (Hess 1982) and/or hypersensitivity reactions (Reider 1999). The two cytochromel were identified as CYP2D6 and CYP2C19, part of the extensive P450 cytichrane enzyme systems found mainly in the liver but also present in other tissues such as guft, lung and brain. Ethnic differences in these two pathway have also been found CYP2D6 enzymes is lacking in 8% of caucasians and 1% of asians. CYP2C19 is lacking in 20% of Asian, 4–8% of Blacks and 3% of Caucasians. These are two of the three commonest first phase, metabolic pathway. The most common CYP3A4 has not demonstrate Ethnic sensitivity.

Perpherazine and over-the-counter (OTC) ingredients codeine and dextromethorphan are metabolized by the debrisoquine–sparteine oxidative pathway. The percentage of an ethnic or racial population poorly metabolizing by this pathway varies greatly; e.g. Switzerland 9–10%, Hungary 10%, USA 7%, Nigeria 3–8%, and Japan 0.5% (Wood and Zhon 1991), but if not will gain no pain relief.

Clinically, this has been shown to make a difference in a small study in males, involving 10 Chinese and nine Caucasian subjects; the Chinese metabolized propranolol more rapidly, clearance was 76% higher, with a lower area under the curve (AUC) and plasma levels lower than the Caucasians at all time points. In this study, when dosage was adjusted upwards to equilibrate to Caucasian therapeutic blood levels, a greater response was noted in the Chinese subjects (lower blood pressure and pulse rate) (Zhou et al 1990). Conversely, the presence of very fast metabolizers in a population may also vary.

The mephenytoin metabolic pathway is utilized by commonly used drugs, such as mephobarbital, hexobarbital, diazepam, imipramine, and omeprazol, but only 3–5% of Caucasians and 8% of Blacks are poor metabolizers of mephenytoin, compared to 15–20% of Chinese and Japanese populations (Kupfer et al 1988). This enzyme's activity is inhibited by floconazole and fluoxetine and induces drugs such as barbiturates and nicotine (smoking).

The lack of digestive enzyme lactase in many Hispanics, especially Mexican-Americans and African-Americans, causes lactose intolerance, with nausea, diarrhea, and occasionally vomiting. It is understandable that lactose is no longer prefered as a filler (non-active excipient) in tablets and capsules.

Some drugs, such as phenothiazines and tricyclic antidepressants, show greater preference for binding and transport on α-1 acid glycoprotein rather than onto albumin. Thus, 44% of Swiss and both US White and Black populations have higher levels of this protein, compared to 15–27% of the Japanese population (Eap et al 1989; Mendoza 1991). This might explain the higher fraction of free drug found in Asians (with a greater volume of distribution and clearance), as well as the fact that the metabolism of some benzodiazepines appears to be slower in Asians than in Caucasians (Kumana et al 1987). One study (Zhang et al 1990) showed that Chinese subjects who were either poor or ex-

tensive mephenytoin metabolizers when taking diazepam (mephenytoin pathway) still metabolized diazepam at the same rate as Caucasian poor metabolizers. The higher proportion of slow metabolizers of mephenytoin pathways is thus not the only difference. However, ethnic differences in the percentage of body fat between the two groups could also account for this. The 'p' protein transport system is also being explored for ethnic drug variations, especially in the maintenance of the blood–brain barrier.

As previously noted, drugs such as propranolol and imipramine each have two major pathways, and even poor metabolizers of any significant pathways usually have alternative pathways, which might be expected to show some increased handling ability over time. Thus, in many cases, plasma levels and clinical differences between poor and good polymorphic metabolizers may be insignificant. In others, especially where the therapeutic index is small, it may be critical—usually these drugs are titrated for efficacy and safety and thus, the effect is avoided. In other cases, such as antihypertensive agents, the clinical effect of genetic differences may not be seen, because the patient's dosage is titrated to blood pressure response (Eichelbaum and Gross 1990) and only a large meta-analysis may show ethnic dosage.

Prescribing Differences

Of great concern are findings that ethnicity may affect prescribing habits. Sleath et al (1998) looked at the patient's ethnicity and the likelihood of a psychotropic being prescribed: they found that Caucasians received medication 20% of the time and non-Whites only 13.5%. A similar finding was made by Khandker et al (1998) concerning any prescription drug. Differences were found at all ages, with Black children receiving 2.7 fewer prescriptions than their Caucasian counterparts. This rose to 4.9 prescriptions in adult Blacks and 6.3 in elderly Blacks. All the patients were on Medicaid, so ability to pay was not a factor. Dinsdale et al (1995) confirmed a similar pattern in prescriptions issued for analgesics for postoperative pain to be self-administered by the patient, with Caucasians receiving prescriptions significantly more frequently than minorities ($p = 0.01$).

Genetic and Ethnic Susceptibility

Therapeutic effects may vary between ethnic populations, due either to a sizeable representation of poor metabolizers present or to a genetic or ethnic-related 'susceptibility'. Clozapine is associated with the development of agranulocytosis in 20% of Ashkenazi Jews, compared to 1% of the general population treated for schizophrenia. This was found to be highly associated with specific linked genes, agranulocystosis and especially those of Ashkenazi Jewish origin (100%) (Leiberman et al 1990). Yet again, the best known example was the sensitivity to quinine and its derivatives in Blacks given to prevent malaria, resulted in many deaths in World War II.

Another example of pharmacodynamic differences is that of reports on lithium in the manic phase of bipolar depression. Asian patients, including Japanese, are reported to have therapeutic blood levels at 0.5–0.8 m.eg/l compared to required levels in US Caucasian patients of 0.8–1.2 m.eg/l (Jefferson et al 1987; Yang 1987; Takahashi 1979); these findings, however, are disputed by Chang et al (1985). African-Americans require less drug, but this is because of higher levels due to a slower clearance rate than Caucasians (Jefferson et al 1987; Lin et al 1986).

Asians have been reported to require smaller doses of neuroleptic drugs and to suffer adverse events at lower doses than Caucasians, even after body weight was accounted for (Wood and Zhou 1991; Poland 1991). With tricyclic agents, the picture is more confusing between Asians and Caucasians, but Asians appear to show more variability overall and African-Americans tend to have higher plasma levels, faster therapeutic effect, but more side effects than either (Strickland et al 1991).

Essential hypertension is a disease of modern society, and its treatment accounts for a sizeable portion of global prescriptions. As a result, there is a great interest in reported ethnic and racial differences reported in the literature. The use of appropriate therapy in Black patients has been best studied. As monotherapy, calcium channel blockers and diuretics appear to be most effective in Blacks, while β-blockers and ACE inhibitors produce smaller reductions in blood pressure (Hall 1990; Freis 1986; Kiowiski et al 1985). However, this may more reflect the lower plasma renin, salt and water retention and intercellular sodium and calcium in Blacks, compared to other groups (Kiowiski et al 1988). There are individual exceptions amongst patients and among drugs, even within these classes; e.g. labetalol, a combined α- and β-blockers, can be equally effective in both African-Americans and Caucasians and, as mentioned previously, the Chinese appear twice as sensitive as Caucasians to propranolol (Oster et al 1987; Zhou et al 1990)

Receptor Sensitivity

Salzman described a downregulation of benzodiazepine and β-blocker receptors linked to aging. It has been postulated that Asians have fewer benzodiazepine and β-blocker receptors than Caucasians. Downregulation of these receptors with age (Salzman 1982) has been described and postulated by Zhou et al (1990), but hard evidence of racial or ethnic differences is still awaited. If the Chinese are more sensitive to propranolol in spite of their high catabolic rate, it might be linked to adrenergic receptor sensitivity.

Looking at the broader picture, part of today's discovery process is the incorporation of iso-enzyme detector screens and computer predictor modeling, to eliminate potential drugs posing major metabolic and ethnic problems or interference patterns. This is being done as part of the screening process for lead candidates prior to preclinical screening. Drugs such as terfenidine and mibefradil would not pass these screens today.

In-depth Drug Case Studies

The European Federation Pharmaceutical Association (EFFPA) commissioned a third party, the Centre for Medicines Research (CMR, UK), to collect data on a small number of targeted drugs. By direct appeal to manufacturers through an independent third party, compliance information between regions was made available, as well as pharmacokinetic data. In addition, data on efficacy and safety were also requested from firms operating in the three major areas.

The CMR conducted this study amongst European and American companies to assess the significance of inter-ethnic differences in clinical responsiveness, and to determine the implications of such differences for international clinical development. Information was collected for all three phases of clinical development. Data from 21 compounds developed since 1985 in the West and Japan, and covering a wide range of therapeutic categories, were analysed. Overall, there was no indication that the metabolism of any of these drugs was affected by genetic polymorphism. One compound is known to be eliminated by an enzyme which is polymorphic, but there was no evidence of altered phenotype or subset population within any ethnic group. Although three compounds displayed some regional variability in pharmacokinetics, further analysis of the data provided rational explanations for all such perceived differences. All the regional variations were attributable to different pharmaceutical formulations, reduction of initial doses, and alteration in sampling times and techniques, and none of these differences had any significant impact on clinical development.

There was considerable regional variation in dosing or frequency of dosing, with a tendency towards lower Japanese doses, due to cultural differences in medical practice. The type and frequency of adverse reactions observed during clinical trials was generally lower in Japanese subjects, although there was no correlation between reduced adverse reactions and lower doses. Cultural attitudes relating to the use of preferred terms, different assessment methods and reporting differences were provided as explanations for the lower incidence of Japanese adverse reactions. More Western subjects were included in trials for a given indication than Japanese adverse reactions. More Western subjects were included in trials for a given indication than Japanese subjects, and Japanese dose-ranging trials were frequently of an open design. Phase III trials were controlled, although regional differences in the numbers of subjects and the use of placebos and reference drugs were observed, placebo controls being more frequent in the USA.

The only apparent difference in clinical effectiveness between the West and Japan was not considered to be significant, for all 21 compounds displayed no geographic differences in risk–benefit assessment (for further details, see Harvey and Walker 1993).

Other Ethnic Factors with Pharmacologic Implications

Differences seen across regions and nations, both in reports of efficacy and incidence of adverse reactions, are much greater than can be accounted for by ethnic variations of pharmacokinetics and pharmacodynamics. Other objective differences are now discussed.

Alcohol

Even modest amounts of alcohol may induce enzyme activity of many hepatic-metabolized drugs; thus, it is conceivable that data derived from a French, Italian, or Spanish European population, who regard wine or beer as a 'digestive' and part of the daily diet, might enhance, albeit slightly, a higher metabolism of some drugs, thus requiring higher dosages to achieve efficacy. Contrast this with the same drug developed in a Moslem or Mormon society, or in populations who have less tolerance of alcohol, because of poor metabolism due to a reduction or absence of either aldehyde dehydrogese or gastric alcoholic dehydrogenase. This reduction or absence of enzyme occurs in Japanese (44%), Eskimos (43%) or South American Indians (41–43%) and to a much lesser degree in other ethnic groups (Mendoza 1991). Initially, this reduced enzyme might exaggerate possible adverse events with drugs competing for the same metabolic pathway.

Other Influences on Drug Differences

Some curiosities, such as prolongation of ductus arteriosus closure in the neonate at high altitudes and its resistance to indomethacin closure, are interesting but hardly relevant to most populations. Of greater impact is the effect of ultraviolet light on skin. Black pigment gives about 30% protection from sunburn, but Caucasian populations living in tropical areas not only suffer exaggerated sunburn and photosensitivity when ingesting some classes of drugs, e.g. tetracyclines and quinolones, but also develop a higher incidence of skin cancers.

Concurrent presence of diseases dominating in a region, e.g. chronic hepatitis B, which is endemic in Asia and may affect up to 30% of the population, might distort laboratory normals of liver enzyme responses to drugs and population baseline measurements. Heterozygous sickle cell anemia gene confers immunity against falciparum malaria to Africans (Medawar 1961), but in African-Americans this benefit is unneeded in malaria-free USA, and homozygous genes (two sets) confer illness and sickle cell anemia episodes may confuse drug assessment. Indeed, drugs such as chloroquine give rise to occasional fulmanent hepatitis in these patients and diltiazam has been shown to produce greater sensitization of the PR interval in sickle cell C and S patients (Weintraub and Rubio 1992).

While nutritional status is good in Japan, much of Asia lives on less than optimal nutrition, and it might be argued that the USA and Europe suffer from nutritional excess, with about 30% of their populations overweight. Either status has implications regarding lipophilic drug storage, metabolism, and tissue distribution.

Ethnic variations in diet, additives, or salt content, may alter metabolism rates. Lin et al (1986) and Henry et al (1987) report that antipyrine metabolism was different in rural Asian Indians than in Asian Indian immigrants resident in England for some years. Dietary environmental differences may also account for the findings of Gould et al (1972) and Kato et al (1973) of a gradation of heart and stroke incidence, lowest in residents of rural Japan, higher in Japanese in Hawaii, and highest in Japanese in California.

High- or low-fat diets can affect ingestion of drugs, as can a high intake of salt affect diuretic efficacy. Findings that some spices may influence metabolism have been reported. Baily et al (1991) showed that enhanced bioavailability of felodipine can be more than doubled, and to a lesser extent, nifedipine, with concurrent consumption with grapefruit juice compared to water (an effect not seen with orange juice), and many other drugs (Rau 1997).

Age, Height and Weight Differences

Currently, there is an obvious difference in average height–weight of US/European citizens vs. the Japanese. This reflects in a difference in blood/tissue volume which alone probably accounts for more real drug differences than pharmacogenetics

and other factors previously discussed. In the USA and Europe, from the largest normal to the smallest normal males in terms of height and weight, there is a 70% difference (Metropolitan Life Insurance Tables, 1999). Add to this 30% lower height–weight for the smallest normal-sized female.

To compound this, the Japanese small normal female is 20% smaller than her European counterpart. Despite this, in general, blood level differences are not as great as might be supposed. However, these regional size differences appear to be decreasing as the average increase of height in the USA is slowing, while in other nations, such as Japan, they are increasing.

A final physiologic population difference to be considered is the relative ages of the three populations: USA 32.9, Europe 34–38, and Japan 38.2 years (World Almanac 1992; and World Population [WHO] 1992). The differences between the average age of the three populations may cause a slight 'age effect' change in the average function of organs such as kidney and liver and the metabolism and excretion of drugs. Japan and Sweden have a greater proportion of their population over 80 years compared to the other regions and this segment, while generally increasing worldwide, is increasing faster in Japan.

SUBJECTIVE FACTORS

The previous *objective* factors can produce, on occasion, a real although usually small/difference in drug levels and effect. The next group of factors to be discussed are largely *subjective*, but still have an even more profound effect on protocol design, execution, measurement, outcome, recording and interpretation of the data collected. The subjective biases of doctors, patients, study monitors, experts, investigators and regulatory assessors are affected in different ways by variations of the three regional medical cultures and practices, and their population cultural values. It is also an area which is poorly researched by comparative studies. Many of the observations reported in this next section came from the experiences of the author or from the literature of anthropology and social biology.

Medical Practice

Physicians in Japan try to achieve effectiveness with no adverse effects with what, by US standards, appear to be almost homeopathic doses at times. In Europe, the aim is to achieve effectiveness with some minimal side effects, often by titrating the dose upwards. In the USA, the aim is to achieve optimal effectiveness with acceptable adverse effects and then titrate downwards. Thus, the highest total daily dosage tends to be greater in the USA than in the other two regions.

The pressure to prescribe is greater in the USA than in Europe; e.g. antibiotic usage per capita is twice as great in the USA compared to the UK, and four times more than in Germany. Defensive medicine is only part of the story; the need for an aggressive approach, with the need to cure as opposed to treatment, is a major factor in the USA. Less litigation may reduce this pressure, but this is unlikely to occur. Conversely, fear of litigation also increases drug attribution and reporting of adverse events.

In Japan, concurrent prescribing of different drugs of the same class in small doses is not unusual. Disclosure of cancer diagnosis to the patient is frowned upon in Japan, and reporting of GI side effects by the patient may be discouraged by the culture.

Differences in preferred dose form, availability of suppositories in France, injections in Italy, pills in the UK, and polypharmacy in Japan, reflect medical practice, education and practice conditions. There is great emphasis and concern in Germany over the heart and diet; in France, over the liver; in the UK, over viruses; and in the USA, over hypertension and obesity. Only in 1999 were oral contraceptives approved in Japan, a brave action, for it may increase the falling rate of Japanese population replacement, shared with Italy and Western nations (excluding the USA). All reflect different small emphases on drug development.

In the different regions, the physicians and investigators are held in varying degrees of esteem by their patients. In Japan, the ability to depend on others, to lean and to be leaned on, is considered healthy (Doi 1973). The doctor is held in great respect by the patient, and both the doctor and patient regard the chief investigator with even greater respect. This can interfere with adverse event reporting (avoidance of offense) by the patient, and perhaps lack of critical observation by their subinvestigators. These factors can influence the use of placebo, and 'informed consent format' in clinical studies. However, great strides are being made in Japan to share the responsibility with the patient for mutual benefit.

Physicians in the three regions deal differently with failure to achieve the desired clinical effect. In the USA, the tendency is to change medications. In other countries, dose titrations of the same medication may be used more frequently. The different approaches reflect both medical school teaching and expectation of the results of therapy. In many areas of Europe, the physicians and investigators are free, to a certain extent, from suspicion of monetary influence because of extensive socialized or government-backed health schemes. This has its pitfalls, but allows a degree of benevolent, autocratic meritocracy to emerge, which resulted in the evolution of the 'expert system' for regulation in Europe and the 'doctor knows best' for the patient in Japan, which works quite well in those cultures. Again, the reporting, anticipation, or recognition of adverse effects may be diminished. This contrasts with the USA, where frequently almost twice the number of adverse events are reported compared to European studies (except Sweden) and, not infrequently, placebo response rates are also increased. It has been postulated that these increased effects spring from both the aggression of American medical practice in search of *cure* and from the higher doses used. In addition, US physicians often focus on extensive data gathering in an attempt to achieve diagnostic certainty. This leads to increased search for, and investigation of, adverse reactions and their causality. This may also be due to the litigious nature of the US system. The diagnostic approach 'blitz' has been heavily impacted by the inroads of managed care to reduce costs.

Ethnic Effects on European Adverse Event Reporting

As part of an ongoing effort by the EC's General Directorate for Scientific Research, the European 'concertation' procedure's impact on the ability to monitor and detect changes in clinical safety was studied. Some of the information gathered on spontaneous adverse event reporting (ADRs) was made available to the ICH EC Working Party by Dr M. Papaluca.

The nature and incidence of serious spontaneous ADRs on three different new agents approved by the 11 EEC, at that time member states (1989–1991) was examined. As expected, the reporting rate varied between regions, according to the reporting framework and regulatory requirements, but qualitatively, the same serious adverse events were reported appropriately per capita in all member states where the drug was available. It thus appears, for serious ADRs, that ethnic variation in Europe does not influence the pattern of adverse events or its reporting. Other preliminary findings also showed a similarity of serious ADRs in multinational, multicenter European studies, provided that similar methodology and reporting formats are used. These observations did not apply to non-serious ADRs, where marked national differences were seen.

For further discussion, see sections on Evolution of ICH Topics and Ethnic Factors and Clinical Responsiveness (Papaluca 1993).

National Socioeconomic Influences

National reimbursement policies, therapeutic policies on patients, and third-party reimbursement differences between nations and national or private insurers, can all have an impact on how drugs are used. Obvious examples are the 1999 refusal of the UK government to reimburse the Glaxo Wellcome antiflu drug Relanza™ Advice National Institute for Clinical Excellence except now "at risk" patients (Nov 2000), because relief of 1 day of illness (out of an average of 6 days) did not justify the price. Another example, Germany, France and Italy's policy on pricing, grants only 'improved' drugs a higher price than the advertised therapy, even to the denial of some 'me-too' drugs. The pricing policy in Japan, with the compulsory dropping of a company's drug price after a few years, irrespective of patent life, is a further example. Lastly, the lately rescinded Canadian legislation, basically denying research costs against developers' taxes and shortening patent life nearly crippled research in Canada and slowed the applications until a price

structure had emerged for drugs in the USA and Europe.

Finally, the US population and US third-party insurance, both government and private industry, all pay 30–50% higher prices for the same medicines than Canada, Mexico or Europe. Pressures on the US manufacturers to reduce US prices will have a chilling effect on the development of new medicines and, hence, on the availability of new medicine globally (the USA is the origin of about 60% of the world's new chemical entities).

Terminology, Diagnosis and Other Subjective Factors

As previously mentioned, some diseases and syndromes are not universally recognized in the three regions. Until recently, neither AIDS nor depression was diagnosed in Japan. Conditions such as 'cardiac fatigue' and 'postural hypotension' in Germany; 'liver crisis' in France; 'heavy leg syndrome' (pre-varicose-vein development) in Switzerland; and 'anxiety neurosis' in the USA are unique to these regions. The endpoints for treatment may also be different, e.g. that for blood pressure in Japan is 160/95; in Europe 140/90; and in the USA 130/80. Indeed, even in the same language, 'I am in the pink' and 'I feel blue' have opposite meanings, and used in self-rating scales but have no or different meanings for the USA and UK, respectively.

The end result of these differences, although apparent rather than real, may be why the recommended dose of captopril (an ACE Inhibitor, antihypertensive drug) is 75–450 mg/day in the USA and 37.5–122.5 mg/day in Japan (with overall adverse events of 39% and 3.8% respectively). With a non-steroidal anti-inflammatory agent, overall adverse events were 45–51% in the USA and 24% in Japan at the same dosage; however, efficacy was the same (Dziewanowska, 1992). In general, the British, Dutch, and Scandinavian data are closer to those observed in the USA, with the German and Swiss data 'least reactive' and French, Italian and Spanish in between. As mentioned previously, severe ADRs in clinical studies tend to be the same; the major difference was in 'minor' adverse events, such as nausea, headache, etc. Thus, national temperament also may play a part in the expectation of efficacy and adverse event reporting. This finding was reflected in a study of attitudes of 4000 nurses from 13 countries to ethnic tolerance of pain (Davitz and Davits 1981), that Jews, Hispanics, and Italians appear to suffer more than Germans, Anglo-Saxons, and Asians, but such difference may simply appear to be the socially acceptable level of expression of pain vs. the actual pain severity itself.

In many African animist cultures, Western medicine may cure the disease but not the patient, who continues to languish. Western medicine is regarded in Africa in the same way that the Western world regards naturopathy—as ineffective, and this can cause the reverse placebo effect. This can be seen to the extreme in the severe mental function and physiologic systemic shutdown produced by a witch doctor's curses, which seem totally unresponsive to antidepressant medication (Cannon 1957) and the first author of this chapter has witnessed and successfully treated such an episode, but had to use unconventional methods.

In addition, Third World patients who report seeing spirits and ghosts may not be equated to 'hallucinating patients', as in a Western culture, for they may be experiencing the prevailing expectations of their culture (Hartog and Hartog 1993). Even within the USA, 70–90% of self-recognized episodes of sickness are managed outside the formal health care system (Zola 1972). Thus, the incorporation of clinical social sciences is essential if physicians are to understand, respond to and help patients (Eisenberg 1973); this is also applicable to the interpretation of clinical results.

THE EVOLUTION OF ICH TOPIC E5

Background

In November 1991, in Brussels, the International Conference on Harmonization of Technical Requirements for Registration of Pharmaceuticals for Human Use (ICH) was held. A new topic was proposed to, and accepted by, the ICH Steering Committee. This was the thorny issue of tripartite mutual acceptance of 'foreign' data. It was assigned the prefix E5 (efficacy, fifth topic approved) but was to be one of the slowest to be resolved—as the reader by now will appreciate,

slowly resolved because of its complexity, not because of ill-will. It is true that initially, mutual suspicion reigned, with regional rights and pride. This was quickly replaced by mutual respect, first amongst the regulators and then between the regulators and the pharmaceutical industry representatives. At a meeting in Washington in 1992, Professor Chikayuki Naito from Teikyo University, Japan, was handed perhaps the toughest job of ICH. He was appointed chairman of the E5 working party. He selected his working party members from the three regions, including this chapter's first author. He then immediately set us to work. One of the most interesting discussions was the topic's title; should it be 'ethnic' or 'racial?'—so interwoven were these descriptors with cultural, religious and language differences. Eventually, 'ethnic' was selected, for it allowed more regional incursion than 'racial', which was too restrictive. Then tasks were assigned on a regional basis; the USA representative (the first author) to a literature search, review and compilation; Japanese members were to research the dosing differences between the three regions on the 80 common drugs, backed up where available by matching pharmacokinetics data; Europe was assigned two tasks, first to review of the European adverse event database (national variations) and second, through an independent third party (Center for Medical Research), dosage, efficacy and safety differences. The reports were issued in October 1993 at the ICH 2 Orlando meeting. Professor Naito reported for the Japanese delegation that, amongst 42 drugs examined, daily doses of β-blockers and ACE inhibitors in the USA and Europe were twice as high as in Japan. Hypolipidemic drugs were similar in all the regions but, surprisingly, the highest doses were in the EC. Similarly with antibiotics: higher maximum doses were prescribed in EC and also in the USA, than in Japan.

H_2 blockers, a protein pump inhibitor and NSAIDs showed no difference in daily doses in the three regions, but again, maximum and lowest doses allowed were all lower in Japan. They had also reviewed the pharmacokinetic factors in 80 drugs approved in the three regions but largely concluded that intra-ethnic variation in drug metabolism was as large or larger than inter-ethnic differences; however, this variability was greater in the Japanese population. Professor Naito concluded that, if the metabolism of a new drug was influenced by genetic polymorphism, then additional regional pharmacokinetic and dose-ranging studies might be required.

Dr S. Walker of CMR approached European and US companies for information on 21 drugs savailable in the three regions. Within this narrow sample, only one drug had genetic polymorphism, but even this did not translate to ethnic variations. Three other drugs showed regional variability in pharmacokinetics, but these were attributable to different formulations, different sample times and reduction of the initial dose. The CMR survey confirmed that the reported levels of adverse events were lower in Japanese patients, even when adjusted for dose—a cultural variation.

The US report on findings in the literature were given by the first author of this chapter and R. Williams of the FDA. Much of the earlier part of this chapter was drawn from these reports.

Deciding what to do about this complex issue took another 4 years! Two more conferences were needed to resolve the issue, but finally in July 1997, Step 3 was concluded, Europe and Japan referred it to their governmental bodies and the USA published the draft guidelines in the *Federal Register*. Phase 4 acceptance by the ICH Steering Committee occurred in February 1998, and the final guidance document was implemented in the USA in June 1998 (Step 5) (*Fed Reg* 63 1998).

Outline of the *'Guidance'*—E5

Overall, it will not be necessary to repeat the entire clinical drug program in each of the other two regions. Each regional authority will judge whether the clinical data fulfill their regulatory regional requirements (i.e. are a complete package). If so, can they be extrapolated to their population? If the authority is concerned that a drug could be subject to ethnic factors impacting on efficacy or safety, then limited clinical data gathered in people of that region may be required to 'bridge' the clinical data between the data generated in one region to those of the area in which the data were generated. If new data are required by the new region anyway (inadequate for regional requirements), the study could also do dual duty as a bridging study.

What is a Complete Package?

Studies should be adequately well-controlled endpoints and medical and diagnostic definitions appropriate to the region. The specific needs are mostly covered in other ICH guidances Good Clinical Practice [(GCPs) (E6), dose response (E4), adequacy of safety data (E1 and E2), studies in elderly (E7), reports (E3), clinical trials (E8) and statistics (E9)]. Occasionally a region may feel that other studies are needed in areas that other regions are less concerned with; a different 'golden' standard as comparator, or at a dosage as approved in that region, as well as patients with renal or hepatic insufficiency, are given as examples.

Ethnic Factors and Population Extrapolation of a Drug

Some properties of a drug or its class may make it insensitive to ethnic factors. This will make it easier for extrapolation to different regions and reduce the need for 'bridging' clinical data. Properties that make it susceptible to ethnic influences see likelihood Ethnic Sensitive/Insensitive in Table 29.1 will require bridging studies, sometimes of pharmacokinetics/dynamics studies or safety and efficacy either or both.

Assessing the Potential Sensitivity of a Drug to Ethnic Factors

If a drug is of a known class, the sensitivity may already be determined, but by the end of Phase I most of the pharmacokinetics (PK) and pharmacodynamics (PD) of a drug will be known. The properties of the compound that may indicate potential ethnic variation (ethnically sensitive) are:

- Non-linear pharmacokinetics.
- A steep efficacy and safety pharmacokinetics dose curve.
- Narrow therapeutic dose range.
- Highly metabolized, especially if through just one pathway (potential for drug–drug interaction).
- Metabolism by enzymes known to show genetic polymorphism.

Table 29.1   Classification of intrinsic and extrinsic ethnic factors (ICH Guidance 1997)

INTRINSIC		EXTRINSIC
Genetic	Physiological and pathological conditions	Environmental
Gender	Age (children-elderly)	Climate Sunlight Pollution
Height Bodyweight		
	Liver Kidney Cardiovascular functions	Culture Socioeconomic factors Educational status Language
RACE		
ADME Receptor sensitivity		Medical practice Disease definition/Diagnostic Therapeutic approach Drug compliance
Genetic polymorphism of the drug metabolism		
		Smoking Alcohol
Genetic diseases	Diseases	Food habits Stress
		Regulatory practice/GCP Methodology/Endpoints

- A pro-drug relying on enzyme conversion subject to ethnic variation.
- Low bioavailability (ethnic dietary effects).
- Projected common use in multiple co-medication.
- Potential for inappropriate use.

Properties that reduce a drug's potential for ethnic variation (ethnically sensitive) are the converse of the above, with the addition of low potential for protein binding and non-systemic use.

Bridging Data Package

This consists of information from the complete clinical data package selected for its relevance to the new region. Pharmacokinetic (PK), pharmacodynamic (PD) and early dose-response date should all be included. If a bridging clinical study between the foreign data and the new region's population is needed, this may be a pharmacokinetic study, or pharmacodynamic demonstration of efficiency or a full clinical efficacy and safety study, with perhaps one center running a pharmacokinetic study add-itionally on volunteer patients. A bridging clinical study may not be needed (a regional regulatory decision). This is most likely where: (a) the medicine is ethnically sensitive and medical practice and conduct of trials are similar; and (b) if ethnically sensitive but the two regions have similar clinical make-up of populations; and (c) when extrapolation from drugs of a similar class can be made. If the drug is ethnically sensitive and clinical data are derived from dissimilar ethnic populations, provided that other non-physiological factors are similar, a simple pharmacodynamic dose–response study may suffice. This could utilize an endpoint predictive of clinical value (surrogate), e.g. blood pressure. If pharmacokinetics were also undertaken in the same study, dynamic effects may be directly reflected by the blood levels.

If the bridging study shows similarity to the dose–response study in safety and efficacy, this is usually sufficient, even if this study shows that a different dose is indicated. That is especially so if at that new dose (range) a similar safety and efficacy profile has been demonstrated.

Where the differences are greater (medical practice, a new drug class to the region, different concurrent medicines, and clinical study design varies from that of the region standard, a controlled, randomized clinical study for efficacy will be required. This might utilize shorter duration surrogate end-points, rather than the clinical end-points common to Phase III studies.

Bridging Safety Studies

The new region may also have concerns regarding the relevance of the safety data of common serious adverse events and their incidence to their ethnic population. The guidance recommends that the clinical efficacy study should be powered to capture a 1% incidence of an event, namely 300 patients for 6 months on the new medicine. Additional patients will be needed for the control group in a controlled trial, given an expected dropout rate of 15–30%, dependent on disease and severity of efficacy depends on the balance of the groups (1:1, 1:2, 1:3). A small safety study might be done initially to assure the sponsor and the region that a high incidence of serious events is unlikely to be seen in the larger study.

Practical Implications to Sponsors of New Medicines

Most major clinical pharmaceutical manufacturers recognize that it is not profitable to develop a drug just for one region. In the past, most drugs were introduced first in Europe, even by USA-based firms for pricing reasons, often country by country, and in Japan even later. This has dramatically changed since the Prescription Drug User Fee Act, which speeded up US approvals and the introduction of the 'centralized procedure' of Application for Europe. Frequently firms will conduct multicenter studies in both the USA and Europe and submit them almost simultaneously to the FDA and European Medical Evaluation Agency (EMEA). This was not possible to do for Japan; now it is! Indeed, Japan now can conduct studies in other regions on their drugs and combine them with confidence into their own more extensive clinical data package for foreign submission. Differences of Japan's chemical manufacturing and quality control section (CMC)

still have to be resolved before full interchange-ability (mutual recognition) of their Common Technical Documents occurs. Many firms now do pharmacokinetic and pharmacodynamic dose–response studies on Japanese patients in Japan. In addition, even if not needed, they conduct a controlled local comparison clinical study to expand the database, and for sound marketing reasons.

In the USA, because of legislation previously discussed, data on major ethnic groups is collected and analyzed and may in general provide reassurance that the most obvious ethnic differences are observed. This is of less concern to the other regions.

For many years, the FDA has encouraged a wide geographic distribution of Phase III multicenter studies. This can be used to enroll minority and cultural ethnic groups, because they tend to congregate in regional clusters, e.g. Hispanics in Miami and New York. Placement with a physician investigator of different ethnic origin can enhance the enrollment, for frequently they will attract patients of that group. It should be noted that "hispanic" analysis has been dropped as a requirement unless culturally relevant.

The current regulatory position of the three regions has been outlined in the notes for *The Guidance for the Mutual Use of Foreign Data in the EC, Japan, and US, Part 1*. The ADME concern has been well defined and quantified in separate reports.

Does It Matter? The Reality

Despite this huge list of possible factors influencing the drug development and assessment process, the reality is emerging that:

- For most drugs the therapeutic range is broad, and rarely is an optimal dose so critical for effective treatment. Exceptions, such as cardiac glycosides, anticonvulsants, anticoagulants, etc., have a narrow therapeutic window and must be individualized by titration. Such drugs, if not useful, are soon discarded (Benet 1992). Despite the presence of multiple conflicting factors, the global dosage trend is towards a global 'mean'. Over time, the same dosage range emerges in many countries, adjusting to the 'real world' as opposed to the narrow demographics of research or cultural expectations.

- Generally, where dosages are the same, the incidence of *serious* adverse events tends to be the same in the three regions (Edwards 1993; Papaluca 1993.).

- Objective differences, when found, are largely due to physiologic influences (blood/body volume and metabolic intrapopulation differences) and less commonly due to ethnic variation. In the USA, an estimate of less than 5% of drugs subject to significant clinical ethnic variation was reported by participating companies in a USA/PMA Survey (Edwards, 1991) and confirmed by the retrospective surveys undertaken for ICH 2. (Naito and Yasuitata 1993; Harvey and Walker 1993).

- Data are more interchangeable between the USA and Europe than between Japan and the USA, or between Japan and Europe, but this is less often due to pharmacokinetic differences, body size and diet but more often to the even larger differences in medical and cultural attitudes of Japan and to Europe and the USA which influenc dose selection and data compatibility.

THE FUTURE

Technology, television, transcontinental travel and international scientific and medical conferences continue to narrow the subjective variations. Differences in diagnosis, data measurement and interpretation will diminish with such exchanges. It is possible that methodology, study design and case report forms can be constructed that correct for culture, diet, and at least some subjective factors, which will allow comparability of efficacy and adverse events on dose/mg/kg body weight measured between European, US and Japanese data.

In conclusion, most but not all differences will disappear and indeed, from such diversity there may spring new understanding of both clinical and therapeutic mechanisms for the development and applicability of better medications.

RECOMMENDED FURTHER READING

Walker S, Lumley C, McAuslane N (1994) *The Relevance of Ethnic Factors in the Clinical Evaluation of Medicines.* Kluwer Academic: Hingham, MA.
Fed Reg (1999) Ethnic factors in the acceptability of foreign clinical data. *Fed Reg* 63(111), June 10: 31790–94.

REFERENCES

Agarwal DP, Goedde HW (1990) *Alcohol Metabolism, Alcohol Intolerance and Alcoholism.* Springer-Verlag: Berlin.
Apple P, Weintraub M (1993) *Notes for Guidance: the Use of Foreign Clinical Data in the EEC, Japan and USA.* ICH: Orlando, FL.
Baily DG, Arnold JM, Munoz C, Spence JD (1991) Interaction of citrus juices with felodipine and nifedipine. *Lancet* 337 (8736): 268–9.
Benet L (1992) IOM Workshop.
Cannon W (1957) Voodoo death. *Psychosom Med* 19: 182–90.
Chang SS, Davis JM, Ku NF, Pandey GN, Zhang MY (1985) Racial differences in plasma and RBC lithium levels. Paper presented at the Annual Meeting of the American Psychiatric Association. *Continuing Medical Education Syllabus and Scientific Proceedings*: 239–240.
Chen., Poth (1929) *J Pharmacol Ther* 36.

Code of Federal Regulations 21 Foreign data. Section 314.106. Application for FDA approval to market a new drug or antibiotic.
Davitz JR, Davits LL (1981) *Interferences of Patients' Pain and Psychological Distress: Studies of Nursing Behaviors.* Springer: New York.
Dinsdale JE, Rollnik JD, Shapiro H (1995) The effect of ethnicity on prescriptions for patient-controlled analgesia for postoperative pain. *Pain* 66(1): 9–12.
Doi T (1973) The anatomy of dependence. *Tokyo Kadansha International.*
Drayer DE, Reidenberg MM (1977) Clinical consequences of polymorphic acetylation. *Clin Pharmacol Ther* 22: 251–8.
Dziewanowska ZE (1992) International harmonization of clinical trials. Fifth World Conference on Clinical Pharmacology and Therapeutics, Yokahara, Japan, July.
Eap CB, Bauman P (1989) The generic polymorphism of human α-1-acid glycoprotein: genetics, biochemistry, physiological functions and pharmacology. *Prog Clin Biol Res* 300: 111–25.
Edwards LD (1992) *Gender and Ethnic Monitoring* Survey, Pharmaceutical Manufacturers' Association. Reported PERI Workshop.
Edwards LD (1991) Most Major Companies Test Medicines in Women, Monitor Data for Gender Differences. New Medicines in Development for Women (1991 Survey). *Pharmaceutical Manufacturers Association*: Washington, 27–8.

Eichelbaum M, Gross AS (1990) The genetic polymorphism of debrisoquine/sparteine clinical Aspects. *Pharmacol Therapeut* 46: 377–94.

Eisenberg L (1973) The future of psychiatry. *Lancet* 2: 1371–3.

Fed Reg (1998) Ethnic factors in the acceptability of foreign clinical data (E5). *Fed Reg* 63(111): 31790–96.

Fairburn WD (1989) Japan drug regulations—a United States industrial perspective. *Regulatory Affairs* 1: 25–33.

Folsom AR, Rosamond WD, Shahar E, Cooper LS et al (1999). Prospectual study of markers of hemostatic function with risk of ischemic stroke. The Athero Sclerosis Risk in communities (ARIC) study investigators *Circulation* 100(7): 736–42.

Food and Drug Administration (1975) New drugs for investigational use: adoption of informational clinical research standards: acceptance of foreign data. *Fed Reg* 40(69): 16052–7.

Food and Drug Administration (1985) New drug and metabolic regulations; final rule. *Fed Reg* 50(36): 7452, 7483–7485, 7505.

Freis ED (1986) Antihypertensive agents. In Kalow W, Goedde HW, Agarwal DP (eds), *Ethnic Differences in Reactions to Drugs and Xenobiotics.* Alan R. Liss: New York, 313–22.

Gibaldi M (1992a) Pharmacogenetics: Part I. *Ann Pharmacother* 26: 121–6.

Gibaldi M (1992b) Pharmacogenetics: Part II. *Ann Pharmacother* 26: 255–61.

Gould SE, Hayashi T, Nakashima T, Shohoji T et al (1972) Coronary heart disease and stroke. Atherosclerosis in Japanese men in Hiroshima, Japan and Honolulu, Hawaii. *Arch Pathol* 93(2): 98–102.

Hall DH (1990) Pathophysiology of hypertension in Blacks. *Am J Hyperten* 3: 366–71S.

Hartog J, Hartog EA (1983) Cultural aspects of health and illness behavior in hospitals. *West J Med* 139(6): 910–26.

Harvey C, Walker S (1993) Review of European CMR database for 21 drugs common to the 'West' and Japan. E5 Workshop Report ICH-2, Orlando.

Henry CJ, Emery B, Piggot S (1987) Basal metabolic rate and diet-induced thermogenesis in Asians living in Britain. *Hum Nutrit Clin Nutrit* 41(5): 397–402.

Hess EV (1982) Drug-related lupus. *Arthrit Rheumat* 25(7).

Homma M (1991) Ministry of Health and Welfare Report. Proceedings of First International Conference on Harmonization. ICH-I, Brussels.

Jefferson JW, Ackerman DL, Carol JA, Greisi JH (1987) *Lithium Encyclopedia for Clinical Practice.* American Psychiatric Press: Washington, DC.

Kalow W (1989) Race and therapeutic drug response. *N Engl J Med* 320: 588–9.

Kato H, Tillotson J, Hamilton HB, Nichaman MZ et al (1973) Epidemiologic Studies of coronary heart disease and stroke in Japanese men living in Japan, Hawaii and California. *Am J Epidemiol* 97: (6): 372–85.

Khandker R, Simoni-Wastilia LJ (1998) Differences in prescription drug utilization and expenditures between Blacks and Whites in the Georgia Medicaid population. *Inquiry* 35(1): 78–87.

Kiowiski N, Bolli P, Bühler FR, Ernep P et al (1985) Age, race, blood pressure, and renin predictions for hypertensive treatment with calcium antagonist. *Am J Cardiol* 16: 81–5H.

Kumana CR, Chan M, Ko W, Lauder J, Lin HJ (1987) Differences in diazepam pharmacokinetics in Chinese and White caucasians: relationship to body lipid stores. *Eur J Clin Pharmacol* 32: 211–15.

Kupfer A, Preisig R, Zeugin T (1988) Pharmacogenetic aspects of biological variability. *J Gastroenterol Hepatol* 3: 623–33.

Leiberman JA, Canoso RT, Egea E, Kane JM, Yunis J (1990) HLA-B38, DR4, DQW3 and clozapine-induced agranulocytosis in Jewish patients with schizophrenia. *Arch Gen Psychiat* 47: 945–8.

Lin KM, Lesser JM, Poland RE (1986) Ethnicity and psychopharmacology culture. *Med Psychiat* 10: 151–65.

Lin KM, Mendoza R, Poland RE et al (1991) Pharmacokinetic and other related factors affecting psychotropic responses in Asians. *Psychopharmacol Bull* 27(4): 427–39.

Metropolitan Life Insurance (1999) (www.metlife) *Male, Female, Height and Weight Tables.*

Medawar PB (1961) Immunological tolerance. *Nature* 189: 14–17.

Mendoza R (1991) *Psychopharmacol Bull* 27: 449–60.

Ministry of Health and Welfare Notification 660 (June 1985); and *Notification of PAB Director General: Acceptance of Data on Clinical Trials Conducted in Foreign Countries* (June 29, 1987) Japan.

Natio C, Yasuhova H (1993) Retrospective survey of pharmacokinetics: dosage of 80 drugs approved in the EC, Japan, and US. E5 Workshop Reports, ICH-2, Orlando.

Oster G, Huse DM, Deles TE et al (1987) Cost-effectiveness of labetalol and propranolol in the treatment of hypertension among Blacks. *J Nat Med Assoc* 79: 1049–55.

Payer L (1988) *Medicine and Culture.* H. Holt: New York.

Pemberton J (1989) Does constitutional hypotension exist? *Br Med J* 298: 660–62.

Papaluca M (1993) Ethnic factors and clinical responsiveness: basic concepts of the retrospective survey. ES Workshop Report, ICH-2, Orlando.

Rieder MJ, Sheer NH, Kanee A et al (1991) Prominence of slow acetylator phenotype among patients with sulfonamide hypersensitivity reactions. *Clin Pharm Ther* 49: 13–17.

Salzman C (1982) Increased receptor sensitivity, psychoactive drugs, and analgesics. A prime of geriatric psychopharmacology. *Am J Psychiat* 139: 67–74.

Sleath B, Svarstad B, Rotes D (1998) Patient race and psychotropic prescribing during medical encounters. *Patient Educ Counsel* 34(3): 227–58.

Strickland TL, Lin KM, Mendoza R et al (1991) Psychopharmacologic considerations in the treatment of Black American populations. *Psychopharmacol Bull* 27(4): 441–8.

Takahashi R (1979) Lithium treatment in affective disorders: therapeutic plasma level. *Psychopharmacol Bull* 15: 32–5.

US Bureau of the Census (1991) Press release C891–100.

Uchida K (1988) Acceptability of foreign clinical trial data in Japan. *Drug Inf J* 22: 103–8.

Vessell E (1989) Ethnic differences in reactions to drugs and xenobiotics. *Progr Clin Biol Res* 214: 21–37.

Weintraub M, Rubio A (1992) Scoring system in a pilot effectiveness study of patients with sickle cell anemia. *J Clin Res Pharmacoepidemiol* 6: 47–54.

Wood AJJ, Koshakji RP, Silberstein DJ (1989) Racial differences in drug response-altered sensitivity to and clearance of propranolol in men of Chinese descent as compared with American Whites. *N Engl J Med* 320: 565–70.

Wood AJJ, Zhou HH (1991) Ethnic differences in drug disposition and responsiveness. *N Engl J Med* 320: 565–70 *Clin Pharmacokinet* 20: 350–73.

World Population Prospects (1990) United Nations Publications: New York.

Yang YY (1987) Prophylactic efficacy of lithium and its effective plasma levels in Chinese bipolar patients. *Acta Psychiat Scand* 71: 171–5.

Zhang Y, Bertilsson L, Lou T et al (1990) Diazepam metabolism in native Chinese, poor and extensive hydroxylators of S-mephenytoin: inter-ethnic differences in comparison with White subjects. *Clin Pharmacol Therapeut* 48: 496–502.

Zhou HH, Adeloyin A, Wilkinson GR (1990) Differences in plasma-binding of drugs between caucasians and Chinese subjects. *Clin Pharmacol Therapeut* 489: 10–17.

Zola IK (1972) Studying the decision to see a doctor. In Lipowski Z (ed.), *Advances in Psychosomatic Medicine*, vol. 8. Karger: Basel, 216–36.

Section VI

Medical Services

Introduction to Section VI

Anthony W. Fox

EBD Group Inc, Carlsbad, CA, USA

This section covers the area that, in most companies, is called 'medical affairs'. The chapters cover the specific areas of knowledge and capability that those working in such departments should possess, but perhaps a few words on less concrete aspects of this type of role could be added here.

The pharmaceutical physician/pharmacist/nurse/scientist working in medical affairs is likely to be faced with perhaps the greatest diversity of tasks in any department. Anything that has any clinical implications at all, and that is not strictly related to the development of an investigational drug, is likely to end up in medical affairs. Such matters range from marketing and promotion, to Phase IV clinical trials, to pharmacovigilance and even to legal issues, such as litigation and patent implications (see Section V for the latter).

However, such an opportunity also comes with responsibility. Very often, for a matter involving a marketed product, the medical affairs specialist becomes the company's ombudsman. It is medical affairs that often must resolve the inevitable conflicts that arise between ebullience in the marketing department and conservatism in pharmacovigilance matters. If the company must defend itself in litigation, then it is the responsibility of the medical affairs specialist to provide the attorneys with a realistic assessment of all the facts, in an appropriate context, even when these might not be the most advantageous 'spin' from a commercial point of view. This can sometimes be a lonely role, and the medical affairs specialist must be acutely aware how properly to take and defend a position without casting a shadow over his/her own career within the company!

Such a role is, of course, best exercised after long experience. None of these chapters, while containing valuable information, can replace several years 'in the trenches' of a vigorous medical affairs department. This role can be amongst the most stimulating of any in the industry, and it is truly the preserve of the generalist.

30

An Introduction to Medical Affairs

Gil Price

Medimmune Gaitherburg, MA, US

OVERVIEW

The scope of responsibilities of a medical affairs department varies significantly among companies. In general, 'medical affairs' is an interface between clinical development, regulatory affairs, and sales and marketing. The medical affairs professional has been described as an 'orchestra conductor'. By working effectively across intradepartmental groups, the medical affairs professional helps to ensure a successful product launch, label expansion and, ultimately, product sales growth. The sections of this chapter will outline the core organizational functions and basic information important for the success of a medical affairs department.

ORGANIZATION

The function and responsibilities of a medical affairs group is related to the reporting structure for the department (clinical vs. marketing). Medical affairs departments that reside under the clinical development umbrella are more likely to participate in the company's broader product-related activities, such as safety surveillance, Phase IIIb/IV studies, and small center-specific clinical projects used primarily to introduce thought leaders to products they may not, historically, have prescribed. Medical affairs departments that reside under the marketing umbrella are generally more focused on customer-related issues, such as drug information, pharmacoeconomics, current literature bulletins, and disease management activities. Staff size is a function of corporate size, specific departmental objectives, expectations, and overall responsibilities. Regardless of the reporting environment, the fully integrated medical affairs

department will consist of the following types of personnel:

- Medical science liaisons
- Medical communications
- Pharmacoeconomics
- Competitor intelligence
- Postmarketing safety and surveillance

The interface that often occurs between medical affairs personnel and the three previously mentioned functional groups (clinical development, regulatory affairs, and sales and marketing) is depicted overleaf.

Medical Science Liaisons

These health care professionals (MD, PhD, PharmD) provide a link between marketing, clinical development, and healthcare professionals. Medical science liaisons often direct key Phase IIIb/IV product development through the use of IND clinical studies, center-specific clinical projects, and the distribution of educational grants. As a result, they are required to have a thorough understanding of protocol design and study implementation. Also important is an understanding of regulatory procedures, including postmarketing reporting requirements, adverse drug experience (adverse drug reactions; ADRs) reporting requirements, and good clinical practices (GCPs). Typically, medical science liaisons create their greatest value by identifying and communicating clinical and research issues from practising thought leaders in the field, prior to journal publications or new product introductions.

Principles and Practice of Pharmaceutical Medicine. Edited by A. J. Fletcher, Lionel D. Edwards, Anthony W. Fox and Peter Stonier © 2002 John Wiley & Sons Ltd.

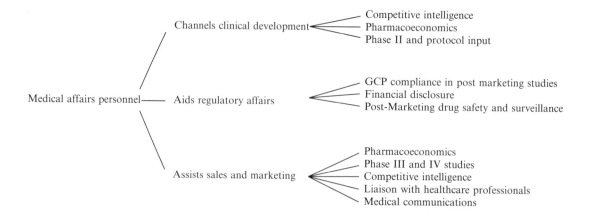

Medical Communications

As early as 1962, the Pharmaceutical Manufacturers' Association Commission on Drug Safety identified as the two main responsibilities of the pharmaceutical industry: (a) to provide therapeutic agents of uniformly high quality; and (b) to supply the medical profession with the best available information pertaining to their use. Pharmaceutical industry involvement in information services is well documented, and has been increasing in sophistication and influence over the past several years. Delivery of product information occurs via several different mechanisms, including the sales force, advertising, and professional meetings. To support the complex and varied product information needs of a healthcare professional, most pharmaceutical companies have organized drug information services, with the primary function of answering unique product inquiries. Methodological approaches to drug information, including the flow of a specific request from the field to resolution, have been published. In general, labeled information is considered to be within the public domain and requires very little oversight in terms of its delivery to a customer. Most drug information requests regard non-label issues. The FDA has issued several guidances regarding the distribution of non-labeled information. The essence of these instructions are:

- Requests must be non-solicited.
- Response information must be balanced.

- Company responses should be accompanied by an approved package insert.

Evaluation of the scientific literature is the drug information service's most distinguishing characteristic relative to services provided by other groups within medical affairs. The drug information/medical writing/medical library specialist is generally a pharmacist who specializes in drug information practice. He/she utilizes his/her training and experience to evaluate the clinical relevance of the literature relative to a given query, and formulates that information into an understandable, appropriately formated response. These responses are compiled and archived as standard letters for future inquiries. Responses may be sorted into categories such as (AE = adverse events; CT = clinical therapy; DI = drug interactions, etc.). Responses may be further sorted into performance categories, such as:

- Number of contacts.
- Average number of questions per contact.
- Number of questions asked.
- Average response time.

The current month's numbers may be compared to numbers from the previous month, the same month last year, year-to-date, or the previous year.

The number of drug information requests is often predictable, based on the product life cycle. The first 6 months following launch generally represent the heaviest call volume.

Pharmacoeconomics

Cost-effectiveness is a method used to evaluate the outcomes and costs of interventions designed to improve healthcare. It has been used to compare costs and years of life gained for a variety of diagnostic screening, vaccine prophylaxis, and drug treatment interventions. The results of analyses are generally summarized in a series of cost–effectiveness ratios that show the cost of achieving one unit of health outcome (e.g. the cost of a life-year saved) (Eddy 1989). By providing estimates of outcomes and costs, pharmacoeconomic studies show the tradeoffs involved in choosing among interventions. This relatively new tool of pharmacoeconomics has proven a valuable partner to the historic method of medical decision making based on 'medical necessity'. Medical affairs professionals will increasingly be called upon to review, evaluate, and conduct pharmacoeconomic studies to facilitate cost-effective healthcare decision making. Before undertaking a cost–effectiveness study, the medical affairs professional should have a clear understanding of the study objectives, target audience, various types of economic analyses, including the prospective of analysis to be considered, such as societal, institutional, third-party payer, or family and patient (Torrance 1996). A pharmacoeconomist is typically an individual with an advanced degree in health economics and experience in developing economic models that clearly demonstrate the burden of disease and the benefit of the given product as it relates to cost.

Competitor Intelligence (CI) Specialist

Competitor intelligence (CI) is a widely practised formal discipline in the pharmaceutical/biotech industry and is a key to rational decision-making on tactical and strategic issues. Numerous articles and books describe the array of information and analysis activities that CI departments commonly provide to their organizations. Leonard Fuld (1995), a well-known expert in the field, has stated that 'competitive intelligence can be simply defined as gathering raw data and information about your competitor, and then using your experience and common sense to figure out what it really means'. The key to this statement is the last portion, sug-

gesting analysis of information being the most critical component of competitor intelligence. According to Desai and Bawden (1993):

> Competitor intelligence may help a business in several ways (Creer 1989): in making strategic decisions and plans '[stimulating] strategic thinking and behaviour'; in developing its resources; in directing innovation and change; and in entering into new ventures (Anon 1989). It should specifically help to identify competitors in the marketplace, track and assess their market thrusts, products, strengths, and weaknesses, with consequent identification of marketing opportunities (Ghoshal and Westney 1991; Herring 1988). It should act as an early warning system: preventing surprises, and identifying threats, changes, and opportunities in time for action to be taken. It has a forecasting component, providing predictions on how external forces will disrupt or enhance business plans, and reducing uncertainty. Finally, CI makes a major contribution to organizational learning, teaching lessons about the marketplace which may be of use in the future.

In general, it is the medical affairs professional who is responsible for the analysis of gathered information, whether the information was derived through sales and marketing or any of the research and development branches of a sponsor company. Within the competitive intelligence community, there are four generally recognized levels of activity. Level 1 is routine vigilance and surveillance of published sources or commercially available databases. Level 2 is customized briefings/reports for *ad hoc* questions for ongoing issues (the use of advanced databases). Level 3 is associated with the capture of soft information, usually discovered at professional meetings through seminar handouts or poster presentations. Level 4 is primary research involved with interviews, freedom of information requests, funded research grants, and trend testing. Each of the various levels requires a significant financial and human resource commitment. Effectiveness and efficiency may be enhanced when the competitor intelligence program is successfully integrated within a wider corporate information system.

It is generally held that 90–95% of the information sought is freely available if only one knows where to look (Tyson 1989; Ljungberg 1983). Potentially useful sources of information are

Information source available to the competetive intelligence professional

Sales figures	IMS MIDAS service
	Brokers/investment analysts reports
Product portfolios	IMS product monographs
	Data sheet compendium and drug lists
R&D portfolios	*IMS Drug Licensing Opportunities*
	Pharmaprojects
Market information	*PJB Scrip*
	IMS Marketletter
Company information	Annual/broker/investment analysts reports
	PJB Scrip
	IMS Marketletter
	Predicast's Prompt
	Dun & Bradstreet Services
Economic data	*Datastream*
Medical information	*Medline*
	Excerpta Medica
Press sources	*Financial Times*
Patents information	*Current Patents Fast Alert*
	Patents Previews

numerous and diverse. Sources are categorized in divisions, according to their perceived usefulness. In general, categories relate to: (a) current awareness; (b) specific product information; or (c) related research and development information. The above table is an example of the multiple sources available to the competitive intelligence professional (Desai and Bawden 1993).

The successful CI professional has an advanced science degree with experience in business development and strategic planning.

Postmarketing Safety Surveillance

Sponsor companies must collect, analyze, and submit data on postmarketing adverse drug experiences (AE), so that the company and the FDA can continue to reassess the product's risk–benefit relationship and the conditions under which the drug should be marketed and used. Adverse experiences are generally reported by healthcare professionals. The accepted form to report such experiences is the FDA's MedWatch program, which is designed to facilitate the reporting of adverse events and product problems for all FDA-regulated products. Clinical trials are not enough, especially when considering rare events that are difficult to detect and confirm. Additionally, clinical trial populations often have narrow demographics, due to inclusion and exclusion criteria. Finally, the short duration of clinical trials does not allow for the long-term consequences of a therapeutic intervention to be exposed. It is important to remember that product development is a continuum, extending beyond product licensure. New information about product safety may continue to be added by additional studies or spontaneous reports of adverse events. This new information may change the labeling or use of a product. Product labeling changes are an important public health aspect of postmarketing surveillance. FDA receives and analyzes pharmacovigilance information in order to ensure the safe and effective use of drugs and biologics. In general, 90% of AE reports to FDA are submitted through the manufacturer; fewer than 10% are direct reports.

It is important to have an historical perspective on postmarketing safety and surveillance. FDA acts as public health protector by ensuring that all drugs on the market are safe and effective. Authority to do this comes from the 1938 Federal Food, Drug, and Cosmetic Act, a law that has undergone many changes over the years, just as it changed earlier drug regulation. Some major milestones in the evolution of US drug law (FDA 1999) are:

- *Food and Drugs Act (1906).* This first drug law required only that drugs meet standards of strength and purity. The burden of proof was on FDA to show that a drug's labeling was false and fraudulent before it could be taken off the market.
- *Federal Food, Drug, and Cosmetic Act (1938).* A bill was introduced into the Senate in 1933 to completely revise the 1906 drug law—then widely recognized as being obsolete. However, congressional action was stalled. It took a tragedy in which 107 people died from a poisonous ingredient in 'Elixir Sulfanilamide' to prompt passage of revised legislation that, for the first time, required a manufacturer to prove the safety of a drug before it could be marketed.
- *Durham–Humphrey Amendment (1951).* Until this law, there was no requirement that any drug be labeled for sale by prescription only. The amendment defined prescription drugs

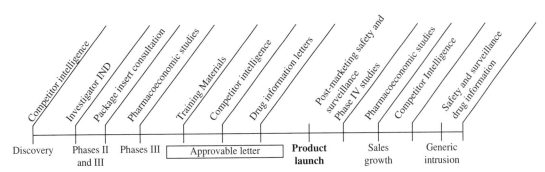

Figure 30.2 Medical affairs phase activities

as those unsafe for self-medication, and which should therefore be used only under a doctor's supervision.

- *Kefauver–Harris Drug Amendments (1962).* News reports about the role of an FDA medical officer in keeping the drug thalidomide off the US market aroused public interest in drug regulation. Thalidomide had been associated with the birth of thousands of malformed babies in Western Europe. In October 1962, Congress passed these amendments to tighten control over drugs. Before marketing a drug, firms now had to prove not only safety but also effectiveness for the product's intended use. In addition, firms were required to send ADR reports to the FDA, and drug advertising in medical journals was required to provide complete information to doctors—the risks, as well as the benefits. The amendments also required that informed consent be obtained from study subjects. (Note: In July 1998, thalidomide was approved by the FDA with significant restrictions; because of thalidomide's potential to cause birth defects, FDA invoked unprecedented regulatory authority to tightly control the marketing of the product in the USA.) FDA recently acted on these restrictions, with a warning to the manufacturer that their marketing practices had exceeded the previously agreed-upon boundaries. By not complying, penalties, including corrective action and product seizure, may be invoked.

The pharmacovigilance specialist is responsible for recording, reporting, and analyzing all collected data. The successful candidate has an advanced

science degree (MD, RPh, RN) with experience in regulatory safety report requirements.

PHASELINE

The phaseline shown in Figure 30.2 suggests appropriate intervals for medical affairs activities during the corresponding phases of product development. This chapter is intended to illustrate the potential corporate structure and personal responsibilities for medical affairs professionals. On their own, each function is deserving of greater detail. This suggestion may be fulfilled in a future text.

REFERENCES

Creer J (1989) Business intelligence—relevance to the pharmaceutical industry. *Pharmaceut Times*: 18–20.

Desai, Bawden (1993) Competitor intelligence in the pharmaceutical industry; the role of the information professional. *J Inform Sci* 19: 327–38.

Eddy DM (1989) Screening for breast cancer. *Ann Intern Med.* 111: 389–99.

FDA (1999) *From Test Tube to Patient.* US Food and Drug Administration Center for Drug Evaluation and Research Special Report.

Fuld LM (1995) *The New Competitor Intelligence.* Wiley: New York.

Ghoshal S, Westney DE (1991) Organizing competitor analysis systems. *Strateg Managem J* 12: 17–31.

Herring JP (1988) Building a business intelligence system. *J Bus Strategy* 4–9.

Ljungberg S (1983) Intelligence service—a tool for decision markers. *Int Forum Inform Document* 8: 23–26.

Torrance GW (1996) Framing and designing the cost effectiveness analysis. In Gold et al (eds), *Cost-Effectiveness in Health and Medicine.* Oxford University Press: New York.

31

Drug Labeling

Anthony W. Fox

EBD Group, Carlsbad, California

The purpose of the drug label has been stated succinctly in the Japanese guidelines:

> Package insert statements should generally contain information essential to using the specified drug for approved indications and within the range of approved dosage and [route of] administration. However, other important data regarding any use of the drug should also be evaluated and described (PAB Notification No. 606, April 25 1997).

In other words, the drug label is the summary of all that is learned during drug development, plus that which is inevitably discovered during postmarketing surveillance. The terms 'drug label' and 'package insert' (the former in common use in North America, the latter in Europe and Japan) are used interchangeably in this chapter.

The intent of this chapter is to review drug labels in North America, Europe and Japan. The philosophy of these differing types of labeling will be explored. The reader can easily access local examples of current, approved labeling; these will not be reproduced here, and could, in any case, rapidly become out of date. Much of the content of drug labeling is the subject of other chapters in this book; the approach here will avoid redundancy.

DRUG LABELING IN JAPAN[1]

The Ministry of Health and Welfare has a subordinate organization known as the Pharmaceutical and Medical Safety Bureau, which supervises drug labeling in Japan. This bureau has prescribed a standard set of subtitles for drug labeling which must always appear (Table 31.1).

Table 31.1 Subtitles that must appear in Japanese drug labeling, and the order in which they appear (after Article 52, Item 1 of the Pharmaceutical Affairs Law).

1. Date of preparation or revision of label
2. Japanese Standard Commodity Number
3. Therapeutic category (e.g. bronchodilator)
4. Regulatory classification (e.g. 'Designated Drug')
5. Brand name
6. Warning(s)
7. Contraindications
8. Composition and description
9. Indications
10. Dosage and administration
11. Precautions
12. Pharmacokinetics
13. Clinical studies
14. Pharmacology
15. Physicochemistry
16. Precautions for handling
17. Conditions for approval
18. Packaging
19. References and how to order
20. Identity of manufacturer, etc.

As can be seen, the structure of a Japanese drug label is a standard format that would also be familiar to physicians in Europe or North America. The one major difference, however, is that a separate regulation (PAB Notification No. 607, April 25 1997) governs how precautions should be displayed in drug labels, and is quite elaborate in comparison to its European or North American counterparts. The Warnings and Contraindications sections of the drug label (items 6 and 7 in Table 31.1), are required to contain, under this regulation, the subsections shown in Table 31.2. While most of these subtopics would have stand-alone counterparts in drug labeling elsewhere in the world, this regulation

---

[1] With acknowledgments to Dr Hiroko Sakai, Yamanouchi Pharmaceuticals, Tokyo, Japan.

Principles and Practice of Pharmaceutical Medicine. Edited by A. J. Fletcher, Lionel D. Edwards, Anthony W. Fox and Peter Stonier © 2002 John Wiley & Sons Ltd.

Table 31.2 Sub-sections of 'precautions' in Japanese drug labeling

1. Warnings
2. Contraindications ('do not administer to the following types of patients')
3. Careful administration ('administer with care to the following patients')
4. Important precautions
5. Drug interactions:
   (a) Contraindicated co-administrations
   (b) Precautions for co-administration
6. (a) Clinically significant adverse events
   (b) Other adverse events
7. Use in the elderly
8. Use in pregnancy, delivery and lactation
9. Pediatric use
10. Eects on clinical laboratory tests
11. Overdosage
12. Precautions concerning use
13. Other precautions

emphasizes drug tolerability. The visual presentation of the precautions subsections goes further to make this point: warnings are printed in red within a red box, while contraindications are printed in black, and again within a red box. Lastly, contraindications for co-administered drugs must be printed as a table within a red box.

Japanese labeling regulations require that animal data and data from other members of the same chemical or pharmacological class of drugs should be included, even when these allude to adverse drug reactions (ADR) that have not actually been observed for the product that is labeled. When direct drug attributability of an ADR has not been established, it remains a requirement that other indirectly obtained information must still be included; this would include epidemiological information or pharmacodynamic effects observed in normal volunteer studies. ADR frequencies (section 4, Table 1) may be presented in a table, usually for all adverse event types reported with frequencies > 5%, between 0.1–5%, and < 0.1%.

DRUG LABELING IN THE USA

The US Food and Drug Administration (FDA) is, among other things, probably the most stringent controller of drug labeling of all the world's regulatory authorities. Typically, drug labels are agreed with pharmaceutical companies at meetings shortly before product approval, where the proposed label is debated line by line. Such meetings often include not only Division Directors but also Center Directors. The relevant parts of the Code of Federal Regulations (CFR) are authorized by the Food, Drugs and Cosmetics Act (21 US Code 321). While the licensing of drug products (21 CFR 310 and 314) and biologicals (21 CFR 601) are different, their labels are governed in a similar manner. The general principles that apply to all US drug labeling (whether a package insert or an advertisement) are:

- Consistency with approved package insert.
- Absence of misleading information.
- Fair balance.
- Absence of relevant omissions.
- Defensibility from the clinical trials database.

Promotional materials in the USA are also viewed as a form of labeling (21 CFR 201.1). All magazine advertisements, etc., have to be accompanied by a complete copy of the approved package insert. Unlike any other jurisdiction in the world, initial promotional materials have to be specifically approved by the FDA before product launch. Thereafter, a specific division of FDA (the Division of Drug Marketing, Advertising and Communications; DDMAC) must be provided with all further promotional materials, although they are presumptively assumed to be satisfactory for use. Promotional materials can be ordered to be recalled by FDA, and companies can be forced into prescriptive corrective measures for advertising that the FDA views as misleading. Any drug that is 'black-boxed' in the USA usually remains on the market pending the sponsor's compliance not to engage in any further promotion of the product (this does not apply to certain opioids and muscle relaxants, where black-boxing is designed to deter all except anesthesiologists from using the product).

Drugs that are extemporaneously compounded from legally obtained starting materials, by individual pharmacists per physician's prescription, are also subject to different regulations (21 CFR 216). These regulations nonetheless contain a list of drugs which are prohibited from compounding, usually in response to corresponding product withdrawals under the orthodox regulations (e.g. dexfenfluramine, chlorhexidine, tetracycline, for any, topical, and pediatric uses, respectively).

It is surprising that these strict regulations and their energetic enforcement apply only to approved drugs. The USA currently has a vigorous market in so-called 'natural products'. Thus, oral proteoglycans 'to repair joint cartilage', *Gingko biloba* extracts 'to improve memory', or the 'anti-aging effect' of oral, powdered, shark cartilage may still be advertised to the general public with impunity; these drugs may also be purchased without prescription. Legally, this creates a paradox, because manufacturers want people to believe that these drugs are effective, and yet therapeutic effectiveness is tantamount to one criterion for bringing drugs under the jurisdiction of the Food, Drugs and Cosmetics Act (1983). However, at present, there is strong political resistance to extending FDA jurisdiction over such products.

The components of US drug labels are provided in 21 CFR 201–202, and various related matters (e.g. imprinting of tablets, labeling of controlled drugs, use of official and trade names, etc.) are governed by regulations scattered between 21 CFR 206–299. Spanish translations of drug labels are permitted (especially for products sold in California, Florida, New York, and Puerto Rico), and some mandatory, equivalent Spanish vocabulary appears in the regulations (e.g. 21 CFR 201.16). The various sections of a US drug label will not be replicated here: the reader is advised to look in the current edition of the *Physician's Desk Reference* for a model to follow, when writing a new drug label. Most European physicians comment on the greater technical detail and length of US labels, in comparison to those in Europe.

A central legal term in the USA is when a drug is alleged to be 'misbranded'. A misbranded drug attracts enforcement actions. Misbranding is usually alleged when the provisions of the NDA have been breached. Such breaches may include: (a) when FDA has determined that the drug is being promoted for indications, dose sizes, or routes of administration that are outside the approved labeling; (b) unapproved ingredients have been used in manufacture, or approved ingredients have failed some quality control that is specified in the NDA; or (c) the sponsor has violated some previous agreement with FDA about how the drug product should be marketed. Almost any infraction perceived by FDA will be termed misbranding.

Comparative statements ('Drug X was better than drug Y'), and active comparator clinical trials data in a proposed package insert, are especially likely to meet with disapproval by FDA. This is a general characteristic of American law: e.g. the registration of motor vehicles and the marketing of wines, are both regulated under the aegis of compliance with a set of standards for product labeling.

The degrees of FDA enforcement may be summarized in escalating order of severity:

1. Warning letter from FDA to the manufacturer, requiring a specified corrective action within a reasonable time frame.
2. Mandatory issuance of a 'Dear Doctor' letter.
3. Black boxing of drug product (usually with agreement not to promote)
4. Product recall (although, in practice, most of these are voluntary on the part of the sponsor).
5. NDA withdrawal.
6. Product seizure and establishment closure.

While all such enforcement actions may be appealed in the Federal Court, it is usually only the last of these, forced product withdrawal, that justifies the time, expense, and uncertainty of such legal action. Drug products usually remain off the market under temporary injunction while such proceedings take place, and this prolonged period *per se* is often sufficient to kill the product for economic reasons. The more serious of these enforcement actions is also punishable with prison terms and fines under the Food, Drugs and Cosmetics Act. A large inspectorate is distributed throughout the USA and around the world as part of FDA's enforcement arm.

Typically, FDA requires that postmarketing surveillance of new drugs is reported at less than annual intervals. Usually, after 3 or 4 years of market experience, annual reports can then be made. A review of the labeling is made on these occasions, which, for non-urgent matters, would be when a Sponsor or FDA might suggest changes. All advertising materials that have been used during the year must also be filed with these annual reports, even though they were sent to DDMAC at the time of their introduction.

EUROPEAN DRUG LABELING

There is reasonable similarity across the countries of the European Union (EU), and these labels are collated into national compendia such as the *Rotte Liste* in Germany or the *Data Sheet Compendium* in the UK, to which the reader is referred. Consistency between countries is likely to increase now that drug licensing has been centralized at the European Medicines Evaluation Agency (EMEA). Many of the headings within European labeling correspond to those shown for Japan (Table 31.1, above), and the USA.

American or Japanese physicians are frequently surprised at European drug labels. The brevity and (usually) the absence of quantitative data (such as adverse event rates or statistical analyses of efficacy end-points) reflects a very different philosophy. Such labels arise from a regulatory *milieu* which itself has a different philosophy, expecting product manufacturers to assume responsibilities that would be accepted by the regulatory authorities in the USA and Japan. There is no European equivalent of the worldwide enforcement arm of the FDA.

There can be no doubt that the principles that underlie European labeling are the same as those enumerated above in other jurisdictions. Consistency of promotional materials with the approved package insert, the absence of misleading information in package inserts, fair balance, absence of relevant omissions, and defensibility of all statements from the clinical trials database are also characteristic of good European labeling. However, there is a sentiment widely expressed in Europe that the long and technical labels promulgated by FDA are unlikely to be read by the ordinary prescriber. Thus, European labeling provides well-balanced summary information, in a much more succinct manner. For this reason, European labels are usually more difficult to write than, say, US labels, and are much more likely to be debated among the physicians in a company's medical department, and between the company and the regulatory authority on subjective, interpretative grounds.

These fundamental differences between European and US drug labels also leads to unexpected tangential difficulties, especially for international corporations. The corporate lawyers in the USA live in a more litigious environment than their European or Japanese colleagues. In the USA, these lawyers will be quite properly concerned about the potential for litigation after the launch of a new drug. Such litigation might result when a patient experiences an ADR that does not appear in labeling, even though at the time of NDA approval it might have been an ADR type that had not yet been identified as associated with use of the new drug. Companies are sued in the USA for adverse events that occur in Europe, and plaintiff's counsel will often wish to exploit differences in drug labels in different jurisdictions. Thus, the company lawyers in the USA would usually like two things: (a) any and all ADR types to appear in labeling, so that the company cannot be accused of failing to disclose any relevant information; and (b) consistency of such information in all drug labels around the world, so that a picture cannot be painted suggesting to a jury that the company was willing to warn Americans but not Europeans of such-and-such an ADR type. Given the typical inability to assign drug attributability to low-frequency ADRs, and the philosophy of European labeling, foreign subsidiaries often object to the inclusion of (probably irrelevant) minutiae in their labeling.

FINAL WORDS

The real key to understanding drug labeling is to scrimmage with it for real. Almost all entry-level medical affairs positions can provide this if the post-holder expresses appropriate interest. Similarly, almost all successful drug development (i.e. Phases I–III) positions are guided by draft labeling. When writing labeling, the first thing to do is to seek out a recent model that is already approved (indeed, such models can also serve as guides to clinical development plans at the very start of drug development). When making judgments about how to amend labeling and what may or may not be an acceptable précis when converting a US label to a European label, remember to seek the advice of those with experience within the medical, regulatory, and legal departments.

32

Organizing and Planning Local, Regional, National and International Meetings and Conferences

Zofia Dziewanowska,[1] Linda Packard[1] and Lionel D. Edwards[2]

[1]La Jolla, CA, and [2]Basking Ridge, NJ, USA

One of the most important vehicles of communication about a company's products and, indeed, its own scientific image is to utilize scientific meetings effectively. As a result, most scientists (and as medicine is now a science, physicians are included) working in the industry are encouraged to participate in scientific organizations and to present their work at scientific meetings. This, over time, usually results in the frequent speaker being asked to chair and help organize professional scientific meetings in his/her discipline. In addition, many firms will organize satellite meetings around a major conference, often a half-day or evening meeting. This can be a 'non-commercial', sponsored meeting, attracting education credits, discussing diseases or events in areas in which the company has a product franchise. Alternatively, it may be a promotional meeting whose agenda addresses issues, diseases, clinical and other scientific material around one of the company products. Inevitably, the ultimate aim of scientific organizations and pharmaceutical companies is to attain a further major vehicle or communication, that of publication.

Most scientists, including physicians, have never been trained to organize, let alone achieve, publication of scientific meetings, conferences, or seminars. Pharmaceutical scientists are even more frequently expected to organize company meetings, such as company briefings (e.g. on entry into a new therapeutic area), investigator meetings and other meetings not intended for publication. While hands-on experience is the best tutor, this chapter is aimed at helping the initial effort and also giving a framework around which planning can occur.

GOALS, TYPES OF MEETINGS AND PARTICIPANTS

The goal of the meeting usually determines the type of meeting, moderators and speakers, and the audience. It is critical that this be clearly defined by the company or obtained from the organization. Table 32.1 lists some examples of the most common goals of conferences and working meetings organized by professionals in the pharmaceutical medicines area.

Once the goal or goals of the meeting are determined and agreed, then the type of conference or meeting will determine its format. Table 32.2 shows some of the most frequent types of meetings and Table 32.3, typical participants.

Table 32.1 Typical goals of conferences and meetings

- To secure consistency of clinical trial conduct and evaluation
- To obtain peer and/or opinion leaders' review input
- To obtain drug approval
- To present a new drug/project to a broad audience
- To promote new treatment
- To exchange scientific information
- To educate

Table 32.2 Types of conferences

- Multicenter investigators meeting
- Advisory board/consultants
- Special meeting to introduce new drug
- Regulatory presentations
- Therapeutic review conferences
- Special subjects, e.g. safety, HMOs, globalization, etc.

Principles and Practice of Pharmaceutical Medicine. Edited by A. J. Fletcher, Lionel D. Edwards, Anthony W. Fox and Peter Stonier © 2002 John Wiley & Sons Ltd.

Table 32.3 Participants—who?

- Chairman of scientific program
- Chairman of social activities
- Collaborators and members of advisory board, some specialty vs. multifunctional
- Moderators: balanced international participation
- Speakers/panelists
- Audience

After the decision is made regarding the goals of the meeting, the next action is to select a chairperson or organizational person for the meeting. This person is the key to the overall success of the meeting and should have a general overview responsibility for the scientific as well as the social program. If the meeting will have a large number of participants and the staff/volunteer support appears to be inadequate, hiring a professional meeting/event planner may be the proper direction to take. The meeting planner can help select the site, negotiate with the facility and caterers, compile a database of prospective participants, arrange for printed materials, manage the registration, and organize social and companion events, amongst the many meeting planner's activities. If a meeting planner is selected who is familiar with the location of the meeting, he/she can offer invaluable insight into activities, facilities, and site selection in that area.

A chairperson should be selected for the scientific program. This is the person who will determine the subjects for the meeting, lay out the program, and line up the speakers. This person must be extremely knowledgeable on the subject, be well known and know other experts on the meeting subject, and he/she must be willing to work hard. All these are key to successful meetings.

The program chairman usually circulates the draft of a program to either the conference organizers or the Scientific Program Advisory Board, if one exists. He/she can break major topics into subsections/tracks and recommend appropriate chairs and speakers. It is not unusual to have eight to ten or more drafts of the program circulating to a wide advisory group for major international meetings before agreement to cover all the relevant topics, as well as the most appropriate speakers and participants. It is also often very important to secure appropriate balanced participation of different functions or countries. It is advisable to be very sensitive to national differences between countries and regions. In Europe and Japan, it is very important to select and match the chairs of the sessions and the speakers by their professional and/or social status.

Enough time must be allowed to organize the meeting. A large-scale conference involving section chairs, speakers and other participants (not including the audience) of 100 or more requires approximately 1 year to plan and organize properly. For these large conferences, staff and/or volunteer support is a necessity. Both have to be adequate for the tasks, as it will require a lot of administrational and organizational work. Early on one needs to secure an up-to-date mailing list to reach the prospective participants and audience for your meeting. If one must be compiled, be sure to leave adequate time for this task and regularly update it. It is surprising how many scientific people frequently move their homes or change offices or firms.

A decision must be made as soon as possible as to the site selection and general administrative/budget planning for the meeting. In selecting a location for the meeting, one needs to be attentive to where the prospective participants are concentrated. If the meeting is to be fairly short in duration (3 days or less), the objective for the meeting may require that the meeting be located in the area of the most participants. If the meeting is to run for more than 3 days, the participants may be interested in attending a meeting that combines sightseeing

Table 32.4 Steps in organization of the program

- Agree on main subject
- Decide on duration of meeting
- Outline overall program
- Decide on sequential or concomitant sessions
- Divide into logical subsections
- Decide on style—interactive or classroom type
- How much time to be spent on science vs. social activities
- Decide on the balance of domestic vs. international issues

Table 32.5 Information exchange

Before	After
Circulation of flyers	Summary and minutes
Professional magazines	Transcripts
Direct mail/invitation	Proceedings/publications/ supplements
Program and documentation	Conclusions/bulletins

and recreational activities with educational aspects. One needs to look back to the objective of the meeting (which is the number one priority) and make the decision on location accordingly.

The next step is to select a facility (hotel, convention center, resort) for the meeting and obtain preliminary estimates of costs. It is best to initiate the search for a facility at least *1 year or more before the event for a 100-participant meeting* that includes a block of hotel rooms, several meeting rooms and catering facilities. For larger meetings, 3–5 years advance facility selection may be required to lock in favorable rates.

This is also the time to prepare budgets and sign contracts with the facility and catering providers. Table 32.6 shows the essential information required and the major costs involved for a fairly simple 100-participant meeting. It may be more or less elaborate, depending on the scope and objective for the meeting. After completing the budget, it should be possible to estimate the cost per participant. This will pinpoint the registration charge for each participant and will allow the calculation of the total cost of the meeting in order to get approval from the firm or sponsoring organization. Using a track record for similar previous events will be of great assistance when filling in the budget items. It is crucial to decide how the meeting will be underwritten, by registration fees, sponsorship or a combination of both. A determination of the timing and pattern of spending must be made, as well as a calculation of when money will be released and acquired.

At least 8–12 months prior to the most major conferences, one needs to plan and begin to implement the promotional campaign for the meeting. This includes printed materials, announcements, press releases, and mailing.

Eight months before the meeting, the preliminary meeting program should be mailed out with registration information. It should include all

Table 32.6 Budgets

Currency	Key costs
How much needed?	Facilities
Who would pay?	Accommodation (food and lodging)
When money needed?	Transportation
How to secure?	Honoraria
	Social events

the registration information necessary (participant information as well as workshop, program and social event selection, as required). Again, if registration fees are applicable, there is a need to implement accounting procedures for funds received and funds dispensed; in addition, procedures should be developed confirming participants' registration.

Six months before the event, one needs to check that all required permits and licenses have been obtained and to discuss menus, audiovisual requirements, and general meeting layout with the conference facility. It should be decided if security persons should be hired for the event.

Five months before the event, one should decide on procedures for the registration table at the meeting and plan timetables to print all materials and handouts for registration, as well as making sure that the registration table at the meeting will be adequately staffed.

Four months before the event, arrangements with all speakers need to be checked as to special needs, audiovisual requirements, hotel reservations, and transportation, and also to mail out the final meeting program brochure and registration information. As listed in Table 32.5, one needs to decide at this time the most appropriate follow-up to each meeting. Depending on the type and the purpose of the conference, one can opt for a simple summary with key conclusions to be circulated to all the participants and company managers, or one can arrange for a full transcript, with the possibility of converting it subsequently to the supplement which will be published in the professional press.

One month before the event, all programs should be finalized, meetings scheduled, audiovisual requirements and menus ready. If a block of rooms has been reserved at the hotel for overnight meeting participants, check weekly to be sure that the meeting block is being filled according to schedule. If the block is filling up rapidly, increase the block with the hotel. If overnight reservations are slow, one could release some rooms to the hotel so as not to be charged for rooms that go unused. It is a good idea to send out reminder postcards to prospective attendentees on the list.

Two weeks before the event, one needs to finalize with the hotel the attendance numbers for meals and preferably even the events. Familiarize your staff with facility layout and business services offered at the facility. Prior to the meeting, lay out materials, train all the registration table staff for registration and set up a message board at the registration desk. During the meeting, staff should be available to deal with equipment failure and booking problems, man the telephone desk, and be ready to assist both speaker and audience. For large meetings/conferences, it may be necessary to retain staff afterwards to settle the final bills of caterers, vendors, site charges, and lodging/travel

charges acquired by sponsored speakers and, lastly, to arrange publication of the 'proceedings' and to close the book accounts.

In conclusion, helping to organize a scientific meeting is a time-consuming and a tough job requiring patience and an ability to take timely decisions and actions. It tests an individual's communication skills; it can also be very rewarding, bringing the respect of colleagues and a rapid development of professional contacts.

33

Drug Surveillance

Howard J. Dreskin and Win M. Castle

Glaxo SmithKline, Philadelphia, PA, USA

The primary duty of a drug monitoring system is less to demonstrate dangers or to estimate incidences than to initiate suspicions... (Finney 1982)

Who do we monitor safety for (e.g. lawyers, regulators, patients, prescribers)? The monitoring of safety has relevance for a wide audience. Patients gain most from enhanced prescribing information or removal of products no longer considered to be safe, as a result of pharmacovigilance by companies and regulatory agencies. Physicians benefit by being able to prescribe the most appropriate medicine for a given patient. Regulators continuously watch over the adverse events reported by manufacturers and independent reporters, and add newly reported events to existing safety databases for analysis. Finally, lawyers require, in some countries such as the USA, that reported events be listed in the local prescribing information, in an effort to inform patients and prescribers of any possible known adverse events, although it is important that the clinically most important information is not lost in the information added for legal liability considerations.

Safety monitoring is a shared responsibility. Monitoring the safety of medicines is a shared responsibility involving, among others, the pharmaceutical industry, physicians, and regulatory authorities. The primary responsibility must belong to the individual pharmaceutical company, which knows the most about the drugs and has the greatest interest in the proper and safe use of the drugs and in maximizing the usefulness of their products to patients.

REASONS FOR MONITORING SAFETY POSTMARKETING

Despite the rigors of clinical testing, the safety profile of a drug is in its early stages of evolution after the drug is approved for marketing. It can change over time as increased numbers of patients have been prescribed a drug and new adverse drug reactions (ADRs) are reported. In order to ensure continued patient protection, it is therefore necessary to monitor the safety profile of marketed drugs continuously for new signals of concern that might prompt revisions in prescribing information.

ADRs are generally classified as Type A or Type B (Venning 1983; Rawlins and Thompson 1977). Type A reactions are usually pharmacologically predictable, relatively frequent, seldom fatal, and usually identified during clinical trials, whilst the drug is in development. Type B reactions are unpredictable idiosyncratic reactions which are usually infrequent but can be very serious or fatal. Postmarketing ADR monitoring usually identifies the more serious, Type B reactions.

Spontaneous or unsolicited ADRs reported postmarketing may contain limited, unclear, or imperfect information. It is the responsibility of the manufacturer to try to obtain as much relevant information as possible so that they can be clinically assessed, particularly those that are serious.

Sample Size

Clinical trials designed to prove the safety and efficacy of drugs are limited by sample size and

Principles and Practice of Pharmaceutical Medicine. Edited by A. J. Fletcher, Lionel D. Edwards, Anthony W. Fox and Peter Stonier © 2002 John Wiley & Sons Ltd.

strict enrollment criteria. As such, ADRs occurring at fairly low rates (e.g. 1/1000) or those occurring in patient subpopulations not studied during clinical investigations may not be identified during clinical trials and can only be identified postmarketing. New rare, serious events may be reported only after large numbers of patients take a new drug, often after several years of marketing experience (Gerald et al 1990; Kessler 1993).

Calculations estimating sample size needed in clinical trials to detect differences between an incidence rate of 1/10 000 and 2/10 000 indicate that 306 000 subjects would need to be enrolled into each group (i.e. placebo, drug) to detect these differences. For such serious ADRs as chloramphenicol-induced aplastic anemia, which occur in 1/30 000 (Lasagna 1983); studies large enough to detect these differences would be prohibitively large.

Potential for Drug Interactions

Potentially harmful drug interactions may not be identified during controlled clinical trials, due to the exclusion of patients taking concomitant medications, which are not allowed to be taken during a study. For example, terfenadine, a novel non-sedating antihistamine which was found to cause a serious and potentially fatal cardiac arrhythmia, torsades de pointes, when administered along with ketoconazole or erythromycin, could not realistically have been expected to be identified in the clinical trial setting. The mechanism of this adverse drug interaction was found to be due to inhibition of cytochrome P-450 by ketoconazole or erythromycin, leading to the build-up of native terfenadine, which is toxic but is normally metabolized very rapidly (Reck et al 1993; Fed Reg 1997).

In order to identify new events or signals manufacturers need to have in place systems for monitoring newly reported events—'pharmacovigilance'. They need to analyze events in an aggregate fashion, such as formalized periodic safety update reports, increased frequency reports, or other types of safety analysis. Pharmaceutical manufacturers must have pharmacovigilance monitoring systems in place, and many countries throughout the world require formalized reporting of serious ADRs and aggregate periodic safety update reports

in an effort to detect new signals. Even so, there are many hurdles to overcome, as history shows.

CIOMS INITIATIVES

In 1986 the Council for International Organizations of Medical Sciences (CIOMS) of the World Health Organization (WHO) began meeting to discuss worldwide harmonization and standardization of ADR reporting of marketed products (Gerald et al 1990; CIOMS Working Group I 1990). The original CIOMS I working party consisted of representatives from six regulatory authorities and seven multinational pharmaceutical manufacturers, and discussed how the reporting of individual ADRs from marketed products should be done by manufacturers to regulators. The goal was to develop a single reporting form (the CIOMS I form), which would be accepted in all countries. It was felt that if there were a more consistent, uniform approach to reporting ADRs, there would be more efficient reporting to, and enhanced communication among, regulators. While the group had no official authority, it was hoped that the members would influence their respective government agencies to enact regulations which would improve safety reporting, based upon the CIOMS initiatives.

The CIOMS I working party proposed, and regulatory authorities subsequently endorsed, that serious unexpected ADRs should be routinely reported to regulatory agencies, and what minimal information was required for reporting. Any report of serious, unexpected adverse drug reactions was to be submitted to regulators within 15 working days of receipt by the company.

In 1989, the CIOMS II working group was formed to develop a uniform approach to aggregate periodic safety update reporting, which would be harmonized throughout the world (CIOMS Working Group II 1992). Like CIOMS I, the second working party consisted of representatives from regulatory agencies and multinational pharmaceutical companies, which could only suggest changes in local country regulations. The CIOMS II Working Group (1992) developed a standardized periodic safety update report which could be used by all countries with periodic reporting requirements. The International Conference on Harmonization (1994; ICH E2C, see below) later adopted the CIOMS II report format with minor modifications and proposed that it be used globally.

Building on the work of CIOMS I and II, a third CIOMS working group was established to propose guidelines for preparing core clinical safety information on drugs (CIOMS Working Group III 1995). The Core Data Sheet (CDS) was defined as:

> A document prepared by the pharmaceutical manufacturer, containing [among other things] all relevant safety information, such as adverse drug reactions, which the manufacturer requires to be listed for the drug in all countries where the drug is marketed. It is the reference document by which 'labelled' and 'unlabelled' are determined [for the purpose of international ADR reporting]...

Safety information was noted to be described in various sections of a CDS, including ADRs (undesirable effects), warnings, precautions, and contraindications. As there were questions pertaining to what information should be included in a CDS, and how the information should be updated, along with no internationally agreed standards for preparing this information, the CIOMS III working party proposed several guidelines for production of core safety information. Topics such as the first core safety information, updating safety information, different presentations, and uses of medicinal products, excipients and other substances, national differences in data-sheets, what to include, and what not to include, were described.

Benefit–Risk Evaluation

The comparative evaluation or balancing of risks and benefits of pharmaceutical products is inevitable, although there are no standard, widely accepted definitions used in medicine. Definitions and terms depend on the context in which they are used, or on the user. Patients, physicians, formularies, pharmaceutical companies, ethics committees, regulatory authorities, and other public health bodies, insurers, consumer groups, and others may have very different perspectives, e.g. the perspective of regulators and companies usually in-

volves aggregate data, whereas physicians tend to focus on benefit–risk evaluations, which may affect treatment of an individual patient. Factors influencing benefit–risk assessments include the audience of the information, the nature of the problem, the nature of the indication and population under treatment, and, to be realistic, economic issues.

The CIOMS IV working group discussed benefit–risk evaluations for use where there is a significant safety issue with a drug. The benefits of the subject drug are described, compared to alternative therapies (medical and surgical) and no treatment at all. Similarly, after discussing the new safety issue, the risks are compared between the subject drug and alternative therapies. Methods are suggested by the CIOMS IV working group for balancing the benefits against the risks for each of these therapies. If specially planned studies can help, the protocols should be outlined. The final selection should be based on a review of the 'pros' and 'cons' and likely consequences of each option, including the quality and qantity of any subsequent evidence that would influence the decision.

CIOMS V, to some extent, is a revisit of earlier CIOMS initiatives, particularly focusing on pragmatic approaches to good case management, follow-up, and generating periodic safety updates.

ICH INITIATIVES

The International Conference on Harmonization (ICH) was formed in 1989 (Secard International Conference on Harmonization 1994; Worden 1995) to provide a forum for discussions regarding differences in technical requirements for product registration, to identify where technical modifications or mutual acceptance of research and development procedures could lead to more economical use of resources, and to make recommendations on practical ways to achieve greater harmonization. The ICH E2 working group was formed with the goal of harmonizing ADR reporting requirements between manufacturers and regulatory agencies in the USA, Europe, and Japan. This working group split off three subgroups: ICH E2A discussed reporting of individual adverse experience reports; ICH E2C discussed electronic transmission of individual case reports; and ICH E2C discussed periodic safety update reporting (PSUR). Whereas the CIOMS initiatives were 'suggestions', the vision of ICH is to lead to the enactment of specific local regulations. ICH expanded on many of the initiatives started by CIOMS, in an effort to make them 'official'.

The ICH review process proceeds through five steps:

Step 1   Preliminary discussion and draft report.
Step 2   Draft is submitted to three regulatory agencies (USA, EU, and Japan) and industry representatives for consultation and comment.
Step 3   Comments are collected and incorporated and drafts referred to the ICH steering committee.
Step 4   Final draft is discussed within the ICH steering committee and adopted by the three regulatory parties.
Step 5   The full recommendations are incorporated into domestic regulations.

ICH E2 (1994) described clinical safety data management and included definitions and standards for expedited reporting of individual case reports describing serious, unexpected ADRs. ICH E2 defined an *adverse event* (or *adverse experience*) as 'any untoward medical occurrence in a patient or clinical investigation subject administered a pharmaceutical product which does not necessarily have a causal relationship with this treatment'. An *adverse drug reaction* (ADR) reported in the post-approval phase was defined as 'a response to a drug which is noxious and unintended and which occurs at doses normally used in man for prophylaxis, diagnosis, or therapy of disease, or for modification of physiological function'. A *serious adverse event* (or experience, or reaction) was defined as any untoward medical occurrence that at any dose results in death, is life-threatening, requires inpatient hospitalization or prolongation of existing hospitalization, results in persistent or significant disability/incapacity, or is a congenital anomaly/birth defect.

Expectedness is viewed as synonymous with listedness: an 'unexpected adverse reaction is one, the nature or severity of which is not consistent with information in the relevant source document(s)'. Relevant source documents include the investiga-

tor's brochure for drugs under clinical development, and the master data sheet or core safety data sheet, or local product labeling for marketed drugs.

Causality of clinical investigation cases is determined by the reporting healthcare professional or the sponsor, and is based on a 'reasonable suspected' causal relationship. Spontaneous reports always have implied causality, and are therefore always considered ADRs.

ICH indicated that fatal or life-threatening unexpected ADRs should be expedited to regulatory agencies as soon as possible, but no later than 7 calendar days after the first knowledge by the sponsor, followed by as complete a report as possible within 8 additional calendar days. All other serious unexpected ADRs should be expedited within 15 calendar days.

Minimum reporting criteria defined by ICH for initial reports are: an identifiable patient; a suspect medicinal product; an identifiable reporting source; and an event or outcome that is serious, unexpected, and a reasonably suspected causal relationship.

SPONTANEOUS CASE REPORTS

Spontaneous case reports are unsolicited cases reported to the company after the drug is on the market, by a consumer, his/her relative, a nurse, a pharmacist, a lawyer, a prescriber, or even a sales person from another company! Although in isolation a source of information of limited value, these reports can be important—perhaps more so if clinically confirmed by the patient's prescribing physician. By definition, spontaneously reported adverse events are considered possibly drug-related by the reporter, even if the motivation is only an inquiry into the possibility that the subject drug could be associated with the event in a particular patient. Occasionally a case report, even from a patient, will describe fully his/her adverse event, including positive rechallenge, and this is very important information in relation to the safety profile of the drug.

In general, spontaneous case reports describe Type B reactions (rare, serious, allergic) rather than pharmacological side effects (Type A) detected in clinical trials.

Spontaneous case reports can reassure a company if a report describes a large accidental overdose with no serious adverse effects. They can also provide reassurance, when reviewed as a whole set, that no reports for drug x causing event y have been received. Clusters of similar spontaneous reports should be meaningfully analyzed for consistency in time to onset, pattern of presentation and dechallenge, to identify a signal and to get a feel for its significance.

The spontaneous case report database cannot be used to give an accurate incidence rate of even the Type B adverse reactions, as not all cases are reported, either because someone who should act as the reporter is not sufficiently motivated, or he/she does not recognize the event as an adverse reaction in that patient (Kessler 1993; Fletcher 1991). Nor do spontaneous case reports lend themselves to meaningful comparisons between different drugs. Not only are all cases not reported for either drug, but the reporting pattern varies with the time from launch (the reporting rate generally peaks 1–2 years after marketing (Sachs and Bortnichak 1986; Weber 1984)), and also the reporting rate for a particular adverse reaction tends to increase after publication of a signal.

The main advantage of spontaneous case reports is that they can provide important signals when reviewed collectively. Although it would be wrong to underestimate their occasional individual importance, it is the consistency of time to onset and pattern of presentation that is important. Pharmaceutical companies, individual regulatory authorities and the World Health Organization (WHO) have databases which facilitate this overview. Modern technology, including imaging, will soon eliminate the need for paper transmission of spontaneous case reports, and there may be a day when all cases will be entered electronically by the initial responsible recipient into a 'shared' database. The use of a standard coding dictionary of adverse event terms is essential for analysis, and one, MedDRA (Medical Dictionary for Regulatory Activities) has been accepted as the 'gold standard' to be used. Nevertheless, routine review of individual cases by responsible, experienced reviewers is the most essential factor in identifying new signals and ensuring patient protection.

The denominator is also known with insufficient precision to allow valid comparison. Although it is important to know whether a serious Type B reaction occurs in 1/1000 or 1/10 000 or 1/100 000, it is often not possible to be more specific. Does it matter, though, to the patient or prescriber to know the incidence more specifically, e.g. 1/9000 or 1/11 000? Accepting that comparisons between drugs are not meaningful based on spontaneous case reports, the authors believe that the answer is *no*, and that a good 'ball park' estimate is usually sufficient. For spontaneous case reports in general, the specific incidence is less important than diligent open-minded review of the data, looking for patterns.

CAUSALITY ASSESSMENT

It is often difficult to assess causality, both for individual patients and in relation to the drug itself. In individual patients, factors such as polypharmacy and multiple events occurring during therapy can interfere with the causality assessment of ADRs. In one study, three clinical pharmacologies independently evaluated 500 untoward clinical events reported by physicians as ADRs (Koch-Weser et al 1977). There were broad differences in interpretation of causality of adverse events, representing the difficulties in assessing causality of individual events.

There are questions that can be asked to help determine causality in relation to the drug, i.e. does drug x cause adverse reaction y? What is the background incidence of the event independent of any treatment? Is there evidence that the incidence in users of the drug is greater than the background incidence? What is the chronology of the occurrence of the reaction? Is it consistent between reports? Is the reaction biologically plausible, based on what is known about the pharmacodynamics and pharmacokinetics of the drug? Is there evidence of a drug–drug interaction? Is there an alternative or more plausible explanation (e.g. natural history of disease, concurrent conditions, other therapies, other exposures)? Is the reaction known to occur with other drugs in the same class or with similar structure? Is the reaction commonly associated with drugs in general? Is there any supporting evidence from clinical trials, postmarketing surveillance studies, or animal studies? Are there any cases which reoccurred on rechallenge?

LABELING

Product labeling describes currently known relevant information about a drug and is intended to aid a prescriber in evaluating the risk vs. benefit of a drug. Labeling includes chemistry, mechanisms of action, warnings, side effects, known drug interactions, precautions, and drug formulation and administration. The labeling is often in the form of a package insert or compendium of information, such as the *Physicians' Desk Reference* in the USA, and serves the basis for prescribing physicians to make risk–benefit decisions when prescribing drugs to patients. As the safety profile of a drug changes over time, the product labeling needs to be modified in order to relay current information.

POPULATIONS

Different subpopulations may react differently to drugs, due to a variety of reasons affecting metabolism. However, differences are not always clearly defined. Factors that could influence patient susceptibility include multiple drug therapies, multiple disorders and severity of disease, types of drugs prescribed, altered pharmacokinetics, altered pharmacodynamics, and the age of the population treated (Nolan and O'Malley 1988).

Differences in metabolism among patients can lead to differences in susceptibility to ADRs e.g. patients with abnormal pseudocholinesterase levels have prolonged apnea after receiving succinylcholine; patients with low activity of *N*-acetyl transferase are more likely to develop lupus-like reactions to procainamide, hydralazine, and isoniazid; and variants of the cytochrome P-450 family of enzymes can lead to altered metabolism of a variety of drugs, including antidepressants, antiarrhythmic agents, codeine, metoprolol terfenadine, cyclosporine, calcium channel blockers, and others (Peck et al 1993).

The pharmacological action of drugs in children may differ from adults, and may invoke a different pattern of ADRs (Colline et al 1974; Gustafson 1969). However, there is little epidemiological data on ADRs in young patients, and the surveillance of ADRs in children presents a challenge, due to the limited number of postmarketing surveillance studies (Bruppacher and Gelzer 1991). Postmarketing safety surveillance may be the only way new signals can be detected in this population.

There may be ethnic differences in susceptibility to ADRs. Corzo et al (1995) identified an association of alleles of the HLA-B and DR loci with increased risk of clozapine-induced agranulocytosis. Patients with abnormal pscudocholinesterase levels have prolonged apnea after receiving succinylcholine. Patients with low activity on N-acetyl transferase are more likely to develop lupus-like reactions to procainamide, hydralazine and isoniazid (Peck et al 1993).

PREGNANCY

Fetal injury and death can result from the use of certain drugs by the mother, and decisions regarding risk vs. benefit must be made when no alternative treatment is available. Certain drugs are specifically contraindicated during pregnancy, e.g. angiotensin converting enzyme (ACE) inhibitors, used by a mother during the second and third trimesters of pregnancy to treat hypertension or congestive heart failure, can lead to fetal injury and death (FDA 1992). Thalidomide was found in the early 1960s to cause fetal limb abnormalities (phocomelia) in the children of mothers who took thalidomide as a sleep aid during pregnancy.

POSTMARKETING SURVEILLANCES STUDIES

During clinical trials, investigators are instructed to collect all ADRs reported by patients enrolled in the study, which are tabulated. During final study reports or product marketing applications, ADR data are analyzed by treatment arm. Overall analyses of results are restricted to statements regarding the specific patient populations studied.

Postmarketing surveillance studies attempt to study a drug's toxicity under conditions of actual use. These studies differ from early phase investigations in several ways (Wardell et al 1979): larger sample size, lower cost, non-random assignment, lack of control over subgroups, long-term open-ended studies; and no formal regulation. Cohort studies investigate non-randomized groups(s) on a specific drug, followed through time to see if a specific event occurs. Case-control studies investigate non-randomized groups of subjects with and without an adverse event, reviewed retrospectively to determine which drugs the subjects took. While some types of postmarketing surveillance studies (cohort studies, case-control surveys) may not be as scientifically thorough as the double-blind randomized controlled studies performed during preclinical development, especially if the clinical details are fully known, they can be used to investigate suspicions.

COULD POSTMARKETING SURVEILLANCE HAVE AVOIDED THESE TWO DRUG SAFETY DISASTERS?

Thalidomide and Phocomelia

It is unlikely that the association of thalidomide taken by the pregnant female and phocomelia in the fetus would have been detected via the spontaneous reporting system, because they were unsuspected. Therefore, why would prescribers report cases in association to thalidomide when there had been no suspicion? Vital statistics probably would not have been useful, because thalidomide was not sufficiently widely prescribed. Since there was no hypothesis about the cause and effect, a case-control study would not have been considered appropriate. In addition, no appropriate control group was available. A cohort study of pregnant women taking thalidomide would not have been helpful, since the background incidence of birth defects is relatively high, and therefore the size of the cohort would have been prohibitive. Furthermore, a cohort study would take far too long. It is questionable if record-linkage studies via computerized databases would have aided in the identification of the problem; only if a specific hypothesis was being tested would it have been likely to be of benefit. Probably the only useful tool would have been a case registry of birth defects, which might have enabled researchers to identify the association.

Oral Contraceptives and Gall Bladder Disease

Oral contraceptives and gall bladder disease posed a difficult problem, since early studies inconsistently demonstrated the association between the drug and the event. There is a high incidence of gall bladder disease in the USA and approximately 445 000 cholecystectomies are performed each year. In order to clarify the association or lack thereof, Strom et al (1986) conducted a retrospective cohort study using the Medicaid billing data from Michigan and Minnesota. Based on data from approximately 1.5 million individuals, a relative risk of 1.14 [Cl 1.09–1.20] (users vs. non-users) was observed. A clear dose–response effect was observed, as was an age-related effect. The authors concluded that oral contraceptives are risk factors for gall bladder disease, although the risk is probably of sufficient magnitude to be of clinical importance in younger women only. Vital statistics and case registries would not have been useful or applicable in this example. A case-control study would have been a possibility if the specific gall bladder disorder could have been specified, but it is not immediately obvious what would have constituted an unbiased control group.

WHAT IS THE IMPACT ON PHARMACOVIGILANCE OF THE PROBLEMS CURRENTLY FACING INDUSTRY?

Modern technology presents several opportunities and challenges to ADR reporting. With the increased use of technology, paper reporting of individual case reports will be replaced by electronic reporting via transmission of selected data fields. Standards for data fields, dictionaries, data codes, and security have been discussed and agreed upon within ICH. However, not all databases are compatible with the data sets defined by ICH, and as companies upgrade their safety reporting databases they will need to ensure that new systems are compatible with ICH E2B data transmission guidelines.

Some companies prefer to build their own ADR database, based on unique company specifications, while others prefer to buy 'off-the-shelf' databases from one of several companies specializing in this area. Whichever route is chosen, a company should decide on is own set of requirements for a database, and determine the best course of action to meet the goals set.

Downsizing

Many pharmaceutical companies are experiencing strains on resources due to budget constraints and resource reallocation (or downsizing). This affects safety departments in particular, in that there is usually no decrease in the amount of work presented. In fact, with new drugs more ADR may be reported to a company. Fewer safety professionals need to process more cases and in less time, due to changing regulatory reporting timelines. Computers have an increasingly important role. This added strain needs to be monitored to ensure that regulatory reporting timelines are not missed.

Licensing In and Licensing Out

Many companies in- and out-licence drugs at various stages of development. Company licensing agreements should describe processes for the safety departments of each company to share safety data, to ensure that at least one company has a complete safety database for each drug. Agreements should include wording describing how individual reports will be reported and transmitted between companies, which company (in which countries) has regulatory reporting obligations, which company will prepare and submit aggregate periodic safety update reports, and how core data sheets and product information will be kept consistent between both companies for each licensed product.

THE NEED FOR BETTER COMMUNICATION TO THE PRESCRIBERS AND PATIENTS

The most important responsibility of the pharmaceutical industry is to ensure that any safety messages are communicated clearly and effectively to prescribers and patients. It is insufficient to add new important messages to the core safety information if it is known that these messages do not reach prescribing physicians. This is particularly relevant to contraindications, precautions, and warnings. It is also presumably the responsibility of the regulatory authorities to identify and counsel any prescriber who they identify may have misprescribed a drug to the detriment of a patient. These mistakes are not deliberate, but in view of the volume of literature received by busy physicians, it is essential that important information concerning the administration and safety of drugs is read and understood.

Modern technology should help. For example, pharmacists are developing databases that help them to identify drug interactions. In the future, the medical history of a patient could be added to a card which could be used by a pharmacist to ensure that the patient's prescribed medicine is appropriate. It would also be possible to input safety data on drugs to computer systems already used by prescribing physicians to store their patients' records. The physician would then be alerted to any contraindications, warnings or precautions that may be relevant to individual patients if prescribed the drug.

REFERENCES

Bruppacher R, Gelzer J (1991) Identifying, evaluating, and quantifying adverse drug reactions in children: opportunities and obstacles for the manufacturer. *Bratisl Lek Listy* 92: 549–53.

Castle WM, Cook SF (2001) Pharmaceutical packaging to prescribing of drugs. In Swarbrick J, Boylan JC (eds), *Encyclopedia of Pharmaceutical Technology*, vol 12. Marcel Dekker: New York; 327.

CIOMS Working Group I (1990) *International Reporting of Adverse Drug Reactions. Final Report of CIOMS Working Group.* CIOMS: Geneva.

CIOMS Working Group II (1992) *International Reporting of Periodic Drug-safety Update Summaries.* CIOMS: Geneva.

CIOMS Working Group III (1995) *Guidelines for Preparing Core Clinical-safety Information on Drugs.* CIOMS: Geneva.

Collins GE, Clay MM, Falletta JM (1974) A prospective study of the epidemiology of adverse drug reactions in paediatric hematology and oncology patients. *Am J Hosp Pharm* 31: 968–75.

Corzo D et al (1995) The major histocompatibility complex region marked by HSP70-1 and HSP70-2 variants is associated with clozapine-induced agranulocytosis in two different ethnic groups. *Blood* 86: 3835–40.

Faich GA, Castle W, Bankowski Z, and the Council for International Organizations of Medical Sciences (CIOMS) ADR Working Group (1990) International adverse drug reporting. The CIOMS project. *J Clin Res Pharmacoepidemiol* 4: 83–90.

FDA (1992) *FDA Med Bulletin* 22(1).

Federal Register (1997) *J Am Med Assoc*. Terfenadine withdrawal proposal from FDA. *Fed Reg* Jan 14.

Finney DJ (1982) The detection of adverse reactions to therapeutic drugs. *Statist Med* 1: 153–61.

Fletcher AP (1991) Spontaneous adverse drug reaction reporting vs. event monitoring: a comparison. *J R Soc Med* 84: 341–4.

Gustafson SR (ed.) (1969) *The Pediatric Patient*, J.F. Lipworth: Philadelphia, PA: 112–15.

Kessler DA (1993) Introducing MEDWatch. A new approach to reporting medication and device adverse effects and product problems. *J Am Med Assoc* 269: 183–9.

Koch-Weser J, Sellers EM, Zacest R (1977) The ambiguity of adverse drug reactions. *Eur J Clin Pharmacol* 11: 75–8.

Lasagna L (1983) Discovering adverse drug reactions. *J Am Med Assoc* 249: 2224–5.

Nolan L, O'Malley K (1988) Prescribing for the elderly, Part 1: Sensitivity of the elderly to adverse drug reactions. *J Am Geriat Soc* 36: 142–9.

Peck CC, Temple R, Collins JM (1993) Understanding consequences of concurrent therapies. *J Am Med Assoc* 269: 1550–52.

Rawlins MD, Thompson JW (1977) Pathogenesis of adverse drug reactions. In Davies DM (ed.), *Textbook of Adverse Drug Reactions*. Oxford: Oxford University Press.

Sachs RM, Bortnichak EA (1986) An evaluation of spontaneous adverse drug reaction monitoring systems. *Am J Med* 81 (suppl 5B): 49–55.

Second International Conference on Harmonization (1994) Topic E2. Clinical safety data management: definitions and standards for expedited reporting. Step 4.

Strom BL, Tamragouri RN, Morse ML et al (1986) Oral contraceptives and other risk factors for gall bladder disease. *Clin Pharmacol Ther* 39: 335.

Venning GR (1983) Identification of adverse reactions to new drugs. II. How were 18 important adverse reactions discovered and with what delays? *Br Med J* 286: 289–92.

Wardell WM et al (1979) Postmarketing surveillance of new drugs: I Review of objectives and methodology. *J Clin Pharmacol* Feb–Mar: 85–94.

Weber JCP (1984) Epidemiology of adverse reactions to nonsteroidal antiinflammatory drugs. In Rainsford KD. Velo EP (eds), *Advances in Inflammation Research*, vol 6. Raven: New York, 1–7.

Worden DE (1995) The drive toward regulatory harmonization: what is harmonization and how will it impact the global development of new drugs? *Drug Inform J* 29: 1663–79S.

34

Disease Management—What Does It Mean?

Roy Lilley

Independent Health Analyst, former NHS Trust chairman, and Camberley, Surrey, UK

Any discussion of disease management (DM) must start with a definition. What does it mean? It shouldn't be difficult. The words in themselves are not complex or confusing; they are self-defining. Disease management means the management of disease. Simple? Not quite. Defining how much management, by whom and whose disease, are just some of the further considerations. There are a host of complications based around the wide-ranging perceptions of what DM is and what it should and could deliver. DM has become a complicated concept. While the majority of this chapter concentrates on the practical aspects of DM in the United Kingdom, those working elsewhere will doubtless see local analogies to the underlying concepts.

Why has it become so complicated? Partly from a lack of understanding, partly political interference that has made DM a 'politically unacceptable' topic, and partly from a defensiveness from those with the most to lose should DM become mainstream in the UK.

DM excites considerable sensibilities. Defensiveness on the part of clinicians is commonly concerned with the potential for DM to be used as a lever for change, reducing their power and influence. Political defensiveness arises out of the misconception that because DM can produce closer working relationships with pharmaceutical companies, the inevitable charge would arise that, in the UK, the much-loved NHS was, in some way, being dismantled or 'privatized'—an allegation that no political party is keen to encourage or sustain, but which change is nonetheless taking place. It is the power that DM has to change practice, change attitudes, and change outcomes that has made it something of an orphan policy alternative. DM is a powerful change mechanism that can

eliminate the endemic scourge of the NHS—the fragmentation of services. All management students learn, in their first lesson that it is the interfaces between services that cause the problems. To put this another way: however flat and level a newly laid patio may be, someone always manages to trip up at the point where two slabs abut—the interface, the gap where one service abuts another and takes over from the next. Health service patios are dangerous places! For instance, the interface between diagnosis, pathology testing, X-ray examination and making records—this translates into out of date tests, lost X-ray films, and missing health records. All these interfaces represent an unnecessary interruption of care for patients.

So, to define DM? It is the management of the entire process along the pathway of the disease, focused around the needs of the patient. In this context it can be seen how powerful a tool for change DM may be, and also how threatening it can be to a service and its employees, stuck in their traditions.

If DM really is such a powerful tool for change, why is it not in daily use in every NHS unit up and down the country? The goal of seamless service delivery has eluded health managers for years. Why aren't all suitable patients not benefiting from a DM programme, focused on improving quality, efficiency and the patient experience? The key issues to address in assessing the relative failure of DM services to ignite any enthusiasm in the NHS are three-fold.

First, the NHS works in a paper-driven slum. Its use of technology to manage information is comparable with most Third World post offices. For DM to succeed, it needs easy access to good information about patient groups. There is little that is easily accessible to improve our knowledge of dis-

Principles and Practice of Pharmaceutical Medicine. Edited by A. J. Fletcher, Lionel D. Edwards, Anthony W. Fox and Peter Stonier © 2002 John Wiley & Sons Ltd.

ease prevalence, severity or outcome. Without good outcome data it is impossible to assess the worth of any treatement modality. There is some hope that this might change. The Department of Health White Paper, *Information for Health*, opens a variety of possibilities to make greater use of technology in the understanding and management of information (IM&T). The roll-out of new IM&T programmes are, potentially, funded from within the Government's Health Innovation Fund. However, implementation of the recommendations contained in *Information for Health* is part of a 7-year programme. Progress will not be quick. Other countries fare broadly the same in the way in which they have valued data and sought to store it and use it.

Second, at the heart of DM, is the need to ensure that patients are treated along tightly defined guidelines and protocols. Most health systems demonstrate a wide variety in approach to even simple conditions. In the USA the emergence of health management organizations (HMOs; sometimes called 'payers', or insurers) has gone some way to correct this, although there are still differences between HMOs. The more complex the condition, the greater the likelihood of variations in approach. In the UK, neighbouring hospitals have been shown to use entirely different approaches to treating cancer and other serious disease.

In England and Wales the National Institute for Clinical Excellence (NICE) and its sister organization, the Commission for Health Improvement (CHImp), have been established and will go some way to correcting this. NICE is charged with the evaluation of the new and existing pharma-products and technologies, the assessment of referral protocols and the development of treatment guidelines. CHImp will, through a system of national audits, ensure compliance with NICE's recommendations. However, in primary care, GPs' terms and conditions of service protect their clinical freedom. Indeed, the obligation placed upon a doctor to do, for the patient, what he/she sees as being the best for the patient, may put universal compliance with guidelines out of reach.

Third, the contractual framework within which DM is designed to work creates a difficult interface with the health service. In this instance DM's strength becomes its weakness. A tight contract for DM services, based on clear treatment protocols with defined outcomes, would be seen by many as contracting-out an NHS service. This ignites the charge that services are being *privatized*. Furthermore, because most existing services are fragmented between departmental 'suppliers', where there is no single department or component that is pre-eminent, no-one may be in a position to initiate a DM contract.

So, back to the primary task; how to define DM? It is a radical policy and not for the faint-hearted. It has far-reaching consequences for the health services and its employees and for the politicians whose policies are the ultimate sanction for all publicly-funded services.

For the pharma-industry, the definition might be around the identification of a new product to promote at a time when pressures on margins and difficulties in research and development spell out an uncertain future. For health providers it might be a management-based approach to what has been traditionally a clinical-based service—and that spells erosion of power and influence. For politicians it can mean decoupling from the traditional path of healthcare delivery, spelling out patients' worries, voter concerns, and re-election uncertainty.

Speaking at a conference on DM in London in October 1995, Roger Holstein used the following definition:

> A coordinated approach to ongoing patient care that influences the behaviour of providers to achieve the best measured outcomes at the lowest possible cost.

Speaking at the same conference, David Hill said:

> The detection and treatment of a disease on the basis of the total cost of all inputs, and measurement of the resulting outcomes, in contrast to the independent management of the various component activities.

Andy McKean, whilst Under-secretary at the Department of Health, UK, speaking at the same event, said:

> DM involves single budgets covering all aspects of care, accounting systems that are based on disease rather than inputs, so that care is managed by 'disease' rather than by inputs, with that care based on protocols agreed between clinicians.

For my part, as good as the definitions are, only Holstein comes close to the pivotal ingredient—the payer–provider relationship. My belief is that DM functions best when it is the product of a binding contract that is based on whole treatment protocols that have regard to quality and efficiency and that are delivered in a way most appropriate for patients. They are also founded in rewards for success and penalties for failure. I see DM as more than a management tool. I believe it to be a management lever—for change.

POLITICS AND HISTORY

It seems it is the politicians who have the greatest difficulty in coming to terms with DM. Since its inception, in the late 1940s, all governments have been keen to identify with the successes of the UK's health services. The NHS is a much-loved British institution. Despite a good deal of voter ambivalence around just how much of their taxes citizens are prepared to pay for their NHS, the Service occupies a special place in public sector services, meaning that changing it is very difficult. Other nations, where health services are less of a national institution, face less voter resistance to change. Nevertheless, it is generally true that public skepticism and concerns around the reconfiguration of any part of *their* health services always meets resistance, and politicians are always conscious of where their votes and their salaries come from!

DM is a powerful tool for change and so far, no post-war British government has made it part of a manifesto commitment or operational policy. The implication that DM will involve the private sector or some part of the pharmaceutical industry is difficult for service managers and strategists, wedded to a publicly-funded, universally accessed service. However, the political landscape may be changing. Speaking at the Corn Exchange in the Spring of 1997, the man who was to be swept into Downing Street with the biggest post-war majority, Labour leader Tony Blair, said:

> What counts is what works. There should be no dogmatic belief that the private sector should do everything or that the public sector should do everything. It is the public interest that is important. What works is what counts.

The present UK government appears open-minded about 'what works'. There is evidence to suggest that, in other parts of Whitehall, government departments are going out of their way to encourage closer cooperation and working with the private sector. The prison service works with the private sector; some schools are now run by the private sector; transport is in the hands of the private sector; even the Downing Street catering is 'outsourced'! So, why not the NHS? Given that DM might depend on close working relationships with the private sector, is DM more or less likely to find a permanent place in the managerial repertoire in solving modern UK healthcare problems?

DM as a delivery tool was developed in the USA, first in renal services initiated by a health visionary, Bernie Salick. Salick's son suffered renal failure and could only dialyse during the day. This meant he was unable to work, and no work meant no income to pay for the dialysis. Salik opened dialysis suites in the evening. The rest is history and part of the folklore of modern healthcare. Salik later opened services for cancer patients and now for a whole raft of services, focusing on chronic illnesses.

The foundation of DM is in well-honed contracts for service, a model that suits the US healthcare delivery mechanism and business methodology well. It is precisely because of its US antecedents that many NHS policy makers see DM taking us closer to a US model of healthcare that is, in the UK, widely perceived to have failed. This is a prejudice that is not without some foundation, when taking into account the concept of universality of access to healthcare that is a cornerstone of the UK system, and substantially missing in its US counterpart.

It was the UK Conservative governments of the 1970s, 1980s and 1990s that took many public services closer to a market-driven system. However, apart from the Thatcher government's experiments and reforms of the healthcare system in the late 1980s, which introduced what became a largely dysfunctional internally *managed market* (a contradiction in terms and in operation), no-one has attempted to create closer working relationships between the British NHS and the private sector.

Pharmaceutical companies have tried modest experiments, but have not seen many of their efforts sustained. In many cases they have been rebuffed entirely.

During 1994 the UK government addressed the prospect of a greater private sector involvement in the NHS. Guidance was issued (Executive Letter 94/94) that, whilst not making DM projects impossible, made them next to impossible. In brief, the guidance highlighted the following areas of concern:

1. Patients should always receive the most clinically appropriate treatment. DM contracts might place restrictions on the use of some drugs which might not be in the patient's best interest.
2. Patient medical records would have to be available to DM companies and this would raise questions about patient confidentiality.
3. Treatment for patients with multiple or complex diseases would be difficult to provide for, e.g. in the case of some older patients suffering diabetes.
4. What would happen if the DM company ran into difficulties and ceased to trade?
5. Who would the DM company be accountable to? The patient or the contracting parties?
6. Who would be the employer of staff working in the DM company and who would they be accountable to—the patient, the company, the contracting authority, or their professional body?

These six questions do not present insurmountable problems. Proponents of DM argued that:

1. DM contracts would only be let on the basis of treatment choices, e.g. where it means services or products being supplied by more than one company, so-called 'bundling'—so be it.
2. Patients' clinical notes are the property of the Secretary of State and, with the consent of the patient, can be available to anyone.
3. In complex cases, it is obvious that a DM approach will not be appropriate. DM is not a universal panacea to the problems of creaking healthcare systems! It can, however, play a part where appropriate.
4. Company insurance for performance bonding is a common private-sector practice that ensures there is money in the system to ensure continuity of supplies or services if problems should arise.

5. Staff would be subject to the same rigors and professional criteria as when they are working in the NHS.

Despite the obvious answers to the concerns expressed in Government guidance, few companies or health service units appeared to have had the enthusiasm to take on the inevitable obstacles and bureaucracy involved. Few saw the rewards outstripping the effort.

PHARMA-PARTNERSHIPS AND WIDER BENEFITS

At the heart of most DM initiatives is a redefined relationship with the pharmaceutical industry. The pharma-company becomes the predominant partner in providing care, instead of merely providing the components of it, such as pharmaceutical products, drugs and the like. The relationship between the British NHS and pharmaceutical companies has never been really close in the same way that non-healthcare private sector manufacturers and service providers get close to their suppliers and see them as part of the value chain.

The implementation of NICE, with its powers to recommend the use (or not) of new products in the healthcare system, and its duties to define treatment referrals, protocols and guidelines, has produced a new tension in an already troubled relationship.

There are those who are uncomfortable with, and sometimes downright hostile to, the pharma-industry, whose profits and ostentatious displays of wealth go against the grain of the not-for-profit public sector healthcare systems. Indeed, many argue that the reimbursement arrangement that UK pharma-suppliers to the NHS enjoy are designed to keep the pharma-companies rich and the NHS poor. The spate of pharma-mergers, the pressures on share price and boardroom practice, are of themselves redefining pressures. However, add to this mix the likelihood of a major pharma-company having a key new drug denied access to the nation's medicine cabinet (as in the case of Glaxo-Wellcome's anti-flu drug, Relenza), and the pressure mounts. If these difficulties are overcome and there is a renaissance in the pharma-

NHS relationship, there is a great deal to be gained for all sides.

There appear to be five principle areas:

1. DM provides an opportunity to be able to understand better the true cost of healthcare. The NHS has a poor record of unit costing, and some parts of it still see accounting for where money has been spent as an unwarranted intrusion of the care process. Many clinicians remain convinced that costs should never be a determinant the type of treatment on offer to their patients. Confusion over the role of capital charges and labour costs, derived from multi-professional participation, makes NHS calculations of the cost of an episode of care unfathomable! The private sector, or the DM partner, will have a different attitude and approach to costs and accounting for them. The DM model is based on a tight and specific contract arrangement, at the heart of which is the unit cost of treatment. DM could accelerate the NHS's journey into proper, business-like accounting.

2. Risk and cost sharing. Contracts may be drawn up in such a way that DM is rewarded for keeping the patient out of hospital and penalised in the event of an unplanned admission. Asthma is an obvious example of disease where good patient compliance with treatment regimes and careful monitoring can reduce the number of symptom-debilitating days. Relapses or acute episodes, resulting in unplanned hospital admissions, are expensive and the costs could be set against the DM contract payments.

3. The NHS focuses its attention almost entirely on dealing with the consequences of sickness. Grouping or 'bundling' services, such as preventative medicine, scanning, and monitoring, could prevent the need for expensive treatment later in the patient's life. This might result in huge long-term savings to the health budget.

4. Where long-term arrangements with pharma-partners mean an assured market, the pharma-company may come to place less reliance on the need to promote particular products. The cost of marketing and promoting products is not small. Savings in the marketing budget could be expected to be reflected in the contract price.

5. Pharmaceutical companies argue they are research- and innovation-led. The difficulty for its principle customer, the NHS, is that it is the cost of innovation that busts their budgets. A new approach to managing the entry of new medicines into the NHS is being defined in the work of NICE. Their concern is that medicines of value enter the system. By value, they mean not just medicines that work at a technical level or are safe—they mean 'work' in the sense of value for money. For a pharma-industry unused to dealing with questions of what constitutes cost-effectiveness in the use of their products, this is starting to look like a difficulty. However, DM allows a pharma-company to demonstrate, for example, that the use of a product may keep a patient out of hospital. This could represent significant cost and resource savings. The cost reduction is equal to a cash saving that should be available to reward both sides of the partnership.

WHO BENEFITS FROM DM?

Modern management tells us to look for a 'win–win' in every deal. Is DM a win–win? Who are the participants and what can they hope to win? There are three 'P's who stand to win; patients, health service providers, and pharmaceutical companies.

Patients

How can patients benefit? A seamless pathway from the loss of function back to wellness is optimal. Sadly, all too often the patient experience is characterized by delays, misunderstandings, fragmentation of services, travel, inconvenience, inappropriate treatment, mistakes, errors, and poor outcomes. Does DM have anything to offer?

Most citizens in developed European nations feel that their health services are world beating. This is a myth the politicians who are responsible for delivering tax-funded health care systems encourage us to believe. In the UK, at least, it is far from true.

As far back as the late 1980s commentators and others were pointing to shortcomings in UK cancer services. This precipitated the report by the Chief

Medical Officer on cancer (known as the Calman–Hine Report). The report acknowledged the shortcomings in performance and variations in clinical outcomes and treatment regimes. The report called for the concentration of professional excellence in cancer centers, arriving at a consensus amongst professionals about which treatment approaches were best and the development of so-called 'cancer pathways' to map the patient's experience from diagnosis to best-practice treatment, and long-term support where it was needed; at the heart of the pathway, a clear clinical protocol—one clinical record, consistency of advice to prevent duplication and confusion, with events and outcomes logged for the clinical audit process.

To any manager working in any other field of service or manufacturing, such approaches are 'everyday' and would not be worth commenting upon. In the British NHS they were regarded as revolutionary, and as the century has turned the NHS still has difficulty in delivering the Calman–Hine system. Indeed, the NHS still has some of the worst cancer outcomes in Europe.

From the patient's point of view, the pathway model opens the possibility of delayed mortality, longer periods of symptom-free life, even complete recovery. All of this could be delivered by a DM approach to care. This would require what is known in the USA as a 'carve-out', the treatment of patients with common conditions, 'carved-out' of the mainstream system, and passed to an outside organization to deliver. The Salick organization did this in the USA. Following a confirmed diagnosis, the cancer patient would be handed over to Salick, who would follow precise treatment protocols to provide care for the patient. Salick was able to claim lower costs and improved outcomes. Would it work in the NHS? Cancer treatments may be too complex a starting point. However, simpler conditions are well suited to a DM approach and the benefits to patients are obvious.

Take, for example, the management of diabetes mellitus. Since the introduction of the NHS 50 years ago, the pattern of treatment for diabetes has been the same. A patient would present with weight loss, pronounced thirst, or excessive urination, perhaps abdominal pain and recurrent infections or unexplained tiredness. The doctor's response would be the same: blood sugar tests, diet advice medication, monitoring (at home and

in the surgery) and, if the case was more severe, referral to hospital for specialist management. Almost nothing has changed in 50 years. For the patient there is still the anxiety, waits for test results, trips to hospital and visits to the surgery. For the working diabetic the services are generally accessed between 9 a.m. and 5 p.m. and his/her working day is disrupted.

With diseases such as diabetes there is huge scope for DM to improve the service to patients. DM diabetic providers are set up to focus on the specific task of managing the patient with the most appropriate staff; doctor, nurse, optician, and chiropodist. Better organized, they could expect higher standards of outcome and clinics open at times that do not interrupt the working or lifestyle pattern of the patient. Overall cost-effectiveness is improved, agreed protocols can be shown to have been adhered to, and detailed contract provision makes the collection of data a pivotal part. In this way the patient's experience is bound to improve.

Health Service Providers

Health service providers can gain under DM. The UK system of healthcare is dependent on the middle-ranking management layer, at health authority level, determining the healthcare commissioning requirements for its geographical area. Recently the commissioning environment has been complicated by the emergence of Primary Care Groups. These groups are syndicates of locality GP practices which acquire various levels of responsibility for running and commissioning healthcare. Whilst the current picture is evolving, in the longer run the policy intention is that the former health authorities will give way to primary care trusts, who will emerge at the top of the management pyramid, with powers over budgets and healthcare provision. As the progress into this model is not time-staged, for the foreseeable future, there is likely to be a variation in commissioning models. However, whatever the final model of commissioning is to look like, the problems remain the same. Whoever commissions healthcare will be beset with the traditional problems of juggling demand and resources, whilst attempting to improve quality.

It is possible that DM could assist those who commission health care, whomever it turns out to be. Contracts between commissioners of healthcare for particular tranches of service, tightly bound with contractual requirements, rewards for achievement, and penalties for under-achievement may help commissioners to stay in budget and improve the quality of care. They may even use the model to attack an often overlooked part of the agenda; health and wellness promotion.

In the present model of healthcare the commissioners have few carrots and even fewer sticks to employ. A DM contract can provide for excellent performance, such as disease reduction and savings, to provide the rewards. Penalties for poor performance, such as unplanned admission to hospital or quality failures, become the stick.

Pharmaceutical Companies

Pharmaceutical companies may also find DM a winner. The difficult future faced by pharma-companies is well known and recognized by most commentators. Pressures from shareholders for profits and dividends, the complexity of modern product development, the costs of research, and the obstacles of managed entry into the system because of NICE (not a purely UK phenomenon, as other countries have or are proposing similar systems; indeed, there are world-wide strategies for cost-containment), are just some of the challenges they face.

Hitherto the standard response has been for pharma-companies to acquire merger partners. Some of the mergers have been marriages of convenience, others appear to have been far more of a shot-gun affair. One thing is certain; to survive, pharma-companies must change.

All healthcare systems face the challenge of aging populations, the increase in chronic disease, and technology fuelling public expectations. In the UK, pharma-companies are fighting for about 10% of the UK healthcare budget. Although there is some evidence that this percentage is slowly increasing, there is no evidence that the increase is enough to sustain the growth expectations shareholders and investors have for pharma-company performance. They have two options; increase their market share or cut their operating costs.

Mergers are thought to be one way of cutting operating costs. Evidence in other sectors would query this thinking, e.g. studies of the mergers in the banking sector in the early 1980s show, over time, that operating costs were not cut, profits did not increase, and there was no benefit to shareholder value.

Most pharma-companies' strategies limit their participation in the system to the supply of drugs. This precludes their potential to benefit from the wider health service economy. By restricting their activity to being pharmaceutical product suppliers, they deny themselves the chance to be considered as providers of the whole treatment.

The pharma-component in general is a small part of the overall costs of providing treatment. Plumridge (1990) found that the rank order of antibiotics costs used in secondary (hospital) care was quite different from a ranking based on the whole drug therapy. Davis and Drummond (1994) showed that the costs of pharmaceutical drugs only accounted for 3% of the total cost of managing schizophrenia; the major costs were for the supervision and hospitalization of the minority of the seriously ill.

From this, two facts emerge. First, it is not the best use of its time for a health service to focus on cutting expenditure on the drugs budget, since this is a tiny proportion of the cost. Second, it is inappropriate for the pharma-company to seek to increase market share in such a tiny market. Pharma-companies would do better to find ways of participating in the wider aspects of healthcare delivery—because that is where the money is! DM, with its multifaceted and comprehensive approach, provides that vehicle.

Why should a pharma-company making pills for the management of diabetes restrict itself to the delivery of the drugs alone? There are far greater profits to be had in managing the patient throughout the whole spectrum of treatment, monitoring, prevention of complications and need.

THE MANAGEMENT OF INFORMATION BY THE USE OF TECHNOLOGY

Information technology (IT) and information systems (IS) play a central role in most modern business and organizations. Indeed, there are industries that, without the use of technology, would not exist at all. Why is it, then, that the British NHS (and many European healthcare systems too)

remain an IT-free zone. Modern healthcare is dependent on technology for diagnostics, testing,
sampling, life support, and even some treatments.
As a percentage of revenue worldwide, healthcare
is estimated to be at the bottom of the list in investment in IT, at less than 2% of spending. Financial
services, about 12%, was at the top of the expenditure league, followed by computer companies
10%, utilities 7.5%, aerospace 7% and insurance
about 5%.

New IM&T strategies in the UK public healthcare arena, planned for the 7 years starting 1999,
are not expected to have a dramatic effect on the
NHS's efficiency. The investment cash, earmarked
for development, is too small to catch up from the
very low starting base. For a seven-year IT project,
by the time the job is finished it is highly likely that
the systems selected in year 1 will be obsolete by
year 7. Outside the NHS, spending on IT growth
continues at an average of about 10%. Current
expenditure projections show that the NHS cannot
catch up.

The NHS appears to have lost sight of the fact
that healthcare delivery is largely about the collection of data—patient records, outcome data, monitoring information, and so on. Health services are
founded on the simple expectation that public
health measures and medical technology provide
the balancing factors of prevention and cure that
are either side of the fulcrum point of 'health'. This
may have been the case in dealing with acute illnesses that are largely curable. However, our ma-
turing society now seems to have collected a raft of
chronic diseases that are not. The balancing act
changes.

In the chronic disease sector, we look for long-
term management of the condition and a cost-effective extension of quality life-years. It is IT-based
solutions that we look to, to track the path of
disease and evaluate the outcomes of care. The
collection of data, the integration of the information, its interpretation, are all open to us. It systems
can support our decisions, schedule our interventions, count the cost of the resources we use, and
evaluate our outcomes. This brings a dramatic improvement in what we know about what we are
doing. DM would expect to use information from
a number of sources to converge on the answer to
the questions, What are we doing? Does it work?
and Do we want it again?

Is it true that *vice versa* DM could advance the
use of IT in the management of information in
health care? The answer is, most definitely. This
conclusion is based on the assumption that the
DM programme will be the consequence of a contract between a health commissioner (or payer) and
the service provider. The contract will call for
a specific treatment protocol or a guideline to be
followed. The contract will include the calculation for payment based on the number of patients
treated, and how, and with what. The contract will certainly call for monitoring and evaluation, and finally will undoubtedly include
some instrument for the calculation and evaluation
of outcomes, including distribution of savings,
or penalties for breakdowns or unexpected
events.

To provide this level of information in a timely
and reliable way is currently almost beyond the
NHS's systems. By providing for this level of information requirement, by the use of IT, the DM
company has ready-made advantages over what
the existing systems offer in terms of knowledge-
base and information. The relationship between
payer and provider changes. Measuring performance becomes possible. The mysterious world of
the medic is revealed and power shifts to the
payer. Because it provides knowledge, IT is a
powerful tool; knowledge about activities, performance, opportunities for improvement, failures
and foul-ups at zero investment for the commissioner or payer, the data routinely collected by DM
and subject to the terms and conditions of a contract, all routinely made available to the payer, who
can command open access to the systems used by
DM. Unquestionable the relationship between IT
and is intimable and reciprocal.

WHERE'S THE EVIDENCE THAT DM WORKS?

DM originated in the USA, where it is sometimes
referred to as Patient Management Strategies. It is
to the US system that we must first turn for evidence. Health insurers exert pressure on clinicians
to perform uniformly and to aim at benchmarked
and similar outcomes at comparable costs. The
payer relationships are visible in the USA, where
systems are funded, for the most part, by premium-

paying customers who want the best possible treatment at the lowest premium cost.

In the UK system, where money in the system is 'invisible', the same pressures do not apply. This may, in part, account for some of the reluctance of UK health commissioners to embrace DM. However, in the USA, DM systems are commonplace, e.g. for the treatment of congestive heart disease and asthma, for which some 470 000 Americans find themselves admitted to hospital for treatment each year.

Health management analyst Paul Gross has stated that using DM to control demand through patient education and a 1 week, patient-centred, multidisciplinary outpatient clinic at the National Jewish Centre (Denver) reduced admissions to hospital by 83%, accident and emergency visits by 45% and inpatient days by 82%. The cost savings are not recorded but can be assumed!

There seem to be four features of an effective DM scheme (based on GRCS 1998):

1. Patients must be treated in a vertically aligned system. This means that the care pathway has to be carefully planned, and unlikely to be found in an existing system. The delivery of a seamless and integrated care program is most likely to be the product of organizational re-engineering.
2. The method of payment, or the contractual base, has to have both carrots and sticks, i.e., an element of risk-sharing between the provider and the payer. Where savings or economies can be found, the proceeds must become available to both parties. Where over-runs or non-budget expenditure occurs, managing the cost implications should be clearly defined, either as a penalty for the provider or a shared risk between the provider and the payer.
3. The management of information must be done by the use of technology. Provision for patient privacy and access factors are vital. However, the collection of data and shared access between the provider and the payer are fundamental.
4. Agreed case management must be based on protocol-driven care, with staff committed and trained in related care such as patient education.

In a telling paragraph from his chapter in the book *Disease Management* (Lilley et al, 1998), Paul Gross writes:

> Successful DM—involving some attempts to link health outcomes with the costs of achieving those outcomes—requires comprehensive processes that are now emerging in best practice DM projects, such as Mayo Clinic's work for the John Deere company, Mayo Clinic's costing studies and clinical practice protocols for specific diseases (including infectious diseases), National Jewish Centre's DM of asthma, City of Hope and Salick's DM of oncology patients, New York's Cardiac Surgery Reporting System and its Department of Health Quality Improvement Initiative, and Australia's embryonic National Hospital Outcomes Programme and Cardiovascular Disease Monitoring System.
>
> Each of these prototypes used valid science to develop clinical practice protocols, test the protocols, and evaluate their impact on both outcomes and costs. They may achieve cost–effective care of specific diseases quicker than all the Cochrane Centres put together, or the panoply of cost-effectiveness studies undertaken by health economists, or the hordes of companies now marketing partial versions of DM, worldwide.

WHERE'S THE EVIDENCE THAT DM DOESN'T WORK?

DM is not without its critics. In Europe the criticism is founded largely on the prejudice that DM is the product of the US healthcare system, a system widely perceived as unsatisfactory in that it is not universally inclusive. Some 37 million Americans have no permanent healthcare cover. Therefore, it is claimed, any product of that system must be bad. However, it is equally true to say that where the US healthcare system 'works', it works well. Outcomes are good, management is good, and satisfaction levels are high.

DM was pioneered by US pharma-companies, working with HMOs keen to extend their influence into patient care beyond the fulfilment of a prescription. As they exhaust themselves in their pursuit of ways to increase their profits, they will find what most other large-scale industries have found—that solutions to increased profitability in a changing market are not to be found in merely getting bigger, or merging simply to carry on doing the same things but on a different scale. DM provides an interesting and potentially profitable extension to their business.

It is also true that the US system, based on a form of purchaser contracting unpopular in the UK system, is an easier environment for DM concepts to flourish. Criticism of DM as a method of healthcare delivery should be based on more than the US experience.

At the heart of a well-managed DM system are protocols and clinical guidance; it is these factors that critics cite most. Tightly-drawn protocols tailored to the needs of particular patient groups can exclude patients who have those diseases but who suffer multiple pathology or complications to their conditions. What happens to these patients? For instance, they may well be obliged to incur the costs and inconvenience of travel to more than one centre for treatment.

It is argued, with some justification, that holding doctors to tight clinical guidelines makes a nonsense of clinical freedoms. This may raise medicolegal issues, particularly for general practitioners. GPs' terms and conditions of service make it clear (Sec 43), that practitioners *must* provide appropriate services to their patients. This gives rise to the opportunity for GPs to set aside guidance and protocols that have no legal status. The celebrated Bolam v Friern Hospital (1957) case adds to the complexity. In short, the judge said that guidelines could be ignored where a responsible body of professional opinion accepted an alternative standard of care as reasonable.

Perhaps the most important limitation on DM is evidence of its effectiveness and the effectiveness of the treatments and protocols it may be based upon. Scientific evidence requires high standards. Meta-analysis of randomized controlled trials, large-sample randomized control trials, small-sample randomized control trials, cohort studies, and case-control studies are all approaches that have varying levels of reliability in proving for a particular approach. Very little work of this nature has been undertaken in relation to DM. The work of the National Institute for Clinical Excellence may go some way to addressing this issue in relation to clinical, therapeutic, and treatment guidelines. However, DM is a whole-system approach.

A further criticism of DM is the issue of cost. Although DM is thought of as a way to reduce costs, there is the factor of transaction costs to take into account; the cost of striking and setting the contract, as well as the cost of monitoring its performance. These costs are inevitably passed on to the healthcare purchaser in the overall contract price. However, they may be mitigated where the DM supplier has more than one contract running and is able to benefit from savings of scale.

If the common US model is replicated, it may be assumed that a pharmaceutical company is involved at some stage. The motivation for the company to be involved is likely to be based on a desire to acquire a monopoly in the market.

Few companies have, in their product listing, all the drugs that may be needed to treat a particular condition, e.g. a company specializing in the manufacture of insulin products for the treatment of diabetes may not have all the drugs needed to treat a hypertensive diabetic. In the competitive environment of the pharma-industry, cooperation is rare and collaboration even rarer. It could be that a monopoly supplier would also attract the attention of the Office of Fair Trading or even the Monopolies and Mergers Commission.

In 1996, Dr Harry Burns, the Director of Public Health for the Glasgow Health Board, said: 'If Disease Management is desirable, then the NHS should adopt its use'; he said this knowing that the pharmaceutical industry has no track record of managing healthcare delivery. Professor Alan Maynard of York University went on to argue; 'If long-term contracts based on cost-effectiveness guidelines were negotiated with key pharmaceutical manufacturers, it may be possible to reduce the costs of pharmaceuticals and remove some of the unhelpful budget boundaries by purchasing disease management services from publicly-owned providers, or franchizing services. However, there is, as yet, no evidence that disease management in the NHS would be efficient'.

IS DM JUST FOR SICKNESS?

What is the opposite of disease management? How about wellness management?

What does it mean? Due definition is that it means maintaining health through integrated planning and the delivery of services for specific conditions. In other words, keeping people well, rather than waiting for them to get sick, or sicker.

In healthcare systems struggling for budget, it does seem obvious commonsense that preventing more people from getting sick or becoming more ill is one way of making available resources go further—in other words, demand management. A quick tour of the Internet will soon reveal that health service demand management is high on the agenda in the USA. HMOs, are contracting with the increasing number of emerging companies to manage the demand for healthcare, for some chronic conditions, by providing lifestyle advice and health maintenance programs.

Wellness management can be a practical way of harnessing the benefits of real collaborative working, creating the opportunity for new initiatives beyond the normal boundaries of hospital and community care, along what Professor Brian Edwards at the University of Sheffield might call a 'care pathway'.

When the concept of wellness management was first mooted in the mid-1990s, the British NHS was struggling to come to terms with the radical Thatcher NHS reforms. A new operational freedom was emerging. NHS Trusts, formerly NHS units such as hospitals and community services, were standing on their own two feet, planning and preparing services in a so-called 'competitive' managed market. The operational freedoms that they enjoyed liberated much of their thinking but, arguably, produced an operational isolation. Their quest for freedom was often at the expense of integration. It was the lack of integration that prompted the work on wellness management. Treating some conditions effectively requires demolition of the operational boundaries that exist, as patients track their path through the system from department to department, from primary to secondary care, and often back again—crossing supplier boundaries that created interface quality problems, communications difficulties and inconvenience.

The Labour reforms of the late 1990s have sought to overcome those problems by developing an NHS model led by an integrated primary care model, where all the stakeholders in service provision—health, social services, local authorities, and the voluntary sector—have a voice. This moves us towards a model we might recognize as wellness management.

However, if healthcare is to ignore service boundaries and the needs of residents, patients, and clients are seen as a horizontal continuum, the flow of money has to produce a high tide of resources and a wave for others to ride on. In England, in part, merging budgets between hospital and primary care services and the prospect of pooling resources between social services and health goes some way to creating the right environment. However, it is in Scotland, where the model is different, and where that the best possibility for wellness management exists.

The so-called 'Tartan Health Paper' of 1998 (the Scottish equivalent of the English White Paper, *Modern and Dependable*), creates a new tool; the Joint Investment Fund (JIF). The JIF invites managers to identify and extract the whole cost of care for a particular disease, from primary, secondary and tertiary care, and to reinvest it, ignoring the system delivery boundaries that bedevil most healthcare planning.

This means that models of care that are genuinely horizontal can be created by shifting funds to where they are most needed or may produce the greatest benefit, either in treating a disease or preventing it. This approach is in its infancy, but is already emerging as a useful way to address the very high incidence of coronary heart disease in Scotland. At the forefront of this work is the Director of Public Health for the Glasgow Health Board, Dr Harry Burns. Burns, a former surgeon, is using the budget stripping and reinvestment opportunities in JIF to reshape services.

The key issue is the facility to take the whole disease area budget and focus it on prevention as well as cure—in other words, wellness management. In England, Health Improvement Programmes are the tool; managers, clinicians, and others will use to focus on local disease and public health problems and address them. It is a strategic and planning tool that might fall into the category of planning for wellness. Time will tell.

So, wellness management, as a component part of disease management, seems a real possibility. How does it work? Can it work? If the approach has a weakness, it is that it depends on good quality data to identify potential sufferers and the usual problems of defining optimal care pathways based on treatment protocols.

Next, it requires resource analysis. At local level, this may not be easy, e.g. the administration of an expensive drug at an early point in the process, may result in the re-engineering of the existing process of care, where an anticipated, subsequent admission to hospital for treatment becomes redundant.

Recent developments in the UK NHS system may make this a possibility. Hospital and community budgets can now be merged with primary care budgets. Hitherto, the administration of an expensive drug in primary care that kept a patient out of secondary care was a cost and a loss for primary care, and a saving and a win for secondary care. There was no mechanism to share the cost or to redistribute the savings. The patient was the biggest loser, in that the best choice of treatment was often not available. There was no incentive to cross bureaucratic boundaries. The new arrangements create the possibility of a win–win situation for both sectors and in the end the patient becomes the biggest winner.

The next component of wellness management is outcome measurement. The assumption is that wellness management creates a better outcome. The next step is to prove it! Experience shows that few of the measures used in research are easily adapted to routine practice. Few measurements exist to compare long-term care settings, and fewer still can be applied in multidisciplinary and multi-agency care. Perhaps the most reliable approach is to be found in patient satisfaction data?

Does it work? Kirby and Peel introduce us to the concept of therapy economics; the comparative analysis of alternative courses of therapy, which is taken to include treatment and drug regimes, in terms of their costs and consequences. The complex calculations include: cost-benefit analysis; cost-effectiveness analysis; cost-minimization analysis; the cost of illness, e.g. the annual cost of cardiovascular disease in the UK; and quality-of-life measurements, the impact of alternative treatments on patient well-being and expectations.

This dynamic modelling approach looks at the subtle interaction between treatment protocols and processes. From that, new protocols can emerge. Wellness management responds to the need to reduce costs and improve quality.

HOW WOULD DM BE PUT INTO PRACTICE?

Practical advice on setting up a DM service is hard to come by. There is little hands-on experience in the UK. However, one former front-line GP Dr Paul Lambden, has given the issue thought and study. Lambden was a Fundholding GP who went on to become the CEO of a large acute NHS hospital. It is his unique experience that provides an interesting perspective on how to set up a service that might cross the boundaries and budgets of primary and secondary care.

He took, as his example, a service for the treatment of diabetics. This is a useful starting point as the approach has implications for many other services. He calls first for a clear definition of the types of patients who will be offered treatment. Some patients will control their symptoms by diet alone; others may need oral or injected insulin replacement; some may have stable disease; and others may be *brittle*, requiring much closer monitoring. Immediately we see the complexities facing the commissioner for DM services. Furthermore, there is the extent to which the chronic patient's regular physician, whom the patient will trust and be used to dealing with, will participate in the care programme. There are other questions: is it likely that the DM programme would manage and maintain patients while they are stable and easy to care for, but as soon as there is a complication, they will be handed back to their GP? This has a number of obvious implications for the continuity of care, out-of-hours care, and budgets.

Provided that these and general information obstacles can be overcome, the next step is constructing a tender, inviting DM companies to offer a service. Identification of the limits of care, the numbers and types of patients to be included, the treatment protocols, and the outcome or success criteria are all vital considerations. Lambden lists 13 key issues:

1. The types of patient to be included in the programme.
2. Referral criteria.
3. The type of investigations to be performed.
4. Frequency and content of regular monitoring appointments.

5. Drugs to be used and the criteria for their usage.
6. Management of acute events, with exclusion arrangements.
7. Information recorded and available for audit purposes.
8. The time over which the contract will operate.
9. Procedures to withdraw patients from the scheme and arrangements to repatriate them to their GP.
10. The quality and format of initial information.
11. Agreed standards of clinical information and governance.
12. Limits of care.
13. Emergency arrangements for risk-sharing, if the number of patients referred exceeds the number contracted for.

Where the DM is a pharma-company a number of other issues emerge. The pressure will be to provide a uniformity of care, centered around a particular drugs regime. The benefits are the cheaper purchase of drugs, better understanding of the treatment regimes by those who are providing the care, and better monitoring of care for comparative purposes. However, the disbenefits are: the infringement of the clinical freedom of the physician; patient choice; the potential to block out new or innovative treatments not included in the contract; and difficulties when the contract comes to an end and it is inherited by another company with a different range of drugs or approach.

Monitoring the contract calls for precise measurements for success criteria. These may include patient throughput in the scheme, cost and budget factors, and general management issues. In addition, there are the medical issues concerning the performance of the clinical regime and how well the patients do. Lambden makes two points. The first is clinical measurement (for diabetes) of, say, a 6 monthly measurement of HbA1C, the yardstick of the success of blood glucose control. It is worth making the point that with other conditions there may be no biochemical markers of success. His second point is patient self-assessment of treatment success. He points out that this is useful in assessing the shortcomings (or otherwise) of service delivery, convenience, approach, attitude, and so on, but that it may not be adequate to measure clinical improve-

ments in outcome. A patient who reports feeling well may not have the whole picture.

Staffing becomes a major factor. In addition to doctors and nurses, in the case of diabetes, for instance, there is the further consideration of the turn-around of blood sample evaluation and access to other services, such as ophthalmology, chiropody, and dietary advice.

The choice of company is, self-evidently, vital. The organization's ability to deliver the service can only be taken against the success of its current activity. The newness of DM in the UK market is likely to make the choice of company, where there is no proven track record, even more difficult. The support of the medical profession, whose cooperation is required, can be a way around the lack of hard evidence. Indeed, the DM company may not be from a single background such as a pharmaceutical company; it could be the result of the merger of a number of companies who have an interest in the disease. For instance, in the case of diabetes, there are three major manufacturers of diabetic medication.

The management of information by the use of technology invites the question, 'could the DM provider be led by an IT company'? Sites, or locations for care, or patient transport, might be required, which means that a facilities management company will be involved. In some disease areas a medical equipment supplier might be pre-eminent, e.g. in the case of dialysis; and where the evaluation of samples is a prominent requirement, a pathology laboratory.

If innovative ideas are to be developed, the companies' willingness to provide services at the patient's home, at week-ends, and during evenings may be a contractual consideration, as would staffing. The repertoire of skills normally associated with a doctor is fast being eroded into the nursing arena. The substitution of doctors for nurses may become a consideration.

PATIENT PERSPECTIVES?

A contract without patients is no use. What is the likely reaction of patients to DM-provided services? In primary care, most GPs will tell you, patients have a remarkable loyalty to their GP.

Patient reaction to the reconfiguration of services brings howls of protest and it is invariably taken as a cut or closure of service. Moving patients, particularly those with chronic conditions who are likely to have an attachment to a practice or doctor, is not easy!

In 1998, Lambden wrote:

> The history of medicine and its provision has been peppered with opposition, unexpected opposition from patients groups who have succeeded in encouraging politicians, managers and others, to take the line of least resistance and advocate the status quo, as a way of calming adverse publicity. Often the real benefits of change have been ignored. The risk of patient backlash is a potential and must be effectively countered through careful patient education before any problems arise.

Moving suitable patients into a DM service takes patience, sensitivity, and care. Patients cannot be treated *en bloc*, and any transfer should come as the result of individual negotiation between the doctor and the patient. The doctor will have to be convinced that what he/she is recommending is in the patients' best interest. Anything short of outright support for the change on the part of the doctor will not do. They have to be convinced.

Demonstrable benefits to the patient are an essential part of the package. There must be clear improvements in terms of quality of care, access to care and the convenience of care. Preparing a patient for transfer may involve literature to explain the benefits and reasons for change, and pre-transfer visits to new facilities and meeting the clinical or care team may underpin patient confidence and create a willingness to change.

Where existing patients are reluctant or unwilling to change, there can be no question of coercion or compulsion. This means that special arrangements must be made for the continuation of services for those unwilling to transfer. The situation of new patients who may present for treatment after DM arrangements are in place, may be different. They are likely to be subsumed into a scheme and accept it as 'the way treatment is provided'.

Attention to patient confidentiality will be a concern for many clinicians. The transfer of patient records to a third-party service supplier has been one of the major concerns put forward by the Government in the UK and the doctors' trades union, the BMA. Patient records are the property of the Secretary of State, and may be divulged to a third party on the consent of the patient. Clear and unequivocal arrangements are needed to ensure that patients understand, and are willing, for their records to be handed over to a DM company. Consideration should be given to whether or not the whole of the record needs to be divulged to a third party.

Patient satisfaction with services must be monitored, and continual sampling, surveying, and questioning will reveal trends in the care profile. Patient satisfaction is often thought of as the first and the last factor. True, but bear in mind that patients may not be aware of the latest developments in treatments, neither is it realistic to expect them to be aware of all of the nuances of the quality of care that they might expect. The truth is that DM is not a way for commissioners to abrogate their responsibilities.

THE DM COMPANY

In the present UK healthcare market, prospective DM companies will need to overcome a great deal of inertia and bureaucracy to establish a service. Apart from the usual requirements of business planning synonymous with all business start-ups, the unique environment of DM adds 10 additional requirements:

1. Identification of a healthcare market niche in which demonstrable cost saving or clinical quality improvements are clearly needed and achievable.
2. Identifying a commissioner who is enthusiastic about the benefits of DM and will stand by his/ her decisions to support such an initiative.
3. Identifying key opinion-formers who may be against the introduction of a DM service and working with them.
4. Identification of clinicians prepared to support the venture and with the initiative to say so.

5. Fully developed care protocols that are endorsed by local clinicians and their appropriate professional bodies and patient associations.
6. Systems for accurately costing episodes of care—understanding that start-up is likely to be the most expensive time.
7. Arrangements for risk-sharing in the event of unplanned-for changes, and formulae for the distribution of any savings that the DM solution may generate.
8. Robust IT systems for the management of information by the use of technology, and a clear understanding about access to it—what information is to be shared with the commissioner and what is private to the company.
9. Staffing levels and skills mix. The cost of staffing will very likely be the highest component of operating costs. The temptation might be to de-skill, or re-skill, tasks wherever possible. The use of experienced and appropriately qualified staff will be vital to the delivery of good quality DM care.
10. A willingness to be innovative in the development of flexible approaches to the delivery of care. DM services should not simply seek to replicate existing care models; they should aim to provide services that are uniquely based around the needs of patients. Out-of-hours services, and services provided at convenient times and locations, are often out of the reach of NHS providers—they must be part of the offer from the prospective DM company.

limiting choice, restricting care, or precluding innovation, have all been vocal against DM.

However, there is evidence from countries where DM services have matured that they work well. As a mechanism to control costs, by modern management methods and the improved use of the management of information by the use of technology (something that defeats most European healthcare systems), DM services can perform well.

Basing DM services on thoughtful and appropriate care protocols used to be seen by many as its unique point of advantage. However, in the UK and other countries, the emergence of clinical governance as an overarching regulatory framework, and the results of the work of organizations such as NICE in the UK (being replicated in other European and Australasian countries) in developing protocols, the evaluation of medicines for cost-effective performance, and therapy guidelines, means that guideline-based medicine is likely to become a permanent feature in the healthcare landscape.

So, is DM a system worth bothering with? Most healthcare systems are running out of solutions. Putting ever more of a nation's gross domestic product into healthcare systems is an unsustainable ambition. When the last taxpayer's pound has been eaten by a health service, it will still demand more. In as much as DM is a way of leveraging quality upwards and cost containment downwards, DM deserves a better airing. The issues of patient choice, clinical freedoms, patient confidentiality, and all the other reservations regularly aired by its detractors, can and should be overcome in the name of better services for patients and a better deal for the tax-payer.

SUMMARY

Disease management services have had few supporters from within the NHS community. Politicians, sensing public concerns over the potential for confusing the outsourcing of some services for some patients with the emergence of a precursor to outright privatization of the NHS, have been reluctant to encourage its use. The medical community, suspecting that DM will restrict clinical freedom, and patient groups nervous that DM might mean

REFERENCES

Bolam v Friern Hospital Management Committee (1957) *All England Reports*, 2, 118–128.

Burns H (1996) Disease Management and the Drug Industry: carve out or carve up? *Lancet*, 347, 1021–2023.

Davies LM and Drummond MF (1994) Economics and Schizophrenia: the real cost. *Br. J. Psychiatry*, 165 (suppl. 25), 18–21.

Gross P (1998) International Overview. In, Lilley R (ed.) *Disease Management*, John Wiley & Sons, Ltd, Chichester, pp. 123–151.

Kirby S and Peel S (1998) Wellness Management. In, Lilley R (ed.) *Disease Management*, John Wiley & Sons, Ltd, Chichester, pp. 71–81.

Lambden P (1998) At the Front Line. In, Lilley R (ed.) *Disease Management*, John Wiley & Sons Ltd, Chichester, pp. 27–45.

Lilley R (ed.) (1998) *Disease Management*, John Wiley & Sons, Ltd, Chichester.

National Health Service General practitioners' terms and conditions.

National Health Service (1994) Executive letter 94/94.

Plumridge RJ (1990) Cost comparison of intravenous antibiotic administration. *Med. J. Australia*, 153(5), 516–518.

35

Publishing Clinical Studies

Anthony W. Fox

EBD Group Inc., Carlsbad, CA, USA

This chapter has three objectives. First, it is necessary to discuss the ethics and desirability of publishing clinical trials, and the biases that may be involved with that process. Second, junior pharmaceutical physicians may benefit from some discussion of classic parts of an orthodox clinical trial report in a peer-reviewed journal, and some clues for effective oral presentations. Third, alternative forms of publication are discussed, including isolated abstracts and posters, electronic publication and press releases. The scope of this chapter is strictly formal publications: regulatory documents (which are typically not published and are a different form of clinical trials reporting) and marketing materials are dealt with elsewhere. A summary and prospectus closes this chapter.

ETHICS IN PUBLISHING CLINICAL TRIALS

For all forms of publication, the objective usually goes beyond the mere reporting of clinical trials data. In some way or another, the pharmaceutical physician will interpret his/her data to reach conclusions, and will want to urge some change in the behaviour of the target audience. These changes might include prescribing habits, healthcare resource utilization, public health policy, or regulatory practices.

Whatever the form of publication, the only tools available to persuade people to make these behavioural changes are the well-created document, audiovisual presentation, press release, etc. Often the actual dissemination of these materials takes place at a time or place remote from the writer's supervision. Publications must be well-made for stand-alone use.

Conclusions that extrapolate beyond the range of available data are as inappropriate in scientific publications as they are in regulatory documents and marketing materials. Omissions of details in methods and results pursuant to a concise presentation will always be subjective, and there is a close link between the appropriateness of this subjectivity and the integrity of the pharmaceutical physician.

The pressures on the pharmaceutical physician, whether writing him/herself or when guiding specialist medical writers, are many, sometimes contrary to common standards of integrity, and often emanate from powerful people who lack the training needed to assess the data objectively. Such people will include journalists, who oversimplify or sensationalize; marketing department staff, wanting to amplify positive messages and silence negative ones; and corporate officers, who want to use publications as vehicles for enhancing the share price or negotiating better financial arrangements on Wall Street. Rarely, even government politicians get involved, whose tactics include those used by journalists, the diligent application of complete ignorance, and the forced fit of technical information to a predetermined political position.

The publication of clinical trials, then, is one example where the pharmaceutical physician (acting as publicist or medical writer) may become an agent for social change (Gray 1994). Even when he/she acts solely as a medical writer, the pharmaceutical physician must understand the ethical responsibility to represent the material in a fair, balanced, and, above all, accurate manner. While an ombudsman-like role may help in finding compromise among the various pressures that are applied to this process from diverse outside parties, the pharmaceutical physician will inevitably (and

Principles and Practice of Pharmaceutical Medicine. Edited by A. J. Fletcher, Lionel D. Edwards, Anthony W. Fox and Peter Stonier © 2002 John Wiley & Sons Ltd.

hopefully consistently) find him/herself as the company's repository of integrity in this process; this can be a lonely place to be, but nobody else is going to fulfill this role.

DESIRABILITY OF, AND BIASES IN, THE PUBLICATION OF CLINICAL TRIALS

Everybody finds the publication of an *ideal* clinical trial to be highly desirable. Clinical development departments find it efficient to mail out reprints in response to clinicians' inquiries and to append them to Investigators' brochures and IND amendments. Regulators controlling promotional practices need only satisfy themselves that the publication accurately reflects the report that has been submitted to the approved dossier or NDA. Marketing departments can use these publications for promotional purposes, knowing that the data is cast-iron, the message is unarguably positive, and that the self-evident benefits of the drug will be understood by the most sceptical clinician meeting the least adept salesperson. Lastly, senior management can bask in the glory of its contribution to the public health, and direct observers on Wall Street to the appearance of its clinical trials in the world's most respected medical journals. For small companies, this might even be life-saving. How on earth could such a laudable activity go wrong?

The answer, of course, lies in the fact that many clinical trials are less than ideal candidates for publication. These poor publication candidates may be trials that did not result in a positive outcome, or those that generated data about some prosaic aspect of drug action (e.g. tolerability in a special population). Studies replicating a positive finding are often a regulatory requirement, but me-too papers do not find homes in prominent journals. Lastly, some good studies are less than ideal publication candidates solely because the manuscript has been drafted badly.

Negative trials are rarely accepted for publication by good journals unless their results seriously dispel some previously-held belief, or contradict previously published studies. Some areas of therapeutics are notorious for the high proportion of negative clinical trials results (e.g. pharmacological treatments for depression). However, the majority of negative clinical trials are those where either drug efficacy is simply not evident or where no difference is found between two active treatments. Negative data are the inevitable result of conducting clinical trials that are true experiments; there is nothing dishonourable in such a result, even if it is disappointing. However, the failure to publish such studies risks waste of further resources, and duplication of the patient hazard, needed for an independent study group to discover later the same negative result. Chalmers (1990), somewhat hyperbolically, has actually characterized under-reporting of clinical trials data as 'scientific misconduct'.

If this under-reporting is suboptimal, then those who publish clinical trials must take their share of the blame. Incongruously, it is the same journal editors who have traditionally been least likely to publish negative data that are making the most noise about how unsatisfactory is the performance of the pharmaceutical industry in failing to publish it (e.g. Horton and Smith 1999; Tonks 1999). This author cannot agree with Dickersin et al (1992), who wrote: 'Contrary to popular opinion, publication bias originates primarily with investigators, not journal editors...', because the busy pharmaceutical physician is unlikely to spend the time writing a paper that he/she knows has little chance of publication.

The establishment of clinical trials registries may be one way to overcome the bias against reporting of negative clinical trials. This is not a new idea (e.g. Simes 1986) and several worthwhile attempts have been made to accomplish this. The National Health Service in the UK (Peckham 1991), an amnesty for the publication of clinical trials offered by some journals (Roberts 1998), and specialized databases (especially in the areas of malignant disease and AIDS) have been partial responses to the many pleas for registration of clinical trials. Two large pharmaceutical companies have taken an initiative to register their own clinical trials (e.g. Sykes 1998), but have been ungratefully criticized for both doing too much and doing too little: some think that the registered information is insufficient, while others believe that this creates a commercial disadvantage (Horton and Smith 1999).

A further bias in clinical trials publishing is the selective reporting of subsets of secondary endpoints. This is usually associated with active-comparator trials having a primary objective of demonstrating the superiority of one treatment over the other. All too often the primary objective of the trial is not achieved: the authors then selectively publish a few of the many secondary end-points that did support their hypothesis. The 'if you have 100 end-points and $\alpha = 0.05$, then, at random, five end-points will be statistically significant' principle supervenes; fallacious treatment differences are claimed after reporting only those five end-points. Solutions to this problem could include an independently-prepared summary of the protocol, with its prospective objectives and complete list of end-points, perhaps in mini-type, at the end of such papers, as well as sensitization of reviewers to this potential problem. Journal editors sometimes approach this ideal by asking for protocols to accompany the submitted manuscripts; some companies view their protocols as confidential, and one wonders whether this is one of the reasons why.

Thus, there are multiple ways in which publication bias may be created by study sponsors, publicists, medical writers, and those who control journal content. Clinical trial registries still do not exist in any comprehensive fashion. Those constructing meta-analyses from published studies should beware.

THE CLASSIC COMPONENTS OF A CLINICAL TRIAL REPORT IN A PEER-REVIEWED JOURNAL

The publication of clinical trials in peer-reviewed journals normally follows the same format as for any other paper: title, authors, sponsorship, abstract, introduction, methods, results, discussion, concluding paragraph, acknowledgments, references, tables, and figure legends, with each figure attached on a separate sheet labeled on the reverse. The overall philosophy is also the same as for any other paper, namely that there should be enough information for the study to be replicated in independent hands, should the need arise. It is beyond the scope of this chapter to teach how to write a scientific paper: there are many other themselves to manuals, and journals that devote enough space for this purpose (succinct examples include Skelton 1994; Bonk 1997; Fromter et al 1999).

All journals publish guidelines describing the formats for the often diverse types of article that

will be considered. The corollary is that the writer should identify the target journal before putting pen to paper, and judge whether the quantity of material supports a whole paper, a brief report, or even more than one paper.

Authorship on papers is a matter of substantial debate. Under some circumstances, literally dozens of co-authors will clamour to be listed, and this phenomenon is not restricted to the publication of huge multicenter clinical trials. Clinical trials are a specific case of this general, perennial problem, to which Rafal (1991) has provided a somewhat humourous guide. There are two solutions.

The first solution is the prospective promulgation of a set of criteria that every author must meet. Many journals publish their own specific guidelines or criteria, and these do not differ greatly in qualitative terms. In the practicality of publishing clinical trials, the following would be typical:

1. The principal investigator(s) is(are) authors, unless so numerous as to require a team designation (see below).
2. The statistician(s) who personally accept(s) responsibility for the statistical analysis in the corresponding document(s) that is/are submitted to regulatory authorities should sign off on the paper and be named as author(s).
3. Key members of the clinical team within the pharmaceutical company may (but not necessarily need to) be authors.
4. All named authors should be able to personally defend the paper after publication, and be familiar with (but not necessarily have personally performed) all the methods employed in the clinical trial.
5. There should be no circumstances where 'guest authorship' or 'gratitude authorship' is awarded; all authors' participation must have been essential to the conduct and success of the clinical trial.
6. All authors should be prepared to disclose all conflicts of interest and the sources of financial support for the clinical trial.

The second solution is to publish the paper under the name of the team that conducted the trial, rather than the personal names of the participants. The acknowledgments can then list all those who took part (e.g. the Subcutaneous Sumatriptan

International Study Group, 1991). A hybrid variant is also sometimes used, where a one (or a few) lead author(s) are named and stated to represent the rest of the team (e.g. Cady et al, 1991). The advantages of this tactic are that there is at least one person who accepts responsibility for defense of the paper after publication. A further advantage is that this can be used to motivate investigators in multisite studies: the protocol can state that the investigator who recruits the most completed patients, without violations, will be the named first author in any publication.

ISOLATED ABSTRACTS AND POSTERS

An argument can be made that the isolated abstract format is not a good vehicle for the publication of clinical trials. Indeed, the inclusion and exclusion criteria in most clinical protocols alone exceed the word limit of most isolated abstracts. Too often, the publication of an abstract or poster is a criterion used by companies to justify the time and expense of sending staff to a conference: authors then generate and submit unimportant abstracts, principally for use as tickets to venues that attract them for ulterior reasons.

There are a few exceptions to this generalization, however. Legitimate retrospective analysis of the database of a clinical trial that has been previously published in full sometimes can make a isolated abstract, provided the full reference is provided, and an educated audience at, say, an academic conference, will be aware of the potential biases of this technique. Similarly, the open-label tolerability extension to a previously published controlled trial might be usefully published as a poster. But these are minor exceptions to the general principle that, in order to assess the validity of a clinical trials report, far more detail is needed than can be published in the small spaces of isolated abstracts and posters.

AUDIOVISUAL PRESENTATIONS AT ACADEMIC MEETINGS

It is an amazing thing that apparently intelligent people regularly attempt to speak to their peers at academic meetings with: (a) disorganized speech (due to disordered thought processes and/or acute episodic dysarthria); and (b) an inability to control a slide projector. This ineptitude is displayed by all medical specialties (including pharmaceutical physicians and clinical trialists), by most other non-medical professions, and shows no sign of declining with time. Some hosts make the talk more challenging by impishly providing slide projectors with various diseases (Fox 2000). One's amazement is all the greater because these incompetent speakers must often have heard equally bad productions, and slide projector controls are simpler than an hotel alarm clock. Again, there are textbooks and courses that teach public speaking, and teaching this art is beyond the scope of this chapter, except for specifics that apply to presenting the results of a clinical trial.

The most important time when making oral publications is before you even begin the talk. You should have the following three things *sine qua non*:

1. An understanding of the audience and the vocabulary needed to communicate with them (the general public, a patient advocacy group, an academic society, and an in-house department seminar all require very different approaches).
2. A slide set that is cogent, organized and familiar.
3. A look at the venue and the various pieces of equipment that will be at your disposal; think about how to match your speaking volume to the open air or to the microphone (if any), and where to stand so that you can see your slides without having your back to the audience.

For the actual talk itself, one useful checklist is as follows:

1. What is the take-home message, in one simple sentence of the language of the conference? (e.g. 'Drug X was superior to placebo in treating disease Y, in a patient population with characteristics A, B, and C, i.e. like the known epidemiology of the disease').
2. State the purpose of the talk at the beginning: usually this will be to explain how one will defend the take-home message ('this talk is to describe the clinical trial that has led us to

conclude that drug X is effective for disease Y in a patient population that is representative of the known epidemiology of this disease').

3. Organize one's slides in a manner that would be used sequentially to illustrate a written paper in a peer-reviewed journal (see above).

4. Make sure that all slides are legible (e.g. a minimum of bold 24-point text for a Microsoft®, Powerpoint® presentation).

5. Avoid tables of data in slides; if you can't graph it, then it is probably not worth showing at all.

6. Make the text of each slide concise (e.g. maximum of 30 words/slide).

7. Create slides to be self-supporting: if you gave your set of slides to someone equipped with a projector, could they, without any further explanation, more or less work out your subject and principal conclusions?

8. Plan to use about one slide per minute of time allotted.

9. Number your slides with bright labels on the plastic holder (so that you can see or feel the bright label in near-darkness). Use a consistent location for your label, and then use that label to orientate the slide when loading the carousel. Usually, but not always, this is 'right way round, wrong way up'. Practice showing one slide before wrongly loading all of them.

10. Relate the middle part of your talk to your take-home message (e.g. if disease Y is type I diabetes, then, 'As shown in this slide, the patient population included 30% adolescents because this group represents a relevant fraction of the whole population with type I diabetes').

11. At the end, repeat the scientific conclusions, briefly review the data that you have presented in their support, and then interpret these conclusions, once again, into your take-home message.

Most people are in an altered psychological state shortly after giving a talk, whether or not it seemed to go well. In this psychological state, they gladly accept thanks and congratulations, but are incapable of hearing constructive feedback. Feedback is essential to either improve the talk the next time round, or to improve one's presentation skills in general. Seek out this learning opportunity from friends, and tell them in advance that you will be asking for this feedback, probably a few days after the event.

NEWER FORMS OF CLINICAL TRIALS PUBLICATION

Electronic publishing is relatively new and is not yet in any standardized form. It is important to understand, however, the main classes of electronic publication, before taking the big step of committing your clinical trial report to it. Only then can the central question be answered for that clinical trial: would electronic publication make these data more easily available to the audience that can best use them (Geddes 1999)?

The CD-ROM vs. the textbook is probably the most primordial form of the digital vs. analogue debate. This battle has probably now been fought to a standstill, with winners and losers on both sides. Example replacements include the approximately two dozen annual volumes of *Index Medicus*, or both 37 annual volumes of *Headache* and 17 annual volumes of *Cephalalgia*, by single CD-ROM disks. This replacement saves trees, speeds search times, and has lower production and shipping expenses, but requires readers to have access to a computer at the same place as the disk. Clinical trial databases can be usefully placed on CD-ROM, and this can facilitate explorations beyond the prospective trial objectives. Epidemiological studies, where huge numbers of patients are often studied, may be especially suited to this form of publication.

Many traditional journals have sprouted electronic limbs. The most common form at present is probably the distribution of electronic facsimiles of printed papers, usually in .pdf format, which can be read using Adobe® Acrobat® software that can be downloaded without charge. Access to these facsimiles is usually restricted to those who also have a subscription to the paper version of the journal, and thus represents a duplication of, or extension to, paper publication, rather than its replacement. In some cases, journals publish electronically a wider selection of submitted papers than can be accommodated in their paper versions, or restrict new electronic material to correspondence that does not appear in print (Chalmers 1999; Delamothe and Smith 1999; McConnell and Horton 1999).

Song et al (1999) have suggested that electronic journals can reduce publication bias (see above), principally by accommodating and providing access to greater quantities of published information. Chalmers (1999 and see above) is an enthusiast, so presumably this is correct. Chalmers and Altman (1999) have even proposed that not only will publication bias be reduced, but also the intrinsic quality of clinical trials themselves could be improved as a result of electronic publication; this is unproven at present. However, this enlarged volume of publications also mandates a different peer-review system, or even no peer-review at all. It is possible that electronic publications may come to be suspected as both providing higher quantities of information but possibly with lower quality than more orthodox publications.

PRESS RELEASES

Pharmaceutical physicians in large pharmaceutical companies will only very rarely be exposed to the need for press releases concerning their clinical trials. In contrast, the small entrepreneurial pharmaceutical company may live or die on the outcome of a single clinical trial. The rapid dissemination of the results of such a clinical trial to the appropriate audience (shareholders and investment community) is legally required when material to the prospects of a small, public company. The press release then becomes an important tool for publishing clinical trial results.

When writing press releases, absolutely no technical knowledge can be assumed on the part of the recipient. Often their questions parse simply to 'Did the drug work or not'? Extended detailed explanations can actually create the false impression that the drug did not work, when in fact the trial outcome was quite satisfactory for product registration purposes. Equally, when clinical trials fail, ingenious but scientifically meaningless explanations by corporate officers can create the false impression that the outcome was better than it was. A good example is the often-used: 'We still have confidence in our ability to register Drug X; Drug X performed as we expected, but it was just

that the placebo response rate in this [pivotal] study was unexpectedly high'.

Pharmaceutical physicians may often want to avoid involvement in the drafting of press releases altogether. However, this creates a liability that one's independent comments may not then dovetail with the company's press releases, causing harm not only to the company but also to one's longevity within it!

The best advice on press releases may be twofold. First, avoid scientific nuance and technical detail. State clearly whether or not the primary objective of the clinical trial was met. Whichever was the case, then state clearly the implications of these data to the clinical development plan: if it needs redirection, then state what that redirection is, and the implication for the registration timeline.

COPYRIGHT

Copyright exists to prevent the exploitation of a publication (or trademark) by anyone other than the publisher. This protection of the right to exploit a publication is central to the promotion of publishing *per se*, and thus an incentive to disseminate free speech.

In most developed countries, copyright can exist in two forms. First, for a fee, the protected publication can be registered with the national office of copyright. Second, the copyright holder can simply assert in the publication ownership of copyright under the Common Law. Both forms may use the familiar © symbol. The registered copyright is easier to enforce in court because the date of registration and priority of first publisher are on independent record and can be compared to the behavior of the alleged infringer. The Common Law alternative can also be legally enforced, but requires the development of a set of evidence; an infringer usually has at least an initial defence that due search of the national register failed to locate the alleged infringed copyright.

It is a peculiar and remarkable aspect of academic journals that their publishers make a profit while receiving almost all their copy entirely for free. Almost all journals require transfer of copyright from authors to publisher upon acceptance of submitted manuscripts. Technically, this requires that an author needs specific permission from the publisher to use his own manuscript later; in practice, this permission is routinely granted upon written application. A few journals now seek only exclusive licenses from authors, one condition of which preserves the author's right to personally use his/her own work, and which leaves copyright ownership with the author(s); the license can also become void if the publisher fails to exploit it, and can yield royalties to the authors. In practice, this license removes the administrative burden of granting routine permissions by the publisher, and royalties on journal reprints are either nominal or absent.

Reprints disseminated for medical information or marketing purposes should be those purchased from the publisher. Alternatively, photocopying license fees can be paid, and in the USA a national clearing house exists for this purpose.

Copyright for publications is not universal. In the USA, manuscripts from federal employees cannot be claimed as proprietary; most journals operate a copyright exemption system for this purpose. In many Third World countries, copyright, if it exists at all, is unenforceable.

Every website page can potentially be copyrighted. Few are actually registered, although assertion of Common Law copyright is common. So far, there has been insufficient litigation to delimit the copyright aspects of electronic publishing.

SUMMARY AND PROSPECTUS

In summary, the construction of a clinical trial report for use in the peer-reviewed literature is much like that for any other scientific paper; it must contain most of the things that would appear in the executive summary of a clinical report used for regulatory purposes. Clues for effective oral presentations are also provided. Systems for publication of clinical trials are currently neither comprehensive nor universally available to the relevant target audiences. Pharmaceutical companies and journal editors both introduce publication bias; the former are likely only to expend resources in reporting, and the latter are likely only to publish, clinical trials with positive outcomes. Registration of clinical trials was suggested more than 15 years ago, as one method for avoiding the bias against

publication of negative trials. Some pharmaceutical companies are beginning to provide such registries for their own work, but no internationally coordinated or funded agency has yet emerged, except in specialized areas with relatively small academic audiences. It is possible that electronic publication can improve this situation, but, at present, there is more optimism than proof that this is the case.

REFERENCES

Bonk RJ (1997) *Medical Writing in Drug Development*. Pharmaceutical Products Press/Haworth Press: Binghamton, NY; 77–81.

Cady RK, Wendt JK, Kirchner JR et al (1991) Treatment of acute migraine with subcutaneous sumatriptan. *JAM Med Assoc* 265: 2831–5 (see especially the footnote to the first column on p. 2831, and the acknowledgments).

Chalmers I (1990) Underreporting research is scientific misconduct. *JAM Med Assoc* 338: 367–71.

Chalmers I (1999) A symbiosis of paper and electronic publishing, serving the interests of the journal's readers. *Br J Psychiat* 175: 1–2.

Chalmers I, Altman DG (1999) How can medical journals help prevent poor medical research? Some opportunities presented by electronic publishing. *Lancet* 1999; 353: 490–493.

Delamothe T, Smith R (1999) The joy of being electronic. The BMJ's website is mushrooming. *Br Med J* 319: 465–466.

Dickersin K, Min YL, Meinert CL (1992) Factors influencing publication of research results: follow-up of applications submitted to two institutional review boards. *J Am Med Assoc* 267: 374–8.

Fox AW (2000) The morbid anatomy and pathophysiology of the slide projector (forthcoming).

Fromter E, Brahler E, Langenbeck U et al (1999) Das AWMF-Modell zur Evaluierung publizierter Forschungsbeitrage in der Medizin. *Dtsch Med Wochenschr* 124: 910–15.

Geddes JR (1999) The contribution of information technology to improving clinicians' access to high quality evidence. *Int J Psychiatr Med* 29: 287–92.

Gray BS (1994) Health communicators as agents for social change. *Am Med Writers Assoc J* 9: 11–14.

Horton R, Smith R (1999) Time to register randomised trials. *Br J Med* 319: 865–6.

McConnell J, Horton R (1999) Lancet electronic research archive in international health and eprint server. *Lancet* 354: 2–3.

Peckham M (1991) Research and development for the National Health Service. *Lancet* 338: 367–71.

Rafal RB (1991) A standardized method for determination of who should be listed as authors on scholarly papers. *Chest* 99: 786.

Roberts I (1998) An amnesty for unpublished trials. *Br Med J* 317: 763–4.

Simes RJ (1986) Publication bias: the case for an international registry of clinical trials. *J Clin Oncol* 4: 1529–41.

Skelton J (1994) Analysis of the structure of original research papers: an aid to writing original papers for publication. *Br J Gen Pract* 44: 455–9.

Song F, Eastwood A, Gilbody S, Duley L (1999) The role of electronic journals in reducing publication bias. *Med Inform Internet Med* 24: 223–9.

Sykes R (1998) Being a modern pharmaceutical company. *Br Med J* 317: 1172–80.

The Subcutaneous Sumatriptan International Study Group (1991) Treatment of migraine attacks with sumatriptan. *New Eng J Med* 325: 316–21.

Tonks A (1999) Registering clinical trials. *Br Med J* 319: 1565–8.

Section VII

Legal and Ethical Aspects

Introduction to Section VII

Sara Croft[1] and Timothy Pratt[2]

[1]Shook, Hardy and Bacon MNP, London, UK and [2]Shook, Hardy and Bacon LLP, Kansas City, Missouri, US

BASIC LEGAL PRINCIPLES

A range of laws and regulations affect pharmaceutical physicians in different aspects of their working lives. We discuss here how these principles may apply to the pharmaceutical physician in practice, introducing themes that will be developed in more detail in subsequent chapters.

CRIMINAL AND CIVIL LAW DISTINGUISHED

Law is broken down generally into two separate components—criminal law and civil law. A crime is an offence or wrongdoing against the State and punishable by the State. Civil law concerns the breach of a private right or duty. Thus, in contrast to criminal cases, most civil actions are not brought by the State, but by private individuals or other legal entities, such as corporations. In some instances, an individual's actions can give rise to both a criminal offence and a civil liability, e.g., an assault can result in a prosecution by the State and a claim by the victim for damages for personal injury.

Another important distinction between criminal and civil cases is the threshold 'burden of proof' that must be reached in order to prove the case against the defendant. In a criminal case, the State must prove its case 'beyond a reasonable doubt'. In civil actions the plaintiff must prove his/her case 'on a balance of probabilities'. The standard of proof for criminal matters is higher, essentially because an individual's life or liberty may be at risk.

CRIMINAL LAW

Fortunately, instances where pharmaceutical physicians face criminal prosecution are rare. However, there are a number of specific ways in which the criminal law can affect pharmaceutical companies and their physicians. One significant area is in the regulatory context, which may vary from country to country. For example, in the UK, the Medicines Act 1968 creates some statutory offences, such as providing false information when applying to licence a product. In the USA, the Food Drug and Cosmetics Act[1] (FD&CA) also creates statutory offences for certain actions or inactions. For example, it is impermissible to sell a misbranded drug or device, or one with labeling that is false, misleading or fails to bear adequate directions for use. Additionally, one may not introduce an adulterated product, such as one that has been modified from its intended use[2]. The US Supreme Court has observed that an offence is committed 'by all who do have such a responsible share in the furtherance of the transaction which the statute outlaws'[3]. Another area where potential criminal liability may occasionally emerge is fraud or forgery during the course of a clinical trial. Pharmaceutical physicians designing and monitoring clinical trials should build in various safeguards to protect against this possibility.

CIVIL LAW

The two main areas of civil law that may affect the pharmaceutical physician are the law of contract and the law of tort. Essentially, a contract is a legally binding agreement between individuals (or other legal entities such as corporations), where one of the parties assumes an obligation or makes a promise to, the other. Usually, the parties to the contract owe obligations and gain rights under the agreement. The law of contract regulates the enforceability of such agreements and the steps that can be taken if the contract is broken. Perhaps the most fundamental feature of contractual liability is that it is strict and not fault-based[4]. This means, broadly speaking, that it does not matter whether a party to the contract acted reasonably or not; what matters is whether the contract has been broken.

The pharmaceutical physician will be very familiar with certain types of contracts, depending on his/her role within the company. Examples include agreements with contract research organizations, contracts for the sale of the finished pharmaceutical product, and licensing or distribution agreements.

Generally, there is no contract between the pharmaceutical company and the patient who is prescribed the product by a doctor. In the UK, it has been held that where a product is prescribed under a National Health Service scheme, it is not prescribed as a result of a contract between pharmaceutical company and patient because legislation exists that requires a pharmacist to supply the product on the production of a valid prescription[5]. For non-prescription, 'over-the-counter' (OTC) products, there is a contract between the retailer and the consumer who purchases the pharmaceutical product, but there is still usually no direct link in contractural terms to the maker of the product. However, it may be that the contract between the manufacturer and the retailer contains an indemnity provision. The indemnity may provide that, in the event of a successful claim for breach of contract being made against the retailer by the customer, the manufacturer will pay the retailer the amount the retailer is ordered to pay in compensation to the customer.

In the USA, as in the UK, a contractual right of action generally exists only between parties to the contract. This is known as the rule of privity. Courts in the USA have recognized, however, that in a mass-consumption society, there is little real privity between manufacturers and consumers. Manufacturers are remote to the ultimate consumer, sales are accomplished through intermediaries, and products are marketed through the use of advertising media. Therefore, some courts have carved out an exception to the privity rule for contract claims, such as breach of warranty. Accordingly, some courts have recognized that consumers may bring breach of express warranty claims against pharmaceutical companies, based on statements made in the package insert as well as promotional literature and advertisements[6].

For the individual pharmaceutical physician, arguably the most important contract will be his/her own contract of employment with the company. This is likely to contain terms which, if broken by the individual, could give rise to a claim being made against him/her and, of course, *vice versa*. The contract of employment may cover matters such as confidentiality and restrictive covenants, as well as defining the individual's role and responsibilities within the company.

Distinct from the law of contract, the law of tort serves to regulate standards of behaviour, operating to deter conduct that may cause injury or damage and to remedy the consequences of such actions[7]. This area of law includes the tort of negligence. An important case in the development of the tort of negligence in the UK is the case of Donoghue v Stevenson, which involved a woman, Mrs Donoghue, who was unfortunate enough to drink from a bottle of ginger beer containing the remains of a snail[8]. There was no contract between Mrs. Donoghue and the manufacturer of the ginger beer, so she could not claim a breach of contract. However, the court held that the company actually had a *duty of care* to the ultimate consumer of its product to take reasonable care in the manufacture of its product[9].

The main elements of negligence have been distilled from this statement in various cases over time. In order for a person (the 'plaintiff') to prove negligence by another (the 'defendant'), he/she must show:

1. That the defendant owes the plaintiff a *duty of care*; and
2. The defendant has *breached* the duty of care; and
3. The breach of duty actually *caused* damage that the plaintiff alleges he suffered[10].

In order to succeed in a claim of negligence, a plaintiff must prove *all three* elements. It is not enough to show that the defendant had a duty of care and was in breach of it. It must also be shown that the breach caused the plaintiff's alleged injury, often the most difficult task for a plaintiff, especially in claims concerning pharmaceutical products, where there may be other possible causes of the plaintiff's condition.

In the law of tort, including negligence, liability is fault-based. It must be proved that the defendant was at fault in that he/she acted wrongfully and as a result violated a right of the plaintiff, causing harm to him/her. The requirement of fault differentiates a genuine accident from a negligent act for which the injured person can be compensated.

To complicate matters, however, in some countries, liability may also arise in tort *without* proof of fault. This is known as *strict liability*. An important example of strict liability for pharmaceutical companies is what is commonly referred to as the 'European Products Liability Directive', which introduced a European-wide scheme of strict liability for defective products[11]. The Directive has to be implemented in each European country through national legislation and, as a result, the law in each country may differ. Since liability is strict, the defences that are in the Directive and in national legislation are most important. The UK legislation, for example, includes a 'development risk defence'[12]. This essentially means that, if the state of scientific knowledge was such that the producer could not have discovered the defect, this will provide a defence to the claim. However, the individual doctor or pharmaceutical physician does not fall within the definition of a 'producer', although the pharmaceutical company usually will. Therefore, the individual pharmaceutical physician is unlikely to have proceedings brought against him or her personally.

The USA has also adopted a theory of strict liability. This theory imposes liability on the seller of a product that is unreasonably dangerous because of a defect in its design, manufacture, or warnings. There are special provisions carved out for pharmaceutical products because of their value to society and the fact they are 'unavoidably unsafe'. Such products need to be accompanied by an adequate warning. Under this theory, a pharmaceutical company is unquestionably subject to strict liability as a 'seller' of a pharmaceutical product. A pharmaceutical physician, however, is generally not.

THE LEGAL FRAMEWORK FOR REGULATING PHARMACEUTICAL PRODUCTS

As any pharmaceutical physician is well aware, the development, manufacture, marketing and safety of pharmaceutical products are subject to close governmental control in most countries. The government exercises control through specific regulations on the sale of medicines and medical devices. Pharmaceutical physicians play a key role in ensuring that, at each stage in the life of a pharmaceutical product, the regulatory requirements have been met. As discussed above, there may be criminal implications for the applicant for a licence if certain of the requirements are not fulfilled. Also, in a negligence action against the pharmaceutical company, the failure by the company or one or more individual employees to comply with the regulations may be relevant to the question of whether or not a company had acted reasonably. In the USA, some courts have held that a company failing to comply with government regulations may be presumed to be negligent.

In the UK, regulation is derived from the Medicines Act of 1968, which provides a comprehensive system of licensing affecting most aspects of the sale of medicinal products. It also contains provisions on related matters, such as pharmacovigilance and the requirements for the reporting of adverse events. The Medicines Act encompasses measures contained in European Community Directives, including the first on the control of medicines, introduced in 1965[13]. The Medicines Act led to the creation of various regulatory bodies to carry out the functions outlined in it, including: (a) The Licensing Authority, which decides whether licences for medical products should be granted; (b) The Medicines Commission and the Committee on the Safety of Medicines, which are examples of independent bodies set up under the Act to advise the Licensing Authority; and (c) The Medicines Control Agency, which is the government agency that regulates the pharmaceutical sector in the UK

The European Community, through a series of Directives, has introduced measures to try to harmonize the regulation of medicines throughout Europe[14]. These directives established the Committee for Proprietary Medicinal Products (CPMP), as well as mechanisms to 'harmonize' procedures for licensing products within Europe. A new body, the European Medicines Evaluation Agency (EMEA), was established in February 1995, and further procedures were established for the regulatory harmonization of pharmaceutical products throughout Europe[15]. They are:

- The 'centralized procedure', which involves one application made to the EMEA. This has been mandatory for biotechnology products since January 1995 and for other products since January 1998.
- The 'mutual recognition' procedure (or the 'decentralized procedure'), which is in essence a national registration recognized by the other Member States.

The UK Medicines Act (1968) places responsibility on the applicant for a licence, which in most cases is a company, not on an individual within the company. The legal responsibility is thus that of the company to comply with the various regulations under the Act. Under certain circumstances, the regulatory authority (i.e. the government), may be sued if it was allegedly somehow at fault in granting or failing to withdraw a licence for the product that supposedly caused harm[16].

In 2001, all European Community Directives adopted between 1965 and 1999 on the regulation of medicines have been consolidated into a 'Community Code'[18]. The codification did not change the content of the legislation. The Code was finalized too late to incorporate the Clinical Trials Directive (2001/2002) which is to be implemented in 2003. The European Commission has also published proposals to change European pharmaceutical legislation including the regulatory framework set out above. Before taking effect any such changes will have to be adopted by the Commission and then implemented by the European Member States.

In the USA, pharmaceutical products are the most federally regulated of all consumer products. The Food and Drug Administration (FDA) is the primary regulatory agency and the FD&CA[17] is the principal statute governing pharmaceutical products. Regulations relating to pharmaceutical products address the safety and efficacy of pharmaceuticals and range from initial testing of a drug to postmarketing surveillance.

Government oversight for drugs begins with (potentially) audit of GCP and GMP facilities prior to the manufacturer filing an investigational new drug (IND) application. The IND application includes, among other things, a detailed analysis of the drug's chemical properties, a summary of preclinical tests showing the safety and effectiveness in humans, and detailed protocols for proposed clinical investigators.

The preclinical tests reported in the IND generally include both animal and *in vitro* tests. Once safety and efficacy information is developed for a drug through preclinical laboratory and animal studies, as reported in the IND, the next step in the drug approval process is clinical testing, which may not be conducted without FDA approval.

After a manufacturer submits an IND application, there is a 30 day time period in which the FDA evaluates the submission. If the FDA does not act on the IND within the 30 day period, the manufacturer may begin clinical testing. If, however, the FDA finds that the IND contains insufficient evidence or the proposed clinical protocols do not protect research subjects, it may place a 'clinical hold' on the IND. A manufacturer cannot go forward with clinical research within the United States until it corrects the deficiencies identified by the FDA.

Once the manufacturer completes the IND clinical trials, it submits a New Drug Application (NDA). Although a significant portion of the information contained in an NDA is similar to that required in an IND application, the scope of an NDA is broader and includes greater and more detailed technical data. In theory, the FDA has 180 days in which to approve or disapprove the NDA. But typically, the FDA requests additional information, thereby extending the approval period beyond 180 days.

After the FDA determines that the NDA is 'approvable', but not yet 'approved', it will ask the manufacturer to submit labeling and planned marketing materials. Labeling, which contains information for the physician who prescribes the drug, must comply with the FDA's specific labeling requirements (see Chapter 31). The FDA's regulation over 'labeling' includes all written materials attached to or accompanying the product or container, as well as journal, television and radio advertising.

When product labeling is adequate and not misleading, the FDA will formally approve the NDA. Theoretically, the FDA issues a Summary Basis of Approval detailing the safety and effectiveness data the FDA reviewed in approving the drug, but in practice these are written by NDA sponsors for FDA review, amendment, and approval. After FDA approval, a manufacturer may sell and market the drug in accordance with the approved uses contained in the drug labeling.

Federal regulation of a drug does not end with NDA approval. The FDA requires drug manufacturers to engage in postmarket surveillance of approved drugs. A manufacturer must report to the FDA and further investigate any adverse drug experiences in accordance with FDA regulations.

THE PHARMACEUTICAL INDUSTRY'S VOLUNTARY CODES

In addition to the provisions of the UK Medicines Act (1962) and European Directives, and other similar mandates, the pharmaceutical industry also carries out a measure of self-regulation through its own industry bodies. For example, in the UK, the Association of British Pharmaceutical Industries (ABPI) operates codes of practice concerning, for example, the promotion of prescription only and OTC products.

Voluntary codes are not legally enforceable in the same way as a statute. However, such codes are an important part of the overall picture, as they play a part in setting the standards of behavior for the pharmaceutical company and may be used as evidence in civil cases. The ABPI code of practice on promotion of prescription medicine ('the Code') is operated by the Prescription Medicines Code of Practice Authority (PMCPA), which was established by the ABPI as an independent authority. It is a condition of membership of the ABPI that the pharmaceutical companies abide by the Code. In addition, the Code contains a number of sanctions that may be imposed against member companies. Complaints are made to the PMCPA, and if it is decided that there has been a breach of the Code, the company concerned has 10 working days to provide a written undertaking to discontinue the promotional activity in question, with an 'adminis-

trative charge' levied. The amount depends on the breach. There are also other sanctions available to the PMCPA, such as reporting to the Board of the ABPI, which has the authority to remove the company from membership or publish the complaint report in a quarterly bulletin.

Some provisions of the Code are of particular importance to pharmaceutical physicians, e.g., Clause 14 requires that promotional material be certified by two persons in the company, one of whom must be a doctor. The other must be a pharmacist, or another person 'appropriately qualified'; or a senior official in the company or an appropriately qualified person whose services are retained for that purpose. The promotion must be certified to be in accordance with the Code, including the relevant advertising requirements. It must also be consistent with the marketing authorization and summary of product characteristics and be a fair and truthful representation of the facts about the medicine.

INDIVIDUAL OR CORPORATE RESPONSIBILITY?

As noted above, the circumstances in which a pharmaceutical physician will personally be sued under the civil law are relatively rare. It is much more likely that the company will be a defendant to an action by an individual patient or by another company, whether in tort or in contract. The deeper pockets of the company, in comparsion to the individual pharmaceutical physician, practically guarantee that this is also the case in the USA. It is more likely that criminal sanctions could be applied to the individual. As discussed above, the UK Medicines Act (1968) makes it an offence for an applicant (i.e., the company) to give false information in connection with an application for a licence for a pharmaceutical product. However, the Act also provides that where a company commits the offence under the Act, but it can also be shown that it was committed with the consent and connivance of, or attributable to the neglect of any director, manager, or similar officer of the company, those individuals may also be personally liable. This may obviously affect the pharmaceutical physician, who is a director or equivalent in the company, on the signatory to advertising materials.

It is sometimes the case that the company *and* the pharmaceutical physician are sued for negligence, where the allegations include specific acts for which the pharmaceutical physician is responsible, such as the warnings in a data sheet.

CONCLUSION

Caution and compliance are the bywords for pharmaceutical physicians. One must be knowledgeable about the many laws and regulations that directly affect pharmaceutical manufacturers and their employees. Sanctions for failing to comply with these requirements may be severe, both for the pharmaceutical manufacturer and for its physicians. The following chapters will more specifically address the rights and responsibilities of pharmaceutical physicians.

NOTES AND REFERENCES

1 21 USC § § 301–393.
2 21 USC § § 501(f), 331, 351(f), 352(a) and 352(f).
3 United States v. Dotterweich, 320 US 277 (1943).
4 Someone is liable if the court finds the law has been broken.
5 Pfizer Corporation v. Ministry of Health (1965) 1All ER 450, HL.
6 See Overstreet v. Norden Labs., Inc., 669 F.2d 1286, 1289–90 (6th Cir. 1982); Morris v. Parke Davis & Co., 667 F. Supp. 1332, 1347–48 (CD Cal. 1987); Tinnerholm v. Parke Davis & Co., 285 F. Suppl. 432, 442–43 (SDNY 1968).
7 See generally Clerk JF, Brazier M, Lindsell WH, Brazier M (Eds) *Clerk & Lindsell on Torts*. London: Sweet & Maxwell 17th Edn., 1998 with supplements. Chapter 1 pages 1–38. The French word for 'tort' literally means 'wrong'.
8 Donoghue v. Stevenson (1932) A.C. 562.
9 '...a manufacturer of products which he sells in such a form as to show that he intends them to reach the ultimate consumer in the form in which they have left him with no possibility of intermediate examination and with the knowledge that the absence of reasonable care in the preparation or putting up of the products will result in an injury to the consumer's life or property, owes a duty to the consumer to take that reasonable care' (*per Lord Atkin at p. 599*).
10 This is a simplification of a complex area of the law for the purposes of this introduction. These themes are explained more fully in subsequent chapters.
11 European Community Directive 85/374.
12 The Consumer Protection Act (1987).
13 European Community Directive 65/65/EEC Now codified into Community Code 2001/83/EC.
14 See, for example, European Community Directives 65/65/EEC, 75/391/EEC and 83/570/EEC See Community Code 2001/83/EC.
15 Council Regulation 2309/93.
16 For example, in the UK the government was a defendant in actions brought by hemophiliacs alleging contamination with the HIV virus through use of blood products.
17 21 USC § § 301–393.
18 Directive 2001/83/EC

36

Pharmaceutical Product Liability

Han W. Choi and Howard B. Yeon

Product liability has become one of the fastest-growing, and perhaps the most economically significant, applications of tort law. Pharmaceutical companies have been defendants in some of the most widely publicized and costly product liability lawsuits in the USA and Europe, prompting many companies to lobby vigorously for tort reform and prepare years in advance for the possibility of litigation (Nace et al, 1997). The liability burden of pharmaceutical companies has been described as extremely disproportionate to their sales when compared with other manufacturing industries (The Progress and Freedom Foundation 1996, p. 101). However, direct comparisons are difficult because the market for ethical pharmaceuticals is unlike ordinary markets, where consumers can be left to buy from competing producers on the basis of quality and price. Rather, in the case of ethical pharmaceuticals, a physician selects the drug and the consumer only pays a fraction of the price, while a third-party payer can pay for the majority of the drug's actual price (Mossialos et al, 1994). Nevertheless, and most disturbing of all is that these high-liability costs occur under a regulatory regime that is extremely stringent, especially compared with those in place for other consumer products. In the presence of such stringent regulatory criteria, one wonders why the pharmaceutical industry has been the object of such extensive litigation. This chapter will introduce the basic concepts of pharmaceutical product liability law, review the landmark cases and statutory provisions in the major markets, discuss the emerging trends among pharmaceutical companies and product liability lawyers in recent cases, and show how they might impact the industry as a whole in the future.

PRINCIPLES OF PRODUCT LIABILITY LAW

In general terms, 'product liability' refers to the liability of a seller of a product which, because of a defect, causes damage to its purchaser, user, or sometimes a bystander. The origins of product liability law can be traced to cases brought before British courts shortly after the onset of the Industrial Revolution in the first half of the nineteenth century. Since then, an ever-increasing volume of product liability cases have been brought before the courts in industrialized countries. In the USA alone, product liability lawsuits have increased from over 2000 cases in 1975, which marked the first crisis in the product liability insurance market, to over 13 000 cases in the late 1980s (Epstein, 1995). Although approximately 60% of this increase resulted from cases involving exposure to asbestos, a large fraction of the remainder have been brought against pharmaceutical companies.

Product liability law is broadly based upon legal principles involving contract law, the Law of Torts, and the relevant statutory provisions of the country or jurisdiction where the action is brought (Jones, 1993). However, in general terms, there are three legal principles under which a seller of a product can be liable for damage incurred from the use of that product: strict liability, warranty, and negligence.

Strict Liability

Strict liability is a principle of both tort law and contract law (i.e. purely under the civil law), which provides that a seller of a product is liable without fault for damage caused by that product if it is sold

Principles and Practice of Pharmaceutical Medicine. Edited by A. J. Fletcher, Lionel D. Edwards, Anthony W. Fox and Peter Stonier © 2002 John Wiley & Sons Ltd.

in a defective condition that is unreasonably dangerous to the user or consumer. Thus, strict liability would mean that pharmaceutical companies would have to pay damages in some cases, even when they had researched their drugs impeccably (Hunter, 1993). Strict product liability similarly applies not only to the product's manufacturer, but also to its retailer, as well as to any other party in the distributive chain. However, in the UK it should be noted that a product would not give rise to strict liability if it is found to be 'unavoidably unsafe'. This has direct relevance to pharmaceutical companies, in that most courts have agreed that a product will not give rise to strict liability if it is unavoidably unsafe, as described by labeled descriptions of adverse events, and its benefits can outweigh its dangers. Furthermore, most courts have also held that the existence of 'unreasonable danger' and 'defectiveness' should be based upon the state of scientific knowledge and technology at the time when the product is sold, and not on the date when the resulting product liability case comes to trial. The courts have taken a similar approach to 'failure to warn' claims: if the state of scientific knowledge and technology at the time of manufacture is such that the defect or danger is neither known nor knowable, not only is the manufacturer protected from ordinary strict liability, but the manufacturer is also relieved of his duty to warn of the unknowable danger.

These legal principles regarding strict liability have been codified in the UK and other European countries. In the UK, Parliament passed the Consumer Protection Act of 1987, partly to give effect to the EC Directive of 1985, which required harmonization of the law regarding product liability actions throughout the European Community. According to Section 2(2) of the Consumer Protection Act of 1987, liable parties may include the producer of the product, any party who holds him/herself out as the producer by putting his/her name, trademark, or other distinguishing mark on the product, or an importer of the product into a Member State from a place outside of the European Community in order to supply it to another in the course of his/her business. Section 3(2) of the Act further provides that, in determining liability, account will be taken of all the surrounding circumstances of the case, including the purposes for which the product has been marketed as well as its

warnings and instructions for its use. In overview, subject to certain defenses, the Act created a regime of strict liability, although existing common law rights have remained unaffected, so that if the Act does not apply to a particular case, a plaintiff may still have a cause of action under the principles of negligence (Heuston and Buckley, 1992).

Warranty

Warranty is also a principle of both tort law and contract law, that allows a purchaser of a product to bring a cause of action against the immediate seller of that product if he/she can demonstrate that the seller expressly or implicitly made representations or warranties about the quality of the product that were ultimately false or misleading, without the need to demonstrate negligence on the part of the seller. Thus, the seller may have reasonably and honestly believed that his/her representations or warranties were true, and could not possibly have discovered the defect in the product, and yet the plaintiff may nonetheless recover. Many countries, including the USA, have enacted statutes that apply to such warranties and resulting product liability actions. In the USA, the Uniform Commercial Code (UCC), which is in effect in every state except Louisiana, includes provisions regarding warranties and forms the legal basis for product liability actions brought under the principle of warranty. UCC § 2–313 provides that an express warranty may be produced by an 'affirmation of fact or promise' about a product by a description of that product or by the use of a sample or model. The existence of a warranty as to the quality of a product may also be inferred from the fact that the seller has offered the product for sale. The UCC also imposes several implied warranties as a matter of law. The most important of these is the warranty of merchantability under UCC § 2–314; the warranty that goods shall be merchantable is implied in a contract for their sale if the seller is a merchant with respect to goods of that kind. Similarly, a retailer who did not manufacture a product is nonetheless held to have impliedly warranted its merchantability by virtue of the fact that he has sold it, assuming he deals in goods of that kind. In addition, under UCC § 2–315, a seller of goods may also implicitly warrant that goods are 'fit for a particular purpose' if the seller knows that the purchaser wants the goods for a particular purpose and the purchaser relies on the seller's judgment to purchase the goods in question.

Negligence

Negligence is a principle of tort law that may be defined as the *breach of a duty of care* owed by one party, the defendant, to another party, the plaintiff, which results in damage to the plaintiff. The concept of a duty of care serves to define the interests protected by the tort of negligence, by determining whether the type of damage suffered by the plaintiff is actionable. The plaintiff must also demonstrate that there is a sufficiently proximate causal connection between the defendant's negligence and the damage incurred. The damage in question may arise through mis-feasance or non-feasance and may consist of personal injury or damage to property, which are categorized as pure economic loss under civil law. It should also be noted that manufacturers, but also retailers, bailers, and other suppliers may be liable to plaintiffs under the principles of negligence if they are found to have breached a duty of care.

TYPES OF PRODUCT DEFECTS

With regard to product liability claims, there are two fundamental types of product defects: manufacturing defects and design defects. Manufacturing defects involve a product where the particular item that causes damage to the plaintiff is different from other similar items manufactured by the defendant, and that the difference is attributable to the manufacturing process for the item in question (e.g. an intravenous a fluid mislabeled as 'sterile'). In contrast, design defects involve a product where all similar items manufactured by the defendant are the same, and they all bear a feature whose design is it defective and unreasonably dangerous. It should also be noted that most design defect claims could be categorized as involving either structural defects, absence of safety features, or suitability for unusual purposes. These design defect claims often involve allegations of negligence on the part of the defendant, even though they may be based upon

strict liability principles, in that the plaintiff often alleges that the manufacturer should have been aware of the safety attributes of his/her design and, in failing to do so, breached his/her duty of care.

LEGAL DEFENSES IN PRODUCT LIABILITY CASES

The defenses available to manufacturers in product liability actions vary, based upon the respective common law or statutory provisions of jurisdiction in which the action is filed. However, certain legal principles commonly constitute a full or partial defense to product liability actions.

Regulatory Compliance

The issue of regulatory compliance as a defense in product liability actions, especially those involving pharmaceutical companies, generally arises in connection with allegations of design or manufacturing defects or of failure to comply with federal labeling requirements. In the USA, the general rule is that, unless Congress intended to pre-empt the states from requiring stricter or different warnings, the defendant's compliance with regulatory requirements does not preclude liability (McCartney 1996). However, several states, such as New Jersey, have enacted statutes that allow regulatory compliance as a valid defense in pharmaceutical product liability actions (N.J Code § 2A: 58C-4). Similarly, in the UK, Section 4(1) of the Consumer Protection Act of 1987 provides a valid defense if the defect is attributable to compliance, either with a domestic enactment or with European Community law (Heuston and Buckley 1992).

Disclaimers

With regard to product liability actions brought under the principles of warranty, a defendant may assert a defense based upon a disclaimer from a warranty associated with the purchase or use of the product in question. For example, in the USA under UCC § 2–316(2), a seller of a product may make a written disclaimer of the warranty of merchantability if it is conspicuous. However, it should also be noted that the Magnuson–Moss Federal Trade Commission Improvement Act of 1974, 15 USC § 2301, et seq., provides that, if a written warranty is given to a consumer, there cannot be any disclaimer of any implied warranty.

Contributory Negligence

A defense of contributory negligence asserts that a plaintiff who is him/herself negligent in that he/she does not take reasonable care to protect him/herself from damage, and whose negligence contributes proximately to his/her injuries, is either entitled only to reduced recovery from his/her damages, or in some countries, including the USA and the UK under section 6(4) of the Consumer Protection Act of 1987, is totally barred from recovery (Heuston and Buckley 1992). In these cases, the plaintiff is held to the same standard of care as the defendant, which is that of a similar reasonable party under similar circumstances. Although a plaintiff's contributory negligence will, in most cases, be a defense in product liability actions brought under the principles of negligence, virtually all courts have agreed that in some actions brought under the principles of warranty or strict liability, contributory negligence may not be a viable defense. For example, if a plaintiff's contributory negligence lies in a failure to inspect the product, or a failure to become aware of the danger from that product, virtually all courts agree that this is not a defense. However, if the plaintiff learns of the risk and voluntarily assumes the risk in purchasing and using the product, contributory negligence may be a defense to strict liability. Similarly, if the plaintiff's contributory negligence consists of his/her abnormal use or misuse of the product in question, this may be a defense to strict liability, depending upon the degree of foreseeability of the abnormal use or misuse.

CONCLUSIONS

In overview, courts in various countries have interpreted pharmaceutical product liability law in various ways. The inconsistent court interpretations may be partially responsible for the increased

number of product liability lawsuits against prescription drug makers. However, most courts have allowed an exception to strict liability for products that are beneficial but unavoidably unsafe. However, these courts have adopted this exception on a case-by-case basis. Therefore, to avoid liability, prescription drug makers need to ensure that information is provided promptly to physicians when an adverse drug reaction is discovered with one of their products (DeConinck 1994).

INTERNATIONAL ISSUES

Pharmaceutical companies are facing increased litigation from overseas claimants because of the international differences in product liability laws that make then easier targets. Such differences include the absence of discovery mechanisms, jury trials, legal contingency fees, and the presence of 'informed' or 'learned' intermediary doctrines in many foreign jurisdictions. Lawsuits are also being filed in the USA because foreign parties are not able to get justice in their own country. This represents a marked reversal in the 'foreign non-convenience rule', which was originally adopted to protect defendant companies from being sued in some distant location where it had a small operation. Now, the very rules that used to help multistate or multinational corporations are being turned against them, on the theory that it is not convenient for these foreigners to sue in their own country because they do not have a claim there, or they are not able to have their case heard for many years. Similarly, the US plaintiffs' bar has become increasingly sophisticated in using global regulatory inconsistencies, to their clients' advantage during discovery and at trial. During the course of litigation, pharmaceutical companies are now routinely faced with discovery requests, designed to identify documents and data relating to their dealings with foreign regulatory agencies. Plaintiffs' counsel regularly point to differences in labeling and product design resulting from a pharmaceutical companies' compliance with foreign regulations as evidence of 'defectiveness' in similar or identical products marketed in the USA (Moore 1999). Thus, in overview, the global marketing of pharmaceuticals may have several product liability implications resulting from jurisdictional issues, maintaining records for different regulatory agencies, and compliance or non-compliance with regulatory requirements in different marketing venues.

Accordingly, from the perspective of global pharmaceutical companies, it is in their interest to realize that all documents and witnesses located within their company may be subject to discovery during the course of litigation. Therefore, safety issues should be handled on a global basis or at least with the understanding that inconsistencies in a company's response to regulatory inquiries about safety issues in one country may be used as evidence of what the company 'should have done' in another country. Similarly, pharmaceutical companies should be encouraged to adopt 'core' global labeling, document generation, and postmarket surveillance systems and protocols, so that the most critical information concerning drug safety and efficacy is consistent throughout the world (Moore 1999).

LANDMARK CASES

In contrast to the ostensibly uniform framework of product liability law that defines drug-induced tort, the history of high-profile pharmaceutical injury litigation shows that the practical prosecution of drug-related injury claims is broadly varied as it reflects the many possible types of drug-induced injuries. Although the breadth of potential harms from the use of pharmaceuticals is, in theory, limitless, adverse drug effects generally fall into one of seven groups: (a) *toxic effects*, where the drug causes an undesired pharmacologic effect on the body; (b) *allergic effects*, where the drug has an unpredictably severe or harmful effect on hypersensitive individuals; (c) *dependence*, where users of the drug develop a psychological or physiologic need for the drug; (d) *indirect injury*, where the drug interferes with mental or physical functions, resulting in collateral injuries; (e) *interactions*, where ingesting the drug in the context of other drugs or foods causes injury; (f) *inefficacy*, where the drug fails to perform its intended function; and (g) *socially adverse effects*, where a drug (usually an antibiotic) is overused by a population of patients, resulting in the rise and spread of resistant microorganisms (Dukes et al 1998). The follow-

ing discussion of two now-notorious pharmaceuticals, thalidomide and diethylstilbestrol, shows how plaintiffs, corporations, attorneys, and courts have applied product liability jurisprudence to varied types of pharmacologic injury.

Thalidomide

The drug thalidomide caused one of the most appalling and widely publicized tragedies in the history of medicine (Bernstein 1997).[1] Thalidomide is a piperidinedione hypnotic derived from a naturally occurring amino acid, glutamic acid. Thalidomide was first synthesized in West Germany in 1953 by the drug company, Ciba, but it was initially abandoned after tests in laboratory animals revealed neither a beneficial nor a toxic effect. A few years later, chemists at another West German pharmaceutical company, Chemie Grunenthal, deduced from thalidomide's piperidinedione structure that it might have an anticonvulsant effect, and they experimented with giving thalidomide to epileptics. The ensuing studies revealed that thalidomide was ineffective as an anticonvulsant, but that it acted as a mild hypnotic or sedative. On the basis of these data, Chemie Grunenthal brought thalidomide to market under the trade name Contergan on October 1 1957 (Robertson 1972). Thalidomide was an early success; it acted quickly to cause deep, natural-feeling sleep, and the drug soon became a favorite sleeping tablet for over-the-counter consumers and for institutions. Promoted as a perfectly safe tranquilizer, suggested uses of thalidomide mushroomed to include mild depression, 'flu, stomach disorders, menstrual tension, and even stage-fright (Allen, 1997). Also an antiemetic, Contergan was commonly prescribed for the nausea of pregnancy (Sherman 1986; cf. Burley 1986).[2] Although thalidomide showed no toxicity to laboratory animals when tested by Ciba and Chemie Grunenthal, potentially irreversible peripheral polyneuritis was soon identified in patients following long-term use of thalidomide. Symptoms included burning pain in the feet, cramping pain in the calves, loss of ankle and knee reflexes, and tingling hands (Crawford 1994). Other reported toxicity symptoms included severe constipation, dizziness, hangover, loss of memory, and hypotension (D'Arcy 1994). Against the surging tide of reported adverse drug effects, Chemie Grunenthal initially defended thalidomide as a safe product and attributed the reports to overdosage and prolonged use. Reported toxicities in human patients not previously observed in laboratory animals should have been a reminder that animal and human metabolism differ materially, and that safety assurances from Ciba and Chemie Grunenthal based on studies involving only laboratory animals might be suspect. Fortunately, an astute young physician pharmacologist at the FDA, named Dr Frances Kelsey, noticed this discrepancy and requested more data from the drug's manufacturers to show that it was safe (see D'Arcy 1994).[3] In what has been heralded as 'one of the FDA's finest hours' (see D'Arcy 1994), Dr Kelsey stubbornly withheld FDA approval of thalidomide until it became clear that the reports on neurotoxicity were valid and that, in addition, thalidomide was adversely affecting unborn children. In 1961, physicians in Germany realized with alarm that the growing number of otherwise rare severe congenital malformations, including phocomelia (defective development of limbs) and amelia (absence of limbs), could be attributed to the ingestion by women of even a single dose of thalidomide during the critical first few weeks of their pregnancy (Weidemann 1961).[4] This was shocking news about a popular drug that was, at the time, marketed throughout Europe and Asia as a mild, safe sedative and anti-emetic; alarmingly, thalidomide was specifically targeted to pregnant women as a remedy for the morning sickness that accompanies early pregnancy (Allen 1997). Over the next years, it became clear that thalidomide was one of the most potent teratogens in the medical pharmacopoiea. Almost 100% of women who took thalidomide during the sensitive period (days 21–36 of gestation) produced malformed infants (D'Arcy 1994). The spectrum of malformations was also notable for its breadth. In addition to phocomelia, thalidomide babies suffered from spinal cord defects, cleft lip or palate, absent or abnormal external ears, and heart, renal, gastrointestinal or urogenital malformations (D'Arcy 1994; See also US HHS 1997[5]). Before the epidemic was finished, over 12 000 infants were born with deformities attributable to thalidomide (Sherman 1968; see also Szeinberg 1968[6]; see also Flaherty 1984[7]). In 1971, 62 of the estimated 430 British children injured by

thalidomide sued Distillers Co., the British marketer of the drug (Dworkin 1979[8]). The pathognomic physical signs of *in utero* thalidomide exposure, phocomelia or amelia, made the plaintiffs' products liability claims seem initially quite convincing; however, novel and thorny legal questions regarding the applicable duty of care and issues of proximate causation soon made the recovery of damages from Distillers uncertain. The thalidomide plaintiffs' strongest argument under strict product liability was that thalidomide was defective in its design (Cook et al 1991). To prevail on this theory, plaintiffs had the burden of showing that, based on testing procedures and scientific knowledge available at the time of manufacture, the drug's danger to unborn fetuses was known or knowable by the defendant.[9] In the 1950s, though, it was not common practice for drug companies to test new drugs on pregnant animals (Ferguson 1996); also, even if tests on pregnant animals had been conducted, differences between animal and human metabolism of the drug would likely have hidden the drug's teratogenic effects.[10]

Realizing the difficulties in establishing the elements of a design defect case against Distillers Co., the thalidomide plaintiffs pled in the alternative that Distillers had negligently breached a duty of care it owed to all potential consumers of the drug, including the then-unborn plaintiffs. This claim, too, was questionable, however, in light of the contemporaneous Hamilton v. Fife Health Board (1993) decision, holding that a child could not suffer 'personal injuries' while still a fetus. Reasoning that unborn children are not 'legal persons', Lord Prosser ruled that antenatal personal injuries did not give rise to a cause of action for damages. Although the Hamilton case was subsequently overruled by the legislature in the Congenital Disabilities (Civil Liability) Act of 1976, additional uncertainty would certainly have arisen from the empirical difficulty in proving that thalidomide was the teratogenic cause for each plaintiff given the spontaneous risk of abnormality inherent in human embryonic development (See Ferguson 1992). Indeed, proof of causation would most likely have rested on the notoriously shaky statistical analysis of epidemiological data. One German physician even testified that, in his opinion, the injuries sustained by the plaintiffs could not have been caused by thalidomide (Allen et al 1979).

In light of the clear hurdles to establishing a successful strict liability or negligence claim, the thalidomide plaintiffs' lead counsel advised that the plaintiffs' chance of success at trial was, 'slightly less than even' (*The Sunday Times* 1973). Upon this advice, the thalidomide plaintiffs initially agreed to a £3.5 million settlement. Over the next decade, public pressure forced Distillers to increase the settlement amount to £20 million, but it is estimated that this fund will be exhausted by 2012 (Waterhouse 1995). Although the settlement agreement provided some timely compensation to the thalidomide plaintiffs, the fact that the case was settled out of court made it impossible to determine which, if any, of the plaintiffs' claims would have been successful at trial. The legacy of the thalidomide tragedy thus was not a clarification of drug product liability law. Instead, thalidomide focused the attention of lawmakers and scientists on the potential risks of all medications; this legislative mandate ultimately led to stronger and more effective drug regulations worldwide, including in the USA.[11] Foreign legislatures responded similarly (see Bernstein 1997). Bernstein quotes various sources stating that the German Pharmaceutical Law of 1976 and the Japanese Drug Side-Effect Injury Relief Fund Act of 1979 were indirect products of the thalidomide experience. Drug manufacturers in Sweden adopted voluntary regulations and drug legislation in Canada, already strict, was tightened in sympathy with the new US law (which set up the framework for FDA regulations regarding now drugs).

Diethylstilbestrol (DES)

Diethylstilbestrol (DES) is a synthetic analogue of estrogen, first manufactured in the UK in 1937. The inventor's altruistic decision not to patent DES led to the drug's manufacture by more than 300 companies (Ferguson 1996). Arguments in favor of the use of DES at the time of its introduction were largely theoretical, but although few rigorous clinical trials were performed to evaluate its efficacy, physicians began to promote the use of DES in pregnancy to treat threatened abortion or to prevent habitual abortion. Also ignoring the dearth of scientific proof of efficacy, the American Food and Drug Administration (FDA) in 1947

licensed DES for the prevention of early miscarriage. Due to vigorous support by physicians, acceptance by the FDA, and low cost, 3–4 million women in the USA ingested DES; and between 20 000 and 100 000 pregnancies were exposed to DES *in utero*, each year, for 20 years (Dutton 1988).

In retrospect, it is doubtful whether DES had any therapeutic effect whatsoever. In fact, DES may actually have increased the incidence of complications during pregnancy. Beginning approximately 15 years after the peak of DES use, doctors found that female children of mothers who had taken DES during their gestation tended to develop preneoplastic vaginal and cervical changes in adolescence or adulthood. Male and female DES children also showed an increased incidence of fertility disturbances after puberty (Duker et al 1998). DES, sometimes described as 'America's thalidomide' was a tragedy of much broader scope; in 1984, the World Health Organization estimated that hundreds of thousands of pregnancies, especially in the USA and The Netherlands, were potentially affected (Buctendijk 1984).

Since the early 1980s, thousands of pharmaceutical liability cases have been brought against the manufacturers of DES. These plaintiffs had a stronger strict liability design defect claim than those for thalidomide because DES, marketed to prevent miscarriages, had no demonstrable benefit whatsoever. In Barker v. Lull Engineering Co. (1978), a California court adopted a 'risks–benefits' test to assess whether a product is defective. Simply put, this test for defectiveness requires a court to weigh a drug's benefits against its potential risks, in light of evidence that the drug could have been designed more safely, or that other drugs were available that confer the similar benefits with less risk. A drug with no therapeutic benefit, like DES, would, under the risks–benefits test, be held defective in design.

Although drug manufacturer liability under a theory of design defect products tort was relatively easy to prove, especially in courts adopting the Barker risks–benefits test, some DES plaintiffs were barred from recovery by limitations placed on the unborn plaintiff liability doctrine that originated with the thalidomide cases. While thalidomide's teratogenicity affected only fetuses exposed during gestation, the second generation, increasing evidence showed that DES could cause injury to third-generation plaintiffs, the grandchildren of the woman who originally ingested the drug. In one such case, Enright v. Eli Lilly & Co. (1991), the plaintiff claimed that her cerebral palsy resulted from deformities in the reproductive system of her mother, which had been caused by her grandmother's ingestion of DES during pregnancy. Stressing the need to limit manufacturers' exposure to tort liability, the New York State Court of Appeals decided that a cause of action could be brought only by 'those who ingested the drug or were exposed to it *in utero*' (Brahams 1991).

Although the two-generation limitation excluded a relatively few plaintiffs outright, the most important hurdle facing the remaining DES plaintiffs was establishing specific causation—that one specific manufacturer of DES, among the more than 300 companies that produced DES, produced the pills that were ingested by their mothers. This burden of proof created difficult logistical problems, because of the two to three decade delay between ingestion of the drug and manifestation of injury. The loss of medical and pharmacy records due to death or other causes made it difficult in most cases for plaintiffs to establish their mothers' use of a DES preparation made by a specific manufacturer among the more than 300 drug companies that produced DES. Also, anecdotal evidence suggested that pharmacists commonly dispensed DES from different manufacturers fungibly (Schreiber and Hirsch 1985).

A lasting legacy of the thousands of DES cases litigated in the USA are novel theories of causation invented by activist courts to allow plaintiffs who could not prove specific causation to hold one or more of the manufacturers of DES liable for their injuries. Among these theories, the four most commonly and successfully invoked are: (a) *alternative liability*, where a plaintiff sued all of the manufacturers of DES and the court placed the burden on the defendants to prove that they were *not* the manufacturer of the injuring drug[12]; (b) *concerted action*, where the plaintiff showed express or implicit agreement among defendants to commit the tort, all defendants are equally liable[13]; (c) *market share liability*, where the plaintiff is required only to show that the defendants benefited from a substantial share of the drug market, to shift the burden to

the defendants to show that they did not produce the particular injuring drug[14]; and (d) *Hymowitz theory*, where the court focused on the fact that all manufacturers of an injurious product increase the risk to the general public, and thus held each defendant liable in proportion to its share of the drug's nationwide market, regardless of whether the defendant could prove that it did not make the actual preparation that injured the plaintiff.[15]

CONCLUSIONS

This chapter has provided a brief overview of the doctrinal framework of products liability law that is applied in pharmaceutical injury cases. Though the drug industry is heavily regulated in the USA by the Food and Drug Administration (FDA), and abroad by analogous agencies, tort liability in the forms discussed here constitutes a parallel, powerful, regulatory means by which defective products can be removed from the market and negligent manufacturers can be censured. In practice, as demonstrated by the thalidomide and DES litigation, plaintiffs frequently face unpredictable and difficult hurdles to recovery under strict liability, warranty, or negligence theories. Today, product liability issues related to pharmaceuticals continue to capture national attention. Most recently, the continuing saga around the mass tort litigation arising from the diet drug combination, "fen-phen", demonstrates the continuing significance of these issues as they affect patients, physicians, pharmaceutical companies, consumer advocacy groups, and the nation's courts. Ultimately, it is the responsibility of courts to raise or lower these hurdles, to strike the right balance between deterring irresponsible drug manufacturers and encouraging beneficial drug development.

NOTES

1 Bernstein notes that thalidomide quickly entered the lexicon as metaphor for poison and evil. 'For years I have heard the word Wait!', wrote Martin Luther King Jr. in his famous Letter from Birmingham City Jail (1963). 'It rings in the ear of every Negro with a piercing familiarity. This "Wait" has almost always meant "Never". It has been a tranquilizing *thalidomide*, relieving the emotional stress for a moment, only to give birth to an ill-formed infant of frustration'.

2 Burley argues that there is no evidence that thalidomide was neither useful nor prescribed as an antiemetic and thus it had no place in the management of the nausea of pregnancy.

3 Dr Kelsey was also particularly conscious of the potentially harmful effects of drugs on a fetus having been involved with a malaria project during World War II in which quinine (another teratogen) was studied.

4 During the 1960s, virtually every pediatric clinic in Germany had at least one child born with phocomelia or amelia.

5 While it is possible that thalidomide caused this heterogeneous group of deformities by acting through several different toxic mechanisms each targeting a different organ system, it is more likely that thalidomide has a single or few disruptive effects that can manifest themselves pleiotropically, depending on what stage the embryo had reached when the drug was introduced.

6 Szeinberg estimates that 10 000 deformed babies were born in Germany, 1000 in Japan, 400 in England, and 280 in Scandinavian countries.

7 Flaherty estimates that approximately 20 thalidomide babies were born in the USA; most of these were born to women who had received thalidomide from their husbands who were stationed in Europe.

8 Distillers advertized thalidomide as a treatment for morning-sickness that could be given 'with complete safety to pregnant women...without adverse effect on mother or child'.

9 This rule is embodied in the Restatement (Second) of Torts § 402A, comment k, which provides that the supplier of an 'unavoidably unsafe product' is liable only if it was not accompanied by a warning of dangers that the manufacturer knew or should have known about.

10 This conundrum of adequate drug testing persists even today; although more complete and rigorous laboratory testing protocols are now required by pharmaceutical regulatory agencies, many drug dangers like the action of thalidomide as a teratogen can be uncovered only postmarketing monitoring of drug toxicity because of the obvious ethical bar on drug testing using human subjects.

11 Public outcry over thalidomide is credited for the 1962 amendments to the Federal Food, Drug, and Cosmetic Act (FFDCA).

12 Alternative liability originated in the landmark case, Summers v. Tice, (1948), where the plaintiff was shot in the eye by one of two negligent hunters who had shot in his direction. The doctrine is now memorialized in the Second Restatement of Torts: 'Where the conduct of two or more actors is tortious, and it is proved that harm has been caused to the plaintiff by only one of them, but there is uncertainty as to which one has caused it, the burden is upon each actor to prove that he has not caused the harm' (Second Restatement of Torts § 433 B (3).

13 See e.g. Bichler v. Eli Lilly & Co. (1982); concert of action found among DES defendants who pooled information on the basic chemical formula and model package inserts.

14 See Sindell v. Abbott Laboratories (1980); market share liability introduced by the California court specifically in response to the difficulties in proving causation faced by DES plaintiffs.

15 See Hymowitz v. Eli Lilly & Co. (1989); this decision by the highest court of New York State is considered by many to be radical.

REFERENCES

Allen (1997) The return of thalidomide: are we ready to forget images like this and give the drug another chance? St. Louis Post-Dispatch: 28 September; 01B.

Allen, Bourne, Holyoak (eds) (1979) Accident Compensation after Pearson. Sweet & Maxwell: London; Chapter 3, p. 161

Barker v. Lull Engineering (1978) 20 Cal. 3d 413, 573 p. 2d 443, 143 Cal. Rptr. 225.

Bernstein S (1997) Formed by thalidomide: mass torts as a false cure for toxic exposure. Colum L Rev 97: 2153.

Bichler v. Ru Lilly & Co., (1982) 79 App. Div. 2d 317, 436 N.Y.S. 2d 625 (App. Div. 1981); 55 N.Y. 2d 571, 450 N.Y.S. 2d 776, 436 N.E. 2d 182.

Brahams (1991) Diethylstilbestrol: [sic] third-generation injury claims. Medico-Legal J 59: 126.

Buitendijk S (1984) DES—The Time Bomb Drug. In Report of the 13th European Symposium on Clinical Pharmacological Evaluation in Drug Control. World Health Organization: Regional Office for Europe, Copenhagen.

Burley (1986) The decline and fall of thalidomide. In Scheinberg (ed.), Orphan Diseases and Orphan Drugs. Manchester University Press, in association with The Fulbright Commission: London.

Cook, Doyle and Jabbari (1991) Pharmaceuticals, Biotechnology and the Law. Macmillan: Basingstoke, 364.

Crawford (1994) Use of thalidomide in leprosy. Adverse Drug React Toxicol Rev 13: 177.

D'Arcy (1994) Thalidomide revisited. Thirteen adverse drug reactions. Toxicol Rev 13: 65.

DeConinck J (1994) The impact of product liability on the marketing of prescription drugs. Am Business Rev 12(1): 79–85.

Enright v. Eli Lilly & Co. (1991) 77 N.Y. 2d 377, 570 N.E. 2d 198 (1991).

Dukes G, Mildred M, Swartz B (1998) Responsibility for Drug-induced Injury a Reference Book for Health Professions and Manufacturers. IOS Press: Oxford.

Dutton (1988) Worse than the Disease: Pitfalls of Medical Progress. Cambridge University Press: Cambridge, 87.

Dworkin (1979) Pearson: implications for severely handicapped children and products liability. In Allen, Bourne and Holyoak, Accident Compensation after Pearson. Sweet & Maxwell: London.

Epstein RA (1995) Cases and Materials on Torts, 6th edn. Little, Brown: Boston, 727–30.

Ferguson (1992) Pharmaceutical products liability: 30 years of law reform? Juridical Rev 3: 226–39.

Ferguson PR (1996) Drug Injuries and the Pursuit of Compensation. Sweet & Maxwell: London.

Flaherty (1984) Last Thalidomide Suits Settle to End Legal Era. Natl Law J 6: 32.

Hamilton v. Fife Health Board (1993) 4 Med. L.R. 201; 1993 S.L.T. 624; 1993 S.C.L.R. 408.

Heuston RFV, Buckley RA (1992) *Salmond & Heuston on the Law of Torts* 20th edn. Sweet & Maxwell: London, 310–12.

Hunter R (1993) Product liability: dangerous to development. *Int Corporate Law* 27: 27–8.

Hymowitz v. Eli Lilly & Co (1989) 73 N.Y. 2d 487, 539 N.E. 2d 1069, 541 N.Y.S 2d 941.

Jones MA (1993) *Textbook on Torts*, 4th edn. Blackstone: London, 302–13.

McCartney TE, Rheingold PD (1996) From prescription to over-the-counter: watered-down warnings. *Trial* 32(34): 24.

Moore TM, Cullen SA (1999) Impact of global pharmaceutical regulations on US products liability exposure. *Defense Counsel J* 66(1): 101–8.

Mossialos E, Ranos C, Abel-Smith B (1994) *Cost Containment, Pricing and Financing of Pharmaceuticals in the European Community: The Policy-Maker's View*. LSE Health and Pharmetrica: Athens, 18–19.

Nace BJ, Robb GC, Rogers JS et al (1997) Products liability: tips and tactics. *Trial* 33(11): 38.

Robertson G (1972) Thalidomide revisited. *Okla St Med Assoc J* 65: 45.

Schreiber, Hirssh (1985) Theories of liability applied to overcome the unique 'identification problem' in DES cases. *Med Law* 4: 337.

Sherman (1986) Thalidomide: a twenty-five year perspective. *Food Drug Cosmetic Law J* 41: 458–66.

Sindell v. Abbott Laboratories (1980) 26 Cal. 3d 588, 607 p. 2d 924, 163 Cal. Rptr. 132.

Szeinberg (1968) Pharmacogenetics. *Israel J Med Sci* 4(3): 488.

The Progress & Freedom Foundation (1996) *Advancing Medical Innovation: Health, Safety and the Role of Government in the 21st Century*. The Progress & Freedom Foundation: Washington, DC.

Summers v. Tice (1948) 33 Cal. 2d 80, 199 P. 2d 1.

The Sunday Times (1973) *The Thalidomide Children and the Law*. Andre Deutsch: London.

US HHS (1997) MIH will hold public Scientific workshop on thalidomide—potential benefits and risks. August 9 1997 M2 Presswire.

Waterhouse (1995) Thalidomide victims given £3.75 million bail-out. *The Independent*, May 4, 1995; 2.

Wiedemann (1961) Hinweis auf eine derzeitige Haufung hypo- und aplastischer Fehlbildungen der Gliedmassen. *Med Welt* 37: 1864.

37

Patents

Gabriel Lopez

Basking Ridge, NJ, USA

Although the discussion to follow is largely US-centered, many references are made herein to international patent concepts. The realities of modern international corporations and marketing make this more global view inevitable. Because patents are territorial, i.e. they only protect an invention within the borders of the issuing country, the inventor must think of protecting an invention in countries other than in the home country.

This discussion cannot be a learned treatise on patent law, given the enormity of the subject. It is biased toward pharmaceutical patent practice; meaning that issues different from those discussed herein might arise if the invention were a computer program, an electric switch, or a device for milking yaks. Also, as in most fields of law, both the substantive and procedural aspects of the subject are always changing, either by legislative act or judicial ruling, and will make today's statements on substance and procedure, not obsolete, but certainly dated in the not-too-distant future. As a simple example, the lifespan of a US patent used to be easy to calculate: US patents used to last 17 years from their date of issue. Now, a form of tax known as a maintenance fee is imposed. If the patentee does not pay each fee as it becomes due, the patent lapses. Further, US patents for which applications were filed after June 7 1995 will last 20 years from filing, not 17 years from issuance. Lastly, through a mechanism known as 'patent term extension', certain patents, mostly pharmaceutical ones, can now be extended for up to 5 years. The theory is that the patentee has suffered an injustice in that the patentee was essentially denied a portion of the patent's life, and thus not allowed to profit from the invention, because of the proscription against marketing certain products unless regula-tory (i.e. FDA) approval is first obtained. Extensions can also be obtained for certain procedural delays during the prosecution of a patent application. The actual term extension for each patent is determined by its specific facts: 'When does this patent expire?' used to be a trivial question to answer.

INTELLECTUAL PROPERTY

Patents are one of a class of intellectual property rights; i.e. rights to intangible property. These are patents, copyrights, trademarks, trade secrets, and seeds. Each 'right' differs from the others primarily in the type of property it protects, how it is obtained, and the length of protection:

1. *Copyrights*—these protect the expression of an idea. Protection may be obtained by marking the work, as with the symbol ©. The term is typically for the life of the creator, plus a number of years.
2. *Trademarks* (and the related *service marks*)—these protect logos, company names, container shapes, color patterns, etc.
3. *Seed protection*—these protect agricultural seeds.
4. *Trade secrets*—these protect subject matter which is not divulged to anyone unless there is a confidentiality relationship therewith. Trade secret protection has no statutory lifespan; protection lasts as long as divulgation is prevented. Whether divulgation occurs through error or malice is irrelevant; once the secret is out, it is out. There may be monetary recovery through court action against a malicious divulger, who

Principles and Practice of Pharmaceutical Medicine. Edited by A. J. Fletcher, Lionel D. Edwards, Anthony W. Fox and Peter Stonier © 2002 John Wiley & Sons Ltd.

may also be punished under the penal codes, but this is usually small comfort to the previous trade secret owner.

5. *Patents*—these protect designs, asexually produced plants, things, and processes (design and plant patents are not further discussed). Protection is obtained by filing, and then successfully prosecuting, a patent application which discloses the invention. Patents and trade secrets are antithetical protections. To protect by trade secret, the invention must not be disclosed; whereas to protect by patent, disclosure is essential. The patent applicant receives a monopolistic right for a period of years in exchange for putting the invention in the hands of the public (For 'public' read 'competitors'). *This exchange of monopoly for divulgation is at the core of the patent concept.* Failure of the inventor to fully disclose an invention has led to patent invalidation.

Although the subject matter to be protected largely dictates what type of protection is available (e.g. one would not seek trademark protection for a new song), there is an overlap between patents and trade secrets. If an invention can be commercialized without divulging the invention and without risk of being back-engineered, then the innovator should consider not seeking a patent at all, but rather keeping the invention secret. Possibly the longest-kept such secret is the formula for Coca-Cola® , which to this day has been neither stolen, divulged, nor back-engineered. Of course, it is not always easy to make the correct decision. The inventor who decides on trade secret protection may regret that decision in a few years, when the secret is inadvertently revealed, or when some analytical tool is developed which allows back-engineering of the invention. In the area of pharmaceuticals, trade secret protection is not likely to be sought by the innovator, since a new chemical entity is often the invention that needs protection and such an invention necessarily must be publicly divulged. Two types of pharmaceutical inventions, however, are often kept as trade secrets: manufacturing process improvements, and screening assays.

PATENT HISTORY

Patents are not a new concept. They were granted at least as far back as ancient Greece and Babylon. Neither are they the product of only one form of government. Essentially, every country has some form of patent protection, albeit not necessarily as strong as that in the USA and the other industrialized countries. Patent laws can exist even in non-capitalist systems, such as the former USSR. That intellectual property is a highly valued concept can be no better demonstrated than by the observation that there are only two rights (patents and copyrights) that are specifically mentioned in the US Constitution. Sect. 8, para. 8 reads:

> To promote the progress of science and the useful arts by securing for limited times to authors and inventors the exclusive rights to their respective writings and discoveries.

Patents, however, are not free of their detractors. Since they are a form of monopoly, and because monopolies have been subject to abuse (e.g., granting the king's cousin a monopoly on the local water well), antimonopoly laws (e.g., restraint of trade, antitrust, etc.) exist that can be used to limit a patentee's rights. Another severe limitation on patent rights is simply prohibiting the grant of patents on certain types of inventions. There are, of course, the current arguments against 'patenting life', as a result of which some types of 'biotech' inventions are, or may become, unpatentable. Among these can be included transgenic mammals, pieces of the human genome, and, of course, human clones. Another, older prohibition is that against granting patents to pharmaceuticals *per se*. Although their numbers are diminishing, many countries have allowed only limited patent protection on pharmaceuticals; typically, what can be patented is the processes to synthesize the compounds, but not on the compounds *per se*. These so-called 'process countries' are mostly non-industrialized. They argue that they would be at an economic disadvantage if they were to grant compound *per se* protection, because they do not have the in-house infrastructure to invent/patent such compounds themselves. Thus, all such patents would be granted to foreign, international pharmaceutical houses, as a consequence of which, moneys would always be flowing out of these countries to pay for pharmaceutical drugs. The subtleties of this essentially economic debate are beyond the scope of this discussion. However, many 'process countries' already have, or have agreed to amend, their laws to include compound *per se* protection.

PATENT PROTECTION

A patent is a monopoly for a period of time (e.g., 17–20 years, see above) which gives the patentee *the right to exclude others* from making, using, selling, or offering to sell the patented invention. Patents are limited geographically, temporally, and by the rights of others. A patent does not necessarily give the inventor the right to practice the invention. Hence the often-heard, 'We just licensed in the right to make Compound X', when a patent license has been negotiated is incorrect. The right conveyed in the license clearly could not be greater than that which the licensor has, and the licensor does not have the right to make Compound X. What is conveyed by a patent license, and depending on the wording thereof, is: (a) protection from a patent infringement suit by the licensor; or (b) the right to sue others for patent infringement. A relatively simple example explains this concept. A manufacturer has obtained a patent for, and wishes to sell, a chair with two armrests and a wheel under each of its four legs. However, he cannot make such a chair because there is already a patent which, very broadly, claims a chair having a flat sitting surface mounted atop four legs. Although the earlier patent does not claim the armrests and wheels, it will 'dominate' the later patent, assuming that the later chair has a flat sitting surface atop four legs. The first patentee has the right to exclude others, including the later patentee, from making a four-legged chair with a flat sitting surface, *but* it cannot itself make a chair with two armrests which has a wheel under each of its four legs, since this is the subject of the later patent. In this case, the manufacturer can attempt to negotiate a license from the first patentee, which will protect it from patent infringement suit by the patentee. If armrests and wheels produce a much more marketable product, it might be in both patentees' interests to cross-license their respective patents, since neither patentee could sell the more desirable chair without an accommodation with the other. (The manufacturer could also buy chairs from the first patentee and then modify them by adding armrests and wheels, since the sale exhausts the patentee's patent rights in the goods sold. However, this may be economically unfeasible if these added manufacturing costs cannot be passed on to the consumer by charging a higher price.) The situation can quickly become more complicated if we add a third party who also has an earlier patent, this one on a chair with two armrests but no wheels. The license negotiated, as described above between the first patentee and the manufacturer, does not protect the manufacturer from suit by this third patentee, who is not a party to the license. If this third patentee attempts to sell a green, two-armed, wheeled, four-legged chair with a flat sitting surface, both the first patentee and the manufacturer could sue for patent infringement under their own patents, although neither of which mentioned 'green'.

PATENTABLE SUBJECT MATTER

Clearly the terms 'things' and 'processes' cover a broad range of patentable subject matter. It is easier to define what is unpatentable. Generally, unpatentable subject matter includes products of nature, i.e. naturally occurring articles, scientific principles, and some inventions related to atomic energy and nuclear material. In the 'process countries' (see above) patents can be obtained on a process to make a compound, but not on the chemical entity itself. Inherently, this is a more limited patent right, since (a) it may be very difficult to prove that a particular process is being used by the alleged infringer; and (b) other manufacturing processes may have been developed which do not infringe.

Patentable things include compounds *per se* (i.e. new chemical entities), compositions (e.g. a new chemical entity and a pharmaceutically acceptable carrier or two chemical entities), life forms (e.g. a newly discovered microorganism or a region of DNA), and devices (e.g. a new surgical appliance).

Patentable processes include chemical syntheses, screening assays, and methods of using a compound or composition.

CRITERIA FOR OBTAINING A PATENT

There are three criteria for obtaining a patent. The invention must be: (a) novel, (b) unobvious, and (c) useful. Of these, novelty and utility are usually the easiest criteria to deal with.

An invention is *novel* if it was not part of the 'prior art' before the priority date (*vide infra*) of the patent application that claims the invention. The 'prior art' comprises all oral or written information publicly available before the priority date of the application (in some countries the 'prior art' must be publicly available in those countries). This criterion is essentially absolute everywhere except in the USA, where there is a 'grace period' of 1 year, within which one can file a patent application even if the invention has been earlier divulged, either by the applicant or by another. Novelty is fairly strictly interpreted; thus, one can obtain a patent on a compound which is within the scope of an earlier publication, which teaches a generic formula with multiple substituents on a core structural element, but which does not specifically show the now-claimed compound. Thus, to determine novelty, one compares the date of invention (US law) or priority filing date with the divulgation date of the supposed prior art. If the subject matter is the same and the divulgation date of the publication precedes the invention/filing date, then the invention fails the first test and cannot be patented.

One further twist on divulgation dates is that, in the USA a patent is a reference as of its earliest US filing date. Since a US patent application is not publicly available until the patent issues, and since the allowance of a patent may be delayed, either by a prolonged prosecution in the Patent Office (which may include appealing an adverse determination to the Examiner, both within the Patent Office and to the courts) or by the filing of one or more continuation applications, a US patent can become a reference as of its earliest US filing date many, many years later. Such patents (sometimes referred to as submarine patents) can be used as weapons in litigation to invalidate competitors' patents, the applications for which were filed after the said earliest reference date, because the Patent Examiners did not know of, and consequently were not able to cite, the patents during prosecution of the later filed patent applications.

An invention is *utile* (i.e., has utility or is useful) if it has a practical end-use. The requirement can be met by a statement of what the invention can be used for and how to use it; e.g. 'This compound is useful for the treatment of asthma when administered at a dose of 0.1–$5.0\,\mu g/kg/day$'. A more complete teaching would include modes of administration, dosage forms, delivery systems, etc. The utility must be currently available. Although commercial availability is not necessary, mere assertions such as, 'these are therapeutic agents', or 'they are for pharmaceutical purposes', are generally insufficient. If the asserted utility is believable at face value to persons skilled in the art, or in the view of contemporary knowledge in the art, then the burden is upon the Examiner to give adequate support for rejections for lack of utility. As stated by Commissioner Lehman at a hearing on Oct. 17 1994: 'In other words, if an applicant presents a scientifically plausible use for the claimed invention, it will be sufficient to satisfy the utility requirement'. Two types of invention that tend to fail the utility test are perpetual motion machines (the Patent and Trademark Office wants to see working models of these) and 'unbelievable' cures (e.g., a cure for AIDS).

The third, and most difficult, criterion is *unobviousness*, or inventive step. The process for deciding whether or not an invention is 'obvious' was succinctly stated in the Deere case. According to the Court's decision, the Patent Examiner should:

1. Determine the scope and content of the prior art.
2. Ascertain the differences between the prior art and the claims.
3. Resolve the level of ordinary skill in the pertinent art.

Of course, this three-pronged approach is much easier to enunciate than to practice, and much effort is typically spent, during the prosecution of a patent application, in trying to convince the Examiner that the rejection of the claims on the basis of obviousness is incorrect because one or more of the Deere prongs has failed. Steps (1) and

(2) of the Deere analysis tend to be fairly straightforward. However, it is in the third step that the judgment call must be made by the Examiner which presents the most problems. Even if the applicant and Examiner agree on steps (1) and (2), the conclusion to be drawn therefrom is rarely easily agreed upon. Obviousness, like beauty, appears to be more often than not in the eye of the Examiner-beholder. The matter is made worse by the organization of patent applications, which are usually drafted by first stating the background of the invention, which may include a description of the closest prior art and some unresolved problem therewith, followed by a statement of the invention. It should not be too surprising that an Examiner, presented with both a statement of a problem and the solution to the problem, would respond by concluding that the solution is obvious. Most of us have probably had a similar response upon being shown the solution to a trivial geometric puzzle, which of course, up to that moment, had completely baffled us. Hindsight in deciding the question of obviousness, as in many other endeavors, is 20/20.

The task, then, is to convince the Examiner to reconsider the obviousness rejection. Many approaches are possible; in the following examples, the claimed invention is a compound and the prior art discloses structurally similar compounds.

The simplest arguments are based on structural differences, e.g., the reference compound contains an alkyl substituent at the position where the claimed compound contains an aryl group and alkyl does not suggest aryl. Similarly, arguments can be made that 'C' does not suggest 'S'; '2-phenyl' does not suggest '3-phenyl'; 'S' does not suggest 'O'; 'S' does not suggest 'SO$_2$', etc.

An argument based on structural differences becomes more compelling if related to physical properties, such as biological activity, e.g., the reference compound had no activity, had a different activity, had the same but less activity, or had a side effect not exhibited by the claimed compound. Note that, since the rejection is based on what is disclosed in the prior art, the applicant can use what is disclosed in the art to construct an argument. Thus, if the reference discloses that the compound has an ED_{50} of 100 µg/kg and the patent application shows an ED_{50} of 10 µg/kg for the claimed compound, an argument based on unobvious properties can be made without actually determining the ED_{50} of the reference compound.

Another argument may be that the prior art actually taught away from the invention; e.g. the compounds were known to be toxic or unstable, or there was a progression in the references away from the invention (e.g., the claimed compound contains a methyl substituent, whereas the earliest of three references cited against the applicant teaches an alkyl group at the same position of 4–7 carbons, the second reference teaches 10–15 carbons, and the latest reference teaches 20–30 carbons).

Another approach is to argue from 'secondary considerations'. This approach tends to be weak. It brings in such secondary considerations as the commercial success of the invention, that there was a long-felt need in the art, the failure of others to solve whatever problem the invention solves, etc. Failing to convince by mere argumentation, the applicant may choose to introduce tangible evidence, which is typically in the form of a signed declaration which presents the results of comparative testing, i.e., a side-by-side comparison in some assay of the prior art and claimed compounds.

INTERNATIONAL TREATIES

Although patents are territorial, i.e., they are granted by and enforced in individual countries, several international treaties have had a major impact on patent practice on a global scale. Although the lists of signatory countries are not identical for all treaties, essentially all major countries are signatories, except for the European Patent Convention (EPC), which is limited to European countries.

The Paris Convention

The first and most important of these treaties is the Paris Convention for the Protection of Industrial Property of 1883. 'The Convention' allows an applicant to file a patent application in any of the Convention countries and then, no more than 1 year after the filing, to file corresponding patent applications in any, or all, of the other Convention countries and to claim the benefit of the filing date of said earlier patent application. The significance of this cannot be overstated. The first filing date, 'the priority date', shuts off the prior art, not only in the country of original filing but in all the other countries. Since absolute novelty is the rule everywhere except the USA, it is very advantageous to the applicant to be able to fix a date after which no later publicly available information can be cited as prior art, either by a Patent Examiner during prosecution (meaning the give-and-take between the applicant and the Examiner, usually in the form of written communications, which results in granting or denying the grant of a patent), or by opposing counsel in litigation (i.e., in a courtroom), in any Convention country. Actually, multiple patent applications (typically, each an expansion or a more detailed version of the prior one) could be filed within the 'Convention Year'. Each of these could establish a different priority date for whatever is disclosed therein. However, it is simpler to confine this discussion to a single priority filing and a single priority date. There is also a great economic advantage to this arrangement, since the applicant need only file one application to stop the prior art. The applicant then has 1 year in which to evaluate the invention and decide whether additional, i.e. 'foreign', filings are warranted. The foreign filing decision-making process within a pharmaceutical company varies from organization to organization but is often in the form of a committee comprising members from research, marketing, and patents and a tiered country list. An extremely potent new drug, marketable worldwide, with a high likelihood of being patented, is a candidate for global foreign filings. An invention of lesser value might be filed on a more limited basis (e.g. USA, EC, and Japan), while still protecting a significant amount of sales. An invention of very little continued interest might either be made publicly available, as by filing in any non-USA country,* since they all publish patent applications 18 months after the priority date, or not published at all, as by expressly abandoning the pending application. (This paragraph refers to applicants, not inventors. In the USA, patent applications can only be filed by inventors and patents are only granted to inventors. Outside the USA, however, non-inventors can be applicants. These applicants are usually the organizations that hired the inventors, but they could be others.)

The European Patent Convention (EPC)

This is a treaty under which the EC countries created the European Patent Office (EPO) to receive and prosecute patent applications. This system works in parallel with the European national patent offices, which have not been closed. In fact, on filing an EPO patent application, the applicant designates in which of the EC countries patent protection is sought. If the application is successfully prosecuted, the applicant is then granted a patent by each of the designated countries; i.e., each signatory country has agreed to have the EPO determine patentable subject matter and then grant patents based on the EPO's favorable decisions. If one wishes to file a patent application in Europe, there are three routes one must choose among: (a) file nationally; (b) file in the EPO; and (c) simultaneously file nationally and in the EPO. Unless the country list is very small, EPO filing has several advantages. Procedurally, it is the simplest, since there is only one filing, one prosecution, and essentially one set of allowed claims. The entire proceeding can be handled in English. Thus, the cost of translating into the non-English languages can be deferred until the end of the prosecution. If there is an adverse decision, or if the subject matter of the application is no longer of interest, there are no translation costs. The EPO route does suffer from the 'all your eggs in one basket' problem, which, of course, does not exist if one files nationally. This is not viewed by most as a significant impediment. Route c is an expensive alternative to routes a and b and is little used.

The PCT

The Patent Cooperation Treaty (PCT) of 1970 created a mechanism for worldwide patent filing which has been steadily gaining in popularity. The treaty is administered by the World Intellectual Property Organization (WIPO) in Geneva. As with an EPO application, when filing a PCT application one initially designates those countries, or regional patent offices such as the EPO, in which patents are to be sought during the 'national phase'. The PCT application is itself not a patent application. Instead, it reserves the right to file national patent applications in the future in the designated countries. Thus, a PCT filing comprises both an international phase and a national phase.

International Phase

The PCT filing results in an International Search and the issuance of an International Search Report. WIPO will also publish the patent application 18 months after the priority date. The designation 'WO...' in the upper right-hand of a 'patent' indicates that the document is a published PCT patent application. However, unlike an EPO patent application, the PCT patent application is itself not prosecuted to allowance. The filing allows an applicant to defer further action (and cost) until either 20 months or 30 months from the priority date, giving the applicant some time to consider the value of the invention (Does it work? Is it marketable?), and review the contents of the Search Report (How close is the prior art, and can it be overcome?). The timing is the applicant's choice. However, the maximum advantage, in both time and cost, results from deferring national filing until 30 months after the priority date. If the applicant decides to defer national filing to 30 months, he/she must file a Demand for International Preliminary Examination, the result of which is a Written Opinion, which comments on the three aspects of patentability (novelty, obviousness, and utility) as they apply to the claims, and possibly comments on other matters. The Written Opinion, which can be commented on by the applicant, is eventually sent by WIPO to the national patent offices, but it is not binding thereon.

National Phase

Mechanically, the 'National Phase' means filing a patent application in each country initially designated, and still of interest, and advising each national patent office that the application is based on a PCT filing. Prosecution of each application is then handled by each country independently of what any other country may be doing with a corresponding application. Since each national patent office must act in conformity with the patent laws of that country, the Written Opinion cannot control, and there can be a broad range of reactions from the national patent offices to the Written Opinion during the prosecution stage. Some offices appear to totally abdicate responsibility and incorporate the Written Opinion into their own decisions, whereas others appear to disregard it. In any case, the applicant is in a much more desirable position if the Written Opinion is favorable and well reasoned.

The Budapest Treaty on the International Recognition of the Deposit of Micro-organisms for the Purposes of Patent Procedure

There is an inherent problem with many biotech inventions, which was eloquently, if somewhat presciently, stated by Mr Joyce Kilmer: '...But only God can make a tree'. This is not a theological argument against 'patenting life', but rather a recognition that present-day science has its limitations. Until the better microscope is built (and patented), we simply cannot describe every atom in, e.g., an *E. coli* cell and, thus, cannot teach how to make one. If an invention requires such a cell, the applicant cannot meet the obligation to disclose the invention in a patent specification; i.e., there is no way to put the invention in the hands of the public without also giving the cell to the public. However, the cell is likely to be a valuable asset and the applicant will probably not wish to divulge it unless a patent has issued. A solution to this problem is to make a restricted deposit of the cell in a public depository, which will provide an accession number identifying the deposit. The restriction is lifted in the future, e.g., when a patent issues referring to the cell. The applicant can then meet the disclosure requirement by providing the deposit's accession number in the specification. This approach works best if only one country is involved. It works less well with multiple international filings, since the patent office in each country may have its own rules as to what constitutes an acceptable depository, what may be acceptable restrictions on access to the public, etc. The Budapest Treaty resolves these issues by providing a list of approved depositories throughout the world and one set of deposit conditions, including restricted access to a deposit by the public prior to patent grant. The inventor need make only one deposit under one set of rules to enable the invention, and the public gets disclosure of the invention under certain restricted conditions prior to patent grant.

The General Agreement on Tariffs and Trades GATT

GATT is the latest attempt at global patent harmonization, i.e., amending patent laws everywhere so that they are more alike. For example, as a result of GATT, many 'process countries' have agreed to granting compound *per se* patents. This recent (1994) treaty has had significant impacts on US patent practice, most of which are procedural and too arcane for discussion herein. However, a very obvious change is the length of a patent's life and how it is calculated (see above). According to US Patent and Trademark Office figures, the average chemical patent application is pending slightly less than 2 years. Therefore, the 20 year patent has a slightly longer (by about 1 year) patent life than the former 17 year patent term. However, this computation ignores the practical reality that many pharmaceutical patent applications are rarely simply filed and then granted in 2 years. Rather, many of these are just the first of a string of related filings, the last of which may occur 5 or more years after the first. Under the new rules, patents issued from these later-filed applications would expire 20 years from first filing, with a considerably reduced patent life vs. a comparable 17 year patent. GATT did not remove two peculiarities of US patent law: interference practice (see below) and the secrecy of pending applications. There is ongoing discussion to publish US patent application 18 months after the priority date, as essentially every other country does, but at present the US Patent and Trademark Office reveals nothing about pending applications.* GATT did bring about one change, concerning the place of invention, that affects interference practice. Prior to GATT, one could only prove the date of invention by reference to acts committed in the USA. Non-US inventors have complained about the favoritism of this rule, since it gives US inventors a clear advantage. Under GATT, non-US acts can now be used as part of the proof of the date of invention, thus leveling the international playing field.

INTERFERENCE PRACTICE

Unlike the rest of the world, US patent practice is a 'first-to-invent' rather than 'first-to-file' system.

The argument for this was that the Constitutional basis for the patent system was to secure rights for inventors, not for hasty filers. This occasionally leads to a quasi-judicial proceeding known as an 'interference'. An interference arises when two (or more, but this complicates matters even further) patent applications are filed in the US Patent and Trademark Office at about the same time and the same subject matter is determined by the Examiner in each application to be allowable. In the first-to-file countries, the second application is rejected over the first. This ends the matter, unless the second applicant can successfully argue that the Examiner has misunderstood either of the inventions, i.e., that in fact there is no overlapping subject matter or that there is some fundamental error in the first application, e.g., that the first application does not actually teach what it appears to teach.) Usually the determination of overlapping subject matter occurs while both of the applications are still in prosecution, but it can also occur if one has already been granted and a patient has issued. The declaration of an interference can either be the result of an internal check at the US Patent Office of pending applications, or as the result of the provocation of an applicant. This occurs when the applicant sees a patent issue with overlapping subject matter, based on an application filed within certain time limits. The applicant then 'copies claims' from the patent for purposes of having an interference declared. Since the Examiner must first determine that the applications contain otherwise allowable subject matter, interferences take place only at the end of the prosecution stage. There does not have to a complete overlap in allowable subject matter, merely some overlap. The interference is referred to as quasi-judicial because, as in a trial, two opposing sides argue against each other and present evidence, either in support of their side or to contradict the other. The US Patent Office sets up a schedule for exchanging proofs, calling witnesses, etc. Ultimately, a decision is made by a panel of Administrative Patent Judges as to which party is the first to invent and is be to granted a patent. While this decision is binding on both parties, however, it can be appealed to the civil courts.

Interference practice is defended by many as the only way to ensure that the true (read 'first') inventor is granted a patent in accord with the Constitutional intent. It is attacked by many as a costly and time-consuming proceeding that serves no real purpose, since 'inventor' can just as easily be defined as the one who files first, independently of when the invention actually is made. There is pressure from the international community for the USA to adopt a first-to-file system but, for now, interferences will continue.

BIOTECHNOLOGY

Biotechnology (hereinafter, biotech) can loosely be defined as the science of very large and very complicated biological molecules. The patent concepts that have developed over the decades to deal with a myriad of inventions covering organic compounds (i.e. 'small molecules') generally can be, and have been, adapted to cover biotech inventions. However, biotech inventions have two basic types of problems; one technological, the other societal.

One of the issues on the technological side is the question of enablement. This has been discussed in part in the section dealing with The Budapest Treaty (see above). But even if the inventor tries to put the invention or a precursor of the invention in the hands of the public, as by a Budapest deposit, the public may still not be able to reproduce the invention; e.g., because of an inherent instability in the deposited material. Another technological question is how to fully describe the invention. Analogous to a description of a piece of real property (i.e., land) found in a deed, the 'metes and bounds' of the invention must be described in a patent application in such clear and concise terms that a potential infringer would be able to figure out which acts are infringing and which are not. In the biotech area it is often not easy to fully describe the thing that has been invented. The stick formulas used to describe classical pharmaceutical compounds are rarely of any value. The physical properties of biotech inventions are often 'fuzzy', '...having a molecular weight of 75–95 kDa' may be the best molecular weight value the inventor can provide, but it is not very precise. Each type of biotech invention presents it own technological difficulties, which must be resolved using whatever tools are available when preparing a patent application.

On the societal side is the great concern about 'patenting life'. This is another example of the difficulties that arise when technology races ahead of society's capacity to even understand that there is a potential new problem. Although plant patents had been granted for many years, patent offices had refused to grant patents to cover living, non-plant inventions. This all began to change with the 1980 US Supreme Court decision in the Chakrabarty case, where the invention was a modified microorganism. The sole issue before the Court was whether an invention could be denied patent protection because it was alive. The Court said 'No' and the biotech industry exploded onto the scene. No-one today complains about patenting microbes. However, the intensity of the debate is understandable when the inventions involve human DNA, since these are seen by some as endangering our humanity. Today, the major issues relate to patenting transgenic mammals, pieces of the human genome, and human clones. Tomorrow, the great issue of the day may be patenting cyborgs; i.e., creatures comprising synthetic and human components. Undoubtedly, some of these issues will be resolved soon and some will be hotly debated for a long time, at least until a hotter issue emerges.

BIOGRAPHY OF A PATENT APPLICATION

With the understanding that there is no typical patent application, the following is an attempt to describe its typical and highly simplified lifespan. The setting is an international, pharmaceutical corporation.

The application is written within several months after approval to file by a Patent Committee, which has reviewed the inventor's Disclosure of the Invention and has decided that the invention is worthy of patent protection.

In about 1 year from filing, an Examiner takes up the application and communicates (usually in the form of a Rejection) with the patent attorney handling the application. After about another year, the application is either allowed (in which case an Issue Fee is paid and the patent is granted) or the Examiner issues a Final Rejection, to which the response is an Appeal. Appeals are handled by a three-person Board, which reviews all the arguments presented by the Applicant and the Examiner. Favorable decisions result in an allowance.

Unfavorable decisions can be appealed to the courts. Board decisions are currently taking about 2 years from the time the Applicant's Brief and the Examiner's Answer are submitted.

About 9–10 months after filing the application, a decision is made by the Patent Committee about if, where, and how to foreign file the application, which must be done by the 1 year anniversary date. If national filings are decided, the application is sent to an agent in each country with instructions to file the application by the anniversary date. If a PCT filing is decided, the application can be filed by the applicant in the PCT Receiving Office of the Patent Office. Decisions then have to be made shortly before the 20th and 30th months after the initial filing date with regard to national filings, as described in the section on the PCT. National filings, whether directly or through the PCT, are handled by each country's Patent Office. There are a multitude of statutory, formalistic, and stylistic differences among all the Patent Offices, resolved with the help of a local patent agent. However, typically there is a review by an Examiner, amendments and arguments by the Applicant, and either an Allowance or an Appeal. In the EPO, Japan, and other countries, an Allowance does not automatically result in the granting of a patent. In these countries, when the Examiner decides there is patentable subject matter, the allowed claims are Published for Opposition. During the Opposition Period, anyone can protest the granting of the patent. Opponents present their written arguments, which the Applicant attempts to rebut. If the matter is not resolved after a period of arguments and counterarguments, the matter is orally argued before, and decided by, an Opposition Board. As with a US patent application involved in an Interference, ultimate issuance of a patent may take years in the case of a vigorously contested opposition. Finally, after the patent has been issued, it must be maintained. Periodically, additional fees are paid to the patent offices of various countries. In some cases, late payment can be mitigated by extra fees. But if not maintained by such fees, the patent will be determined to have been abandonned or expired.

38

Fraud and Misconduct in Clinical Research

Frank Wells

Medicolegal Investigations Ltd, Ipswich, UK

The welfare of patients is fundamental to the practice of medicine. That there are so many effective treatments available for the cure or control of so many diseases is largely the outcome of decades of research, stretching throughout the second half of the twentieth century. However, there is still a very long way to go to master many diseases, including cancers, psychoses, dementias and many others, which are currently untreatable. Clinical research must therefore continue, including genetic and biotechnological research, recognizing that the welfare of patients/subjects involved in such research must be safeguarded.

One of the greatest potential hazards to the welfare of patients is their exploitation by fraud in the context of clinical research. Although it remains difficult to quantify the actual likelihood of this occurring. Fraud in any context is deplorable, but if it is primarily prescription, tax, or financial fraud, then the only party at risk is the victim of the fraud—and this may be the Government or, ultimately, the taxpayer. *Research* fraud distorts the database on which many decisions may be made, possibly adversely affecting the health of thousands of others. *Clinical* research fraud is potentially horrifyingly dangerous; if licensing decisions were to be made based on efficacy and safety data that are false, the result could be disastrous. Fortunately there is no strong evidence that such a sequence of events has yet occurred, but the importance of the roles of both the clinical trial monitor and the independent auditor cannot be overemphasized in this regard. Nevertheless, they are inadequate by themselves when a fraudster is determined to cheat and to cover his/her tracks so that auditors are hoodwinked into believing that all is well. There is enough published evidence confirming that fraud in clinical research is ever-present (Campbell, 1997).

Ideally, fraud should not occur. Agreed high standards must be set for clinical research, to which all interested parties should adhere. However, procedures must also be in place if fraud is suspected, despite the existence of these standards. Within the pharmaceutical industry, the standards needed for the conduct of clinical research already exist, and have been adopted by all regulatory bodies licensing medicines, international pharmaceutical companies, and contract research organizations. Both the European Commission (CPMP) good clinical practice (GCP) guidelines (EC 1991) and the requirements of the FDA came first, but GCP guidelines adopted under the International Conference on Harmonization (ICH; 1996) process now take precedence, globally. The Step 5 stage of the ICH process having been reached, there is now global guidance—which means that there are now global standards that have been adopted by the three major sectors of Europe, the USA and Japan. Although the standards referred to at the beginning of this chapter are therefore in place, there is no such harmonization when it comes to dealing with fraud and misconduct in the context of clinical research. Indeed, even within Europe there is as yet no agreed attitude towards tackling the problem. But, whatever its incidence, this unacceptable aspect of clinical research must be tackled if we are to achieve and maintain confidence in scientific integrity and in the clinical research process.

HISTORICAL ASPECTS OF FRAUD

Fraud is much less common than carelessness, although its incidence is difficult to quantify. Nevertheless, it has been estimated (Anon. 1996) at 0.1–0.4%. Based on the work on cases of fraud in

Principles and Practice of Pharmaceutical Medicine. Edited by A. J. Fletcher, Lionel D. Edwards, Anthony W. Fox and Peter Stonier © 2002 John Wiley & Sons Ltd.

which I am currently involved, however, my personal belief is that it is higher, maybe nearer to 1%. If we take this figure of 1% this means that, in the UK where I am based, at any one time maybe 30 studies are being conducted that could be fraudulent. Extrapolating this to the rest of the world—and there is no evidence that the incidence of fraud in clinical research differs across Europe or North America (although we are more open in dealing with it in the UK)—there may be 125–150 clinical trials being conducted now in which some of the data being generated is fraudulent, where investigators are making up some of the data to be submitted to a company and—worst of all—maybe exploiting their patients in the process.

Fraud is best defined as 'the generation of false data with the intent to deceive'. This definition includes all of the components of fraud: the making-up of information that does not exist, and intending to do so flagrantly in order to deceive others into believing that the information is true. Most of the earlier documented cases of fraud in the medical research field are from the USA, and many of these refer to published papers, but the phenomenon is global. Eight examples will suffice, although further details of most of them, and several additional case histories, can be found in the definitive book on the subject edited by Lock and Wells (1996).

The first example is that of John Darsee, a research cardiologist, first at Emory University, then at Harvard Medical School (Lafolette 1992). He committed an extensive series of frauds, including non-existent patients or collaborators as well as fabricated data. During his career, he published over 100 papers and abstracts, many of which have had to be retracted from the prestigious journals in which they first appeared.

Robert Slutsky was a resident in cardiological radiology at the University of California, San Diego, during the course of which he had published 137 articles as either author or co-author, all between 1978 and 1985, most of which were based on data that did not exist (Friedman 1990). Although roundly discredited, interestingly, only some of his fraudulent articles have subsequently been retracted by the editors of the journals in which they were published.

The story of thalidomide is well known—less well known are the attempts of William McBride,

who was one of the first to describe the effects of thalidomide on the developing fetus, to discredit another drug, Debendox—known as Bendectin in the USA—along similar lines (Swah 1996). McBride had never in fact conducted controlled trials to determine the thalidomide effect, but had at least accurately observed its toxicity. The situation was different for Debendox/Bendectin, because McBride was ostensibly responsible for conducting studies during the late 1970s on rabbits, which had shown up its toxicity. It took a decade to demonstrate publicly that such studies did not exist, and almost another decade (1996) before McBride was publicly denounced—all of which was much too late to save what was possibly a valuable therapeutic product. Here was an example of an eminent public figure whose reputation was such that it was unthinkable that he might be telling lies. Furthermore, this case demonstrates the messianic complex occasionally seen in fraudsters, who seem to believe that they have a divine right to state falsehoods as if they were proven facts, because they 'know that they are right'.

Dr Roger Poisson was a researcher at St Luc Hospital, Montreal, Canada. In 1993, he was investigated by the Office of Research Integrity (ORI) and found to have fabricated and falsified patient data submitted to the National Surgical Adjuvant Breast and Bowel Project, regarding a number of multicenter clinical studies on breast and bowel cancer. As a result of the ORI's investigation, Dr Poisson was debarred for 8 years from the receipt of any Federal funding. It took until 1996, however, before he appeared before the Discipline Committee of the Quebec College of Doctors. He pleaded guilty to 13 counts of committing 'acts derogatory to the honour and dignity of the medical profession' and he was subsequently reprimanded, fined and permanently restricted from several activities, including serving as a principal investigator in medical research (Anon. 1997a).

The first extensively documented British case, in 1988, was that of Dr Uzair Siddiqui, a psychiatrist in the city of Durham (Anon. 1988). He was found by an astute pharmaceutical company clinical trial monitor to have invented some of the laboratory data for most of the patients purported to have taken part in the trial and to have invented one complete patient. The laboratories used for this study were located in two hospitals inside and outside the city, and the monitor could not find any evidence, at either laboratory, that specimens had been submitted for analysis. When challenged, the doctor claimed that he had not done the study himself, but had delegated it to his medical registrar (a doctor in training), although he had forgotten her name and did not know where she now worked. The help of the trade association for the UK (ABPI) was sought, and it was not difficult to ascertain the name and location of the junior doctor whom Dr Siddiqui had accused. She, however, very strongly denied any involvement in the study and her evidence was accepted and subsequently confirmed. The case was a strong one to take to the General Medical Council (GMC), but, understandably at the time, the company was very concerned that it might be criticized for making an allegation of fraud. Indeed, it was worried that it would lose the confidence of doctors—and thus prescriptions—if it was seen to be taking such an action. With some misgivings, therefore, the case was submitted to the GMC and eventually the professional conduct committee found Dr Siddiqui guilty of serious professional misconduct, and his name was erased from the medical register.

The reaction of the doctors in Durham was exactly what the company had feared might happen; they reacted furiously that a pharmaceutical company, even though it had been supported by the ABPI, had dared to refer an eminent consultant psychiatrist to the GMC. They imposed a sanction against the company by banning it from the local postgraduate medical center, to which all pharmaceutical companies normally had access for the sponsoring of meetings. Fortunately, within 2 weeks it proved possible to hold an independent meeting in Durham, at which the full facts were explained—the case having been conducted in complete confidence until the actual hearing of the professional conduct committee in public—and the status quo ante was able to be restored.

In some ways this was a pivotal event, because a different situation in the UK thereafter became clear: it was expected of the pharmaceutical industry—and very much still is—that it would take forthright action against any doctor found beyond all shadow of doubt to have committed fraud. This has led to 23 further cases since the Siddiqui case was submitted by companies and the trade associ-

ation within the UK to the General Medical Council, all of whom have been found guilty of serious professional misconduct, the majority of them being struck off the medical register.

These events manifestly demonstrate that clinical research fraud is a problem against which all possible steps should be taken. However, little was done to formalize these steps until relatively recently. Even now, and even within the developed world, little has happened other than: (a) isolated initiatives in the Scandinavian countries and Austria, where there are Committees on Scientific Dishonesty (Andersen et al, 1992); (b) in the UK, where the pharmaceutical industry and a private agency have been very active (Smith, 1997); and in the USA, where both the FDA and the Office of Research Integrity (ORI, which also operates in Canada) are active in this regard. Nevertheless, for some time there has been an impression amongst pharmaceutical physicians, clinical research associates, and quality assurance professionals that a small but significant amount of data supplied by clinical investigators is fraudulent. This view was shared by the Royal College of Physicians (RCP), which in 1990 set up its own working party on fraud and misconduct in clinical research, following the publication of a leading article in the British Medical Journal (Lock, 1989). This initiative of the RCP was an important one, in which it was suspected that several serious instances had occurred that had not been investigated or reported. Sadly, no action followed the publication of its report (Royal College of Physicians of London 1991) and it was consequently left to the Association of the British Pharmaceutical Industry (ABPI) to set up its own working party to produce its own report, on which action was taken (Wells, 1994). Clear agreed guidelines for the UK industry thus exist, from which many actions have followed.

THE PREVENTION OF FRAUD

Outside the discipline of clinical research, there are few who are aware of, or understand, the principles of good clinical (research) practice (GCP)—a fact that those involved in it every day sometimes forget. It is therefore essential to invest time and effort in explaining the principles of GCP not only to individual investigators but also to their colleagues and to the leaders of the medical profession. This is for several reasons, including the prevention of fraud. GCP guidelines specifically underline the rationale of monitoring, and of audit procedures, and it is vitally important that these are clearly understood by all concerned, including the implications that action will be taken if data are falsified. Fraud is more likely to be prevented if investigators, and their colleagues, are fully aware of GCP standards, of the requirement for the industry to abide by them, and of the commitment of companies to act vigorously against any irregularities. Scientific research, outside the context of clinical research, is not subject to any agreed standards, and it is therefore relevant to suggest that the equivalent of GCP standards should equally apply to non-clinical scientific studies.

Until relatively recently, there has been scant mention of clinical research fraud in the literature. Little of this has involved the pharmaceutical industry and that is probably because, other than in the USA and the UK, pharmaceutical companies suspecting fraud remain greatly concerned about the risk of repercussions if they are seen to be critical of the medical profession. This, though, is largely due to the unwillingness of the leaders of the medical profession throughout most of the world to take seriously allegations that fraud is occurring. Indeed, until 1989 this was the situation in the UK as well, but an active decision was taken by the industry there, through ABPI, to invest time in discussing the implications of clinical research fraud with leaders of the medical profession, represented by the medical Royal Colleges, the British Medical Association (BMA), the GMC and the Medical Research Council (MRC), which has yielded a very positive and supportive attitude. As mentioned above, however, the application of the principles of combating research fraud need to be taken into areas other than the pharmaceutical industry to be comprehensively effective in any country.

Quite apart from training them properly, steps should be taken to avoid recruiting any potential investigators who would be inappropriate. This includes those who are too busy, too tired, or too frustrated by the bureaucracy surrounding them, too lazy, too greedy, or too careless. Investigators should be actively rejected when, within the company, anyone has any doubts arising from their past involvement in a research project. This particularly applies when there is pressure from someone at senior level, or from a parent company, to use an investigator about whom such doubts have been raised.

There are a number of reasons why doctors may volunteer to become investigators. Some of these are inappropriate. They include: pressure to publish, which is entirely legitimate, although if the publication becomes an end itself rather than the accurate outcome of the study, there can be problems; sheer boredom of routine clinical practice; greed (and here it is important to have a recognized tariff for the involvement of investigators); emotional disturbance or mental illness; and vanity. Regarding the amount of money that it is reasonable to pay investigators, there should be two safeguards: the first is approval by the local research ethics committee that the amount to be paid to the investigator is acceptable; and the second is to have an agreed figure suggested by a body whose influence is largely accepted by doctors throughout the country concerned. Thus, the BMA, through its Professional Fees Committee, suggests an hourly figure for payment by pharmaceutical companies to investigators taking part in clinical trials which is currently about £120 or US $20 per hour. This is generally accepted by pharmaceutical companies as the benchmark level throughout the UK.

THE DETECTION AND INVESTIGATION OF FRAUD

It must always be in a monitor's mind that fraud could occur, anywhere. The biggest case of fraudulent research in the USA was first investigated after the research team at a pharmaceutical company became suspicious when the data submitted by a specialist physician was found to be 'too perfect'. It was indeed just that—too good to be true. On the other hand, a very few investigators are obsessional and have a fanatical attitude towards neatness and tidiness, and these blameless few must of course be recognized.

It must also be mentioned that cases are known where there has been collusion on the part of the company employee or department with the person perpetrating the fraud, although these do not appear in the published literature and are fortunately few and far between. They can, however, be minimized by having a standard operating procedure in place, clearly requiring anyone within a company who believes that his/her concerns are not being taken seriously to report such concerns to management at the most senior level or to a relevant outside body. Such a body could be the Committee on Scientific Dishonesty in Denmark, Finland, Norway, Sweden or Austria, the ORI in the USA, or Medicolegal Investigations in the UK.

Fraud is most often detected by the clinical trial monitor, who may become suspicious because of patterns or trends in the appearance of case record forms or diary cards. Examples include: the use of one pen for a study involving patients from different centers over a prolonged period; the arrival of data from a number of patients in batches; the way in which the 'patient' has marked visual analogue lines with the consistent use of idiosyncrasies—some of which may be those of the investigator; the appearance of diary cards that are in pristine condition but several of which appear to be written in the same handwriting; follow-up attendances that appear to have taken place on national holidays when clinics would not be expected to be open; and similar handwriting appearing to have been used on several consent forms—either by 'patients' or by 'witnesses'. The regular examination of returned clinical trial materials can also be valuable, either because they show returned medication or clinical report forms (CRFs) in pristine condition, or they reveal similarities that are unexpected. An example of this occurred when tubes of a topical skin application were returned squeezed in exactly the same fashion, all eventually being found to match the palm print of the investigator. Any suspicion raised by a monitor justifies consideration being given to the setting-up of a 'for cause' audit—and it is the report of the auditor, together with that of the monitor, that is pivotal in this context.

Statisticians have an important role to play in providing further evidence, once suspicions have been raised—are there any groups of patients whose data are atypical compared with other patients within the same center, or from the other centers within the study? The expertise of statisticians in applying various specialist techniques to suspect data has been crucial in several cases already dealt with. However, the detection of a single

fraudulent entry, or series of entries, relating to a particular visit is difficult.

It cannot, therefore, be emphasized too strongly that requirements for source documentation verification inherent in GCP, and all the associated audit procedures, are essential components of the processes of both detection and investigation of suspected fraud, and that it requires the utmost vigilance from trial monitors and the consistent application of quality control checks to minimize the risk of fraud going undetected.

THE PROSECUTION OF FRAUD

Once an investigator has been shown beyond all reasonable doubt to have submitted fraudulent data to a pharmaceutical company or contract house, it is essential in the interests of the public, the profession, and the industry that that doctor should be dealt with in a disciplinary fashion. In the UK this is usually by referral to the GMC for possible consideration by the professional conduct committee. A memorandum on the activities of the GMC appears as an Appendix to this chapter. Alternatively, the doctor may be prosecuted for the criminal offence of deception. In the UK, the GMC procedure is preferred, as it works more quickly than the courts of law. However, if a company decides, for whatever reason, that it does not wish to use the GMC procedure, or if, for example, in another European country, a company wishes to prosecute a doctor who is not registered with the GMC, it is always open to that company to use a legal process. The GMC has made it clear that it would not seek to usurp the proper authority of the police or of the Crown Prosecution Service where a criminal offence may have been committed. Alternatively, a company that considered itself fraudulently exploited by a doctor could take out a civil prosecution. A prosecution, however, would take considerably longer to process through to conviction than the GMC procedure, and, if successful, would automatically (in the UK) lead to the GMC disciplinary procedure being invoked. By custom and practice, therefore, it is strongly recommended that companies should consider it most appropriate that offending doctors in the UK should be submitted to the professional disciplinary proceedings laid down by law for the GMC (1996).

SOME RECENT CASES

Malcolm Pearce was an eminent obstetrician and gynecologist at St George's Hospital in London, who, during 1995, claimed to have performed a pioneering operation, when a subsequent enquiry found that he had not done so. He claimed to have transplanted successfully an ectopic pregnancy and achieved a successful full-term vaginal delivery. Had this really happened, it would have been the first time such an operation had been successfully performed. The subsequent history of this case is interesting on several fronts: first, the enquiry into the fabricated operation revealed that Pearce had reported on a study on 191 patients with polycystic ovary disease, which was also found to be fraudulent. Second, both these reports were published in the *British Journal of Obstetrics and Gynaecology*; the article on relocation of the ectopic pregnancy was co-authored by two others, one of whom was Professor Geoffrey Chamberlain, who was also Pearce's head of department. Furthermore, Chamberlain was Editor of the journal in question and President of the Royal College of Obstetricians and Gynaecologists. Obviously, Chamberlain could have had no part in the non-existent operation, and his co-authorship was thus untenable. He subsequently resigned both his editorship and his presidency. Third, there is no question of Pearce conducting these false activities for financial gain; his case demonstrates the objective of some fraudsters, who are usually very vain, of wishing to be seen to be pioneers. Once again, his case was referred to the GMC and his name was erased from the medical register.

Animal research can also be fraudulent, although it may be much more difficult to detect. Mr Yi Li was reported early in 1997 in the ORI Newsletter for having fabricated an experimental study on the behavior of rats during his candidature for a PhD degree in the neuroscience program at the University of Illinois, Urbana-Champaign, USA. It was as a result of a review by ORI that his fraud was found out, and he subsequently entered into a Voluntary Exclusion Agreement, in which he agreed to exclude himself from publicly funded research activity for a period of 3 years (Anon, 1997b).

Dr Geoffrey Fairhurst was an eminent general practitioner in St Helens, Lancashire—a town in the North West of England (Dyer, 1996). On this occasion it was the doctor's partner who acted as 'whistle-blower' and who alerted the authorities to activities that Fairhurst was clearly doing his best to conceal. The partner discovered a number of consent forms that were not signed by the patients in question, and who were not aware of their involvement in a clinical trial. Furthermore, the practice nurse was required to alter the dates printed by the electrocardiograph on tracings taken for clinical trial purposes, sometimes by as much as 9 months, on pain of losing her job. After extensive further enquiries, Fairhurst's case was referred to the GMC and his name was ultimately also erased from the medical register.

The final example is that of Dr John Anderton, a distinguished academic consultant renal physician in Edinburgh who, in his time, had been Secretary of the Royal College of Physicians of Edinburgh (Dyer, 1997). An astute clinical trial monitor discovered that the forms on which Dr Anderton had submitted magnetic resonance and echocardiography data had been discontinued by the laboratories concerned some 6 months prior to a particular study having been commenced. This led to the involvement of an investigational agency, which conducted further enquiries, including the questioning of a number of patients, whose consent to be so questioned had been obtained by the local hospital authorities. These enquiries revealed that Dr Anderton had not obtained consent from a number of patients for their involvement in a clinical trial and, worse, that he had required his personal assistant to sign that she had witnessed non-existent signatures from patients he had purported to have consented. His case went before the GMC during the summer of 1997. He, like the last three doctors mentioned above, was found guilty of serious professional misconduct and his name was erased from the medical register.

Two further cases will never be fully documented, because they involved doctors who died prematurely, one where the coroner recorded that the death was due to suicide, the other where the coroner reached an open verdict. In both cases the fraud discovered was multiple, and on a very extensive scale, where the doctor involved had gone to very great lengths to disguise the nature of his fraudulent activities and had thus hoodwinked clinical trial monitors and auditors, who had not detected anything amiss. Original patient records were themselves fabricated in one case, and a vast 'library' of spare ECGs, presumably performed on a small number of patients over periods of hours and then divided up, were drawn upon in the other. Hundreds of consent forms were forged, with signatures varying considerably, but none of them being the signatures of patients purporting to be involved in the various studies.

Other cases are known where ethics committee (IRB) approval has been forged (Blunt et al, 1998), patients have been put into several studies at once without the sponsors being aware of this, nurses have been required to recruit patients, disregarding the inclusion or exclusion criteria, investigators have sampled blinded material themselves attempting to unblind it; and so on.

CONCLUSION

In a climate that is increasingly critical of research processes, particularly those involving the biosciences, the possibility of fraud occurring must be clearly recognized by those whose responsibility it is to maintain standards. Furthermore, it is essential that those responsible for sponsoring research, at whatever level, and wherever located, should take forthright action to prevent fraud from occurring wherever possible, but also to detect and investigate it if it occurs, and to prosecute anyone who is guilty of fraud.

Every organization responsible for sponsoring clinical research should therefore be reminded of its obligations under the principles of GCP, and asked to state its commitment to reporting all cases of fraud and to taking appropriate action. Every such organization should introduce standard operating procedures for the handling of suspected fraud, which should include at least the following items:

1. A clear statement of the organization's policy towards the handling of suspected fraud.
2. A stated policy that any cause for concern regarding suspected fraud must be referred to the medical director, or other appropriate senior or independent person, at the earliest possible stage.
3. Clear guidelines as to the path to be followed if fraud is suspected, culminating in the appro-

priate prosecution of the investigator if the suspicions are proved to be justified.
4. Clear guidelines as to the right of appeal if a complainant feels that his/her concern is being inappropriately addressed within the Organization, so that the 'whistle-blower' is appropriately protected.

Every person involved in clinical research, be he/she a monitor, an auditor, a statistician, a medical adviser, a medical director, a head of department, a co-investigator, a company or health service chief executive, or a university vice-chancellor, should be committed to such a policy and to its publicity, not least to act as a deterrent, in a determination to stamp out fraud in clinical research if it is humanly possible. Every international company, every regulatory authority, and every individual pharmaceutical physician should strive to ensure that there is an effective mechanism in place, in every country, by which anyone who commits fraud can be summarily dealt with. Only the utmost vigor in applying this policy will be successful, but it is in the ultimate interests of patient safety that this happens.

REFERENCES

Andersen D, Attrup L, Axelsen N, Riis P (1992) *Scientific Honesty and Good Scientific Practice*. Danish Medical Research Council: Copenhagen.

Anon. (1996) Dealing with deception. *Lancet* 347: 843.

Anon. (1997) Case summary. *ORI Newslett* 5(2): 4.

Anon. (1997b) Medical discipline committee takes actions. *ORI Newslett* 5(2): 7.

Anon. (1988) GMC professional conduct committee. *Br Med J* 296: 306.

Blunt J, Savalescu J, Watson AJM (1998) Meeting the challenges facing research ethics committees. *Br Med J* 316: 58–61.

Campbell D (1997) Medicine needs its MI5. *Br Med J* 315: 1677–80.

Court C, Dillner L (1995) Consultant struck off for fraudulent claims. *Br Med J* 310: 1554.

Dyer C (1996) GP struck off for fraud in drug trials. *Br Med J* 312: 798.

Dyer C (1997) Consultant struck off over research fraud. *Br Med J* 315: 205.

EC (1991) European Union Note for Guidance. *Good Clinical Practice for Trials on Medicinal Products*. Brussels: European Commission.

Friedman PJ (1990) Correcting the literature following fraudulent publication. *J Am Med Assoc* 263: 1416–19.

GMC (1996). *Fitness to Practice*. General Medical Council: London.

International Conference on Harmonization (1996) *Good Clinical Practices*. International Federation of Pharmaceutical Manufacturing Associations; Geneva.

Lafolette MC (1992) *Stealing into Print*. University of California: Berkeley, CA.

Lock S (1989) Misconduct in medical research: does it happen in Britain? *Br Med J* 297: 1531–5.

Lock S, Wells F (eds) (1996) *Fraud and Malpractice in Medical Research*. British Medical Journal Publications: London.

Royal College of Physicians of London (1991) *Report on fraud and misconduct in medical research*. Royal College of Physicians: London.

Smith R (1997) Misconduct in research: editors respond. *Br Med J* 315: 201–2.

Swan N (1996) Baron Munchausen at the lab bench? In Lock S, Wells F (eds), *Fraud and Misconduct in Medical Research*. BMJ Publishing Group: London.

Wells F (1994) Fraud and misconduct in clinical research. In Griffin J, O'Grady J, Wells F (eds), *The Textbook of Pharmaceutical Medicine* Queens University: Belfast.

APPENDIX

THE GENERAL MEDICAL COUNCIL

In the UK, disciplinary powers were first conferred on the GMC by the Medical Act 1858, which established the Council and the Medical Register. The Council's jurisdiction in relation to professional misconduct and criminal offences is now regulated by sections 36 and 38 to 45 of, and Schedule 4 to, the Medical Act 1983. This Act provides that, if any medical practitioner registered with the GMC:

1. Is found by the Professional Conduct Committee to have been convicted in the British Isles of a criminal offence; or
2. Is judged by the Professional Conduct Committee to have been guilty of serious professional misconduct,

the Committee may, if it thinks fit, direct that his/her name shall be erased from the Register, or that his/her registration be suspended for a period not exceeding 12 months, or that his/her registration shall be conditional on his/her compliance, during a period not exceeding 3 years, with such requirements as the Committee sees fit to impose for the protection of members of the public or in his/her interests.

Cases submitted to the GMC must be presented in the form of a statutory declaration (Figure 38-1). The majority of cases submitted to the GMC by pharmaceutical companies recently have been mediated through the ABPI. The simple statutory declaration must be accompanied by a report setting out the details of the case, including a description of the clinical study, the method of recruitment of the doctor to whom the report refers, the monitoring process, how suspicions were first raised, how they were investigated, and how the conclusion was reached that led to the case being presented to the GMC. Supporting documents are required, although these best follow the declaration and the report. These supporting documents include the clinical study protocol, the recruitment letter(s) to the doctor

The President
General Medical Council
178 Great Portland Street
London
WIN 6JE

Sir

I /We, the undersigned, Dr (*name*), Medical Director of (*company*), of (*company address*), do solemnly and sincerely declare as follows:

That Dr (*name of defendant*), (*position held, i.e. general practitioner, consultant surgeon, etc.*), of (*address*), has acted in a manner which has brought the medical profession into disrepute. Having considered details of the cases which are summarized in the report, a copy of which is attached to this formal declaration and forms part of it, I/*we* allege that a question of serious professional misconduct is raised by the submission of falsified data to (*company*) with the intent to deceive in the context of a clinical trial.

I/*We* make this Declaration conscientiously believing the same to be true by virtue of the Statutory Declaration Act 1835.

Signed..

Declared at:..

On: ....

Before me: ....
(Justice of the Peace/Solicitor)

Signed..

Declared at:..

On: ....

Before me: ....
(*Justice of the Peace/Solicitor*)

Figure 38.1 Statutory declaration to the GMC when submitting a case

concerned, the formal agreement with the doctor, including details of the financial arrangement, and copies of all the clinical report forms, laboratory or other reports and/or diary cards that may be suspect.

The GMC secretariat will acknowledge receipt of the statutory declaration, and will subsequently request any additional documents considered necessary to process the case before or after it has been considered by the preliminary screener. Every complaint is scrutinized meticulously, and if it appears that the evidence submitted is insufficient, the GMC's lawyers (solicitors) may be asked to make enquiries to establish additional facts. Cases recently submitted by the industry have nearly all provided sufficient evidence for this stage to be unnecessary. Nevertheless, it may not be possible for a pharmaceutical company to obtain access to patients themselves, e.g. to verify whether the patients had completed diary cards submitted by the doctor concerned, before deciding to refer a matter to the GMC. If the GMC considered such verification necessary, it would advise the pharmaceutical company accordingly and do what it could to assist.

A decision on whether action shall be taken on an allegation of serious professional misconduct is then taken by the President or by another member of the GMC appointed for the purpose (the preliminary screener). If it appears to the President that the matter is trivial, or irrelevant to the question of serious professional misconduct, he/she will normally decide that it shall proceed no further. However, to date, none of the cases referred by, or in conjunction with, the ABPI have come into this category. If it is decided to make allegations of serious professional misconduct, the doctor is informed of the allegations against him/her and is invited to submit a written explanation. If the doctor responds to this invitation, the explanation offered, which may include evidence in answer to the allegations, is placed before the Preliminary Proceedings Committee that next considers the case.

After considering a case of alleged serious professional misconduct, the Preliminary Proceedings Committee may decide:

1. To refer the case to the Professional Conduct Committee for inquiry.
2. To send the doctor a letter.
3. To take no further action.

The letter referred to under (b) above may be a warning letter or a letter of advice, when it appears that the conduct of the doctor has fallen below the proper standard but not to have been so serious as to necessitate a public enquiry. A small number of cases referred by the pharmaceutical industry have been dealt with in this way. The names of the doctors concerned remain confidential.

Additionally, if it appears to the Preliminary Proceedings Committee that the doctor may be suffering from a physical or mental illness that seriously impairs his/her fitness to practise, the Committee may refer the case to the Health Committee instead of to the Professional Conduct Committee. This safeguard for the doctor concerned is important, and has been used in at least one case referred to the GMC by the industry.

The rules governing the operation of the Professional Conduct Committee require that any allegation of serious professional misconduct, *unless admitted by the doctor*, must be strictly proved by evidence, and the doctor is free to dispute and rebut the evidence called. This means that it is essential that cases referred by companies to the GMC must be supported by the strongest possible evidence. The doctor is entitled to submit evidence and witnesses to rebut the allegations, to call attention to any mitigating circumstances, and to produce testimonials or other evidence as to character. Pharmaceutical companies may be required to provide witnesses for cross-examination, but the case may be so strong that such witnesses are not needed. This is what has happened in the 23 cases referred by pharmaceutical companies in conjunction with the ABPI that, to date, have been considered by the Professional Conduct Committee (Anon, 1988; Andersen et al, 1992; Smith, 1997; Lock, 1989). If the facts alleged are found by the Committee to have been proved, then it is up to the Committee to determine whether, in relation to those facts, the doctor has indeed been guilty of serious professional misconduct.

At the conclusion of an inquiry in which a doctor is found guilty of serious professional misconduct, the Professional Conduct Committee must decide on one of the following courses:

1. To conclude the case without affecting the doctor's registration, although it may admonish the doctor.
2. To postpone its determination.
3. To direct that the doctor's registration be conditional on his compliance, for a period not exceeding 3 years, with such requirements as the Committee may think to impose for the protection of members of the public, or in the doctor's own interests.
4. To direct that the doctor's registration shall be suspended for a period not exceeding 12 months. or
5. To direct the erasure of the doctor's name from the Register.

Doctors who are suspended or erased have 28 days in which to give notice of appeal against the direction to the Judicial Committee of the Privy Council.

In the 23 cases referred to above, all 23 doctors were found guilty of serious professional misconduct. To date, about half have been erased from the register, and the rest have received lesser disciplinary punishment.

Section VIII

Business Aspects

39

The Multinational Corporations: Cultural Challenges, the Legal/Regulatory Framework and the Medico-commercial Environment

R. Drucker* and R. Graham Hughes*

Technomark Consulting Services, London, UK

CULTURAL CHALLENGES

'Culture' has been defined as the 'totality of so-cially transmitted behaviour patterns, arts, beliefs, institutions, and all other products of human work and thought typical of a population or community at a given time' (Webster's Dictionary, 1984). With respect to the multinational pharmaceutical cor-poration, culture can be thought of at three levels: (a) societal; (b) medical; and (c) corporate. At each level, culture has an omnipresent impact on drug development, prior to and after regulatory ap-proval. Sensitivity to cultural considerations will help identify, conceive, present, and respond to issues in drug development. It may also help to identify sources of competitive advantage.

Societal Culture

Societal culture describes those attributes of cul-ture pervading a population or community inhabit-ing a given geographical area. Individuals from the same societal culture share common values. A multinational corporation has to deal with many societal cultures, even, sometimes, within a single nation. Differences in societal culture will result in different responses to key issues. Table 39.1 indi-cates a range of culturally determined responses to important questions.

One can apply the concepts in this table to the pharmaceutical industry, e.g., to management prac-tices originating from one culture being applied in a different cultural setting. For example, companies

Table 39.1 Cultural influences on life issues

Cultural approaches	1	2	3
What is the character of human nature?	Man is evil	Man is a mixture of good and evil	Man is good
What is the relationship of man to nature?	Man is subject to nature	Man is in harmony with nature	Man is master of nature
What is the temporal focus of life?	To the past	To the present	To the future
What is the modality of man's activities?	Activity that gives spontaneous expression to impulse and desires	Activity that emphasizes as a goal the development of all aspects of the self	Activity that is motivated primarily toward measurable accomplishments
What is the relationship of man to man?	Lineal—group goals are primary and an important goal is continuity through time	Collateral—group goals are primary. Well-regulated continuity of group relationships through time is not critical	Individual—the individual goals are most important

Modified from Kluckhohn and Strodtbeck (1961).

Principles and Practice of Pharmaceutical Medicine. Edited by A. J. Fletcher, Lionel D. Edwards, Anthony W. Fox and Peter Stonier © 2002 John Wiley & Sons Ltd.

in the USA tend to use control systems that exert more checks and balances on personnel than do European companies, possibly reflecting America's puritan heritage (embodying the belief that man is intrinsically evil). In a recent merger of a European and an American pharmaceutical company, some of the European executives initially expressed resentment (man is intrinsically good), when subjected to American control systems. Similarly, companies with development programs involving contraceptive drugs have sometimes aroused criticisms among their personnel, depending on country, religious background, and personal beliefs.

Group goals are emphasized by those who see a lineal relationship of man to man as important. This is in stark contrast to those cultures of an individualistic disposition that emphasize individual goals. Concern for the welfare of the extended family might result in the hiring of a close relative in one culture, but cause accusations of nepotism in another.

Medical Culture

Differing perceptions of health and disease by patients, health care providers, and governing and regulatory bodies, are the primary elements of medical culture (Riphagen, 1992). Aspects of medical culture of particular importance to the pharmaceutical industry are those affecting drug development, approval, and marketing, including those that may determine whether a drug should have prescription or over-the-counter status. Other aspects of concern are the type of healthcare funding favored by a particular culture—private insurance or public funding through taxation.

An attempted convergence of medical cultures is currently under way in the area of drug development and regulatory approval, under the auspices of the International Committee on Harmonization (ICH). It remains to be seen whether regulatory harmonization will produce increasing uniformity of prescribing behavior. Convergent thinking is also seen in a worldwide effort to control healthcare expenditure. The various cost-cutting approaches have included:

- Reduced prescribing volume.
- Decreased price of medicines.
- Decreased reimbursement for medicines.
- Delisting of medicines from reimbursement lists.
- Encouragement to parallel trade.
- Control of overall company profitability.
- Drug formularies.
- Encouragement of generic substitution.
- Encouragement of therapeutic substitution.
- Assignment of pharmaceutical budgets to institutions and individuals.
- Encouragement of self-medication.

Despite the calls for cultural convergence in medicine, there are major differences in the incidence and prevalence of many diseases between countries. Even in a relatively homogeneous region such as Western Europe, the incidence of adverse drug reactions to a standard therapy varies dramatically from country to country. The perception of the nature and significance of given disease states varies by country, and the trigger to seek professional assistance also varies. The ensuing doctor–patient relationships reflect not only the national medical culture but also broader societal culture in such practical matters as the patient's 'right to know', freedom of information, tendency to litigation for malpractice, etc.

Corporate Culture

The principal concern of the multinational corporation is the extent to which corporate culture conflicts with societal and medical culture in each country in which the company operates. Corporate culture is evidenced by shared values about the conduct of business. A culture may be strong or weak. An example of a strong corporate culture that crosses business and geographical boundaries is that of Procter and Gamble. In any company, the corporate culture permeates every aspect of the company's activities, affecting promotion prospects, risk propensity, and individual and group behavior.

The most successful corporate culture can foster leadership that is responsive to potential conflict arising in multinational operations from cultural diversity. Organizations with such a culture express a clear vision that is understood and supported internationally. Such organizations benefit from an alignment of business values among employees worldwide, despite varied national and cultural backgrounds.

Complexities can arise when a multinational pharmaceutical company engages the services of another organization, such as a multinational contract research organization (CRO), with potentially different corporate cultures. In each country where the two multinationals collaborate, there is a need to reconcile their corporate cultures, whilst simultaneously being responsive to local societal and medical cultural considerations.

Languages

A multinational corporation necessarily conducts its business in many different languages, presenting challenges of internal and external communications. Companies with a weak corporate culture are paradoxically more likely to cause local tensions by insisting on a rigid mode of operation. Companies with a strong corporate culture are more likely to operate according to local cultural norms under the guidance of local management.

Societal, Medical and Corporate Culture Interplay

Figure 39.1 depicts how the cultural responsiveness of a company in a given country is determined by the overlap of its corporate culture with local societal and medical cultures. The more that the circle corresponding with corporate culture overlaps those of societal and medical culture, the more the area available for culturally appropriate behavior is increased. Figure 39.1 also provides a framework for comparing central with peripheral control of national affiliates. There are many determinants of the balance between the two. However, if a corporate culture is dissonant with the societal and medical cultural imperatives of a subsidiary or affiliate organization, yet is imposed upon that organization because of a policy of 'centralization', then a suboptimal outcome is likely. Conversely, a strong, responsive corporate culture that is consonant with local societal and medical values increases the likelihood of success. A locally responsive corporate culture favors neither centralization nor

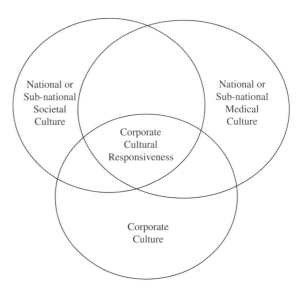

Figure 39.1 Venn diagram identifying area available for culturally appropriate behavior

decentralization—this will depend upon many other considerations (e.g. size of operations, in-country management capability, etc.). However, it facilitates an appropriate devolution of managerial power, which might otherwise be difficult or even impossible. The challenge to the multinational corporation, therefore, is to have a strong corporate culture that is compatible with diverse societal and medical cultures.

THE LEGAL/REGULATORY FRAMEWORK FOR DRUG DEVELOPMENT IN EUROPE AND THE USA

In the USA, the Code of Federal Regulations (CFR), as interpreted by the Food and Drug Administration (FDA), determines the conduct of drug-related activities, including clinical trials. Its two principal medicinal product evaluation arms are CDER (Center for Drug Evaluation and Research), which evaluates drugs, and CBER (Center for Biologicals Evaluation and Research), which evaluates biologicals (vaccines, recombinant products, antibodies, etc). Companies have a statutory right to convene meetings with the FDA at a variety of stages, even before the first human studies, to reduce some of the uncertainties of the process.

In Europe, the European Commission (EC), through its Directorate General, DG III, responsible for trade including pharmaceuticals, and the Committee for Proprietary Medicinal products (CPMP), issued, on November 20 1996, draft notes for guidance, with a 6 month consultation period, on (a) non-clinical safety studies for the conduct of human clinical trials for pharmaceuticals (CPMP/ICH/286/95); and (b) general considerations for clinical trials (CPMP/ICH/291/95). Further revisons are expected. A directive on good clinical practices (GCP) will follow.

Both notes for guidance are derived from the International Conference on Harmonization (ICH) document *General Considerations for Clinical Trials*, which seeks to:

- Describe the internationally accepted principles and practices in the conduct of both individual clinical trials and the overall development strategy for new medicinal products.
- Facilitate the evaluation and acceptance of foreign clinical trial data by promoting common understanding of general principles and approaches, and also the definition of relevant terms.
- Present an overview of the ICH clinical safety and efficacy documents and facilitate the user's access to guidance pertinent to clinical trials within these documents.

Until a harmonized system for the approval of clinical trials is adopted in the European Union (EU) (and probably other non-EU European countries at about the same time), the fragmented national systems will continue to operate.

In Western Europe, there is no uniformity in the order of approval/submission of documentation by the various parties involved. In some countries, approval of a study by the local or national ethics committee is required before documentation is submitted to the competent national authorities, whilst in others this order is reversed.

Some countries vary the procedures depending on the phase of the study. For instance, in the UK, Ethics Committee Approval only is required for Phase I studies, while for Phases II–III a clinical trial exemption (CTX) is required. Some countries, e.g. Belgium and Germany, require only notification of intended studies, sent to the Competent Authorities, while others require advance approval. These different requirements are set out in Table 39.2. The documentation that is required to be submitted to the authorities is also quite variable (Table 39.3). Some countries require brief summaries of available information, while others require detailed information on the preclinical, pharmacy, chemistry, and other clinical data to be submitted. All European countries require, in common with the USA, and in conformity with the Declaration of Helsinki, that ethics committees (the European version of institutional review boards in the USA)

Table 39.2 European regulatory clearance procedures for initiation of clinical trials

Clearance Procedure
Authorization all clinical phases: A, DK, E, IRL, GR, I, N, P, S, SF, USA
Authorization phases II & III only: UK
Notification all clinical phases: B, CH, D, F, L
Notification phases II & III only: NL

Key: A, Austria; B, Belgium; CH, Switzerland; D, Germany; DK, Denmark; E, Spain; F, France; GR, Greece; I, Italy; IRL, Ireland; L, Luxemburg; NL, The Netherlands; N, Norway; P, Portugal; S, Sweden; SF, Finland; UK, United Kingdom. N. B. European Uniformity will increase with a further Directive in 2001.

Table 39.3 European requirements for submissions to competent authorities to obtain clearance for initiation of clinical trials

	Protocol and supporting documents	EC (IRB) approval	Insurance certificate
Austria	X		
Belgium		X	
Denmark	X		X
Finland	X		
France		X	X
Germany	X	X	
Greece	X		X
Ireland	X		
Italy	X		
The Netherlands	X		
Norway	X	X	X
Portugal	X	X	
Spain	X		
Sweden	X		
UK	X		

review protocols from Phases I–IV and the general conduct of trials outside the formal protocol document. However, there is wide variation in Europe as to how this procedure is enacted. In countries such as France and Germany, there is a national system of ethics committees that work at a local level. Spain has a central committee that approves studies but local approval is also required. In the UK, there are a wide variety of ethics committees, such as commercial comittees, those set up by the Royal College of Physicians, and those run by local area health authorities or hospital trusts.

Local medical and societal cultural factors impact upon the ethics committee approvals, so that a study that is considered to be ethical in one country may be regarded as unethical in another. Examples of this may be the unacceptability of the use of placebo control in depression studies in Germany, while similar studies would be permitted elsewhere. Similarly, the common practice of extensive blood sampling in Belgium, especially in pediatric studies, would be regarded as excessive and hence unethical in other countries.

In the USA, there are private and public institutional review boards (IRBs); all major hospitals and teaching establishments have them. Studies in contract sites or clinics can be approved by either a private or public IRB. The CFR determines the constitution of IRBs. However, as with all matters relating to the investigational new drug (IND) process, a certain flexibility is retained so long as the FDA is kept informed. Thus, it is possible to get a foreign study accepted by the FDA, even if the IRB was not a compliant one according to CFR rules, provided that the FDA is informed first and accepts that the non-compliant IRB is acceptable at the local national level.

In the Central and Eastern Region (CEE) of Europe, the clinical trials approval system continues to evolve rapidly. In general, the regulations are converging towards the EU model of submission and approval, but local practices make interpretation at the national level a necessity for the expedient approval of any clinical trial project or program.

Different administrations have different views on their accessibility to eventual applicants for product approvals. These attitudes vary over the years, but currently the UK and French authorities are regarded as open to discussion on drug development programs, and both encourage early inter-

action. However, the advice given is never binding on the authority but is rather a reflection on the authorities' current views, which may well change in the light of further scientific or medical advances. At the other end of the spectrum, the German authorities are considered less approachable on a face-to-face basis.

The question of insurance for clinical trials is an interesting one. The EU guidelines for patient protection lay down that there should be 'sufficient' insurance provision. However, some countries have taken this requirement a step further by laying down the actual sums for which individual patients, or, in the case of Germany, the total number of patients, must be covered. In the USA, patients and volunteers are in general insured by the institution in which the study is conducted; the fees for this are not directly reimbursed by the sponsor but form part of the overall study cost.

Apart from the administrative burdens and the financial implications of insurance, timing of the approval process is of the essence. There are wide variations from country to country, which depend not only on the approval times from the competent authorities but also on the ethical committee approval times. Estimates of approval times are set out in Table 39.4.

Clearly, Europe needs to be tidied up if a harmonized system is to be introduced. However there

Table 39.4 Approval times for clinical trials

Austria	6 months
Belgium	4–12 weeks (EC and time of acknowledgement of receipt of notification)
Denmark	6–8 weeks
Finland	8–9 weeks
France	4–8 weeks (EC only)
Germany	1–2 months (EC and receipt of notification number)
Greece	3–6 months
Ireland	6–12 weeks
Italy	6–12 months (depends on whether the product is new or known)
The Netherlands	2–4 weeks (import permit time)
Norway	6 weeks
Portugal	1–2 months
Spain	2–12 months (EC and authorization)
Sweden	6 weeks
UK	5–9 weeks (+ 1–2 months for EC approval)
USA	1–6 months [plus IRB times (days to weeks)]

is likely to be significant resistance from some countries, e.g. the UK and The Netherlands, where minimization of bureaucracy allows for the rapid commencement of clinical trials. The EU advocates a streamlining of the ethical and administrative burdens, to accelerate the conduct of clinical trials without jeopardizing the safety and well-being of the subject (volunteer or patient).

The IND application system in the USA is often seen as more problematic for companies than the EU system. However, if the USA is a potential market for the product under investigation, there can be significant advantages to conducting studies under an IND, in parallel perhaps with other studies in Europe. An IND application is required in the USA before any new medicinal product may be introduced into man, or before any established product is used in an experimental or novel way. This applies not only to a commercial sponsor but also to an independent physician wishing to conduct experimental therapy for his/her own purposes. In the USA, an IND application must be accompanied by a completed form FDA 1571, which consists of a number of sections:

- Table of contents.
- Introductory statement.
- General investigational plan.
- Clinical investigator's brochure.
- Protocol(s):
     Study protocol.
     Facilities data.
     Investigator data.
     Ethical committee data.
- Chemistry, manufacturing process, and control data.
- Pharmacology and toxicology data.
- Previous human experience (if any).
- Additional information.

The concepts behind this are straightforward and not dissimilar to those of the CTX system operated in several European countries. However, full reports are generally to be submitted, together with relevant summaries to guide the reviewer through the document. Although the writing involved in the preparation of an IND may be regarded as onerous, because the FDA reviewing staff view the 1571 form as a totality, its preparation should not be regarded as a routine exercise.

Rather, it should be an occasion for a critical internal appraisal of the data available and how they support the proposed protocol. Clearly, this is how the FDA views the document. The FDA peer review is thus not just an administrative hurdle to be jumped but a useful, if not indispensable, aspect of the drug development program.

One aspect of this is the ready, statutory availability of the FDA to study sponsors. The sponsors are encouraged by the FDA to hold well-prepared and structured pre-IND meetings before the IND is filed. Provided that the FDA is well briefed beforehand with summary documents of all the technical/medical data available and a full protocol, such meetings can be very helpful and constructive to sponsors, who can get a good understanding of the FDA's feelings and concerns in particular therapeutic areas. The FDA also encourages sponsors to hold meetings at various points along the development path, which again can be most helpful in continuing the program of development.

Once studies have received IND approval, further protocols can be added with little trouble. Of course, the IND lays down responsibilities for sponsors, which include minimum reporting times for adverse events and completion of qualification forms for investigators, etc. These steps add to the administrative load of the clinical drug development process. It is generally thought that it would be a bold company that submitted a NDA to the FDA without the FDA's prior involvement via an IND. However, this has been done successfully in the past and will probably occur again.

A very important cultural difference between Europe and the USA, that impacts upon drug development, is indirectly expressed at the stage when the regulatory authority examines the final submitted dossier. In the USA, the FDA adopts a bottom-up stance, in which it looks at the basic raw data and sees what conclusions can be drawn from it, using its own criteria for analysis and interpretation. In Europe the authorities adopt an attitude diametrically opposed to that of the FDA, by looking at the conclusions of all the studies, as manifested in the proposed labelling, patient leaflets, and summary of product information, and examining to what extent the data presented justify these conclusions. In Europe, considerable importance is placed on the role of independent experts, whose critical reports on the various sections of the dossier provide a sort of *vade mecum* for the reviewer. It is vitally important to understand in detail that the expert report required in Europe is not the same as the integrated summary required by the FDA.

Whatever some recalcitrant politicians may think, Europe, in the pharmaceutical development sense, is becoming very much a federal system. The EU, consisting of some 15 member states, lays down through directives, decisions, rules and regulations, a basic framework for the conduct of drug development in its member states. However, each of the member states overlays its own special set of laws, which make each country a special case. In addition, other European countries, not EU members, have adopted and adapted the EU system to fit in with their own cultural and political needs. Those Central European countries shortlisted for EU membership have made great strides towards adopting EU practices, but still retain their local idiosyncrasies.

In drug development, therefore, significant differences exist on a country-by-country basis in Europe as well as, to a far lesser extent, on a state-by-state basis in the USA. These differences manifest themselves not only in the legal/regulatory framework but also in the commercial practices that surround the conduct of clinical trials by licensed medical practitioners.

THE MEDICO-COMMERCIAL ENVIRONMENT IN THE USA AND EUROPE

One of the major differences between the USA and Europe, as regards the conduct of clinical trials, is the financing of medical care in the two regions. Throughout Europe, medical care is largely funded by governments. In the USA, medical care is largely funded through private insurance, generally paid by a person's employer. Coverage for many of those less able to pay, such as the indigent and the elderly, is provided by the government through the Medicare and Medicaid programs. Military veterans are eligible for medical treatment through the VA program. However, a significant number of people in the USA do not have private insurance and are not eligible for Medicare, Medicaid, or VA medical care. For patients without ready access to medical care, participation in a clinical trial may provide needed medical care.

Contract investigational sites (CISs) are organizations that run clinical trials, using physicians who are full-time, part-time, or contract employees. The companies employ regulatory staff, for IRB filing, adverse event notification, etc. as well as site coordinators, nurses, and quality control personnel. CISs recruit patients on behalf of their doctors, either from databases built up over the years, or by press and radio/TV advertising, and even by direct telemarketing. Non-physician CIS staff do initial screening of potential subjects on the telephone and in face-to-face interviews. Most CISs exist in conventional treatment centers; others treat only patients who are enrolled into clinical studies, and have no other role than to run clinical trials, rather in the same way as Phase I units.

The advantages for the sponsor are several: recruitment by sites is rapid, they are used to dealing with IRBs, monitoring is straightforward, the quality of data is good and the general service is cost-effective. For the patient, there is free medical care and medication, together with 'compensation' for inconvenience, which can add up to an appreciable sum ($500+).

CISs may be multispecialty or be concentrated on a single therapeutic area around a single investigator or opinion leader. Some of the larger CIS companies, with 50–100 employees, are drifting in the direction of becoming full CROs. Others are becoming site management organizations (SMOs), which offer coordination, recruitment, and the other CIS services via other independent specialists. The total number of CISs in the USA may exceed 200—most major cities have at least one.

Increasingly in the USA, sponsors and CROs are turning to CISs for rapid, quality, patient recruitment. This means that the role of the individual investigator is diminishing, although sponsors still run studies that involve opinion leaders and university professor-level investigators, albeit fewer overall. By contrast, in Europe the CIS concept is more weakly established. A few organizations that are broadly similar to the CIS have sprung up, notably in the UK. Sometimes these have been started by groups of general practitioners already running clinical trials. However, nowhere in the UK is there an organization that carries out the full range of function that a US CIS does: the free access of patients in the UK to medical treatment may be one of the reasons.

Some hospital units in Europe have recently become more commercially minded and have set themselves up as profit centers within their own hospitals. As financial pressures increase, with the increased cost of medical technology and the unfavourable demographics of an ageing population, we would expect more hospitals to go along this route.

This leads to one other clinical development arena that does appear different between the USA and Europe: clinical pharmacology. Europe has a long tradition of high-class, highly scientific clinical pharmacology. This has led to the setting up of a significant number of independent companies, which have been spun-off from, or were formed in association with, departments of clinical pharmacology in hospitals. Such units routinely carry out studies involving first administration to man, rising dose tolerance, pharmacodynamics, and sophisticated pharmacokinetics. In the USA such studies are more likely to be carried out in the university hospitals themselves, with the Phase I CROs, generally not associated with hospitals, carrying out the more routine bioequivalence and bio-availability work.

Thus, we have an interesting contrast in clinical development. In the USA, Phases II–III are exploited more and more by commercial contract investigational sites, under the strict regulation of the IND process. In Europe, CISs are just beginning, while Phase I is much more of a commercial enterprise that is subject to little regulatory control, although ethics committees keep a watchful eye over such studies.

Differences in societal and medical cultures thus impact significantly on the development of novel drugs. The ICH process has, to a major extent, harmonized requirements but cannot and will not of itself influence how the data to fulfill these requirements are generated and collected. For the foreseeable future, the USA will be seen as the more prescriptive, litigious society—suspicious of the results, building conclusions from the evidence. Europe, in so far as it can be regarded as a unity, even today, has yet to accept the ever-present lawyer in all public contexts, so that to the American observer it will continue to look laissez-faire and superficial in its regulation of drug development.

REFERENCES

Kluckhohn F, Strodtbeck F (1961) *Variations in Value Orientation*. Row, Peterson: Evanston, IL.
Payer L (1990) *Medicine and Culture: Notions of Health and Sickness*. Gollancz: London.
Riphagen F (1992) Different practices and perceptions from country to country. In *Conference Proceedings*: *How to Cope with Different Medical Cultures in Europe*. IBC: London.
Webster's (1984) *New Riverside University Dictionary II*. Riverside Publishing co: Baltimore MD Philadelphia PA.

40

Outsourcing Clinical Drug Development Activities to Contract Research Organizations (CROs): Critical Success Factors

John R. Vogel

John R. Vogel Associates, Kihei, HI, USA

The field of drug development has changed markedly since the late 1980s. Biotechnology has created opportunities to diagnose and treat diseases (e.g. Lou Gherig's disease) for which modern medicine had all but given up. Clinical trials may involve novel therapies that are linked with unique delivery systems (e.g. monoclonal antibodies). Regulatory harmonization through the International Committee on Harmonization (the ICH Guidelines) has made it possible to conduct clinical trials on a global scale. But the most dramatic change in modern drug development is the trend toward extensive contracting of drug-development responsibilities to contract research organizations (CROs).

The pressures from without have been matched by the pressures from within. Since 1994, the pharmaceutical industry has eliminated more than 40 000 jobs, many in R&D. The task of developing new products with smaller in-house staffs led pharmaceutical companies to increase their reliance on CROs. It is estimated (Getz and Vogel 1995) that 52% of clinical studies are partly or completely contracted.

As pharmaceutical companies strive to increase productivity and decrease costs, they need to improve their skills in dealing with CROs. This chapter examines the challenges of outsourcing clinical drug development activities and identifies critical success factors for working with CROs.

PHARMACEUTICAL INDUSTRY VIEWS OF CROS

'Traditional' View of a CRO

The view that working with a CRO involves unacceptable risk is often expressed by pharmaceutical industry personnel. One project leader who had successfully developed several drugs commented: 'There is significant risk in relying on CROs. I would rather use my own personnel'. The characteristics of this 'traditional' view of working with a CRO are shown in Table 40.1.

In-house staffing is based on long-term workload projections, which focus on the peaks rather than the valleys. The CRO is used as a back-up, a finger in the dike, when the workload exceeds projections, or when staffing levels fall due to a hiring freeze. The CRO is treated as an extension of in-house staff and may be asked to relocate its

Table 40.1 'Traditional' view of a CRO

In-house staffing is based on expected workload
A CRO is used when in-house resources become inadequate
A crisis management atmosphere exists
The CRO is viewed as an extension of in-house staff
The scope of services was limited
Time is a major concern

Principles and Practice of Pharmaceutical Medicine. Edited by A. J. Fletcher, Lionel D. Edwards, Anthony W. Fox and Peter Stonier © 2002 John Wiley & Sons Ltd.

personnel to the sponsor's site. In order to minimize risk, the sponsor contracts the minimum range of services and retains the critical activities for its own staff. The decision to use a CRO is delayed until all other options are exhausted. CRO evaluation and selection occurs at the eleventh hour in a 'crisis' atmosphere, where time is the major concern, rather than quality or cost.

Using a CRO in such a way often leads to disappointing results. Outsourcing failures can usually be traced to one of three causes:

- The sponsor selects the wrong CRO;
- The sponsor does not articulate its needs clearly; or
- The sponsor does not manage the project.

'Modern' View of a CRO

Success with outsourcing, on the other hand, has led senior executives to express such views as: 'If I can contract out cafeteria and building maintenance, I can contract out clinical research'. Characteristics of this modern view of working with a CRO are illustrated in Table 40.2.

In this view, the composition of in-house staff is determined by 'core' needs—what will be needed to design the study, select the CRO and manage the program. The drug development plan includes a description of which studies and services will be contracted. A list of 'prequalified' CROs is developed by matching the sponsor's anticipated needs with the range of services and therapeutic area expertise various CROs provide. The role of the sponsor's personnel is redefined from conducting the project to managing the CRO. Its staff receive training on how to work with CROs. Advance planning and training enables the sponsor to direct its attention to assessing quality and cost of CRO services.

Table 40.2 'Modern' view of a CRO

In-house staffing is based on 'core' needs
CROs are included in resource planning
CROs are prequalified, based on therapeutic expertise, range of services, and compatibility with the sponsor
Personnel are trained in CRO skills
Quality and cost are the major concerns

The Role of CROs in Drug Development

Surveys of pharmaceutical industry use of CROs (Vogel 1993; Getz and Vogel 1995) have shown that outsourcing is expanding. More studies are being contracted to CROs. Getz and Vogel (1995) reported that the percentage of clinical development projects in which CROs played a role increased from 28% in 1993 to 52% in 1995. In addition, a wider range of services is being contracted. In 1992 sponsors were most likely to contract out site recruitment and study monitoring, while other activities were conducted in house. By 1994, sponsors reported large increases in the use of CROs for data management, statistical analysis, and medical writing. Sponsors are more likely today to contract out large Phase III studies that are critical to regulatory approval. CROs are also more likely to be involved in study design. Sponsors are increasingly using multinational CROs to conduct global drug development programs.

DECIDING WHEN TO USE A CRO

Strategies for using CROs typically fall into three categories:

- Tactical outsourcing.
- Maximal outsourcing.
- Strategic outsourcing.

Tactical Outsourcing

This is essentially the 'traditional' view of outsourcing. A sponsor maintains in-house staff levels capable of performing the projected workload. Individual studies or selected activities within a study are contracted to a CRO only when in-house resources become inadequate because of an unforeseen study or a reduction in staff.

Advantages to tactical outsourcing are that the sponsor can exert maximum control over the project. Risk is limited by outsourcing a minimum scope of services (e.g. study monitoring but not data management and analysis). Many sponsors believe it is less costly to use in-house resources, although Hill (1994) suggests that the costs of contracting out are roughly equivalent. A further advantage is that the sponsor maintains in-house drug development expertise.

However, tactical outsourcing has significant disadvantages. It is likely that in-house staff exceeds needs from time to time. If development of a poorly performing drug is terminated, the result may be lay-offs, severance payments, and relocation costs. A project in a new therapeutic area may require new personnel knowledgeable about that area. Staffing up for large Phase III studies, which typically involve thousands of patients, is expensive. Minimizing the work contracted to CROs provides little opportunity for the sponsor's staff to acquire the necessary skills to work with CROs when they are needed. If the sponsor delays the decision to use a CRO until the last minute, finding and contracting with the CRO may delay the study. The pressure to select a CRO provides inadequate opportunity to define the sponsor's needs and select the right CRO.

Maximum Outsourcing

With this strategy the sponsor outsources nearly all of its clinical development activities to CROs. Some pharmaceutical senior executives have expressed the desire to minimize in-house staff and outsource 'everything'.

This strategy has the advantage of minimizing fixed costs and eliminates the need to acquire detailed expertise when the sponsor enters a new therapeutic area. However, there are many disadvantages to maximal outsourcing. Minimal sponsor involvement in a study may lead to deficiencies in quality, cost, and timing. Contracting early Phase II studies to a CRO reduces contact with investigators and may prevent the sponsor from learning important information about the drug. The sponsor risks losing in-house drug development expertise, which many consider to be a core competency, and has no 'fallback' option if it is dissatisfied with the CRO's performance.

Strategic Outsourcing

This approach uses a mix of in-house and outside resources. It is closest to the modern view outlined earlier. The sponsor conducts Phase I and early Phase II studies, and hires CROs to conduct larger and routine studies (e.g. late Phase II and Phase III). An important corollary of strategic outsourcing is that CROs are prequalified according to projected sponsor needs. Relationships are developed between the sponsor and certain CROs that can perform particular types of studies.

Advantages to strategic outsourcing include quick feedback from investigators during early studies and the focusing of in-house staff on 'core' needs, such as designing the clinical program, conducting initial studies and managing CROs. In-house drug development expertise is maintained. Because the sponsor uses in-house resources for early studies, there is more lead time to select and contract with a CRO. The two difficulties with this approach are (a) that personnel must be trained on how to work with and manage a CRO, and (b) that the sponsor must ensure compatibility between its standards and procedures and those of the CRO (e.g. ensure database compatibility).

FREQUENT CAUSES OF SPONSOR/CRO PROBLEMS

Problems with contracted studies can often be traced to one of three causes:

1. *The wrong CRO is selected.* Sponsors often make the mistake of assuming that a CRO that has performed well on one study will be equally capable of conducting a study in a different therapeutic area. Some sponsors mistakenly assume that all CROs are the same, and that it is not possible to determine which one will be most capable of performing a planned study.
2. *The sponsor fails to articulate its needs clearly.* Sponsors sometimes issue a request for proposal (RFP) with little more than a protocol outline, and expect CROs to guess what services and resources are required. The result of inadequate information is that CROs underestimate the sponsor's needs, assigning insufficient numbers of personnel or inadequately trained staff to the study. This can result in errors, delays, and cost overruns.
3. *The sponsor fails to manage the study.* Sponsors sometimes make the mistake of assuming

that in-house resources are not needed once the study is outsourced. In most cases the sponsor should continue to play a critical role in a contracted study, providing guidance to the CRO and ensuring that agreed standards and timelines are achieved.

Three Critical Steps to Ensure Success with a CRO

In order to ensure successful outsourcing, the sponsor should focus on three critical steps:

1. Determine accurate study specifications.
2. Select the right CRO; and
3. Manage the study.

The remainder of this chapter outlines the benefits of these steps and describes specific activities that sponsors should carry out to ensure successful outsourcing.

DETERMINE STUDY SPECIFICATIONS

Study specifications are a list of activities required to initiate, conduct, analyze, and report the results of a clinical study. They include tasks that will be performed in-house and those to be contracted out to one or more CROs (Vogel and Nelson 1993).

Importance of Accurate Study Specifications

Accurate study specifications are a critical tool for planning a study. They assign responsibility to the various disciplines involved in the study (e.g. clinical research, regulatory affairs, data management, clinical manufacturing, programming, statistics and medical writing). By comparing study specifications with internal capabilities, the sponsor can identify activities that must be contracted out. This analysis also provides useful criteria for selecting the right type of CRO, a niche provider or full-service CRO. Study specifications also enable the sponsor to make more accurate projections of study costs and timing.

Study specifications are an essential element of the sponsor's request for proposal (RFP) and the CRO's proposal. Study specifications should be included in the RFP in order to familiarize CROs with the sponsor's project and goals. Study specifications enable the CRO to break down the individual tasks and materials on which it is asked to quote cost and timing, and provides a useful format for the budget proposal.

Accurate study specifications enable the CRO to perform a 'reality check' on the sponsor's expectations. Often, CROs add items to the study specifications (e.g. activities or materials to be provided by the sponsor or other CRO services) that the sponsor may have overlooked. In rare cases, CROs have declined to submit a proposal because they believe the sponsor's study specifications describe an unachievable study plan. The study specifications also enable the sponsor to conduct a 'reality check' on the CRO's understanding of the study and to determine that the proposal covers the project scope. Study specifications facilitate comparison of proposals from different CROs and help ensure that the sponsor's attention is focused on the resources the CRO will provide, as well as on the proposed budget.

Study specifications are also an important tool for managing the study. They help define the various in-house disciplines that will be interacting with the CRO and to project the level of sponsor involvement required. They help focus the sponsor's attention on the deliverables and provide milestones and timelines to assist the sponsor in measuring study progress. Accurate study specifications promote a thorough evaluation of the CRO's performance during, and on completion of, the study.

The Study Specifications Worksheet

An example of a study specifications worksheet is shown in Figure 40.1. The first page of the worksheet, entitled Study Details, is designed to provide an overview of the study and includes information on key parameters, such as the number of patients, number of visits, expected enrollment rate, and number of sites. It also includes information on the health-care setting (e.g. academic medical center, private practice or managed care) and the regulatory status of the product. The Materials and Actions section of the worksheet is divided into 21

STUDY SPECIFICATIONS WORKSHEET

Study details

1. Project leader:

2. Product name:

3. Dose form:

4. Indication

5. Study objective:

6. Study design:

7. Total number of patients:

8. Age range:

9. Sex:

10. Number of visits (run-in phase):

11. Number of visits (treatment phase):

12. Number of visits (follow-up phase):

13. Expected enrollment rate:

14. Number of study sites:

15. Minimum number of patients/site:

16. Healthcare setting:

 _____ Academic   _____ Managed care

 _____ Private practice   _____ Other (specify)

17. Regulatory status:

 _____ New IND   _____ Phase II

 _____ Phase III   _____ Phase IIIb

 _____ Phase IV   _____ Other (specify):

Figure 40.1   Study specifications worksheet

Figure 40.1 (*continued*)

STUDY SPECIFICATIONS WORKSHEET

Activity	Sponsor's responsibility	CRO's responsibility
Materials and actions		
1. IND reporting		
A. Prepare IND updates		
B. Submit IND updates to regulatory agencies		
2. Protocol preparation		
A. Design study		
B. Write protocol		
C. Draft informed consent		
3. Case report form preparation		
A. Design case report forms		
B. Print case report forms		
4. Pre-study preparation		
A. Propose study sites		
B. Provide site evaluation reports		
C. Select investigators		
D. Provide central IRB		
E. Negotiate site budgets		
5. Investigator meeting		
A. Plan investigator meeting		
B. Conduct investigator meeting		
6. Study initiation		
A. Validate pre-study documents		
B. Set up investigator files		
C. Conduct initiation visit at each site		

STUDY SPECIFICATIONS WORKSHEET

Materials and actions		
Activity	Sponsor's responsibility	CRO's responsibility
7. Site monitoring		
A. Conduct monitoring visits (at intervals of __ weeks)		
B. Maintain telephone contacts with study sites (at intervals of __ weeks)		
C. Provide written monitoring reports to sponsor (at intervals of __ weeks)		
D. Communicate with sponsor via electronic mail		
8. Site closeout		
A. Perform drug accountability audit		
B. Dispose of unused clinical supplies		
C. Provide closeout report		
9. Regulatory auditing		
A. Audit study sites		
B. Provide audit report		
10. Serious adverse event (SAE) reporting		
Submit SAE reports to sponsor		
11. Site management		
A. Negotiate investigator grants/contracts		
B. Manage investigator payments		
C. Provide project status reports to sponsor at intervals of __ weeks)		
12. Project management		
A. Conduct project management meetings		
B. Provide minutes of meetings		
C. Provide project status reports		
D. Provide data management reports		
13. Database design and validation		
A. Design database		
B. Set up data-entry program		
C. Create database		

Figure 40.1   (*continued*)

STUDY SPECIFICATIONS WORKSHEET

Materials and actions		
Activity	Sponsor's responsibility	CRO's responsibility
14. Data cleanup		
A. Write data management guidelines and edit specifications		
B. Run edit checks		
C. Clean up case report forms		
D. Perform Q.C. on __ % of CRFs		
15. Data entry		
A. Enter CRFs		
B. Code adverse events and concomitant medications		
16. Generation and review of tables		
A. Prepare tables and listings		
B. Perform Q.C. on __ % of tables		
17. Statistical plan and analysis		
A. Generate statistical plan		
B. Prepare shell tables and listings		
C. Perform analysis		
D. Write statistical methods		
18. Integrated clinical and statistical report		
A. Prepare integrated tables		
B. Write statistical methods		
C. Provide discussion of the significance of results		
19. Manuscript preparation		
A. Prepare draft manuscript		
B. Prepare up to __ revisions		
C. Prepare abstract		
20. Drug packaging and distribution		
A. Formulate and package drugs		
B. Create randomization schedule		

STUDY SPECIFICATIONS WORKSHEET

Materials and actions			
	Activity	Sponsor's responsibility	CRO's responsibility
21.	Regulatory submissions		
	A. Prepare NDA/PLA		
	B. Prepare SNDA		
	C. Prepare CANDA/CAPLA		
	D. Prepare IND/NDA annual report		
	E. Prepare 120-day safety updates		

categories, chosen after consultation with several CROs and designed to be consistent with activities on which CROs base their bids. In order to facilitate the process, sponsors should use these suggested categories.

Within each category are several specific activities listed as examples. The sponsor may list as many specific activities as appropriate for the study. For each activity the sponsor should indicate whether that activity will be the sponsor's responsibility or the CRO's responsibility by placing a check in the appropriate column. In those cases where the sponsor feels that the activity will be shared with the CRO, sponsors should examine the activity to determine whether it could be broken down into more discrete items. This will minimize confusion over who actually is responsible for the activity. The last section of the study specifications worksheet is entitled Project Timeline. It contains the sponsor's projected dates for completion of study milestones. Twenty-six suggested milestones are listed; the sponsor may wish to modify the list according to its own milestones.

Preparing Study Specifications

Study specifications are typically prepared by the sponsor's project team or the project leader. Small companies may hire a drug development consultant or a CRO to help prepare study specifications. Preparation of study specifications should begin 4–6 months before the study begins. Details of all activities may not be available at this point, but sufficient lead time must be given for identifying the necessary services, evaluating in-house capability, and selecting a CRO. Details can be added as they are identified.

SELECTING THE RIGHT CRO

The Three Cs of CRO Selection

The three most important criteria for selecting a CRO are:

1. Capability.
2. Compatibility.
3. Cost.

The most important criterion is *capability*. Can the CRO provide the needed services? Are the CRO's personnel well qualified and do they have experience in the therapeutic area? If the CRO is not capable of performing the study, it will likely fail to meet the sponsor's expectations. A disastrous outcome could harm the careers of sponsor staff, delay product development, and have a negative impact on the sponsor's economic well-being.

Figure 40.1   (*continued*)

STUDY SPECIFICATIONS WORKSHEET

Project timeline		
	Milestone	Date
1.	Sign contract	
2.	Submit list of proposed study sites	
3.	Submit draft protocol	
4.	Enroll investigators	
5.	Protocol approval	
6.	Case report forms/MOPs approval	
7.	Hold multi-investigator meeting	
8.	Complete IRB approvals	
9.	Ship drugs/CRFs	
10.	First patient enrolled	
11.	Data management guidelines approved	
12.	25% of valid patients completed	
13.	50% of valid patients completed	
14.	75% of valid patients completed	
15.	Last valid patient completed	
16.	Submission of first CRF to data management	
17.	Submission of last CRF to data management	
18.	Lock database	
19.	Transfer database to sponsor	
20.	Analysis plan and shell tables/listings	
21.	Draft statistical tables and listings available	
22.	Final statistical tables and listings available	
23.	Draft integrated study report	
24.	Final study report	
25.	NDA/PLA; SNDA; CANDA/CAPLA	
26.	Publication	
27.	Other (specify):	

The second most important criterion is *compatibility*. Are the CRO's procedures and practices compatible with the sponsor's? Is the chemistry between the CRO and sponsor good? The sponsor should examine the CRO's standard operating procedures and talk with CRO staff, to determine not only whether the CRO is meeting the requirements of good clinical practices (GLP), but whether its practices closely parallel the sponsor's. CROs sometimes claim they can work 'according to the sponsor's SOPs', but the results are likely to be disappointing if the two companies have vastly different approaches or use incompatible technologies.

The third important factor is *cost*. The sponsor must ensure that the CRO's price and terms of agreement are acceptable. Sponsors are sceptical of low bids because they may result from the CRO underestimating the resources required to complete the project. High bids, on the other hand, may indicate that the CRO overvalues its services. Equally important are the business terms. Demands for large advance payment and imposition of severe penalties for cancellation should not be accepted.

Prequalifying CROs

Selecting a CRO requires effort by all sponsor disciplines involved in the study. Evaluating a large number of CROs is costly, time consuming and inefficient. A more practical approach is to prequalify CROs to identify the most appropriate candidates for in-depth evaluation. This approach has several advantages. Not all CROs can perform the same range of services. Different CROs are experienced in particular therapeutic areas. Some CROs have more recent experience in conducting studies similar to that planned by the sponsor, or staff with special expertise. Promotional material received from CROs is often not very informative. Most CRO brochures look similar, make similar claims and do not enable the sponsor to differentiate among the large number of candidates. It is important for a sponsor to distinguish between 'can do' and 'have done'. CROs are prone to claim they 'can do' whatever the sponsor wants. The sponsor should focus on what the CRO 'has done' and make its own predictions about what the CRO can do.

The automobile industry has become highly adept at prequalifying suppliers of major components. Automobile manufacturers are becoming much more design houses. They no longer put out to bid each component for each assembly. Rather, they create specifications for major components, such as transmissions or braking systems, then turn to a small group of prequalified 'first-tier' suppliers to design those components, build them and deliver them to the manufacturer. Those on the cutting edge of drug development are moving in this direction in their relationships with CROs.

The Prequalifiction Process

- *Step 1.* From an in-house database, one of the various commercial directories of CROs, or a consultant's database, the sponsor should select those CROs that offer the desired range of services and claim to have experience in the target therapeutic area.
- *Step 2.* The sponsor should contact each CRO and request the details of experience in the target therapeutic area. The CRO's response should describe specific studies completed. For each study the CRO should provide information on the range of services provided, the number of study sites, project enrollment, actual number of patients completed, and the number of months required to complete the study. The CRO should also describe the expertise of personnel who are likely to be involved in the project.
- *Step 3.* The sponsor should review the responses from the CROs and select several of the most qualified ones for on-site visits.

Leveraging CRO Experience

There are several advantages to prequalifying CROs and placing emphasis on the CRO's expertise in the target therapeutic area. A CRO with such expertise may be able to provide valuable input to the study plan and should have a ready list of qualified investigators, which could save the sponsor time. The CRO will be able to make more accurate predictions of patient enrollment if those estimates are based on recent experience rather than optimistic projections from study sites. In addition, experienced CRO staff will likely be more efficient at study monitoring, problem solving, data clean-up and report writing.

It may be possible to leverage the skills of a number of different CROs with competencies in specific areas to create a 'virtual' drug development process. In this scenario, highly specialized, narrowly focused companies provide their services along the value chain of drug development, leaving the sponsor's role as one of initial discovery of the chemical entity, then management of the drug development process and the value chain. Today, most sponsors contract with full-service CROs and closely manage the project, but some are exploring the advantages of using multiple 'niche providers' as a 'virtual' CRO (Lightfoot and Vogel 1996).

REQUESTING AND EVALUATING PROPOSALS FROM CROS

After conducting on-site visits to prequalified CROs, a sponsor should select three to five CROs who will be invited to submit a proposal.

Contents of the Request for Proposal (RFP)

The RFP consists of a cover letter, detailed instructions to proposers, a copy of the study protocol, the completed study specifications worksheet, a resource allocations worksheet, and a copy of the sponsor's standard CRO agreement. The cover letter should briefly describe the study goal, provide an overview of the clinical plan, specify the proposal due date, indicate that the CRO may be invited to present its proposal orally to the sponsor, and specify timing for the sponsor's reply. The CRO should be given approximately 2 weeks to prepare a proposal, and the sponsor should expect to reply to the proposals within 2 weeks.

Instructions to Bidders

Subjects to be covered in the instructions to bidders are listed in Table 40.3. Under the general requirements section, the sponsor should specify:

Table 40.3 Instructions to bidders

General requirements:
  Confidentiality
  Discrepancies and omissions
  Preparation costs
  Form of proposal
  Modification and withdrawal
  Contract award
  Return of documents
  Subcontracting

CRO's qualifications:
  Capabilities
  Experience
  Key personnel
  Study plan
  Investigator recruitment plan
  Availability of patients
  Project management
  Communication with sponsor
  Business terms
  Insurance

CRO's services and fees:
  Activities to be performed by the sponsor
  Services to be provided by the bidder
  Resource allocations
  Service fees
  Estimated pass-through costs

1. *Confidentiality*: the responder must treat all information in the RFP as confidential.
2. *Discrepancies and omissions*: the responder is responsible for bringing these to the sponsor's attention.
3. *Preparation costs*: the responder bears the cost of preparing and submitting the proposal.
4. *Form of proposal*: the proposal must be in the format prescribed by the sponsor and must address all areas of the RFP.
5. *Modification and withdrawal*: the responder may modify or withdraw the proposal if the sponsor receives notice prior to the proposal due date.
6. *Contract award*: the sponsor has the right to select the successful proposal or not to award the contract.
7. *Return of documents*: the responder must return the RFP if requested.
8. *Subcontracting*: the responder may not subcontract services without the sponsor's permission.

In the section on CRO qualifications, the sponsor should direct CROs to address:

9. *Capabilities*: provide a brief description of the services offered and how they relate to the activities requested.
10. *Experience*: summarize experience in the therapeutic area, including the number of prior studies conducted by personnel who are still on staff (for each study, include: number of study sites, number of subjects, study duration, and range of services) and cite the relevant experience gained by staff while in previous academic, industry or external positions.
11. *Key personnel*: briefly describe the training and experience required for key positions that will be involved in the present study (e.g. project manager, medical director, clinical research associate, data administration manager, database administrator, programmer, statistician, medical writer, and regulatory affairs manager) and provide resumés of typical personnel in these positions.
12. *Study plan*: an overview of the study design and plan for implementation.
13. *Investigator recruitment plan*: how qualified investigators will be identified (e.g. database, previous study) and evaluate their appropriateness for the study.
14. *Availability of subjects*: how subjects will be recruited (e.g. subject database, advertising) and predict the enrollment rate.
15. *Project management*: an overview of the plan to coordinate sites and manage study initiation, execution, data cleanup, analysis, report preparation and regulatory services.
16. *Communication with sponsor*: the frequency and formats for periodic progress/status reports, ability to establish specific electronic links with the sponsor (e.g. e-mail, Lotus Notes) and meetings with the sponsor.
17. *Payment terms*: terms and milestones for sponsor payments.
18. *Insurance*: a copy of insurance certificate.

The section on CRO services and fees should instruct the CRO to describe:

19. *Activities to be performed by the sponsor*: list the materials and activities the CRO expects the sponsor to provide.
20. *Services to be provided by the CRO*: list the materials and services the CRO will provide.
21. *Resource allocations*: list the types of personnel to be involved in the study, the estimated number of hours/FTEs for each skill level and the fee charged for each skill level (see the resource allocations worksheet described below).
22. *Service fees*: identify the cost for each category of service listed in the study specifications.
23. *Estimated pass-through costs*: estimates for costs that will not be subjected to mark-up (e.g. travel, central laboratory, central IRB, investigator grants).

The Resource Allocations Worksheet

The principal criterion for selecting a CRO, *capability*, is determined largely by what skill levels and amount of effort (hours/FTEs) the CRO proposes to use to conduct the study. Cost, which is another important selection criterion, is determined by the rates charged for each skill level. CROs should be required to summarize these data in a resource allocations worksheet (Figure 40.2).

The worksheet lists the same 21 service categories the sponsor addressed in the study specifications worksheet. For each category the bidder should list the types of personnel who will be involved in performing that service. For each type of personnel the CRO should define the number of hours/FTEs, the rate charged per unit of time and the total cost for that person to perform that service.

Figure 40.3 shows two examples of resource allocations for protocol preparation. On the bottom, the CRO proposes a team, consisting of a project physician, project manager, statistician, CRA, medical writer, and secretary, with a total cost of $39,120. The top shows another proposal for the same activity, where the task of writing the protocol is assigned to a physician, who will be billed at $150/h, with a total cost of $39 000.

The resource allocations enable the sponsor to make a more critical evaluation of a proposal than

RESOURCE ALLOCATIONS WORKSHEET - (Part A)

ACTIVITY	PERSONNEL	EFFORT	RATE	TOTAL	ASSUMPTIONS
1. IND reporting					
2. Protocol preparation					
3. Case report form preparation					
4. Pre-study preparation					
5. Investigator meeting					
6. Study initiation					
7. Site monitoring					
8. Site closeout					
9. Regulatory auditing					
10. Serious adverse event (SAE) reporting					
11. Site management					
12. Project management					

RESOURCE ALLOCATIONS WORKSHEET - (Part B)

ACTIVITY	PERSONNEL	EFFORT	RATE	TOTAL	ASSUMPTIONS
13. Database design and validation					
14. Data cleanup					
15. Data entry					
16. Generation and review of tables					
17. Statistical plan and analysis					
18. Integrated clinical and statistical report					
19. Manuscript preparation					
20. Drug packaging and distribution					
21. Regulatory submissions					

Figure 40.2 Resource allocations worksheet

RESOURCE ALLOCATIONS EXAMPLES

ACTIVITY	PERSONNEL	EFFORT	RATE	TOTAL	ASSUMPTIONS
EXAMPLE A Protocol preparation	Project physician	260	150	39 000	Total = $39 000
EXAMPLE B Protocol preparation	Project physician	80	150	12 000	
	Project manager	24	80	1920	
	Statistician	48	100	4800	
	CRA	120	80	9600	
	Medical writer	160	50	8000	
	Secretary	80	35	2800	Total = $39 120

Figure 40.3   Resource allocations examples

if the cost of each service were simply listed. In both these examples, the cost of writing a protocol is about $39 000. However, most sponsors would agree that the 'team approach' is highly preferable to assigning the task to an individual physician. Without the resource allocations data, the sponsor would not have been able to differentiate between the two proposals.

The sponsor should circulate the proposals to staff who represent the disciplines for which the CRO will be expected to provide services. Each staff member should review the proposals and prepare written evaluations. A convenient way to compare several proposals is to use an evaluation form, such as that proposed by Vogel and Schober (1993), seen here as Figure 40.4.

After evaluating the proposals, the sponsor may decide to invite two or three CROs for a face-to-face meeting or a conference call, to provide an opportunity for each to present its proposal and answer questions (Vogel and Resnick 1996).

MANAGING THE SPONSOR–CRO RELATIONSHIP

Defining accurate study specifications and selecting the right CRO are critical to achieving success in an outsourced study. However, careful attention must also be paid to managing the study and the sponsor–CRO relationship. The sponsor may mistakenly assume that, once the study is contracted, its staff can be fully allocated to other projects. In fact, a significant in-house effort is needed to manage the project. While it is estimated that managing an outsourced project requires only 20% of the sponsor's resources that would have been needed to conduct the same project in-house, it is an important effort.

The sponsor should follow three principles for managing an outsourced project:

1. Clarify the roles and responsibilities of the sponsor and CRO.
2. Define and use 'performance metrics' to measure study progress.
3. Ensure efficient communication between the sponsor and CRO.

Sponsor Roles and Responsibilities

It is the sponsor's responsibility to design the study, determine which materials and actions it provides, and define the services it requires from the CRO. Accurate study specifications communicate this to CROs. The sponsor must also ensure that the CRO understands and agrees to its expectations. Evaluation of proposals by a multidisciplinary sponsor team, with special attention paid to proposed resource allocations, helps the sponsor verify that CROs understand its needs and provide a reasonable plan to meet them.

The study specifications and the contract with a selected CRO identify key study milestones and timelines. These help ensure that the study is completed on schedule. However, in practice, the intervals between milestones are too long to enable the sponsor and CRO to make mid-course corrections and keep the study on target.

The sponsor needs to monitor CRO accomplishments using objective outcome measures (see discussion of 'performance metrics', below). The sponsor must recognize red flags that signal the need for corrective action. If requested by the CRO, the sponsor should assist in resolving problems by providing needed information and, if appropriate, making amendment to the study protocol. Such assistance should be provided in timely fashion and should involve the appropriate level of authority at the sponsor.

Despite the sponsor and CRO's best efforts to predict all aspects of the study, there often arise occasions on which the study requires CRO services that exceed expectations. In these cases the sponsor must be prepared to negotiate a 'change order agreement' to cover the expenses of additional CRO services. In certain cases the sponsor may approve a change order that amends the study timeline. Sponsor roles and responsibilities are summarized in Table 40.4.

Table 40.4 Roles and responsibilities of the sponsor

Define the study specifications
Provide information to the CRO
Monitor results
Recognize 'red flags'
Resolve problems
Approve changes in 'scope'

CONTRACT RESEARCH ORGANIZATION BID EVALUATION FORM

Selection parameter	CROs (Score 1–5)			
	CRO A	CRO B	CRO C	CRO D
1. *Bidder's qualifications*—is it likely that the bidder will be able to provide the services required by the study?				
2. *Experience*—does the bidder have adequate experience in the therapeutic area?				
3. *Key personnel*—do the personnel in key positions have adequate training and experience for these positions?				
4. *Study plan*—do the bidder's overview of the study design and plan for its implementation accurately reflect the sponsor's needs?				
5. *Investigator recruitment plan*—has the bidder presented a convincing plan (e.g. investigator database, list from recent study) for recruiting qualified investigators?				
6. *Availability of patients*—does the bidder have a reasonable strategy (e.g. patient database, advertising) for recruiting patients and is the projected enrollment rate realistic?				
7. *Project management*—Has the bidder described an appropriate plan for coordinating sites and managing the study?				
8. *Communication with the sponsor*—are the proposed frequency and formats of written and telephone reports acceptable?				
9. *Activities to be performed by the sponsor*—is the list of the sponsor's obligations accurate?				
10. *Services to be provided by the bidder*—does the list of materials and services to be provided by the bidder agree with the sponsor's study specifications?				
11. *Resource allocations*—for each activity to be performed by the CRO, are the types of personnel appropriate and are the estimated workloads (FTEs) realistic?				
12. *Costs*—are the estimated costs reasonable?				
TOTAL SCORE:				

Figure 40.4　Cartract research organization bid evaluation form. (Reproduced with permission from Vogel and Schober 1993)

CRO Roles and Responsibilities

The CRO should evaluate the feasibility of the sponsor's study plan. If the sponsor has provided detailed study specifications and the CRO is experienced in the target therapeutic area, it will be possible for the CRO to compare its past experiences with the sponsor's projections and to identify any inconsistencies. If the CRO believes it cannot achieve the sponsor's expectation (e.g. enroll three patients/month at each site in an arrhythmia study), it is important to bring it to the sponsor's attention and negotiate a more realistic goal.

The CRO has a responsibility to staff the study with adequate numbers of competent, well-managed personnel. This can present a challenge, especially in areas prone to high turnover, such as clinical research associates (CRAs). The CRO must have an adequate training and evaluation program to ensure staff performance and must not promote inexperienced personnel to critical positions, such as project manager. It is the CRO's responsibility to conduct the study activities as prescribed in the study specifications and sponsor–CRO agreement.

Despite the CRO's best efforts, problems will arise. Too often a CRO tries to solve a problem without bringing it to the sponsor's attention. Valuable time may be lost if the sponsor, which could have provided useful information to the CRO, is not consulted. When a problem cannot be readily resolved, the CRO should bring it to the sponsor's attention and present proposed solutions. The CRO should also ensure that proposed solutions are practical and cost-effective. The CRO's experience with similar studies may be an asset in problem solving. CRO roles and responsibilities are summarized in Table 40.5

Table 40.5 Roles and responsibilities of the CRO

Evaluate feasibility
Provide adequate, competent, well-managed staff
Conduct study activities
Manage processes
Bring problems and proposed solutions to the sponsor's attention
Ensure that solutions are cost-effective

Performance Metrics

Identification and communication of problems requires that the two parties agree on what constitutes a true problem. Often a sponsor identifies what it believes to be a significant variance, yet the CRO fails to respond because experience tells it that the variance will not have an impact on the end result. The result of this miscommunication is that the sponsor loses trust in the CRO and the relationship is harmed.

Performance metrics allow the sponsor and CRO to measure the same thing. Performance metrics are systematic and objective measures of CRO and sponsor performance. Their validity is established by demonstrating that they are related to achieving quality, ensuring timeliness, and managing cost. Performance metrics should be negotiated between the sponsor and CRO prior to the study.

They can be established for the qualifications of CRO personnel (e.g. a senior CRA must have at least 2 years of clinical research experience); timing and content of reports (e.g. the CRA's monitoring report must follow the format of the example given, and a copy of the report must be received by the sponsor within 2 weeks of the monitoring visit); patient enrollment (e.g. each site must enroll a minimum of 10 patients/month for the first 4 months of the study); cycle times (e.g. questions on case report form content, 'queries', must be generated within 1 week of receipt of the data by the CRO); database accuracy (e.g. the error rate as determined by comparing actual case report forms with the CRO database must be no more than 0.01); billing practices (e.g. the CRO will invoice the sponsor for the exact amount paid to investigators without a markup); and compliance audits (e.g. the CRO must have written, detailed, standard operating procedures (SOPs), for various activities and must be able to demonstrate that its staff routinely complies with the SOPs).

Performance metrics enable the sponsor to focus on the outcome (managing the CRO), rather than the process (micromanaging the CRO). Micromanaging the CRO by analyzing and monitoring its internal processes is disruptive and conveys a message of mistrust. Performance metrics help distinguish between the sponsor's role, to verify that the CRO is achieving the agreed-upon standards and timelines, and the CRO's role, to select the most appropriate processes to achieve these objectives. When performance metrics demonstrate that the CRO is failing to meet the objective, the sponsor and CRO have a shared responsibility to examine the process and agree on an appropriate solution. After corrective actions have been taken, the performance metrics help demonstrate that the desired effect has been achieved.

The Sponsor–CRO Communication/ Decision-making Model

The CRO's team members are expected to carry out the study activities, while the sponsor's team functions as a resource to the CRO. Most interactions between the sponsor and the CRO will take place between the individual team members and their technical counterparts. Discussions between sponsor and CRO technical staff should focus on information exchange and issue identification. Team members should inform their respective project managers of all communications between sponsor and CRO personnel. The benefit of informing the project manager of all issues is that the project manager can compare input from different team members, relay information to other team members as necessary, and detect issues that may not yet be apparent to the team.

Project managers are responsible for ensuring that their respective teams perform as expected. This may require them to negotiate with functional department heads to acquire needed resources, or to resolve a performance problem. When a problem arises between the sponsor and CRO, the project managers are responsible for negotiating a mutually acceptable solution and for executing a change order, if appropriate. Technical team members should not independently negotiate changes with their counterparts.

Sponsor–CRO Study Initiation Meeting

The sponsor and CRO teams should hold a 'kick-off' meeting prior to initiation of the study. The goals of the meeting are:

1. To promote camaraderie and ownership of the study among team members.
2. To clarify the roles and responsibilities of the sponsor and CRO.
3. To identify the primary sponsor and CRO contacts.
4. To present the agreed-to performance metrics and audit procedures.
5. To define the approach to problem resolution.
6. To define those changes that can be agreed upon informally and those that require a formal change order.

The meeting should begin with introductions of team members and their respective project managers. It is recommended that both sponsor and CRO senior managers make brief presentations, underscoring the importance of the study and reinforcing that the project managers have 'bottom line' responsibility. Additional activities include a review of the performance metrics, explanation of the responsibilities of the sponsor and CRO project managers, review of the responsibilities of the sponsor and CRO teams, description of the communication/decision-making process, and discussion of problem-solving procedures.

The meeting should include exercises designed to teach team members how to recognize behaviors that enhance and impair sponsor–CRO relationships. Participants should also engage in role-playing designed to teach efficient problem-solving techniques. In order to be most effective, the role-plays should be based on scenarios that are likely to occur in the planned study.

Sponsor–CRO Periodic Oversight Meetings

The sponsor and CRO should meet formally at least once every 3 months. The attendees should include the project managers and their respective team members, as determined by the status of the study and the topics to be discussed. The goals of periodic oversight meetings are:

1. To review the status of the study milestones and timelines.
2. To review the budget in terms of cost-to-date, change orders executed, and the latest projection for total cost.

3. To identify ways in which the sponsor and CRO have each significantly advanced the study.
4. To identify opportunities for improvement.

IDENTIFYING AND RESOLVING PROBLEMS

It is self-evident that problems will occur. They should be identified at an early stage, so that they have minimal impact on study cost, timing, and quality. It is also important to address problems when they are small enough to be easily resolved. Earliest detection of problems will likely take place at the technical level. Members of the sponsor and CRO teams will readily perceive issues in their individual technical areas. It is important for a team member to inform the project manager of any issue before attempting to resolve it. This information will enable the project manager to determine whether the problem is an isolated case, which can be resolved at the technical level, or if it is part of a larger problem that needs to be addressed with the corresponding project manager.

Ten 'Red Flags'

Red flags are early warnings that may not require immediate action, but should be evaluated to determine whether a significant underlying problem exists. Each team member may wish to prepare a list of red flags for his/her individual technical area. Ten typical red flags and the possible significant underlying problems are:

1. *Selection of inexperienced investigators by the CRO*: the CRO monitoring staff may be inexperienced.
2. *Questions from the study site directed to the sponsor*: the CRO may not have provided adequate training to site personnel.
3. *Inadequate monitoring reports from the CRO*: the CRO monitoring staff may not be receiving adequate training and supervision.
4. *Enrollment of patients who do not fit the study criteria*: the investigator may not understand the study protocol.

5. *A higher screening-to-enrollment ratio at one site than others*: the investigator may be 'padding the budget' by performing unnecessary screening procedures.
6. *Failure of the CRO to submit monitoring reports promptly after completing visits*: the CRO may not have adequately staffed this study.
7. *Frequent rescheduling of meetings and reports by the CRO*: the CRO staff may be carrying excessive workloads.
8. *Delays in cleaning up case record forms (CRFs)*: the CRO may be processing CRFs in batches, which can hide monitoring problems and delay study completion.
9. *Changes in CRO personnel*: the CRO may be experiencing labor problems.
10. *Unscheduled request for payment by the CRO*: the CRO may be experiencing financial problems.

Sponsor–CRO End-of-study Meeting

The sponsor and CRO should hold a formal meeting at the end of the study. The goals of this meeting are:

1. To review the actual budget and timeline as compared to the sponsor's and CRO's expectations.
2. To characterize the quality and timing of materials and activities performed by the sponsor and of the services performed by the CRO.
3. To discuss follow-up of any unresolved issues (e.g. cost overruns, incomplete services).

CONCLUSIONS

More effective contracting of clinical drug-development activities to CROs can be achieved by applying the following methods:

1. Use a strategic approach to outsourcing.
2. Follow the three principles for achieving success with CROs: define accurate study specifications; select the right CRO; and manage the study.

3. Select CROs according to the three Cs; capability, compatibility, and cost.
4. Evaluate the CRO's resource allocations.
5. Define the performance metrics.
6. Ensure efficient communication with the CRO.

It is important to recognize that the roles and responsibilities of the sponsor and CRO are complementary. Dedication and skill are required of both the sponsor and CRO team members to achieve successful outsourcing.

REFERENCES

Getz KA, Vogel JR (1995) Achieving results with contract research organizations: their evolving role in clinical development. *Appl Clin Trials* 4 (4): 32–8.

Hill T (1994) Calculating the cost of clinical research. *Scrip Magazine* 3: 28–30.

Lightfoot GD, Vogel JR (1996) Contracting CROs into your organization: new strategies for new challenges. In Welling PG, Lasagna L, Banakar UV (eds), *The Drug Development Process: Increasing Efficiency and Cost-effectiveness.* Marcel Dekker: New York; 317–35.

Vogel JR (1993) Achieving results with contract research organizations: pharmaceutical industry views. *Appl Clin Trials* 2(1): 44–9.

Vogel JR, Nelson SR (1993) Achieving results with contract research organizations: determining the study specifications. *Appl Clin Trials* 2(5): 70–6.

Vogel JR, Resnick N (1996) Achieving results with contract research organizations: a case study in evaluating and selecting a CRO. *Appl Clin Trials* 5(6): 30–6.

Vogel JR, Schober RA (1993) Achieving results with contract research organizations: requesting and evaluating proposals from CROs. *Appl Clin Trials* 2(12): 32–41.

41

The Third World

G. Hammad

Walford, UK

The objective of this chapter is to survey the 'Third World', which actually comprises multiple different environments, and consider how these affect the practice of pharmaceutical medicine. The specific problems are related to fundamental differences from the West: culture, economics, and epidemiology.

Medicine is a cultural activity that varies from country to country. The cultural context in which drugs are used varies among cultures. This is true in the Western world (e.g. the use of low-dose digoxin for cardiac asthenia in Germany), let alone in the Third World (where therapeutics may include, for example, natural products prescribed by alternative practitioners).

The Third World is also different from, for example, the ICH territory, in that the economic resources that can be deployed to healthcare and drug purchases are limited. Factors which commonly encourage investment in the West (availability of skilled manpower, strong patent protections, highly-developed drug distribution systems, socialized medical systems, private medical systems, and affluent populations) are typically absent in the Third World. And yet, there are many physicians in the Third World who may fairly be described as being pharmaceutical physicians. How does their environment change cause their practice to differ from those of us in the West?

Many patients in the tropics have diseases that are familiar to Western-trained physicians, but it is the epidemiology that is often different. Comparing the AIDS populations in Los Angeles and Eastern Africa is an obvious example. Different practices in antiviral therapy prescription, distribution, and drug pricing thus emerge in the two environments.

Thus, pharmaceutical medicine becomes governed by epidemiology. Incidentally, and contrary to the assertions of some journalists and their editors, the pharmaceutical industry has made great and unprofitable efforts to increase such drug supplies to Africa. This is in spite of the fact that epidemics are typically halted by public health measures, not by antibiotics.

The range of pathology may be different when it is related to climate: it is for this reason that American and European universities have, for a long time, established schools and departments of tropical medicine. Probably the area of infectious disease is the best example, and malaria one of the clearest examples within the group. If pathology is specific to the Third World, then clinical trials almost always have to be conducted in those same geographical areas.

One real patient brings all these factors together. A middle-aged man in Nepal has had a diagnosis of pulmonary tuberculosis for about 4 years. He supports his family by subsistence farming. There are no telephones, and he walks about 10 miles for an unscheduled clinic appointment when his breathlessness interferes too much with his work. At each clinic appointment his pleural effusions are drained (thus improving his breathlessness, which he appreciates), and a small supply of antibiotics is prescribed, probably with little effect (at best) because he cannot afford to pay for the prescriptions that he has been given, even if rifampicin is in stock locally. He cannot be admitted to hospital for more intensive treatment: he has no adult children to help him in the fields, and his family would starve. How can the practice of pharmaceutical medicine adapt to this sort of environment?

Principles and Practice of Pharmaceutical Medicine. Edited by A. J. Fletcher, Lionel D. Edwards, Anthony W. Fox and Peter Stonier © 2002 John Wiley & Sons Ltd.

PHARMACEUTICAL BUSINESS IN THE PEOPLE'S REPUBLIC OF CHINA

Currently the Chinese economy is the world's third largest and is heading very rapidly to overtake Japan and the USA. Indeed, most observers strongly believe that, if China can hold its course, it it may surpass the American economy to become the biggest in the world and become the greatest economy in history.

In the year 2025, China's population will reach 1.6 billion, compared with USA's 307 million and Japan's 128 million. China's overall growth rate is now 14%, and the province of Guangdong has even reached the highest growth rate in the world at approximately 28–30%. Foreign investment in China increased 17% from January to September 1993, which indicates investor confidence in the future of China's economy. Greater China (People's Republic of China + Hong Kong + Taiwan) imports in the year 2002, according to the World Bank's prediction, will be US $639 billion compared with US $521 billion for Japan. GNP for China is expected to be US $9.8 trillion compared to US $9.7 trillion for the USA.

China offers a unique business opportunity for pharmaceutical and healthcare companies, including those involved in diagnostics and biotechnology. The following is a summary of the demographic and healthcare situation in China (statistics from China–Britain Trade Group 1993).

- China has a population of 1.158 billion (China–Britain Trade Group 1993).
- China has more than 2 million beds in more than 67 000 hospitals, a major potential purchaser of medical goods and products.
- China is opening its economy to foreign investment and moving towards rejoining GATT.
- The pharmaceutical and medical market of China is growing very quickly. The size of China's pharmaceutical market in 1992 excluding bulk drugs and traditional Chinese medicines, was ¥ 19.3 billion and US$3.5 billion at the official 1992 exchange rate. This reflects overall growth of 92% and 30%, respectively, compared to 5 years previously. The pharmaceutical

market grew by 30% in 1993–1994 and is now worth US $10 billion.
- The liberalization of trade in China has facilitated negotiation and sales for foreign companies, leading to increases in sale volume.
- Chinese exports in 1991 were US$72 billion; imports were US$62 billion; foreign exchange reserves (excluding gold) are currently US$43 billion (China–Britain Trade Group 1993).
- The huge size of China's healthcare system means that demands for imports of medical equipment and pharmaceuticals will continue. China has 200 000 medical centers and institutions, including 67 000 hospitals.
- These hospitals are potential customers. The US Department of Commerce estimates that the Chinese medical import market will be worth US$1.1 billion by 1996. All agree that growth in the sector is approaching 25% a year; the lion's share, an estimated 80%, is controlled by the USA, Germany and Japan. Each large hospital gets an annual global budget of foreign exchange to purchase supplies directly.
- There is no shortage of money to purchase new medical supplies. The state now allocates an estimated RMB 5 billion on the nation's hospitals.
- Pharmaceutical joint ventures started in 1980 with China Otsuka Pharmaceutical Company and there are six planned joint ventures in 1995–1996 (see Table 41.1).

Clinical Trials in China

All prescription-only medicines (POMs) must be subjected to local clinical studies prior to local marketing approval. Exceptions are rarely granted, even for 'breakthrough' drugs. This applies even to cough and cold remedies normally available without prescription in the rest of the world.

There is a system for applying for an IND certificate that allows study of medicines previously unregistered in China, and also a marketing authorization (NDA) process for a drug which is known in the country and which an individual

Table 41.1 Pharmaceutical joint ventures in China

Year operational	Pharmaceutical plant
1980	China Otsuka Pharmaceutical Company
1982	Sino-American Shanghai Squibb Pharmaceutical Ltd
1982	Sino-Swedish Pharmaceutical Corporation
1994	Tianjin Smithkline and French Laboratories
1985	Xian Janssen Pharmaceutical Co. Ltd
1987	Beijing Zhongrui Ciba–Geigy Pharmaceutical Co. Ltd
1989	Chongqin Glaxo Pharmaceuticals Ltd
1989	Pfizer Pharmaceuticals Ltd
1992	Second Ciba plant—joint venture with Beijing Pharmaceutical Factory No. 3
1993–1994	Merck Vaccines Plant
1994	Chugai—joint venture with Shanghai Xin Xing Medicine and Drug Development Centre
1994	Tanabe—joint venture with Tianjin Lisheng Pharmaceutical Factory
1994	Second Otsuka Plant
1996	Takeda—joint venture with Lisheng Pharmaceutical Factory
1996	Upjohn—joint venture with Suzhou Pharmaceutical Factory No. 4
1995	Ranbaxy
1995	Hoechst and Huabei Pharmaceutical Factory
1995	Roche and Shanghai Sun Ve Pharmaceutical Corporation
1995	Zeneca

From *China Economic Review* (May 1994).

company wishes to market. Applications for an IND are made at both provincial and national level, and approval must be granted by both to be able to proceed to clinical studies. There is some rivalry between provincial and national bodies, and plans agreed with one may not be acceptable by the other. Applications may be made in any of the provinces and also in Beijing, Shanghai, and Tianjin, cities that are considered 'provinces' for many administrative purposes.

Requirements for Authorization of Clinical Trials

According to the provisions for an NDA, clinical studies on a new medicinal product in China are classified into two categories: clinical trials, and clinical verification.

Clinical trials are divided into three phases. A Phase I trial is carried out with 10–30 subjects, mostly healthy adults and a few appropriate patients, all on a voluntary basis, to find out the optimum dosage and route of administration. Early Phase II trials are carried out as comparative studies, using double-blind methodology. Late Phase II trials are carried out at medical institutions (not less than three) and more than 300 patients should be

included and validated. Immediately after the new medicinal product has been approved by the Health Authorities for provisional production, Phase III clinical trials should be carried out to conduct a community investigation and evaluation of the product.

Clinical studies in China may only be carried out after an application with supporting data, partly equivalent to those for a marketing authorization in many other countries, and are approved by the Bureau of Drug Policy and Administration, Ministry of Public Health. The application must be in accordance with the provisions of the Rules Governing the Approval of Clinical Trial of Foreign Drugs, and the studies must be conducted in compliance with these rules.

Within 30 days of approval of a clinical trial application, the medical institution in charge must submit a detailed clinical trial protocol to the Bureau of Drug Policy and Administration, with copies to the central Committee of Drug Evaluation and the regional Bureau of Public Health concerned. If no opinion on the draft protocol is expressed by the Bureau of Drug Policy and Administration after 40 days, the medical institution may start the clinical trial.

Clinical trials on new medicinal products in Classes 1, 2 or 3 are required to be approved by

Table 41.2 Chinese classification of Western drugs

Class 1	NCE not registered anywhere in the world
Class 2	NCE for the first filing in China but registered elsewhere
Class 3	Compound and fixed dose combination products
Class 4	NCEs previously registered for import into China
Class 5	Registered products for which a new indication is sought

the central Bureau (see Table 41.2). Clinical verifications, mainly for products in Classes 4 and 5, may be approved by a local Health Bureau.

There are 31 medical institutions designated as clinical pharmacology centers. Medical institutions are designated by the Authorities to conduct clinical trials on a new product, but the applicant may propose the name of the institute(s) to be involved in the studies. The requisite range of studies on a foreign product may vary, depending on its status in foreign countries.

In the case of a foreign product filed by a foreign applicant, the Bureau designates a coordinating agent, who may negotiate and sign the contract on behalf of the institutions performing the clinical studies with the foreign applicant and collaborate with the Bureau (IPMA Compendium 1994). The data that should be submitted to the Registration Authorities for a foreign therapeutic agents are:

- Protocol for the clinical trial.
- GMP Certificate.
- Registration status of the drug in the country of origin or in other countries.
- Technical file re: quality control, manufacturing procedures, pre-clinical and clinical studies.

The clinical investigator should receive the following data:

- Therapeutic indication, dosage and how the product is used.

- Pharmacodynamic and toxicological studies.
- The name of the person responsible and the place of the archives.
- Suspected adverse drug reactions (ADRs) and symptoms of intoxication.
- Sponsor's name.
- Investigators in charge of preclinical studies.

Good clinical practice (GCP) guidelines are published and should be adhered to. Normal precautions should be applied to protect the safety and health of test subjects throughout the trial, with provision for emergency treatment and effective treatment against possible adverse reactions.

Chinese clinicians have the same competencies as any elsewhere in the world, but possibly few have any experience of working to GCP standards, and the administrators of hospitals are also not familiar with the concept. Thus, much time and energy needs to be directed at the training of investigators and those with power to 'sell' the concept of source data verification, and such a task must be done by a Chinese speaker because of the subtlety of the alphabet and the risk of misunderstanding.

All the provinces should hold equal sway in terms of their suitability for conducting studies, but Beijing and Shanghai have the greatest 'value' (see Table 41.3). Beijing, as the capital, has strategic influence, and Shanghai is comparatively wealthy and has value for pricing purposes. This latter is crucial, as the pricing granted at the time of licensing is the price that will remain in place during the selling period of the drug. Price increases are not allowed at all.

Approval of medicines (Table 41.4) is a two-stage, two-level process for both IND and NDA. Local approval is by the Bureau of Public Health and national approval is by the Ministry of Public Health (MOPH) for an IND. The Bureau must see pharmaceutical, chemistry, stability data, summaries of preclinical data, and of clinical data to date. Full registration files will not be reviewed, even if

Table 41.3 Clinical trials in China—value of provinces

All 16 + 3 provinces (Beijing, Shanghai and Tianjin are also treated as provinces) should have equal influence, however:
Beijing carries enormous influence over the rest of the country, thus is a frequently chosen city.
Shanghai has fiscal value; tends to set higher cost limits, thus is crucial from a reimbursement point of view
Tianjin is convenient for Beijing, but has little direct influence, although it has several excellent academic centers

Source: Dr David Blowers.

Table 41.4 Approval of Medicines in China

Two-stage, two-level process for both IND and NDA, i.e. approval to investigate and approval to market
Bureau of Public Health at regional level
Ministry of Public Health at national level

Source: Dr David Blowers.

Table 41.5 IND review process—Bureau of Public Health

Wants: pharmaceuticals, chemistry, stability (some), i.e. summary preclinical data, clinical data to date. NB full registration file will not be reviewed, even if available elsewhere
May well have views about the type of studies and the 'best' investigators—they may decide where the clinical trial is conducted
Wants a say in final study design
Likes to attend investigator meetings (usually unannounced)
Often takes a different view to the Ministry of Public Health (e.g. comparators or placebo control)
Potentially open for discussion/influence

Table 41.6 IND review process—companies

Submit clinical proposals, including protocols
Protocols sent to key opinion leaders for review, then to Bureau of Public Health, and to investigators for clearance
All centers endeavor to follow GCP, but monitoring is a problem
Clinical records are not readily available
Trained staff are few and far between

available. The documents must be in Chinese. The Bureau will have views about the choice of study type(s) and also the investigators who should be used. They also like to attend investigator meetings, often unannounced, and can derail the progress of the meeting. They may well have views about the studies which differ from those expressed by the Ministry, and care must be taken to satisfy both groups. Patience, negotiation, and compromise are some of the skills to be used in the meetings. They are open for discussion/negotiation and time spent at this stage is well worth the effort.

The Ministry meets only three times each year, thus timing is critical if documents are to be reviewed with optimal timing. The Ministry insist on seeing all Class 1, 2 and 3 INDs, i.e. all NCEs not registered elsewhere in the world, NCEs new to China, and any combination products. They also review all NDAs (Tables 41.5, 41.6) and the Minister must issue approval for marketing. The activities of the Ministry (Table 41.7) are somewhat secretive, and they are generally mistrusting of company data, especially data analysis, often seeking another review to ensure the quality of submitted data. The Ministry is mistrusting of

the independence of its own experts and provides them with little lead time to review dossiers. It is often the case that documents are only provided the night before the meeting. In addition, decisions taken at the provincial level may be overridden suddenly, without explanation.

There are a few other minor issues that need to be borne in mind about studies in China. First, adverse events are not dealt with in the same way as in Europe. Complaints are often made by the patient direct to the company (an obvious breach of GCP regulations regarding anonymity of data), and staff feel honour-bound to offer some compensation to the complainant, to save 'face' for

Table 41.7 Ministry of Public Health

Meets only three times/year
Needs several weeks' lead time
Must see all Class 1, 2, and 3 INDs*
Must see all NDAs
Rather secretive
Does not trust company data analysis
Does not trust the independence of its own experts
Often reverses decisions taken by the provinces

* Class 1, NCE not registered anywhere in the world; Class 2, NCE registered somewhere; Class 3, combination products.

the company, even if there is limited merit in the complaint. The recompense offered is usually a small amount of money (for inconvenience caused), medicine (to speed recovery), and some food (to facilitate healing). This presents a nightmare of assumed liability, but is very much the norm in China.

Monitoring of Clinical Trials

External communications have improved immeasurably over the last 5 years, but internally things are not perfect. Monitoring is potentially a problem unless there are staff located near to study centres, and data retrieval from remote sites can be difficult.

Data Entry and Statistical Analysis

There is a dearth of trained staff for either of these tasks in China at present, and many companies either ship data in bulk back to a central processing unit or they may transfer a team to China on a project-specific basis. Both methods have their associated problems and the cost of the second option can be considerable.

Dr David Blowers, an international pharmaceutical physician who has conducted and monitored clinical trials and studies exclusively in China, feels that:

- China is a land of opportunity.
- Studies are necessary and are *possible* to reasonable standards.
- The rewards are probably worth the risks.

For a summary of information as clinical trials in China, see Tables 41.8, 41.9 and 41.10

Useful Addresses in Relation to Clinical Trials and Registration

Bureau of Drug Policy and Administration, Ministry of Public Health, No. 44 Houhai Beiyuan, Beijing, China.
Tel: +86 (1) 401 2873; Fax: +86 (1) 401 2870.

Table 41.8 Summary of the general information on clinical trials in China

Phase I	Total number are normally 10–30 patients (health volunteers)
Phase II	300 patients. This is divided into two stages: *1st stage*: to assess the efficacy, indications and adverse reaction of the new therapeutic agents *2nd stage*: similar to 1st stage, except increase the number of cases and increase the number of units where the clinical trial takes place to not less than three
Phase III	Postmarketing surveillance, i.e. ADRs and evaluate continued efficacy of the drug

Table 41.9 Clinical verification

Number of patients should not be less than 100
Objective is the comparison of the new drug with an established drug by comparing the efficacy and ADRs

Table 41.10 Clinical study requirements

Drug class	Study	Control	Total cases
1	300	300	600
2	300	300	600
3	100	100	200
4	100	100	200
5	100	100	200

Address for documentation:
Laws and Regulations, Bureau of Drugs Policy and Administration, Ministry of Public Health, No. 44 Houhai Beiyuan, Beijing, China.
Tel: +86 (1) 401 2873; Fax: +86 (1) 401 2870.

Application Data for Clinical Study

Documentation of General Information

- Name and related information.
- Purpose of and reason for the selection.
- Current state of research on new drug or a review of its production and usage.

Chemical and Pharmaceutical Documentation

- Structure or composition.
- Method of preparation.

- Control of starting materials and related information.
- Control of drug substance.
- Control of the dosage for clinical use, with authentic specimens as reference control.
- Stability (the first test).

Toxicological and Pharmacological Documentation

- Single-dose toxicity.
- Repeated-dose toxicity.
- Local toxicity.
- Reproduction studies.
- Mutagenicity.
- Carcinogenicity.
- Drug dependence.
- Pharmacodynamics and general pharmacology.
- Pharmacokinetics.
- Impact of each ingredient on efficacy or toxicity of the combination product, where applicable.
- Samples.
- Samples for clinical trials and its analytical report.
- Clinical trial protocols and a review on pharmacodynamic and toxicological studies to be sent to clinical investigators.

Application Data for Manufacturing Approval

Clinical Documentation

- Stability under ambient and severe conditions and expiry data where applicable.
- Quality standards for production.
- Clinical pharmacokinetics.
- Bioavailability and a summary.

Special Particulars

- *Dosage form*
  Packaging material, labeling material and draft package insert.
- *Samples*
  Sample for clinical trials, and three to five batches produced in succession, and their analytical data.

Authentic specimens as reference or control (IFPMA Compendium 1994).

Producer Information

All medical products must be labeled on the container, giving the following detailed instructions:

- Name and strength of product.
- Name of manufacturer.
- Serial number of application data.
- Lot number.
- Active ingredients.
- Therapeutic indications.
- Usage.
- Dosage.
- Contraindications.
- Side effects and adverse drug reactions.
- Warnings and precautions.

Summary of Product Characteristics (SPC), Data Sheet and Package Insert (PI)

Package inserts should be included in each package. The draft leaflet, prepared by the medical profession, is required to be submitted to the authorities as part of the application data. The following information has to be included:

- Name.
- Structural and molecular formulas.
- Composition.
- Pharmocodynamics and indications.
- Directions and dosage.
- Adverse reactions and side effects.
- Contraindications.
- Precautions and warnings.
- Package quantities and strength.
- Storage conditions.
- Expiry date, marked clearly.

Samples

There are no legal requirements regarding samples for the medical profession in government or private practices.

Pharmacovigilance Postmarketing Surveillance and Adverse Drug Reactions Reporting

All pharmaceutical manufacturers and medical institutions are required by law to report any serious ADRs to the Bureau of Drug Policy and Administration or to regional competent authorities. There are central and regional ADR Monitoring Centres associated with the central and regional Health Bureaux. University/college hospitals and major medical institutions designated by the central and regional governments are obliged to conduct ADR reporting. The central Committee of Drug Evaluation undertakes the assessment of ADR reports. Actions and measures are taken by the Bureau.

Price Controls

There is some government control over the price of drugs for domestic products. Pharmaceutical manufacturers may negotiate with the regional price agency concerned, based on a full-cost principle. Imported drugs are free in principle, but are worked out by the Bureau of Commodity Prices of China (BCPC) and the State Pharmaceutical Administration of China (SPAC). In 1991 the SPAC set up a national imported drug pricing balance group.

Reimbursement and Health

The Medicare systems in China are: government-paid medical service for state functionaries and university/college students; labour insurance medical service for employees of industrial, communication, and other enterprises; and various forms adopted on a voluntary basis for rural populations. Under the reforms of the healthcare system proposed by the Ministry of Public Health, co-payments were introduced in 10 provinces and cities for employees of state-owned institutions and enterprises to pay for part of their treatment, including drugs (IFPMA Compendium 1994).

THE MIDDLE EAST—LAND OF PLENTY

The Middle East will generate revenue from oil for the next century at least. Currently, two-thirds of the world's proven oil reserves are from this area and this makes these oil-producing countries some of the wealthiest in the world. With a population of some 270 million, the Middle East is the second largest single market after the European Community. Before we go further we should answer the justified question: why should the Middle East be singled out? The answer is very simple, since for Europe and the USA:

- It is the third largest export market.
- There are considerable trading advantages.
- Their share of the market is rising.
- They have a wide range of goods and services that countries in the Middle East need to import.
- Payment terms can be attractive, normally involving an irrevocable letter of credit (ILOC).
- Opportunities for small firms are growing.

Middle East Pharmaceutical and Healthcare Market

The Middle East is still an exciting market place for pharmaceuticals and healthcare products, and the range of opportunities in the Middle East for healthcare companies is enormous. Countries throughout the region have announced far-reaching development plans for their healthcare infrastructures and they have the ability to fund these developments.

Over much of the Middle East there is a great deal of activity taking place in terms of new hospital construction. Governments are increasing their budget allocations in the healthcare field. In short, the Middle East is currently one of the few places in the world where multinational pharmaceutical companies can expand their activities and make profit. The Iranian government has increased its fiscal year budget for 1992–1993 by 21% (7.15% of the total government budget), and one of the greatest increases in the allocation has been given to healthcare. In Saudi Arabia, the massive King Fahd project calls for the provision of 2000 health centers across the country within the next 5 years and the Ministry of Health has announced plans to build an additional 18 major hospitals. The United Arab Emirates sees Dubai alone constructing 40 new clinics and 12 health centers, and creating almost 2000 extra hospital beds by the year 2005. The medical market for the Middle Eastern countries—Egypt, Turkey, Iran, Bahrain, Jordan, Kuwait, Syria, Saudi Arabia, United Arab Emirates, Oman, and Qatar—represents 2% of the world market. The gross domestic product (GDP) in Turkey was 4% in 1991, rising to 5.5% in 1992. Healthcare expenditure in 1989 was US $3 billion, representing 3.8% of GDP. Healthcare expenditure in 1991 in Iran was estimated at US$ 1.4 billion, representing 7.8% of GDP. Over 30% of the current population is under 13 years old, indicating that pediatric services are likely to be in greater demand. It is obvious from all this activity that the Middle East presents an exciting marketing opportunity.

Healthcare Structure in Saudi Arabia

- Saudi Arabia Health Care is controlled by the Government and is free for all citizens.
- Expatriates working in the Kingdom are not eligible for free healthcare and are treated privately.
- To encourage investors in new private hospitals, Government lends up to 50% of the cost.
- The Ministry of Health rents up to 15% of beds in private hospitals for state use.

Saudi Arabia offers the most attractive marketing opportunity in the Middle East. It is difficult to find another country that is continuously spending large sums of money on healthcare. The market will hopefully remain dynamic for the foreseeable future.

Agency Laws in the Middle East

The agent must be a national of the country concerned, or a company with a majority national shareholding. The agency agreement must be registered. The agreement must specify:

- The rights and obligations of both parties.
- The type of agency.
- The date of signature and length of time for which it is valid.
- The provisions for the renewal.
- The territory to be covered.
- The products and services to be covered.

Typical Agency in the Middle East

- Family-owned.
- Most of the financial power is in the chairman's hands.
- Different departments, e.g. marketing, registration, etc.
- Continuous support needed from the manufacturer to ensure:
  Successful company and product registration.
  Good clinical evaluation to generate local data.

What to look for when selecting an agency

- *Personal rapport*—essential if you are to work well together in the long term.
- *Location*—can the agent cover the right market area for you?
- *Business efficency*—you need information on the agent's reputation and financial position.
- *Adequate facilities*—has good facilities for storage and repairs.
- *Contacts*—has the right contacts in government, purchasing organization, major companies, etc.
- *Administration*—does the agent have a good working knowledge of local laws, standard specifications etc? And is he prepared to make routine arrangements for you—booking hotels, making appointments, etc?
- *Competition*—does the agent carry too many competing lines? Can he devote enough time to promoting your products?

Egypt Pharmaceutical Market

The pharmaceutical industry in Egypt was established in 1933–1934; The Hegazi Pharmaceutical Company was established in 1933, Memphis,

MISR and CID companies followed in 1940, and what was to become a huge nationalized industry was born. The year 1952 was the turning point regarding drug policy in Egypt, as was true for the whole spectrum of socioeconomic development. At that time, the yearly drug consumption totalled US$ 12.5 million an average consumption of 55 cents/person. The local drug industry was in its infancy and constituted only 10% of total consumption. From organizational and historical points of view, there were four important stages that influenced drug policy in Egypt:

1. *1933–1961.* At one stage there were 22 000 products available. The market was liberal, which led to fierce competition between foreign companies. The Directorate of Pharmacy, under the Ministry of Health (MoH), supervised local pharmaceutical companies and distributors.
2. *1962–1975.* Egyptian pharmaceuticals were completely nationalized. The Egyptian Institute for Drug, Chemical and Medical supplies (MHO), had total control over the whole pharmaceutical industry, with the aim of providing protection for the local industry. The value in 1971 was US$ 220m, 86% of which was produced locally. Public sector companies numbered 11 at the time. Several European companies had established manufacturing sites in Cairo. The quality center was set up in 1963.
3. *1976–1984.* The Egyptian Institute was abolished and replaced with the Egyptian Organization for Drug, Chemical and Medical Supplies. Its function included strategic planning, follow-up, and performance evaluation of all pharmaceutical activities in the country. The public centre remained as it was, but Squibb negotiated a deal to establish its own manufacturing site, I Egypt, with annual sales of around 26 million Egyptian pounds (E£).
4. *1985 to date.* The government has adopted and maintained a well-balanced policy, encouraging both the public and private sectors. This policy, plus the level of democracy and freedom that Egypt enjoys (there are three progovernment and seven opposition daily newspapers) has attracted huge foreign investment in pharmaceuticals and paved the way for the establishment of new pharmaceutical companies in the private sector, including EIPICO, Pharco, Amryia, Sedico, and 10th of Ramadan Co.

In the past, only 1% of net profit from the local industry was invested in research and development, but this figure is steadily increasing. If the present policy continues, the future for the pharmaceutical industry, both public and private, looks rosy indeed. The local industry is regaining some of its lost ground, while at the same time, a more reasonable importation policy is ensuring that the private sector is encouraged and protected. Total pharmaceutical production for the public sector in 1991 was E£608 million and among companies enjoying their share of the market are MISR, EI Nile, Kahira, CID, ADCO Memphis, and Alexandria Co.

Private Companies

The private pharmaceutical companies currently operating in Egypt include: Pfizer, Swiss Pharma, Hoechst, Bristol–Myers Squibb, EIPICO, Pharco, Glaxo, ABI, MUP, Amryia, Sedico, 10th Ramadan, Mepaco, APIC, October Pharma and Amoun Pharmaceutical Industries. The total pharmaceutical turnover of the private sector in Egypt in 1991 was E£619 million. The total pharmaceutical turnover for the public and private sectors combined was E£1000 million (rate of exchange: E£ = US$3.3).

Company Registration Requirements in the Middle East

- Application form.
- Letter of agency authorization (legalized).
- Manufacturer's certificate (WHO, GMP, EC).
- List of subsidiaries.
- Capital and turnover (sales).
- Lists of products with active ingredients, and where registered.
- Countries where registered.
- Date of establishment, number of employees.
- Summary of main research and associated products (past 10 years).

- For Bahrain and Qatar—proof of registration in two other GCC states, including either Kuwait or Saudi Arabia.
- Normally the company is registered first, followed by the products.

Tips for Success

- Before travelling to the Middle East, read something about the area you are visiting to avoid culture shock.
- A sense of humour is acceptable in some parts and prohibited in others!
- Arabic is the official language, although English is widely spoken.
- Your investigator will shake hands frequently, may hug and kiss you on the cheek in the second visit. *Do not* be alarmed! This is the *norm*.
- Avoid using initials. People in the Middle East like to use their full names e.g. Ali Sayed Al-Qasimmi, NOT as A.S. Al-Qasimmi.
- Personal contact in the Middle East is of tremendous value.
- Avoid discussing clinical trials in Saudi Arabia at the Ministry of Health level. Leave the discussions to your local investigator.
- Tapes, videos, slides, and even newspapers and magazines could be screened at the airport.
- Drive slowly, and keep a letter in Arabic about yourself, your employer and the purpose of your visit.
- Think positively all the time.
- Watch your body language.
- Don't value people according to their fluency in, say, English or French.
- Avoid generalizations.

THE FAR EAST—THE ASIAN TIGERS

There are several reasons to focus on the Far East as part of our review of opportunities for the pharmaceutical industry abroad. In the Far East there in concrete evidence of continuous rapid economic growth in the region; the Far East is the fastest growing pharmaceutical market in the world; there is an annual increase in healthcare budgets and spending in most of the Far Eastern

countries; and the Far East is politically and economically stable.

SOUTH KOREA

Managing the Culture and Business in Health Care and Pharmaceuticals

The Korean population is 42 million. Its capital, Seoul, is one of the world's 10 largest cities, with a population of nearly 12 million. The general character of the country is mountainous and hilly. All available land is intensively cultivated; 20% of the population is engaged in farming and fishing. Korean economic growth since 1986 has been very impressive. South Koreans are proud of their economic achievement. The emphasis in the economy is on exports. South Korea identifies itself with the giant economic power, Japan, and believes it will be soon on the same level economically. In 1987 there was a surplus of around $10 billion—a remarkable achievement.

Healthcare in South Korea

Traditionally, pharmacies have played a leading role in providing medical advice to patients. Pharmacists dispense 70% of all pharmaceuticals consumed in Korea [ethical and over-the-Counter (OTC)]. Physicians, doctors, and medical practitioners are concentrated in the capital, Seoul, and major big towns and cities. Doctors in Korea are now lobbying to separate prescribing, diagnosis, and treatment from dispensing, so they aim to deprive the pharmacists of the therapeutic role they are playing. The government of Korea extended health and medical insurance to cover almost the whole population. Healthcare is free for those over 65 and under 18 years of age.

Pharmaceutical Industry

300 pharmaceutical companies are active in Korea, including multinationals, some of which operate on a joint venture basis: e.g. Glaxo, Otsuka, Sandoz SK&F (SmithKline Beecham), Sanofi, Ciba-Geigy, Squibb, Rhone-Poulenc, Sterling, Bayer, Roche,

Boehringer, Ingelheim, Janssen, Upjohn, Eli Lilly, Pfizer, Searle, Hoechst, Cyanamid, Schering AG, and Syntex are examples of multinational companies with joint ventures in South Korea: foreign capital investment regulation, which came in 1981, has allowed a foreign company to hold an equity share in a joint venture. Up to 70% have attracted a number of multinationals. However, the pharmaceutical market in Korea is dominated by local companies; 30 of these account for over 75% share of the market. These companies include Korea Green Cross, Chong Kun Dang, Yu Han, Choong Wae, Dong A, II Yang, II Dong, Daewoo, Samsung, Lucky Gold Star.

There is a liberal policy adopted by the Korean government regarding importation of pharmaceutical raw materials; 50% of raw materials are imported and the rest manufactured locally. The South Korean pharmaceutical market is ranked 12th in the world in terms of production value.

The market size is $1700 million; 70% of pharmaceutical products are purchased directly from pharmacies. Koreans prefer locally manufactured medical products over imported foreign drugs. Traditional therapeutic herbal products are still widely popular. This applies possibly to most of the Far Eastern countries. In 1986 the top 20 products on the market were all tonics, vitamins, ginseng, and herbal products.

Distribution of Pharmaceuticals

Most wholesalers are too small, and 37% of total pharmaceutical sales is through direct sale by the manufacturer to pharmacies, with only 26% of sales through wholesalers. 26% of sales are direct to hospitals, 4% to other manufacturers and 4% are exported.

Regulatory Affairs and Registration

The Regulatory Authority is located at the Ministry of Health:

Ministry of Health and Social Affairs, Government Unification Building 1, Choongang-dong Kwa-cheon-myun, Sihoog-gun Kyunggi-do, Republic of Korea.
(Tel: Kyunggi 171–11)

The Ministry of Health in 1987 introduced a requirement for all multinational and other companies seeking approval for new indications for an existing substance, or for registration of a new chemical entity (NCE) to conduct clinical trials locally to support their application.

Pricing of Pharmaceuticals

There is price control in both hospitals and pharmacies. In hospitals, products are eligible for reimbursement under the national health insurance scheme and are price controlled. In pharmacies, a standard retail price system is in force (30% mark-up on manufacturer's plant delivery price). Patent protection has been available since July 1987.

THAILAND

Health Care in Thailand

Thailand operates public and private health care systems. There is free medical care, including pharmaceuticals for Thais earning below US$80–100 month. Village health centers provide essential drugs and basic medical services and there is one medical doctor per 6000 people. Bangkok has one-quarter of Thailand's chemists (drugstores), although population-wise it is one-tenth; 30% of healthcare expenditure is contributed by the government, the remainder by the health insurance scheme. There is a national list of essential drugs sold in government hospitals and clinics at fixed prices.

Pharmaceutical Industry in Thailand

There are 193 registered manufacturing companies, of which 21 are joint ventures or foreign-owned, and 424 pharmaceutical traders (importers). Three are contract manufacturing plants used by overseas companies. Local pharmaceutical companies are engaged in formulating and packing. Analgesics, vitamins, antacids, and antibiotics are the largest categories; 90% of the pharmaceutical raw materials are imported; 30% of the market consists of imported finished products; and 60% of the multinational companies' products are manufactured locally. The Government Pharmaceutical Organization (GPO) manufactures preparations in Thailand's National List of Essential Drugs (130 substances, in approximately 420 presentations). The pharmaceutical market size is approximately US$3300 million; 50% of the population prefer self-medication through drug stores, rather than visiting a medical doctor.

Patents Protection and Intellectual Property

The USA removed Thailand from the priority foreign country list and threatened trade sanctions. Thailand remained on the priority watch list. Currently there is pipeline protection for 5 years for pharmaceuticals.

Business Addresses in Thailand

Thai Pharmaceutical Manufacturers' Association, Rattapaitoon Building, 2884 New Petchburi Road, Bangkok 10310, Thailand.

Government Pharmaceutical Organization, GPO 75/1 Phar-Ram 6 Road, Phayathai, Bangkok 10400, Thailand.

Food and Drug Administration, Devavesm Palace, Samsen Road, Bangkok 10200, Thailand.

Pharmaceutical Products Association, 4th Floor, White Group Building, 75 Soi Rubia, Sukumuit 42, Bangkok 10110, Thailand.

SINGAPORE

Singapore Healthcare

Singapore's population of 2.6 million is provided with a comprehensive medical service by the Ministry of Health and by many private practitioners and hospitals. There are about 10 government hospitals, with a total of 7898 beds. Another 2076 beds are available in 12 private hospitals. The latest state-of-the-art center is the 712-bed National University Hospital, set up at a cost of $18 million. The private 485-bed Mount Elizabeth Hospital, acquired by National Medical Enterprises of Los Angeles, with a specialist cancer unit, is the first of its kind in the region. Four of the government hospitals, namely Alexander Hospital, Singapore General Hospital, Tan Tock-Seng Hospital, and Toa Payoh Hospital are designated as regional general hospitals. Kandang Kerbau Hospital is the largest hospital for obstetric and gynacology services. Woodbridge hospital specializes in psychiatry, and Trafalgar hospital is the only leprosarium in Singapore. The 200-bed Center for Communicable Diseases is the center for the treatment of AIDS and venereal diseases. Currently there are 2700 doctors in Singapore, giving a doctor: population ratio of about 1:1000. Singapore will need a total of 4700 doctors by the year 2000.

Hospital Development Plan

In keeping with the Ministry's policy of expanding and upgrading the quality of public healthcare, a modernization programme was drawn up in 1978. The commissioning of the new Singapore General Hospital marks a new era of medical development in Singapore. This hospital has a total of 1651 beds, was constructed at a cost of US$180 million and was equipped with the latest medical equipment; it was commissioned in 1981.

Another landmark in Singapore's progress towards medical excellence is the newly completed National University Hospital, built in two phases, with a bed complement of 712, and opened in 1985. It is significant that this hospital has been given autonomy in management.

Community Hospitals

The first 200-bed community hospital has been built in Ang Mo Kio and was completed in 1990. It provides rehabilitation services and basic laboratory and X-ray services.

Purchasing of Medical Equipment and Supply

Government hospitals always buy on tender. The purchasing policy has been decentralized, the Pharmaceutical Department, 1 Jalan Bukit Merah, Singapore 0316, would call tenders for consumables; the Biomedical Engineering Dept, c/o Singapore General Hospital, 6 Level 2, 7 Outrum Road, Singapore 0316, for electromedical equipment; and hospitals would issue tenders themselves for capital purchases and replacement parts. Private hospitals and medical practitioners buy independently from local agents, who supply the equipment from their stock.

Privatization

The national University Hospital was privatized in 1986 as a pilot scheme. The experiment was successful and the new system will be extended to the Singapore General Hospital and later to other hospitals. It will result in a substantial upgrade of equipment facilities and services in order to be competitive among autonomous hospitals.

Distribution

Most companies have their marketing, sales and distribution operated through a local agent and distributor. Some companies have their own regional offices. Leading distributors in Singapore are Zuellig, Diethelm, Summit, and Guardian.

Patent protection is available

Foreign investment incentives are affected by Singapore government's Economic Development Board as 5–10% tax-free status for new technology companies or those conducting R&D. An investment allowance of 50% may be used in R&D. There is a cash grant for training local staff, etc.

Tips for Success in the Far East

Before travelling to the Far East, read something about the area you are visiting to avoid culture shock. A reasonable sense of humour is acceptable in most countries in the Far East. English is widely spoken, but learning the basics of the national language can open doors and hearts and possibly minds. Shaking hands is a routine daily ritual before and after business meetings. Personal contact in the Far East is of tremendous value. Think positively at all times. Watch your body language. Don't value people according to their fluency in English, French, etc. Modify your ear to listen to English in a foreign accent and try to see the contrast in a positive way—don't expect English with an Oxford accent.

Tips for Registration Dossier Compilation

Communicate with colleagues in the Far East well in advance. Plan well ahead to investigate whether the product is of significant value to the market. Start with documentation and certificates that need legalization to save time. The index of contents should be accurate and clear. Dossier format must be well-presented, bound and clearly labeled. Health authorities' registration guidelines, if available, should be requested and followed. Organize your work and start with priority markets first. The dossier is first checked for completeness, so do not forget any document needed in the requirement. Do not flood the authorities with unwanted information.

MALAYSIA

Trading with Malaysia holds many attractions. It is the most prosperous country in the Far East after Japan. Economically progressive, it has plenty of natural resources, including timber, tin, rubber, petrol and gas, palm oil products, and spices. Indeed, one can say that Malaysia is also a land of plenty. It enjoys a parliamentary democracy, constitutional monarchy, and freedom of the press. It has a well-structured healthcare system and its registration regulations are tailored to encourage multinationals to invest in the country.

Malaysia imports medicinal and pharmaceutical products worth in the region of £80 million a year. The UK's share of this market is approximately 14%, with competition from the USA, Germany, and Switzerland. Malaysia also has a growing domestic pharmaceutical manufacturing industry, mostly wholly owned subsidiaries or joint venture partnerships with foreign manufacturers, mainly from then UK and the USA.

Under the Control of Drugs and Cosmetics Regulation 1984, which came into force in November 1985, it is mandatory for all pharmaceutical products to be registered with the Drug Control Authority (established at the same time) before they can be imported, manufactured, sold, or supplied. The regulation covers 'a drug in a pharmaceutical dosage form or a cosmetic having a singular identity, composition, characteristic and origin'.

Realistically, it was recognized that it would take some time for the authority to complete processing the registration applications for all types of medicines covered, and so the system is being introduced in stages. The first products required to be registered are prescription drugs, technically classified as poisons under the Malaysian Ordinance 1952. They are to be followed by OTC items and, finally, by traditional medicines and cosmetics.

Through their historic links with the UK, Malaysians are well acquainted with UK goods. The many doctors and pharmacists who completed their training in the UK are consequently well informed on British products and have a high regard for UK manufacturing standards. Glaxo is the leading pharmaceutical company, with a plant in Petaling Jaya, near Kuala Lumpur.

A newcomer to Malaysia can do business in the area through one of the large number of Malaysian companies which function as distributors and agents for overseas pharmaceutical manufacturers and suppliers. When appointing an agent, however, it is important to ascertain the equity structure of the company you are dealing with, or what alternative arrangements are in place for participating in government sector tenders. This is because, under the government's New Economic Policy (NEP), which came into operation in 1970, government departments and agencies are obliged to deal only with Bumiputra companies, defined as those which have at least a 30% Bumiputra-controlled equity. Bumiputra, literally translated, means 'son of the soil'—that is, Malay. The NEP was brought in following serious racial rioting in 1969 to increase the modest Bumiputra share of the corporate sector to about 30% by 1990, principally through economic expansion.

When competing for Ministry of Health pharmaceutical tenders, Bumiputra companies consequently enjoy preferential treatment. However, most non-Bumiputra companies now have a Bumiputra partner or associate who processes the government tender applications on their behalf.

Product Registration

Applications for product registration should be addressed to:

The Secretariat of the Drug Control Authority, National Pharmaceutical Control Laboratory, Ministry of Health, Jalan University, PO Box 319, 46730 Petaling Jaya, Malaysia,

and made by the manufacturer or a locally incorporated firm or authorized by the manufacturer in writing to be the holder of the registration certificate. Application forms and guidelines can be obtained from the Drug Control Authority for a fee of M$250 (Malaysian dollars)

The documents that must accompany the application form are: the applicant company's incorporation certificate; a letter of authorization from the manufacturer; evidence of marketing of 'existing products'; certificate of sale and good manufacturing practice (GMP) for imported products; and product information and data-supporting documentation, sufficient to establish safety, efficacy, and quality.

A separate application is required for each product. Where injectable pharmaceutical products are concerned, a separate registration application must be submitted for different packing or pack sizes.

Registration compilation is expected to be well presented and orderly. Important relevant articles, papers, and reports should be enclosed, especially for new or little-known ingredients that are not subject of the current pharmacopoeias and standard references.

Applications must be in the national language (Bahasa Malaysia). All other data and supporting documentation, labels, package inserts and summary of product characteristics (SPC) must be in Bahasa Malaysia or English.

THE PHILIPPINES

Health Care in The Philippines

PHC Project (Primary Health Care) was introduced in 1981. This provides basic medical care to rural areas through hospitals and health centers. District Hospitals and Provincial Hospitals act as referral hospitals. The Philippines' Department of Health has allocated 60% of its budget to the running of government hospitals. The Government spends US$40 million on pharmaceuticals, amounting to 16% of the Department of Health budget, but only 8% of the total pharmaceutical market. Recently the government of The Philippines has started issuing tenders for the purchase of essential drugs. 35 million people are covered by the Medicare Health Insurance Scheme (government and private sector employees). Other private health insurance schemes also exist.

Pharmaceuticals in The Philippines

There are a number of contract manufacturers, e.g. Interphil (subsidiary of Zuellig), and pharmaceutical manufacturers, which provide for 30% of the market; 95% of the pharmaceutical raw materials are imported, with finishing and packaging carried out locally.

There are 32 pharmaceutical manufacturers in The Philippines:

- Bio, Marsman, Hizon, Metro.
- Drug makers and Interphil (Zuellig), engaged in contract manufacturing.
- United Laboratories.

The multinational companies with local manufacturing plant in The Philippines are: Abbot; Bristol–Myers Squibb; Novartis; Hoechst Marion Roussel; Nicholas Kiwi; Pfizer; Smith Beecham; Sterling; Warner Lambert; and Wyeth.

Chem Field is a government pharmaceutical company with almost a monopoly in antibiotic manufacturing, especially ampicillin, amoxycillin and cloaxacillin.

FFPI (Philippines Pharmaceutical Industry Association) is advising the government to set up raw material manufacturing plant, rather than producing finished products.

The Pharmaceutical Market

The Philippines' pharmaceutical market is a small but lucrative one. There are 50 companies which compete in the market, with a market size of US$300 milllion, and 10 874 preparations are available (9154 branded, 1720 generic). The local Philippine pharmaceutical company, United Laboratories, dominates the market and has 22% of the market share. Foreign companies account for 60% of the market; no-one has more than 5% share. Antibiotics form the largest proportion of imported drugs, followed by vitamins. Pharmaceutical exports from The Philippines are almost negligible.

Regulatory Affairs and Registration

The Bureau of Food and Drugs (BFAD) controls product registration. Their address is:

Bureau of Food and Drugs, Department of Health Compound, Albang. Muntinglupa, Metro Manila, The Philippines.

Pharmaceutical manufacturing retail licenses are issued by BFAD. A local clinical trial must be carried out for new substances (new brands or new drugs), and registration is granted for 1 year initially. Postmarketing surveillance reports must be submitted twice a year to BFAD. Patent protection is available and implemented.

Clinical Trials

Clinical trials can be conducted in The Philippines provided prior permission from the BFAD is granted. The application and protocol are submitted to BFAD. There is an approved list of clinicians from which investigators are selected. Clinical trials must be conducted in accordance with guidelines on

GCP. Patients' informed consent must be obtained, in accordance with the Declaration of Helsinki.

INDONESIA

Indonesia is considered the fourth most populated country after China, India, and USA. Two-thirds of the population is concentrated in Java, 19% in Sumatra, 8% in Sulawesi, 5% in Kalimantan, and 6% on Eastern Islands off Indonesia.

Rural health services are provided through a network of health subcenters, health centers and district hospitals. Urban health services are provided through specialized and provincial hospitals, which are located in large cities. A Health Subcenter is staffed by a full-time nurse who provides simple basic medical care, including maternal/child healthcare, vaccinations and nutrition.

Health Centres (Puskesmas)

There are 5800 centres in Indonesia. Health centers provide basic medical care, maternal and child health services. Some health centers have inpatient facilities (10–bedded wards). They are staffed by GPs and nurses.

Hospitals

District hospitals supports the primary health care facilities provided by the health centers, whilst general hospitals provide specialist services.

Health Workers

There are 284 000 health workers in Indonesia in the government sector. These include physicians, dentists, pharmacists, paramedics, nurses, and technicians. There are 40 000 health workers in the private sector.

Pertamina and Indonesia Armed Forces

Pertamina (State Oil Company) and the Armed Forces have their own medical services. These,

together with the private sector, operate well-equipped hospitals.

Pharmaceutical Industry—Distribution, Pricing and Market Size

There are approximately 900 pharmaceutical wholesales, 340 with limited local activities. Distribution is fragmented, due to Indonesia's geography, thus sales figures are difficult to acquire. The wholesalers' mark-up is 20%, whilst the pharmacy mark-up is 45%. The market size is approximately US$400–500 million. The leading products in sales volume are: antibiotics; vitamins and minerals; respiratory drugs; dermatology drugs; analgesics; hormones; cardiovascular drugs; psychotropics; antiinflamatory drugs; anti-TB drugs; and anti-spasmodics.

Registration in Indonesia

All medical products marketed in Indonesia must be registered and approved by the Ministry of Health through POM (Pengawasan Obat den MaKanan, the Food and Drug Authority). Applications are referred to a special committee, PPOJ (Panitia Penilai Obat Jadi), to examine the documents submitted. There are expert committees to review pharmaceuticals and medical products on behalf of PPOJ. The secretariat of PPOJ then prepares a report to the Directorate General and, if the product is approved, a registration number is issued by the Ministry of Health.

Clinical Research

Clinical trials can be conducted in Indonesia, but prior permission must be obtained from the Ministry of Health in advance.

Pharmaceutical Manufacturers in Indonesia

The Indonesian pharmaceutical industry imports 95% of the pharmaceutical raw materials needed. Importation of finished products is not allowed, except for medical products not manufactured locally, e.g. insulin. There are 280 pharmaceutical manufacturers in Indonesia: (a) 40 large local companies, others small; (b) 40 foreign companies; and (c) State-owned companies. A foreign company must operate through a joint venture with an Indonesian firm. The Indonesian firm must have 30% equity in the shareholding.

Multinational Companies Operating in Indonesia

These are Bristol–Myers Squibb; E.Mark; Bayer; Pfizer; and Glaxo Wellcome. Antibiotics assume the leading therapeutic category in Indonesia (25% of total market). They are followed by vitamins, minerals and tonics.

Regulatory Affairs and Registration

There is a long delay for products to be registered; sometimes it can take 2–3 years. Local companies are able to obtain registration as quickly as 6 months. The Regulatory Authority address is:

Directorate General of Drug and Food Centre, Ministry of Health, DIR. JEN. POM, Department Kesehatan R.I, JI Percetakan Negara 23, Jakarta 10560, Indonesia.

REFERENCES

Hammad G (1993) The Middle East—opportunities for the pharmaceutical industry. *Pharmaceut Physician* 5(5): 56–60.

Hammad G (1994a) Medicines abroad: the Far East—opportunities for the pharmaceutical industry, Part I. *Pharmaceut Physician* 6(5): 70–79.

Hammad G (1994b) Malysia—Land of Plenty *Pharmaceut Vision*, 2(2): 62–67, Published by Highbury House Communications PLC, London).

Hammad G (1995) Medicines abroad: the Far East. Part II. *Pharmaceut Physician* 6(6): 58–64.

Hammad G (1996a) Medicines abroad—China (Part I). Pharmaceuticals in the People's Republic—business opportunities in the twenty first century and beyond *Pharmaceut Physician* 7(6): 70–75.

Hammad G (1996b) Medicines abroad—China (Part II). Pharmaceuticals in the People's Republic—clinical trials. *Pharmaceut Physician* 7(8): 59–68.

IFPMA (1994) *IFPMA Compendium*.

42

Financial Aspects of Clinical Trials

R.G. Hughes[1] and N. Turner[2]

[1]Technomark Consulting Services, London, and [2]Astra-Zeneca Pharmaceuticals, Macclesfield, UK

Clinical trials are major budget items in drug development. The total costs vary according to therapeutic area, indication, duration of the study, and numbers of subjects. Even for rapidly acting drugs in acute conditions (e.g. infections), the cost is unlikely to be below $50 million, while for a slow-acting drug for a chronic condition (e.g., osteoporosis), expenditure of $300 million is possible.

The cost of a clinical trial arises from both internal and external costs. Internal costs are those that are wholly incurred within the organization (personnel, office supplies, etc.); external costs are those incurred on such items as investigators, laboratories, travel, etc. Quantification of the internal costs, especially those associated with personnel, has proved a persistent challenge, as discussed below.

We have grouped the external costs of a clinical trial as follows:

- Investigator fees.
- Laboratory charges.
- Travel.
- Clinical trial medication[1] (when manufactured or packaged by a contractor).
- Ethics committees and institutional review boards (EC/IRBs).
- Regulatory fees.
- Consultancy.
- Patient fees.
- Equipment.
- Finance.
- Meetings.
- Printing and copying.

In addition, we have addressed the issue of internal costs and the use of contract research organizations (CROs), particularly with respect to: (a) obtaining and comparing CRO bids; (b) assessing the financial stability of a CRO; (c) choosing the right type of contract.

INVESTIGATOR FEES

Fees paid to investigators to conduct clinical trials vary according to a number of criteria:

- Therapeutic area.
- Country/continent.
- Protocol
- Phase of protocol.
- Number of patient visits.
- Type and number of procedures.
- Affiliation and eminence of the investigator.

The most important of these is probably the protocol, which governs the amount of time the investigator must devote to the patient and to the organization of the trial. Traditionally, investigators would manage studies on a personal basis, but increasingly they have relied on the assistance of more junior doctors, research nurses, and other staff who may not be medically qualified. A more recent innovation has been the emergence of the managed investigational site. In such organizations the investigator handles only the minimum of administration, while the site organization, which has contracted with the sponsor company, handles issues such as patient recruitment, informed consent, patient records, case record forms, appointment keeping, financial accounting, etc. Such arrangements are widespread in the USA but are only just emerging in Europe, particularly in the UK.

The protocol governs not only the time the doctor spends with the patient, but the quality

Principles and Practice of Pharmaceutical Medicine. Edited by A. J. Fletcher, Lionel D. Edwards, Anthony W. Fox and Peter Stonier © 2002 John Wiley & Sons Ltd.

of it and the various procedures that are associated with the study. Some of these may not be supervised by the investigator, or at least only indirectly (e.g. X-rays, ECG, etc.), whilst others may need specialized medical training to be administered, e.g. endoscopy or surgical investigative procedures. In both Europe and the USA, institutions often have a varying pricing policy, depending on who, or which, organization, requests the procedure. Thus, X-rays arranged via a professor may well cost less than those arranged directly by the sponsor. Increasingly, institutions attempt to separate out the cost of investigative procedures from the 'true' investigator fees, which account solely for the time spent by the investigator.

The therapeutic area or medical speciality also determines costs of studies. Information from DataEdge, PICAS[TM] database, indicates widespread variations (Hovde 1993, 1997) (Figure 42.1).

Compared with Western Europe, the USA consistently trends as the most expensive country. A dominant pattern is that the more expensive the procedure, the greater the US price premium. The price ratios for common research procedures have been reported as in Table 42.1.

Comparisons for total clinical trial costs can also be made among countries (Fig. 42.2) may come as a surprise to many that the UK, on the basis of this evidence, comes out the most expensive, although the relatively lower cost of Italy and Spain is more expected. A wider variation in the relative costs of studies for both Europe and the USA is seen. It should be emphasized that these relative costs do not depend on the length and complexity of the study, but are reflective of the fee levels expected by the physicians running the studies and, to a lesser extent, the cost of the investigative procedures.

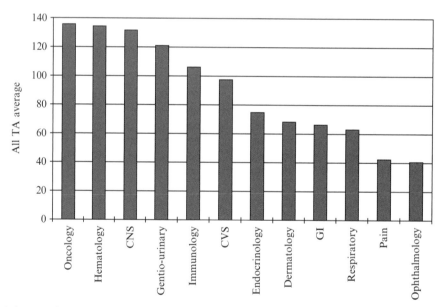

Figure 42.1 Relative costs by therapeutic area

Table 42.1 Price ratios for common research procedures

Procedure	Cost (US $ equivalent)					
	USA	France	UK	Netherlands	Belgium	Denmark
ECG	256	81	100	66	90	96
Chest X-ray	335	114	100	144	121	119

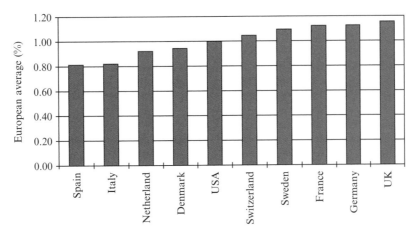

Figure 42.2 Relative costs by country

As recently as 1993 it was widely observed that investigator fees were significantly lower in Eastern and Central Europe (the former communist countries) than in the rest of Europe (Hughes 1994), but now these fees are rapidly increasing to a level approaching that of the West (Hughes 1997). Some sponsors have indicated that, for Europe at least, they will pay the same fee to all investigators, regardless of their country, and this is also now common practice for multicenter studies in various states of the USA. This overcomes the invidious situation of investigators comparing fees at investigator meetings, with the inevitable result that the lower paid feel short-changed. Due to various scandals in Japan, the methods of paying fees to investigators have recently been revised. It is now no longer formally permitted to pay investigator fees to doctors based in National Hospitals directly; all fees now are paid to the institution. Such hospitals typically have a complex calculation chart (Table 42.2), which is used to calculate the fees.

Total clinical costs = subtotal of points (A) × ¥6000 × number of patients + subtotal of points (B) × ¥6000

Such calculations yield fees that are of similar order of magnitude to equivalent studies in North America.

Although not normally regarded as the remit of the ethics committee or IRB (at least in Europe and the USA), such bodies from time to time have indicated to sponsors that they feel that a particular fee paid to investigators for a particular trial is excessive. Such observations have generally been borne out of ignorance of the going rate for investigators and the fact that sponsors compete in a competitive market, in an era of declining government-sponsored research. Indeed, some therapeutic areas are 'fashionable', and when a number of sponsors conduct trials simultaneously in the same, or adjacent, indication, a relative dearth of patients develops, and investigators will tend to raise their fee expectations accordingly. For this reason alone, the sponsor of the first trial in a particular area with a novel drug may gain a financial advantage over its industry competitors with later, me-too, drugs.

The affiliation of an investigator can influence the fees paid in two ways. First, investigators attached to prestigious universities or medical clinics may feel, perhaps justifiably, that they are deserving of higher fees, given that the prestige of their institution adds to the acceptability of the study to the regulators and, more importantly, the value of the study for eventual marketing purposes. Second, institutions now almost uniformly charge an overhead ranging from a few percent to over 100% of the basic investigator fees and procedure fees. In the planning stages of a clinical trial, ignoring such potential up-charges can lead to unpleasant financial surprises at a later date and require revisiting the initial budget.

Table 42.2 Calculation table for clinical fees in Japan

Factors	Weight*	Points			Sum
		I (Weight × 1)	II (Weight × 3)	III (Weight × 5)	
Severity of disease	2	Slight	Moderate	Severe	
Hospitalization	1	Outpatient	Inpatient	–	
Route of administration	1	External use Oral	s.c. or i.m. injection	i.v. Injection	
Study design	2	Open	Single-blind	Double-blind	
Population	1	Adult	Children or elderly	Newborn	
Administration period	2	< 4 weeks	5–24 weeks	> 25 weeks	
Frequency of visit	1	Once in 4 weeks or less	Twice in 4 weeks	More than three times in 4 weeks	
Number of items	2	< 50 items	51–100 items	> 101 items	
Frequency of blood and/or urinary sample	2	Once per visit	2–3 per visit	> 4 per visit	
Non-invasive tests	1	–	< 5 tests	> 6 tests	
Invasive tests	3	–	< 5 tests	> 6 tests	
Subtotal of points (A)					a
Presentation of cases	7	1			
Volume of reports	5	< 30 pages	31–50 pages	> 51 pages	
Subtotal of points (B)					b
Total points					a + b

* Based on numbers of clinical tests, symptoms to be checked per visit.

LABORATORY CHARGES

The cost of laboratory analysis of specimens from patients can be a significant proportion of the overall cost of a clinical trial. For early studies, costs are high for GLP assays of blood, urine or plasma for parent drug and metabolite. Routine hematology and biochemistry at larger scale, then takes over in later trials. The overall cost is not, however, just the cost of analysis; the total cost may include elements such as sample kit design and manufacture, transport of kits to investigator sites, transport of kits to central, analysing laboratories, interpretation of results, customs charges, data processing of results at the laboratory, and transmission of the results to the data management centre, as well as the actual cost of the analysis. Pharmaceutical physicians often miss an opportunity to reduce costs by using local laboratories in multicenter clinical trials. Regulatory authorities have openly stated that much of the laboratory data collected and submitted is superfluous or irrelevant, so that discussion with regulators of what precisely is to be measured in any particular study can result in significant savings.

The cost of the basic hematology and biochemistry varies from country to country, as well as being dependent on the institution carrying out such analysis. Purely commercial central laboratories, which carry out analysis only in connection with clinical trials, may at first sight appear expensive when compared with the cost of a local hospital or doctor's laboratory. However, the additional services provided by the central laboratory, together with the reduced necessity for both qualification and audit of a diverse group of regional laboratories, as well as the not insignificant cost of consolidating the data from these laboratories, should easily compensate for the apparent higher price.

TRAVEL

Few studies are conducted at a single location, and travel by study monitors, CRAs, physicians and auditors can amount to significant expenditure.

Major companies can ameliorate such costs by negotiating special rates with airlines, rental car companies, and hotel chains. Indeed, companies may be able to pass such savings on to CROs working for them. Such savings may amount to 50% of the total travel budget.

Much is made of the savings that can be made by use of regional monitors—either as full-time employees or as exclusive or non-exclusive contract employees. At first sight, such arrangements can result in important savings; however, these can be offset by the need for additional project team meetings and training, greater use of telephone and video conferencing and, not infrequently, by site visits by more senior employees and auditors. It is thus often difficult to determine real savings made by a regional monitor policy.

What is apparent from the recent Central and Eastern European Study (Hughes 1997) is that travel to these countries can be very costly, compared with the cost of travel within, for example, the USA. Likewise, travel to and within Scandinavia still remains a high-cost item.

CLINICAL TRIAL MEDICATION

The sponsor must also account for the cost of preparing and providing appropriately packaged clinical trial medication to be used in its trials. This may include procurement or manufacture of comparator treatments and/or placebo medication.

Clearly, arrangements must be made early in the trial to ensure that an efficient supply chain is set up and the associated costs (which can be significant) taken into account. In recent years, sponsors have utilized methods such as minimization techniques (within the randomization process for controlled randomized trials) to help reduce waste of clinical trial medication and hence reduce the overall cost.

ETHICS COMMITTEES AND INSTITUTIONAL REVIEW BOARDS (EC/IRBS)

IRBs are increasingly requiring payment to evaluate protocols: when a single IRB can be used, this fee is likely to be insignificant. However, in Europe and the USA, multiple local research ethics committees often have to be consulted and, even if their individual fees are modest at rarely more than $2000 per protocol, the effect of dozens of such committees can be quite substantial. In Germany, it is a legal requirement for IRB approval within each State that the study is conducted, since some State IRBs are not constituted in a manner meeting GCP requirements (e.g. they may be composed solely of physicians). Further IRB approval is usually necessary.

REGULATORY FEES

Few developed States currently charge a significant administration fee for a clinical trials approval (Massachusetts is one example). In less developed countries it may prove necessary to pay true fees together with 'consultation' fees to government advisors. Sponsors will, however, need to take into account the costs associated with the effort of their internal regulatory staff in preparing CTX submissions (or their equivalent).

CONSULTANCY

Consultants may be involved in clinical trials at various stages. At the planning stage they may be used to develop, refine, or approve the protocol. Consultants may be used individually to advise during the course of the trial—the 'principal investigator' will often play an important role in the study design, although the distinguished individual usually chosen may not recruit any patients (in Germany the appointment of the principal investigator is a regulatory requirement, and the medical monitor is a signatory on form 1541 in the USA, and the CTX in the UK). Many major studies, particularly those of life-threatening diseases and those with mortality as an endpoint, have steering and advisory committees drawn from the higher scholars of the academic medical world. Such committees add to the prestige and acceptability of such studies, but also add to the cost!

PATIENT FEES

While it is almost universal practice for healthy volunteers to be compensated (paid) for taking part in Phase I studies, to date it is very unusual for European patients to be paid more than token sums for transport and inconvenience, for taking part in studies. In the USA, such practices are common, and advertisements in local newspapers and on radio/TV channels for patients at $500–1000/head are by no means unusual.

In both the USA and Europe, advertising for patients is generally acceptable (although it is much more usual in the USA). Generally, approval of advertisements by local ethics committees is required. Mass marketing techniques and rapid recruitment of qualified patients by external agencies may well be highly cost-effective when clinical trials are planned or under way.

EQUIPMENT

We have already noted that sample kits for clinical samples from patients may have to be designed and manufactured. Additional costs may be incurred, especially in less developed countries, by the need to provide investigators with items of medical equipment. Even in the UK, it is common for sponsors to provide random-zero sphygmomanometers, as well as equipment that would not normally be found in a doctor's office, such as a centrifuge. In Central and Eastern Europe and Latin America, even basic medical equipment may be necessary or appreciated, while communications equipment, such as faxes, modems, or even photocopiers, may markedly improve the logistics of a study.

FINANCE

A multinational trial can be a significant challenge to accounting departments of sponsors, and it is to be strongly advised that accounting/finance and purchasing personnel be involved at an early stage of the project. Such early involvement should allow the efficient financing of the project, not only from the formal budgeting process but also in ensuring that there is an efficient process for investigators and other subcontractors to be paid on time. The added international dimension of large trials can also be a challenge, particularly where fluctuating exchange rates are involved. Finance and purchas-

ing departments should examine the need to hedge against currency variations which, over the life of a study, even in countries with relatively stable currencies, can introduce a variance of ± 30% from the projected out-of-pocket fees.

MEETINGS

One or more investigators' meetings is often regarded as indispensable to the success of a clinical trial. As with so many items, the expenditure on such meetings is far from insignificant. Apart from the hire of an appropriate venue, it is important not to overlook the cost of transportation and investigators' time, as well as the time involved by the sponsor in both organizing and attending such meetings. Such meetings held prior to and during the trial are invaluable, however, for improving conformity of conduct of the study, as well as being strongly motivational for investigators. A final meeting or meetings can also be useful for binding in investigators for subsequent trials, as well as providing strong market promotion when the objectives of the trial have been achieved.

PRINTING AND COPYING

Clinical trials generate paper—at the beginning, during the study, and as a final report. The cost of printing and distribution of printed materials in a large major study should not be ignored, but if undertaken by a sponsor internally, may easily be overlooked. The cost of production of multipart case record forms (CRFs) is only one of the costs involved for a major multinational study. With multiple patients, centers, investigators, and IRB/ECs, many copies of protocols, patient information leaflets, investigator brochures, ethics committee submissions, etc., will add to a printing and copying budget that may be insidiously doubled by these non-CRF printing charges, which are often thought to be insignificant.

INTERNAL COSTS

Apart possibly from investigators' fees, in-house costs represent the greatest single item in a clinical

Table 42.3 Costing categories for a clinical Phase III project

1. Protocol design and development
2. CRF, patient information sheet, informed consent form design and development
3. Investigator identification and qualification
4. Initiation visits to study sites
5. Administration of ethics committee approvals
6. Regulatory approvals
7. Clinical trial supply labeling
8. Translation of study documentation
9. Set-up and attendance at investigators' meetings
10. Study monitoring (including secondary in-house data cleaning and monitoring reports)
11. Administration of investigator payments
12. Identification, qualification and management of central laboratory(ies)
13. Administration of payments to central laboratory(ies)
14. Set-up and administration of central randomization system
15. Reporting of serious ADRs to regulatory authorities and sponsor (including written reports)
16. Distribution of all trial materials (documentation and study medication)
17. Reconciliation of study medication
18. Return of study medication to sponsor
19. Quality Assurance audits:
    (a) Clinical-in-house
    (b) Clinical-on site
    (c) Database
    (d) Central laboratory(ies)
20. Database design (including validation plan and programming)
21. Double data entry and data management (including query generation and resolution)
22. Statistical plan and programming
23. Statistical analysis and reporting
24. Integrated statistical and medical report
25. Archiving of study documentation
26. Project management

trials budget. Table 42.3 lists many of the subdivisions of costing that could be regarded as internal, the vast majority of which could be outsourced to CROs or similar organizations.

In order that the true internal costs of a study can be calculated, it is necessary that a sponsor completes a similar exercise, using its own internal fully overheaded costs for each of the cost center personnel that are used. It should be strongly emphasized that many previous cost estimates produced by sponsors that have seemed at variance with CROs' cost estimates have been based on an inadequate understanding of the sponsors' own fully overheaded costs.

We may observe that the concept of calculating internal sponsor costs, either for executing clinical projects internally or managing such projects through CROs, is a relatively recent one; i.e. it is still not unusual for a sponsor to have little idea about its own internal costs. This was borne out in a recent survey (King 1997) of 27 pharmaceutical companies, 41% of whom reported that they did calculate internal costs, 33% reported that they did not, and, interestingly, 26% didn't know!

Various methods have been and are used for the calculation of internal costs, two of which have been published widely; the Hoechst Marion Roussel model, derived and published by Thom Hill (Hill and Hubbard 1996) and the MSD BARDS model (Papazian and Wise 1995). A reliable and reproducible method must include the calculation of the cost of a full time equivalent (FTE) employee for each function or task involved in executing and managing the project. Hill's model (Table 42.4) provides a useful illustration of how this may translate into sterling or dollars. This exercise is in itself useful (i.e. even if there are no definite plans to outsource), since clinical development functions are working increasingly in an environment of cost containment. Obviously, such calculations also provide a necessary basis for the comparison of internal costs vs. proposed CRO costs for

Table 42.4 Model for FTE cost calculation

Annual base salary + benefits (e.g. 35% of salary) + bonus (e.g. 5% of salary) = Total personnel costs
+ operational costs (e.g. 78% of total personnel costs) includes infrastructure support, overheads and administration = total personnel costs plus operational costs = total or fully overheaded FTE cost

Example calculation of daily FTE cost for an experienced CRA in the UK

Annual base salary	£25 000
Benefits	£8750
Bonus	£2500
Total personnel cost	£36 500
Operational costs (78%)	£28 470
Total FTE Cost	£64 970
Daily FTE Cost (assuming 230 days/year)	£282

Clearly, the calculation of the total cost for completion of a project must rely on good forecasting of resource needs, in terms of number and type of staff required and number of hours/days required.

completion of a project. The sponsor should not forget, however, that there must be a cost associated with the management and overseeing of a CRO, and that this cost must be estimated and included in the overall costs for outsourcing a project (the MSD BARDS group has conducted both a retrospective and a prospective study to quantify the oversight cost, and have suggested adding an average of 15% of the total project cost to cover this) (Papazian and Wise 1995).

USE OF CONTRACT RESEARCH ORGANIZATIONS (CROS)

As mentioned above, it is possible to use CROs to carry out all, or virtually all, the functions of a sponsor in the conduct of a clinical trial X-CROs are no longer being used in emergency—a last resort. CROs are widely regarded as a primary resource by many companies, so much so that preferred provider and strategic alliance relationships have been developed by many of the major multinational companies.

We will now discuss three aspects of CRO involvement in clinical trials that are relevant to the subject of this chapter: (a) obtaining bids; (b) assessing financial stability; and (c) choosing the right contract framework.

Obtaining and Comparing CRO Bids

In comparison with internal cost calculation, this aspect of the contracting process is undoubtedly a much more developed skill within sponsor companies. Although much has been written and presented about the process of requesting CRO proposals (or RFPs, as they have become known), some useful 'rules of thumb' that should facilitate the process are:

- Ideally, bids from no more than five CROs should be requested. The main issues here concern both the difficulty of comparing numerous bids and fairness to the CROs in terms of the probability of winning the business, when considering the degree of effort required on their part to put a proposal together.
- Brief the CROs as comprehensively and consistently as possible. Consistency is key here if bids are to be compared fairly.
- Give the CROs at least 2 weeks to prepare the bid.
- Provide a bid template (Brancaccio 1997) and request that it is used (ask the CROs to estimate their professional fees and the out-of-pocket/pass-through costs). It may be prudent to insist that CROs use a template that can be supplied by the sponsor on disk.

- Request daily rate fees (i.e. FTE rates for each of the functional staff to be involved).
- Ask the CROs to document all assumptions made.
- Prepare yourself for the responses, e.g. construct a master spreadsheet with (internal) costs also inserted in for ease of comparison.
- Be available for clarifying questions from the CRO when making their bid: it is the best way to get an apples vs. apples comparison.

Table 42.5 illustrates the comparative bids received from three CROs who were asked to bid for the partial (2000 patients from 50 centers in the UK) clinical management and complete data management, statistics, and reporting for a 6000 patient multinational cardiovascular mortality study. The study parameters were as follows:

- 4–6 year treatment period.
- 5 year follow-up.
- 250 page CRF.

Despite the relative uniformity of daily rate fees across the three CROs, there are significant variations between the line item (or task) bids, as well as the 'bottom line' or total bids.

The importance of the sponsor having already calculated its internal costs for executing the project cannot be overemphasized in this situation—it allows the sponsor to ask sensible and informed questions of the CROs and, most importantly, it allows the sponsors to assess which of the CROs has provided the most realistic bid; it is not good practice simply to choose the lowest or average bid (i.e. on an empirical basis), since the highest bid may well in fact be the most realistic and based on real experience of performing a similar clinical trial.

Assessing the Financial Stability of a CRO

The financial stability of CROs has commanded more attention than the situation probably deserves. The recent history of CROs shows few business failures and, in comparison with other service suppliers, CROs are remarkably stable and resilient.

The assessment of the financial stability of a CRO is, in general, very difficult to accomplish. In the main, this is due to the fact that the majority of the CRO market is made up of private companies with widely differing, and often secret,

Table 42.5 Comparison of CRO bids (in £ sterling) for a mortality study

	CRO A	CRO B	CRO C
1. Selected daily rates			
CRA	500	550	400
Project manager	650	850	550
Physician	900	900	900
QA auditor	600	650	550
Data entry personnel	250	300	250
Data coordinator	360	350	375
Data manager/programmer	450	450	550
Statistician	450	650	550
2. Selected task bids			
Investigator ID and selection	49 000	110 000	208 000
Monitoring	3 750 783	4 843 875	3 944 350
Auditing	130 604	177 000	110 000
Project management	1 556 824	4 995 535	2 932 160
Database design	11 610	12 000	36 500
Double data entry and management	3 031 824	7 291 000	3 093 750
Secondary CRF review and coding	325 000	1 900 000	2 708 300
Statistical analysis (interim and final)	87 000	56 770	202 900
Integrated report	25 000	25 450	59 000
Total project bid (professional fees)	9 340 945	20 057 380	15 607 660

Table 42.6 Questions designed to elicit the overall picture of a CRO's financial situation

- What are your annual revenues—current and past?
- How are pass-through costs managed (e.g. investigator fees, etc.)?
- How many clients do you have?
- What percentage of your business is accounted for by each of your major clients?
- What is your average size of contract in financial terms?
- How much repeat business (in percentage terms) do you get?
- What is your business breakdown by service?
- Are there any pending legal cases?
- What insurance policies do you have and at what level?

accounting practices. Although most of the large CROs are now publicly quoted, and hence regularly publish their accounts and projection, these account for less than 2% of the total number of CROs worldwide, i.e. there are 20 publicly quoted companies in a total of at least 1200 companies. These 20, however, make up some 50% of the annual revenues of the CRO market sector.

Data on private companies is difficult to assemble and financial checking on the CROs is thus not straightforward. Such companies' accounts, when published at all, are often in abbreviated format, and can be up to 2½ years out of date. Organizations such as Dun & Bradstreet, and even local Chambers of Commerce, may be able to provide useful information. However, it is likely that the best source of reassurance of financial stability of a CRO is via bankers' references, obtained through the sponsor's own finance department.

The data obtained from the aforementioned sources may be difficult for the average functional manager to interpret (this where the finance managers will indeed be helpful, if not essential). However, the importance of asking sensible questions of a CRO cannot be overemphasized; the responses to these questions are essential to completing the overall picture of a CRO's financial situation, and may actually be more revealing than the bald, old audited accounts. Questions to ask would include those listed in Table 42.6. It must be remembered that CROs themselves also have a right to ask questions about their prospective sponsor's financial situation and third-party payment history.

Choosing the Right Type of Contract

An agreement on the overall budget for the project, although clearly an important milestone, does not form the basis of the contractual relationship between sponsor and CRO. The two parties must then agree on the type of contract that best meets the needs of both parties. There are four types of CRO–sponsor contracts that are currently used to any serious degree, and each of these proffers advantages and disadvantages to sponsor and CRO (see Table 42.7).

The choice of contract will depend on a series of factors, including length and complexity of the project, the functions/tasks to be contracted, and the level of trust that has built up between the CRO and sponsor (based on previous contracting experi-

Table 42.7 CRO contracts

Type of contract	Characteristics	Sponsor perspective	CRO perspective
Fixed price	Fixed price for completion of project defined up front. Clearly defined scope of work. Must have mechanism for changes in scope. Typically paid according to predefined tranches	Final price known Pay only for results CRO may have underbid, if making a loss may become lower priority within CRO Pressure to deliver, e.g. final protocol, drug supplies, sample CRFs Renegotiation is almost inevitable, maybe adversarial	Good for documentation and prediction of cash flow and for budgeting Efficiency gains are all profit Price quoted must be accurate in order to realise profit Can become a millstone Blank cheque!

Table 42.7 (*continued*)

Type of contract	Characteristics	Sponsor perspective	CRO perspective
Fee for service	Open-ended. Sponsor billed according to hours spent on project and FTE rate. The so called 'blank cheque' scenario. Must be built on trust through experience. Often used for consultancy projects	Easy to work with Can benefit from CRO efficiency Difficult to control Encourages CRO inefficiency Can create atmosphere of mistrust Blank cheque!	Allows flexibility in budgeting and scheduling of activities No incentive to increase efficiency, i.e. no financial benefit Can create atmosphere of mistrust
Fixed unit price—task-based	Sponsor and CRO agree definitions and dimensions of task (e.g. monitoring visit, database design) and allocate price to the task unit. Sponsor pays according to number of units completed	Can compare CRO activities to internal activities Easy to understand how much additional tasks will cost Renegotiation less adversarial Protracted initial negotiations to agree definition of tasks Does not encourage CRO efficiency	Renegotiation (for extra tasks) easier Protracted initial negotiations to agree definition of tasks Does not encourage CRO efficiency
Fixed unit price—milestone/ deliverable based	Sponsor and CRO agree definitions of milestone (e.g. agreed number of investigators initiated, patients entered, database locked, etc.). Sponsor pays when milestone achieved	Pay only for results Minimal renegotiation Encourages CRO efficiency: get paid quicker if work fast to achieve milestones Longer planning and negotiation phase	Rewards efficiency Longer planning and negotiation phase

ences). The aim should be to create a win – win scenario, whereby the contract is merely a reference document, rather than the controlling factor in the relationship.

Although the decision to outsource a project is not based on purely financial considerations (quality, experience, expertise, and capacity being other key determining factors), it is important for functional managers to understand some of the financial issues that are integral to both the success of an outsourced project and the ability to plan for the future. Thus, we have discussed three of the financial considerations (and associated actions) that a functional manager should and can influence in this regard, that is to:

- Compare internal costs with CRO bids, using the internal costing calculation to ask informed questions about the CRO bid.
- Ask sensible but probing questions of a CRO to help establish whether it is financially stable.

- Decide (with the CRO) on the type of contract that best meets both sponsor and CRO needs.

CONCLUSION

The financial aspects of clinical trials are wide-ranging. The clinical studies, whether managed by in or out of house personnel, represent 30–50% of the total development expenditure on any particular drug. Clinical scientists and research physicians will need much support from their qualified business and financial colleagues in order to manage these complex activities successfully.

REFERENCES

Brancaccio N (1997) The financial aspects of contracting out. *Eur Pharmaceut Contractor* 1(3): 10–22.

Hill T, Hubbard J (1996) Is outsourcing clinical trials really more expensive? *Scrip Magazine* 44 (March).

Hughes RG (1994) Contract Clinical Research in Eastern and Central Europe *Appl Clin Trials* June 3(6) 52–58.

Hughes RG (1997) Drug Information Association (DIA) Workshop—Regulatory Affairs and Clinical Trials in Eastern and Central Europe, Budapest, Hungary, October.

Hovde M (1993) global Costs of Clinical Research Budapest, Hungary, *J Appl Clin Trials* 2(10): 44–55.

Personal Communication Applied Clinical Trials 6(2) 34–42.

King HM (1997) CROs in the 1990s and beyond. Applied Clinical Trials 6(7) 45–49.

Papazian J, Wise A (1995) Comparing the costs of using CRO services to in-house management. *Proceedings of the Drug Information Association (DIA) 5th Annual European workshop on Clinical Data Management*, Nice, France, November.

43

The Impact of Managed Care on the US Pharmaceutical Industry

Robert J. Chaponis[1], Christine Hanson Divers[2] and Marilyn J. Wells[3]

[1]*Pharmacia Corporation, Peapack, New Jersey,* [2]*AstraZeneca, Apex, North Carolina,* [3]*Hampton University, Hampton, Virginia*

After rising sharply during the 1970s and 1980s, overall healthcare costs in the USA have leveled in the 1990s. This control of healthcare costs can be attributed, at least in part, to the dramatic growth of managed care. This paradigm shift from a largely fee-for-service to a managed care environment has affected every aspect of the healthcare system, including the pharmaceutical industry. Managed care organizations have helped to bring healthcare costs under control through a variety of strategies, including controlled access to healthcare providers, health plan benefit limitations, and restrictions, including pharmacy benefits and products, and capitated reimbursement systems. Although satisfied with the results of slowed increases in healthcare costs, purchasers and consumers have been less satisfied with restricted access to providers and benefit limitations and restrictions. As a result, purchasers and consumers are pressuring managed care organizations to improve access to providers and expand benefits and services.

With prescription medications accounting for an increasing proportion of total medical costs, managed care organizations are being forced to implement tighter controls in pharmacy benefit management. Traditionally, managed care impacted pharmaceutical products after reaching the market through pharmacy benefit restrictions, limitations, and product formularies. Today, managed care is influencing pharmaceuticals much earlier in the product life cycle. In many cases, the impact is being felt before a product even enters the market.

Managed care organizations are a major customer to the pharmaceutical industry, with increasing leveraging and purchasing power. Therefore, managed care organizations have had a profound impact on how the pharmaceutical industry develops, markets, distributes, and generates revenue for products. This impact will only increase in the future. This chapter will introduce basic concepts in managed care, discuss the impact of managed care on the pharmaceutical industry, and conclude with a discussion of emerging trends in managed care and how they may impact the pharmaceutical industry in the future.

THE CONCEPTS OF MANAGED CARE

The basic concepts of managed care have evolved and are continuing to evolve over time. To understand this evolution, a brief historical perspective is presented first, followed by discussions of the language and principles of managed care.

Historical Perspectives

Surpassing traditional indemnity, or fee-for-service (FFS) health insurance policies, managed care health plans now represent the largest and fastest growing type of coverage for health and medical care in the USA. From a rather slow initial growth period, which began in 1929 with the establishment of the first prepaid group practice plan, managed healthcare has grown substantially over the last 25 years (Health Insurance Association of America 1996). By the mid-1970s, approximately five million people were enrolled in prepaid group practice plans (MacLeod 1993). As of 1997, over 83 million

Principles and Practice of Pharmaceutical Medicine. Edited by A. J. Fletcher, Lionel D. Edwards, Anthony W. Fox and Peter Stonier © 2002 John Wiley & Sons Ltd.

people were enrolled in health maintenance organizations (HMOs) alone (Hoechst Marion Roussel 1998).

Concern over rapidly rising healthcare costs has been the driving force behind the rapid growth of managed care. Inherently, a FFS system, where reimbursement and compensation for services are directly related to delivery or utilization of services, has the potential to promote overutilization and drive costs upward. Alternatively, a managed care system, where payment for healthcare is typically prepaid or capitated, has more control over the utilization of services, and thereby costs. The potential of managed care to successfully control healthcare costs has long been recognized and supported by the federal government, starting with the HMO Act of 1973 to more recent healthcare reform initiatives, including the introduction, in 1998, of a Medicare Prospective Payment System (PPS) for nursing facilities.

In the managed care system, there are three major market segments—consumers, payers, and providers—each with their own distinct groups. Individual health plan members or patients represent the consumer segment. Payers, who are largely defined by their purchasing power, include employer groups (e.g. larger employers, small employers, small business coalitions, cooperative purchasing arrangements, etc.), the government (e.g. government agencies, public insurance programs—Medicare and Medicaid, etc.), and managed care organizations (e.g. HMOs, preferred provider organizations, etc.). Providers include healthcare organizations (e.g. accredited hospitals, ambulatory care centers, behavioral healthcare facilities, etc.), healthcare professionals (e.g. physicians, pharmacists, nurses, etc.) and, depending on their business model, may include managed care organizations.

While each of these market segments and groups has unique concerns, they also share common goals, through which their collective actions are defining managed care. For example, managed care systems have an intrinsic conflict between prepayment for healthcare and underutilization of needed benefits and services. This conflict has given rise to a greater demand by consumers and providers for managed care to demonstrate quality of care, patient satisfaction, and cost-effectiveness of selected services.

The Language of Managed Care

To further explore the principles of managed care, an accurate knowledge of managed care terminology is essential. Since managed care is an evolving paradigm, with new systems and models emerging continually, no single, universal definition exists for many of even the most basic managed care terms. Certain elements and characteristics, however, are commonly associated with each, in spite of variations in definition and interpretation by the various market segments.

A managed care organization (MCO) is any type of system that integrates the financing and delivery of healthcare to voluntarily enrolled plan members. Common distinguishing characteristics of MCOs include:

- Arrangements with selected providers to deliver a comprehensive package of health plan benefits to enrollees.
- Clear standards for selection of healthcare providers.
- A focus on wellness, preventive care, and disease management to keep plan members healthy, and thereby reduce medical costs.
- Formal quality improvement and utilization review programs.

Based upon how these healthcare delivery and financial management strategies are designed and implemented, MCOs are classified into different types or models—health maintenance organizations, preferred provider organizations, point-of-service plans, and integrated service networks. In addition, pharmacy benefit management organizations provide specialized services to managed care.

A health maintenance organization (HMO) is a type of MCO that offers comprehensive healthcare to voluntarily enrolled members, who pre-pay a fixed amount of money in exchange for access to a clearly defined package of health plan benefits. Generally, HMOs receive a fixed fee from members, regardless of whether healthcare services are utilized or not, i.e. they are prepaid on a capitated basis. A primary distinguishing characteristic of HMOs is that, upon enrollment, members are required to select a primary care physician (PCP), who not only delivers comprehensive care, but also serves as the gatekeeper to specialty services, such as seeing a physician specialist. If a member seeks non-emergency services from an HMO provider without a referral from his/her PCP, or seeks services from a provider who is not affiliated with the HMO, then those services typically will not be covered by the health plan. With these two characteristics in common, HMOs are further characterized into basic models.

A staff model HMO owns its healthcare facilities and employs physicians and other providers to provide the healthcare services to its membership. All premiums and revenues accrue to the HMO, which compensates providers by salary and incentive programs. Alternatively, a group-model HMO contracts with a group of physicians and other providers, who are organized as a partnership or professional corporation. The health plan compensates the medical group for contracted services at a negotiated rate, and then the group is responsible for compensating its physicians and contracting with hospitals and other providers for care of their patients.

A network model HMO is a health plan that contracts with many large physician groups and community pharmacies to provide care to its members. As with group model HMOs, network HMOs do not own their own facilities and typically compensate each provider group at a negotiated, capitated rate. Finally, an individual practice association (IPA) is an HMO model that contracts with independent physicians, pharmacies, and providers in their own practice settings to provide medical services to its enrollees.

Although HMOs are the most common type of MCO, the fastest growing type of MCO is the preferred provider organization (PPO). A PPO is an organization that contracts with providers to deliver healthcare services at a negotiated discount off of their standard fees or the usual and customary rate (UCR), which is the standard for those services in that geographical region. The PPO then encourages plan members to select providers from this network of preferred providers; however, it does not limit members to this closed panel of providers. By selecting network providers, plan members pay lower co-payments and deductibles than if they were to select a non-network provider. Also, unlike HMOs, plan members are not required to select a PCP. Typically, they may seek care from any network provider without penalty.

Another type of MCO is a point-of-service (POS) plan, which is a hybrid between an HMO and PPO. Like HMOs, POS plans typically use PCPs to deliver the comprehensive set of health benefits and to serve as gatekeepers to control access or referrals to specialists. Like PPOs, POS plans also allow health plan members to use non-participating or non-network providers at a reduced level of benefits (e.g. higher co-payments, higher deductibles, etc.). POS plans have emerged in response to needs and desires in both the consumer and payer market segments. Dissatisfied with both restricted access to providers in HMOs and higher premium costs associated with PPOs, consumers have responded favorably to the emergence of POS plans that blend the flexibility of PPOs with the lower-costs of HMOs. HMOs have willingly developed such plans to gain competitive advantage over PPO plans.

A gradually increasing trend in managed care is the emergence of integrated services networks (ISNs). ISNs are large integrated organizations that incorporate facilities, providers, and payers. These organizations provide patients with an array of healthcare services through providers who are affiliated under a single payment structure.

Recent trends in managed care indicate increasing numbers of PPO, POS, and IPA plans. This movement represents a shift from the more restrictive staff and group model HMO plans to the less restrictive types of managed care plans with open-ended coverage. According to 1997 HMO statistics, IPAs have the majority of members with 55.8% of all HMO enrollees, as shown in Figure 43.1 (Hoechst Marion Roussel 1998).

According to 1997 statistics, 92% of HMOs engage a pharmaceutical benefit manager (PBM), i.e. a company to administer all or part of their pharmaceutical benefits and services (Hoechst Marion Roussel 1998). Some of the basic functions provided by PBMs include dispensing, formulary management, mail-order drug dispensing, drug utilization reviews (DURs), prescription claims processing, and academic or counter-detailing. Academic detailing supports formulary adherence through the use of educational interventions, such as telephone calls or letters, to prescribers. Among HMOs, over 90% of IPA and network models contract with PBMs, in contrast to 69.0% of staff model HMOs (Hoechst Marion Roussel 1998).

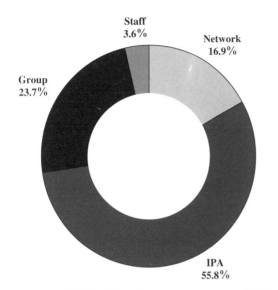

Figure 43.1 1997 Health maintenance organization (HMO) enrollment by model type. Adapted from Hoechst Marion Roussel 1998

Overall, 86.9% of all managed care plans contract with PBMs for their prescription drug benefit claims processing services (Hoechst Marion Roussel 1998).

Key Principles of Managed Care

Successful managed care systems deliver high quality healthcare to their members, while maintaining low operating costs through effective application of basic principles of managed care. Three key issues addressed by these managed care principles include provider compensation, cost containment, and quality of care.

Provider compensation includes the methods by which MCOs financially compensate or pay their providers. Provider compensation varies with the nature of the relationship between the MCO and the provider (e.g. employer–employee, contractual agreements, strategic partnerships, joint ventures, etc.). Typically, payments are negotiated and may include a variety of methods, including the following:

- *Capitation*—The MCO negotiates with the provider, who agrees to provide a clearly defined set of healthcare services to plan members for a fixed amount per member per month (PMPM), regardless of the amount of services delivered.
- *Discounted fee-for-service*—The MCO negotiates with the provider, who agrees to provide services to enrollees at a discount from their UCRs for FFS patients.
- *Per diem*—The MCO negotiates with a provider organization (e.g. accredited hospitals, ambulatory care centers, etc.), who agrees to deliver care for a fixed rate per day that an enrollee receives care.
- *Per case*—The MCO negotiates with the provider who agrees to deliver care for a fixed amount or rate of compensation per case for a specified illness or condition.
- *Risk-sharing*—The MCO negotiates with the provider, who agrees to deliver effective, efficient, and high quality care to all enrollees with some degree of financial risk.

Integral to these payment methods are their administrative methods. For example, two specialized approaches to assessing payment methods are carve-out and global costs. With carve-outs, the MCO negotiates with a specialized provider or service organization, such as a PBM, to provide a narrowly-defined set of specific services. Reimbursement for these carve-out services, however, is usually on a capitated basis. With global costs, an MCO allocates all healthcare costs under one budget. Some MCOs may even negotiate with providers and healthcare facilities, who agree to receive a global fee for all professional services and institutional expenses for a particular episode of care or diagnosis, except optional benefits, such as medications. Typically, this global fee is capitated.

While provider compensation methods are effective in controlling a significant proportion of managed care's costs, they cannot work alone, as there are other priority issues that continually challenge managed care's ability to deliver high quality services, yet control healthcare costs. Cost containment issues that influence business decisions in managed care include medical loss ratios (MLRs) and pharmacoeconomic and outcomes data.

The MLR is a cost:revenue ratio. It is calculated by dividing the total costs of delivering the health and medical care covered by plan benefits (i.e. total costs) by the total revenues received from members in the form of dues or premium payments (i.e. total revenues), and then multiplying by 100%.

$$\text{Medical loss ratio} = \frac{\text{total costs}}{\textit{total revenue}} \times 100\%$$

From a business perspective, MCOs aim for low costs and high revenues, resulting in a small MLR. Managed care executives, however, must continually balance the demands of their various constituents to achieve an acceptable MLR, e.g. members want unlimited access to providers and the very best medical treatments with zero to low annual premium increases, while shareholders and investors want operating costs (e.g. medical costs, provider compensation, etc.) held to a minimum with annual premium increases. According to industry experts, these forces can be significant, as indicated by the sizable differences in MLRs for indemnity health insurance companies vs. HMOs. For indemnity health insurance, the MLR is usually in excess of 90%. For cost-efficient HMOs, it is usually less than 80–85%.

When available, MCOs can use pharmacoeconomic and outcomes information to drive the choice for cost-efficient therapeutic alternatives. For this reason, pharmacoeconomic and outcomes data are becoming increasingly important to MCO decision-makers, including formulary decision-makers. Pharmacoeconomic and outcomes data tend to have the greatest impact on managed care decisions when the novel product or drug under consideration produces positive patient outcomes, or yields substantial cost savings within the first 6–12 months of initiation of therapy, as compared to older, less expensive therapies. If positive pharmacoeconomic or patient outcomes are not seen until 2–5 years after initiating drug therapy, then the economic information tends to have a lesser impact on the MCO's pharmaceutical benefit or drug therapy decisions.

Intrinsic to the principles of managed care is the conflict between the desire to control costs and the desire to promote quality of care. Two common measures of quality of care are health plan member satisfaction and health plan accreditation. Member satisfaction surveys assess the extent to which a managed care plan is able to satisfy the diverse needs of its members. Increasingly, member satisfaction is an important measure for MCOs because it can impact the ability of the plan to attract and retain new members, reduce turnover rates, and achieve accreditation.

Accreditation of managed care plans is a relatively new process, driven by consumer demand for improved quality of care. In recent years, several non-profit entities have developed mechanisms for evaluating and accrediting MCOs. The National Committee for Quality Assurance (NCQA) has emerged as the most recognized and respected among these. NCQA's accreditation process is designed to assess, measure, and report on the quality of care provided by managed care plans. To receive accreditation, a managed care plan must demonstrate the ability to provide consumers with protections required by the accrediting agency, and to continuously monitor and improve the quality of care for its members. Accreditation status is not an absolute guarantee of the quality of care that an individual plan member may receive, or that a network provider may deliver. As competition in the managed care market continues to stiffen, accreditation is becoming increasingly important to MCOs.

THE IMPACT OF MANAGED CARE ON THE PHARMACEUTICAL INDUSTRY

In the late 1970s, pharmaceutical companies developed and marketed new products to physicians with minimal, if any, interference from third-party insurers and payers. Even in the mid-1980s, the pharmaceutical industry paid little attention to group- and staff-model HMOs because they imposed restrictions on sales representatives and demanded price concessions (Pollard 1990). Over the last decade, however, managed care plans have experienced sustained growth and consolidation and, in the process, demonstrated their ability to impact the pharmaceutical industry. For example, managed care plans have driven pharmaceutical costs down by demanding economic proof of a product's cost-effectiveness, by measuring the impact of products on health status (e.g. patient outcomes, quality of life, etc.), and by integrating drug utilization into standard treatment protocols. Managed care plans are now the pharmaceutical industry's largest customer base, and these advancements have had a profound impact on how pharmaceutical manufacturers develop and market products to MCOs.

To more fully understand the impact of managed care on the pharmaceutical industry, a look at managed care's cost containment strategies and continued movement toward multiple payers will be presented first, followed by the influential market dynamics of increased competition and changing demographics. Concluding the section will be a discussion of how these factors have impacted the pharmaceutical industry's research and development priorities and product life cycles.

Managed Care Cost Containment Strategies

According to current managed care industry estimates, prescription medications account for up to 15% of total medical costs for some managed care plans (Meyer 1998). In addition, prescription drug costs are rising by 15–20% each year, much faster than other components of healthcare, for many managed care plans (Meyer 1998). Furthermore, as the pharmaceutical industry introduces a rush of innovative and expensive drugs, MCOs are mounting defensive strategies to control prescription costs, yet maintain quality of care for their members. Managed care plans that have implemented integrated formulary and disease management programs, outcomes assessment, and risk-sharing contracts have been more successful at controlling pharmaceutical costs than plans without such strategies.

Formulary management is the most common strategy used by managed care plans for controlling increasing drug costs and access to prescription medications. A formulary is a list of drug products that have been reviewed and approved for use in a particular medical setting. Typically, normal prescribing is restricted to drugs listed in the formulary. A formulary system is a method of drug-use control that involves a systematic approach to evaluating drug products, providing guidelines for utilization, informing appropriate parties of current formulary status and policies, enforcing adherence to those policies, and implementing the system.

Responsibility for developing, maintaining, and enforcing formulary systems in managed care lies with the pharmacy and therapeutics (P&T) committee, which normally comprises health plan physicians and clinical pharmacists. Additional responsibilities of a managed care P&T committee may include development, implementation, or maintenance of drug utilization policies, drug utilization review (DUR) programs, prescribing protocols, generic drug substitution policies, and educational programs.

The formulary approval process for a new drug is a two-step process in managed care. Reimbursement status is determined in the first step; formulary inclusion in the second step. The decision for reimbursement usually occurs zero to 6 months postlaunch, and its purpose is to determine whether or not a product will be covered by the plan. Typically this decision is made before the product is evaluated for formulary acceptance. An MCO will then determine whether or not the product will be included on the formulary by routing the new product through the plan's formulary evaluation and decision process, which usually occurs 6–12 months after launch. Therefore, under a managed care plan, US Food and Drug Administration (US FDA) approval of a new product is no longer a guarantee of unrestricted access to the product, since evidence of a drug product's economic value is typically required prior to formulary acceptance.

In general, MCOs with formulary programs use a variety of methods to enforce formulary adherence. These methods vary in their restrictions, and typically include financial incentives for both prescribers and patients. Table 43.1 lists and defines typical restriction methods, such as prior authorization and treatment limitations. Table 43.2 lists commonly used enforcement strategies and financial incentives, including switch programs, differentiated/tiered co-payments, and education programs.

The pharmaceutical industry has long challenged the necessity of formularies and related enforcement policies that restrict a prescriber's choice. In response, pharmaceutical companies have engaged a number of their own strategies to counter managed care's cost-containment practices. For example, they are funding pharmacoeconomic, quality-of-life, and other outcomes studies to demonstrate the economic and societal value of a drug product, and thereby influence formulary acceptance by managed care decision makers. In general, MCOs view pharmaceutical industry-

Table 43.1 Drug utilization restrictions used by managed care organizations

Restriction	Definition
Prior authorization	A physician or patient must receive authorization by the plan before the drug will be covered
Quantity limitations	The amount of medications prescribed/dispensed is limited to a prespecified quantity (usually a monthly limit)
Specialist-only	Only specialists are allowed to prescribed medication
Treatment limitations	Treatments are limited on a per-member or per-year basis
Step protocols	Treatments are restricted to a specific step in a protocol (i.e. a second or third-line treatment in a protocol)
Patient criterion	Patient must qualify for treatment by meeting specific criteria (usually used in conjunction with a prior authorization program)

Table 43.2 Formulary enforcement policies used by managed care organizations

Enforcement Policy	Definition
Switch programs	Whereby physicians are called and asked to switch to a specific formulary products
Risk sharing	Policies whereby the physician [usually the primary care provider (PCP)] is placed at financial risk for providing services (including prescription drugs) to the patients
Financial penalties	Physicians are financially penalized for prescribing non-formulary products
Differential/tiered co-payments	Member's prescription co-payments are higher for non-formulary products
Out-of-pocket payments	Members pay for non-formulary drugs (either a fixed amount/co-payment or the fee-for-service cost of the prescription)
Education programs	Education programs for physicians (usually the PCP) to educate physicians on formulary products and selection criteria
Report cards/performance records	Monthly or quarterly reports comparing and evaluating physicians' prescribing patterns are generated and distributed to all participating physicians
Intervention programs	Telephone calls and/or letters are sent to physicians prescribing non-formulary drugs

sponsored economic evaluations as useful in comparing therapeutically similar products; however, sponsor bias and applicability of study results to a plan's population are major concerns (Luce et al 1996). Out of all the research conducted by MCOs, economic studies have the greatest potential to guide formulary decisions.

Another increasingly important strategy for the pharmaceutical industry is assessing whether a new product's therapeutic category is on the MCO's 'radar screen'. Criteria for inclusion of a product's therapeutic category on an MCO's radar screen include the following:

- The current budget and resources allocated for patients with the target disease.
- The ability of the plan to realize a significant return on investment if the disease is managed (i.e. cost–effectiveness) appropriately.

- The ability of the plan to provide staff for development and implementation of disease management programs.
- The ability of the plan to effectively measure the impact of a disease management program.

Because of increased difficulty in getting a new drug on an MCO's formulary, it is now common for pharmaceutical companies to collaborate with managed care decision-makers in 'round table' or 'advisory board' meetings. These discussions, which normally occur before product launch or as early as Phases II and III of clinical development, are helpful in determining reimbursement status and identifying potential barriers and restrictions that may be placed on the product, once approved.

Disease management programs represent another pharmaceutical industry strategy to counter managed care cost-containment efforts. Offered by pharmaceutical manufacturers to MCOs to demonstrate the clinical merit and cost–effectiveness of their drug therapy, disease management is 'a collaborative process which assesses, plans, implements, coordinates, monitors, and evaluates options and services to meet an individual's health needs through communication and available resources to promote quality cost-effective outcomes' (Care Management Society of America 1995, p. 8). MCOs are increasingly adopting disease management programs to provide comprehensive medical care and improve patient outcomes at a lower cost (Schulman et al 1996). Today, virtually all managed care plans offer a disease management program for asthma to prevent costly emergency department visits and hospitalizations.

Some MCOs have even forged partnerships with pharmaceutical manufacturers to allow the sponsoring company to track patient outcomes, to gauge a disease management program's effectiveness, and to access scientific and financial support for the program. Other disease management programs involve risk-sharing contracts between the MCO and the pharmaceutical company, through which both parties share in the financial risks and rewards of doing business. Package pricing (i.e. special discount on a product line) and rebate programs that reward an MCO for achieving a certain market share of the product are two other contracting strategies that have been adopted by the pharmaceutical industry.

In addition to integrated formulary and disease management programs, outcomes assessment, and risk sharing contracts, MCOs are implementing a variety of other services and programs to minimize costs, modify provider behavior, enhance patient outcomes, and differentiate themselves in the marketplace. The pharmaceutical industry has responded to its managed care customer base needs by offering a variety of innovative, value-added services, including medication compliance programs, patient education programs, and call center services.

Multiple Payer Influence in Managed Care

In addition to cost-containment strategies, managed care is impacting the pharmaceutical industry through a continued movement toward multiple payers of healthcare. The make-up of the payer market is changing as increasing numbers of MCOs are doing business with the government and large employers. These payer market segments are exerting a greater influence on the scope of their health plan benefits and treatment decisions.

Both the federal government and state agencies are moving increasing numbers of Medicare and Medicaid recipients, respectively, into managed care plans, to control healthcare expenditures, including drug costs. Clearly, the impetus has been the ability of managed care plans to reduce healthcare expenditures, which is accomplished by shifting the focus of healthcare away from incident-driven delivery to preventive and coordinated care. State Medicaid agencies have been actively promoting managed care plans to recipients. Medicare, in general, does not cover prescription drugs on an outpatient basis, however, many MCOs are offering prescription drug benefits as an incentive to attract Medicare members. Managed care plans, however, must monitor this benefit carefully because of high drug utilization in the elderly. Because of escalating drug costs, some Medicare managed care plans have elected to cap or eliminate drug benefits altogether (Meyer 1998).

Although the effect of employers on the pharmaceutical industry is still unknown, employers are significant purchasers of managed care health plans, and, as such, in a position to significantly impact the pharmaceutical industry. Market dynamics indicate that in the future, large employers or employer groups will work directly with buyers and providers of healthcare, thereby challenging managed care for contracts with employers. In addition, employers may require MCOs to use fewer carve-out services, like PBMs, to encourage a more global perspective in caring for their employees. Responding to the needs of both payers—employers and MCOs—the pharmaceutical industry is positioned to sponsor wellness and preventive care programs to help differentiate MCOs from their competitors and facilitate contracts with employers.

Finally, consumers, or individual health plan members, represent another payer group within managed care. Consumers pay for healthcare through health plan premiums, deductibles, and benefit-specific co-payments, including prescription drug co-payments. To address consumer needs, as well as to expand market share, many pharmaceutical companies have invested significant resources in direct-to-consumer advertising (DTCA) campaigns. Furthermore, since the FDA relaxed advertising regulations in 1997, pharmaceutical companies can now make product-specific health claims and link it to treatment of the indicated disease, as long as they disclose the major risks and side effects of the product. As a result, the pharmaceutical industry spent more than $1.2 billion on DTCA in the USA through November 1998 (IMS Health Web Site 1999).

Consumer advocate groups contend that DTCA has the potential to alert patients to potentially serious medical conditions and available drug therapies. Within the pharmaceutical industry, drug product managers see increased use of their product by better-informed consumers. MCOs have responded less enthusiastically to DTCA, due to its potential to increase drug costs through overutilization of prescription medications. In support of this position, a recent Yankelovic patient awareness survey found that 15% of consumers discussed an advertised drug with their physicians, and 8% visited a doctor specifically to discuss an advertised product (Headden and Melton 1998). Critics further contend that DTCA increases the overall costs of medical care, that therapeutic alternatives and side effects of the medication are often inadequately presented, and that information may be misleading (Gandy 1992). Despite the resistance, DTCA is a powerful tool that the pharmaceutical industry continues to use to increase product awareness and market share in a multiple-payer managed care system.

Managed Care Market Competition

A managed care market dynamic that has impacted the pharmaceutical industry is increased competition. With the managed care market becoming increasingly competitive due to market saturation, many MCOs are employing innovative strategies to recruit and retain members. One such strategy is to offer enrollees multiple products and expanded health plan benefits. In a US national survey of managed care health plans, Gold and Hurley (1997) found that MCOs are providing a selection of benefit programs in response to customer interests and to ease the transition to more traditional managed care, especially in consumer markets with low managed care penetration; 71% of the plans in

their sample offered at least two products, and a majority of plans with multiple products offered three or more options.

In highly penetrated managed care markets, health plans are strategically expanding benefits and services to foster loyalty and improve member retention, largely in response to the realization that it costs five to seven times more to recruit a new health plan member than to keep one (Edlin 1998). Health Net, based in Woodland Hills, California, and a subsidiary of Foundation Health Systems, automatically enrolls members in their WellRewards program, which offers discounts of 20–50% on quality health-related products and services, including vitamins and supplements, sports and fitness equipment, veterinary services, and pet care supplies, and medically supervised weight management (Edlin 1998). Prudential HealthCare of South Florida offers members nicotine patches at a discount through its smoking-cessation program, Committed Quitters, and bicycle helmets for $10 through its bike helmet program for members and non-members (Edlin 1998).

This expansion of health plan benefits and availability of multiple product offerings has created new opportunities for the pharmaceutical industry, e.g. pharmaceutical manufacturers with drug products in therapeutic areas not traditionally covered by managed care, such as smoking cessation, weight loss, and infertility, are now targeting plans with expanded benefits in those areas to promote their products. Another strategy employed by the pharmaceutical industry is to offer a portfolio of value-added services associated with a product, rather than promoting the therapeutic benefits of an individual drug, to help managed health plans achieve market differentiation and a competitive advantage.

Within the managed care industry, increased market competition has led to the emergence of the sales and marketing director and the benefits director as key decision makers, with increasing influence on medical decisions, including pharmacy benefits and formulary coverage. To effectively communicate with and sell to these stakeholders, the pharmaceutical industry has developed specialized sales teams, and expanded the responsibility of the managed care sales force to identify and target these directors for selected sales promotions.

Industry-wide consolidations, acquisitions, and mergers are also affecting managed care market competition. Since the early-1990s, mergers and acquisitions among MCOs and insurers have occurred at a record pace. In late 1998, Aetna US Healthcare, formed by an $8.9 billion acquisition of US Healthcare by Aetna in 1996, announced plans to acquire Prudential Healthcare for $1 billion, making the combined entity the largest managed care company in the USA with 18.4 million members (Aetna US Healthcare Web Site 1998). One evident outcome of consolidation among MCOs and insurers is that the pharmaceutical industry is now dealing with fewer, larger customers, who are gatekeepers for member services. As managed care market consolidation continues, it will become increasingly important for the pharmaceutical industry to identify and understand the role of the gatekeeper in formulary decisions, monitor product utilization through provider pharmacies and health systems, and develop strategies to link inpatient and outpatient drug use to coordinate pharmaceutical care.

In response to consolidations throughout the entire healthcare industry, as well as to increasing drug development costs, the pharmaceutical industry has also experienced a series of mergers and acquisitions in the last decade. Since the late 1990's, horizontal integration in the pharmaceutical industry has produced drug conglomerations, such as Astrazeneca, Aventis, and GlaxoSmithkline. These transactions enable economies of scale in research and marketing to better compete with rival firms. In addition, merging companies claim they will benefit from enhanced research and development capacity and better access to global markets (Bond and Weissman 1997).

Another aspect of market competition that is of even greater concern to managed care and payers than pharmaceutical manufacturer consolidations is the pharmaceutical industry's trend toward vertical integration through the acquisition of PBMs. Because they manage drug benefits for approximately half of the US population, PBMs have significant buying power, and therefore represent a real threat to a pharmaceutical company's market share and profits (Bond and Weissman 1997). In 1993, Merck & Co. paid a record $6.6 billion to purchase Medco, and less than 1 year later, SmithKline Beecham acquired Diversified

Pharmaceutical Services (DPS) and Eli Lilly bought PCS Health Systems. Despite allegations from consumer advocate groups that the transactions were made to preserve each acquirer's market share and profits from brand name products, the pharmaceutical companies contend that vertical integration of a PBM has enabled each to deliver integrated pharmaceutical care and compete more effectively in the managed care arena. While the Merck–Medco alignment has generated robust sales for Merck products that might otherwise have been spent on competitors' products, Lilly has struggled to increase its market share of brand name products on the PCS formulary. Since the acquisitions, federal regulators now pay attention to the PBM practice of switching patients to the parent company's drug. In the fall of 1998, Lilly announced that it was leaving the PBM business and selling PCS to Rite Aid, one of the nation's largest pharmacy chains, who wants to market its drug benefit package and pharmaceutical care services directly to MCOs and payers.

Finally, with increased consolidation in the managed care and pharmaceutical industries, as well as throughout the healthcare industry, comprehensive, integrated data management systems will be needed to enable industry partners to collect, manage, analyze, and disseminate medical and utilization information in a comprehensive and standardized manner. Integrated data management systems are critical for healthcare consumers, payers, and providers, because they enable each group to evaluate treatment selections or use decisions, identify substandard utilization patterns, provide comprehensive and accessible medical records for plan providers, and identify risk factors for chronic and expensive urgent-driven healthcare needs. A complete, integrated management system allows pharmaceutical companies to demonstrate how prescription medications may decrease costs and optimize the quality of care provided to an MCO's members.

Population and Managed Care Market Demographics

The US population and managed care market demographics are changing significantly, largely due to increased life expectancies and an aging 'baby boom' generation (i.e. individuals born 1946–1964). As this generation reaches retirement age, there will be a larger geriatric market than ever before, as an estimated 10 065 Americans turn 50 years old each day, according to US census data.

> Over the next 30 years, the proportion of the population of the United States that is over the age of 65 will grow from 12 percent to 18 percent; fastest growing of all will be the population over the age of 85. Today over one-third of spending for healthcare in the United States is done by and for the elderly, and that proportion will increase (Health Insurance Association of America 1996, pp 98–99).

While Medicare beneficiaries have not enrolled in managed care plans at rates seen in the employer market, Medicare is exploring innovative approaches to encourage managed care enrollment to achieve the cost savings potential of managed care. Cost savings will become increasingly important in this expanding senior market, due to the increasing incidence of chronic diseases, including Alzheimer's disease, arthritis, and osteoporosis. Brumback and Leech (1994) estimate that the number of persons with Alzheimer's disease will double, from 4.5 million currently to 9 million, by the year 2030. Both this growing geriatric population and managed care plans with significant numbers of Medicare enrollees will drive the demand for better treatment options.

The pharmaceutical industry is responding to the increasing geriatric market with increased research and development for products for the treatment of chronic diseases. Some pharmaceutical firms have even established geriatric-focused research departments to identify and address the special needs of the elderly.

Pharmaceutical Research and Development

In addition to the influence of a growing geriatric market segment on pharmaceutical industry research and development, each of the other managed care and market influences—cost containment strategies, multiple payers, and market competition—have collectively impacted pharmaceutical research and development. The pharmaceutical industry is highly competitive and heavily invested in

research and development. For example, recent consolidations among pharmaceutical companies are due, in part, to the enormous risk and expense in bringing a new drug to market and the desire to spread development costs over a larger revenue base (Pollard 1990). Increased global competition has also influenced pharmaceutical industry research and development. Finally, MCOs and PBMs, focused on cost-containment strategies, are resisting expensive drugs that lack explicit advantages over older, less expensive therapies. They are forcing the pharmaceutical industry to focus on drug candidates with the largest potential for financial return, a move that has raised concerns about which drugs get developed. Therefore, there is increasing concern that clinical research in the USA is being threatened by the proliferation of managed care.

One indication of this concern over pharmaceutical research and development, is that pharmaceutical manufacturers are shifting clinical investigations from costly academic medical centers (AMCs) to less-expensive private study centers and third-party contract research organizations (CROs), to reduce both drug development time and costs. Some MCOs are reluctant to refer members to AMC-conducted trials, even if the research is pharmaceutical industry-sponsored, due to concerns of higher patient care costs and litigation over unexpected adverse events. Critics contend that the managed care practice of restricting patient access to AMCs for specialized care has accelerated declining physician revenues, which directly affects the ability of an AMC to engage in clinical research (Burnett 1996). Furthermore, declining AMC patient care revenues and the pharmaceutical industry's cost-saving strategy of shifting studies to CROs are contributing to a lack of funding for training future research investigators.

Despite MCO concerns over patient costs and liability issues, the number of research studies is steadily increasing in the managed care setting. Many investigators believe that the managed care setting is ideal for conducting clinical research, because care is standardized and easier to control, potential study patients can be easily identified through centralized databases, and the population is representative of the real world, especially for postmarketing and safety surveillance studies. In fact, most MCOs are more interested in establishing the effectiveness of a product, i.e. how well the drug performs under real-world conditions, than in determining a product's efficacy through rigorously controlled clinical trials. Although rare, some firms will halt development of a compound as early as Phase II trials if there appears to be no perceived economic value. Conversely, pharmaceutical companies with favorable outcomes and pharmacoeconomic (i.e. cost-effectiveness) data at the launch of a new product have assisted MCOs in their formulary decision processes and have had successful launch campaigns. Indeed, prelaunch research participation may help an MCO gain a competitive edge, by integrating experimental care into clinical practice and offering new treatment options to their members.

Pharmaceutical Product Life Cycles

In addition to its influence on pharmaceutical industry research and development, managed care has significantly impacted product life cycles. Drugs identified as preferred products by managed care health plans have a steeper, or faster, uptake and initial growth period, as shown in Figure 43.2, than products that are covered, non-formulary. MCO-preferred products reach their sales peak earlier and experience a longer, sustained maturation phase. Covered, non-formulary products never reach as high a maturation peak as preferred products. However, once a preferred product's patent expires, there is a rapid decline in sales, since most health plans routinely switch the formu-

lary choice to a generic equivalent. In addition to identifying preferred products for reimbursement, MCOs are implementing disease management programs to foster increased utilization of the preferred product over similar, but competitive, products.

Pharmaceutical companies are adopting a number of strategies to maximize market share of a new product in a managed care environment. Achieving formulary acceptance by MCOs is the first step for ensuring a successful life cycle for a prescription product, as shown in Figure 43.3. To positively influence formulary decisions and gain preferred product status, pharmaceutical companies are generating pharmacoeconomic and outcomes data. Once accepted by the managed care health plan's P&T Committee, pharmaceutical companies may invest in pull-through programs to increase market share and appropriate utilization of the product. Pull-through programs may involve special contracting agreements or comprehensive disease management initiatives to highlight the clinical and economic value of a specific product. In addition to pull-through programs and value-added services, such as patient education materials, pharmaceutical companies are discounting targeted prescription drug products or entire product lines where competition is fierce.

Finally, to maintain a healthy product life cycle until patent expiration, pharmaceutical companies are engaging business strategies, including risk-sharing contracts, DTCA, and co-marketing partnerships. Pharmaceutical companies are developing co-marketing partnerships in record numbers to achieve maximum global market penetration, by

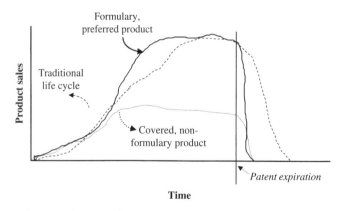

Figure 43.2 Impact of managed care on pharmaceutical product life cycle

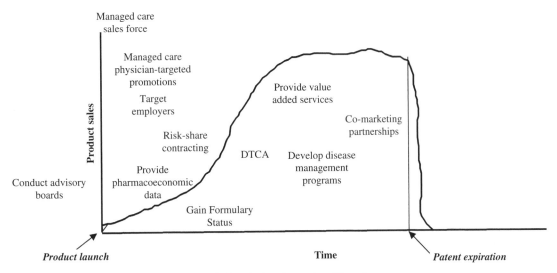

Figure 43.3 Pharmaceutical industry strategic initiatives during the product life cycle

leveraging research and marketing strengths in key therapeutic areas. Co-marketing partnerships are being formed through joint ventures, licensing agreements, strategic alliances, traditional mergers, and acquisitions (Kaniecki and Goldberg-Arnold 1993).

EMERGING TRENDS IN MANAGED CARE AND THEIR IMPACT ON THE PHARMACEUTICAL INDUSTRY

Diverse factors will continue to influence managed care in the future, and subsequently impact the pharmaceutical industry. Managed care consumers, payers, and providers will continue to be the key facilitators of change. Key areas in which these distinct, but interconnected market segments will drive change include the continued integration of information technology into disease management programs, an increased need for pharmacoeconomic and outcomes research, and the repositioning of PBMs.

Integration of Information Technology

Innovations in information technology and its application to disease management will be vital to the future of managed care. Disease management aims to optimize consumer healthcare outcomes, while reducing financial costs, by prolonging the time interval between episodes of acute care and minimizing the severity of these events. At the center of disease management is a specially-trained nurse care manager who functions 'much like an information manager in a patient-centered healthcare environment—receiving, relaying, and imparting information to members, providers, health plan officials, quality assessors, and regulators' (Finch 1998, p. 102). In this capacity, the disease state manager needs a variety of tools (e.g. health risk assessments, clinical guidelines, and preventive care recommendations), which are or can be made available online and are having a profound effect on managed care. Further innovations in information technology will continue to revolutionize disease management (Goldstein 1998; Navarro 1998).

For example, a patient infected with the human immunodeficiency virus who fails to refill his anti-retroviral medication at the expected interval of time can be contacted immediately to determine the level of adherence, perhaps intervening before the emergence of viral resistance.

Case managers can also use push technology to send E-mail reminders or educational information to E-mail addresses of patients with conditions requiring care management...(Finch 1998, p. 102).

The continued integration of information technology into disease management will impact the way the pharmaceutical industry targets its customer segments and their needs, e.g. pharmaceutical companies are beginning to leverage the power of information technology to provide patient access to disease management applications, and treatment information to improve outcomes and compliance. The ability to coordinate pharmaceutical care by linking patients, physicians, pharmacists, and healthcare payers will be critical to deliver cost-effective healthcare.

Increased Need for Pharmacoeconomic and Outcomes Research

To plan and implement successful launch campaigns, the pharmaceutical industry will increasingly need to meet managed care's need for practical pharmacoeconomic and outcomes data to assist in formulary decision-making processes. Therefore, in the future, the pharmaceutical industry may conduct pre-launch clinical trials in MCOs to address the economic and outcomes issues associated with new products in real-world settings. This will provide the added advantage of introducing the product to managed care physicians and providers prior to launch. In the future, the pharmaceutical industry will need to develop MCOs into research-ready sites for gathering and analyzing outcomes data, to address specific managed care clinical and economic issues.

Repositioning of PBMs

As managed care moves toward globalization of all medical care expenditures, including pharmaceutical products, PBMs will be at-risk, since they are typically viewed as a carve-out expenditure. To remain viable and to protect themselves from integration and competition, PBMs will have to reposition themselves in the marketplace. They will need to offer more than pharmacy management services. In response to this emerging trend, a few PBMs are offering additional services, such as managed care-based contract research, to expand their client base to include the pharmaceutical industry and CROs. Other needed services that PBMs may offer include call center-based services, patient compliance programs, and disease management programs.

The repositioning of PBMs in the managed care market could have a tremendous impact on the pharmaceutical industry. Pharmaceutical companies should continue to outsource a larger proportion of their research studies to CROs, due to both corporate downsizing and the lack of specialized expertise. Coupled with the increased demand for managed care-based outcomes research, PBMs could become an important vendor to pharmaceutical companies, especially for tracking long-term outcomes and the costs of disease. A PBM that offers CRO services could be a cost-effective solution to the information gap between what MCOs need and what the pharmaceutical industry can fulfill. To facilitate this process, the pharmaceutical industry will need to establish an information system through which they can enhance their understanding of new PBM services, and develop methods of marketing to this newly positioned customer.

SUMMARY

Managed care has surpassed traditional indemnity or fee-for-service health insurance to become the predominant form of coverage for health and medical care in the USA. Concern over rapidly rising healthcare costs has been the driving force behind the rapid growth of managed care in recent decades. Through effective application of key managed care principles of restricted access to healthcare providers, defined health plan benefits and services, and capitated reimbursement, MCOs have demonstrated their ability to control healthcare costs. In the process, managed care has affected every aspect of the healthcare industry, including the pharmaceutical industry.

With medications accounting for an increasing proportion of total medical costs, MCOs have been forced to implement cost-containment strategies to managed pharmacy benefits, including integrated formulary and disease management programs, pharmacoeconomic and outcomes research, and risk-sharing contracts. In addition, MCOs have become a major customer base to the pharmaceutical industry, with increasing leveraging and purchasing power. Therefore, managed care has had a significant impact on the way the pharmaceutical industry develops, markets, distributes, and generates revenue. Two aspects of the pharmaceutical industry that have been impacted the greatest are pharmaceutical research and development and product life cycles.

Finally, diverse factors will continue to influence managed care into the future, and subsequently, the pharmaceutical industry. Emerging trends include the continued integration of information technology into disease management, increasing need for pharmacoeconomic and outcomes research, and the repositioning of PBMs. Therefore, the pharmaceutical industry must be positioned to maximize sales of targeted products and services and return on investment (ROI) in an increasingly managed healthcare system.

REFERENCES

Aetna US Healthcare Web Site (1998) Aetna to acquire Prudential Healthcare for $1 billion. Available at http://www.aetnaushc.com/about/press/dec10_98.html. Accessed December 10.

Bond P, Weissman R (1997) The cost of mergers and acquisitions in the US healthcare sector. *Int J Health Serv* 27(1): 77–87.

Brumback RA, Leech RW (1994) Alzheimer's disease: pathophysiology and the hope for therapy, *J Okla State Med Assoc* 87: 103–11.

Burnett DA (1996) Evolving market will change clinical research. *Health Affairs* 15(3): 90–92.

Care Management Society of America (1995) *Standards of Practice for Case Management*. Care Management Society of America: Little Rock, AR.

Edlin M (1998) Fostering member loyalty. *Healthplan* 39(5): 73–8.

Finch M (1998) Information technology, best practices, and care management. Part II. *Managed Care Interface* 11(12): 101–3.

Gandy W (1992) Advertising badly to the public. *N Engl J Med* 326:350.

Gold M, Hurley R (1997) The role of managed care 'products' in managed care plans. *Inquiry* 34: 29–37.

Goldstein D (1998) Web-based applications to reduce costs and improve patient care. *Managed Care Interface* 11(10): 60–63.

Headden S, Melton M (1998) Madison Ave. loves drug ads: cures for ulcers, toe fungus, even fleas. *US News World Report* July 20: 56–7.

Health Insurance Association of America (1996) *Managed Care: Integrating the Delivery and Financing of Health Care*, 2nd edn. Health Insurance Association of America: Washington, DC.

Hoechst Marion Roussel (1998) *Managed Care Digest Series*. Hoechst Marion Roussel: Kansas City, MO.

IMS Health Web Site (1999) Prescription drug ad spending in US exceeds $1.2 billion through November 1998. Available at http://www.IMSHealth.com/html/news_arc/02_09_1999_145.htm. Accessed February 9.

Kaniecki DJ, Goldberg-Arnold RJ (1993) Integrating worldwide marketing needs and clinical research. *J Clin Pharmacol* 33(10): 989–92.

Luce BR, Lyles CA, Rentz AM (1996) The view from managed care pharmacy. *Health Affairs* 15(4): 168–76.

MacLeod GK (1993) An overview of managed healthcare. In *The Managed Health Care Handbook* 2nd edn. Aspen: Gaithersburg, MD.

Meyer H (1998) The pills that ate your profits. *Hospitals and Health Networks* 2: 19–22.

Navarro RP (1998) Managing pharmacy benefits through the internet. *Managed Care Interface* 11(2): 65–7.

Pollard MR (1990) Managed care and a changing pharmaceutical industry. *Health Affairs* 9(3): 55–65.

Schulman KA, Rubenstein LE, Abernethy DR et al (1996) The effect of pharmaceutical benefit managers: is it being evaluated? *Ann Intern Med* 124(10): 906–13.

Appendix—Useful Internet Links

While this book has been in preparation, the worldwide web has grown enormously, making a wealth of information available within seconds. While websites change constantly and while the choices are enormous, the following collection is offered as those the editors have found valuable substitute editorial. Note that many of these links offer links to still more sites. While great care has been taken, please accept our apologies for choices with which you disagree and for any outdated links.

REGULATORY LINKS

Australia—Therapeutic Goods Administration:
http://www.health.gov.au/tga/

Canada—Health Protection Branch (HPB):
http://www.hc-sc.gc.ca/hpb/

European Confederation of Medical Devices Associations:
http://www.eucomed.be/

International Conference on Harmonization of Technical Requirements for Registration of Pharmaceuticals for Human Use (ICH):
http://www.ifpma.org/ich1.html

Japan—Ministry of Health and Welfare (Koseisho):
http://www.mhw.go.jp/english/index.html

Pharmaceutical Research and Manufacturers of America (PhRMA) Regulatory Affairs Website:
http://209.52.56.34/index.html

RAPS (Regulatory Affairs Professional Society)
Website: http://www.raps.org/

Regulatory Affairs Website:
http://www.medmarket.com/tenants/rainfo/rainfo.htm

The European Agency for the Evaluation of Medicinal Products (EMEA)
http://www.eudra.org/emea.html

United States —FDA—CBER: http://www.gov.CDPR

WHO—World Health Organization:
http://www.who.ch

PHARMACEUTICAL-RELATED SOCIETIES

American Academy of Pharmaceutical Physicians:
http://www.aapp.org/

Drug Information Association (DIA):
http://www.diahome.org/

Faculty of Pharmaceutical Medicine of the Royal Colleges of Physicians of the United Kingdom:
www.fpm.org.uk

International Federation of Pharmaceutical Manufacturers Associations (IFPMA):
http://www.ifpma.org/

Pharmaceutical Research and Manufacturers of America (PhRMA):
http://www.phrma.org/

The International Federation of Associations of Pharmaceutical Physicians (IFAPP):
www.IFAPP.org

OTHER MEDICAL SOCIETIES

American Medical Association (AMA):
http://www.ama-assn.org/

Association of American Medical Colleges (AAMC):
http://www.aamc.org/

Centers for Disease Control and Prevention (CDC):
http://www.cdc.gov/

National Institutes of Health (NIH):
http://www.nih.gov/

SELECTED PHARMACEUTICAL COMPANIES

Listing of pharmaceutical companies in the UK:
http://www.bbi.co.uk/pharm/alphalist/index.html

Principles and Practice of Pharmaceutical Medicine. Edited by A. J. Fletcher, Lionel D. Edwards, Anthony W. Fox and Peter Stonier © 2002 John Wiley & Sons Ltd.

Pharmaceutical Companies, Worldwide:
http://www.pharma-lexicon.com/zpharmaceutical_companies.htm

SELECTED CONTRACT RESEARCH ORGANIZATIONS

Listing of CROs:
http://www.dataedge.com/cro_info.htm

MISCELLANEOUS

A Dictionary of Pharmaceutical Medicine (and much more):
http://www.pharma-lexicon.com/

PERI Pharmaceutical Medicine Certificate Program:
http://www.peri.org/shtml/pharm/pharm.htm

Postgraduate Programme in Pharmacology and Pharmaceutical Medicine:
http://medinfo.ulb.ac.be/pharmed/index.html

Pharmacy Information on the Internet:
http://www.pharmweb.net/

The Cochrane Collaboration: www.cochrane.org

ETHICS IN CLINICAL RESEARCH

Bioethics information (from the University of Pennsylvania Center for Bioethics):
http://www.bioethics.net/

Federal Policies and Guidelines (numerous links):
http://www.uthscsa.edu/irb/fedlinks.html

Guidelines for the Conduct of Research Involving Human Subjects at the National Institutes of Health (revised 3/2/95):
http://ohsr.od.nih.gov/guidelines.php3

ICH Guideline for Good Clinical Practice:
http://www.ifpma.org/pdfifpma/e6.pdf

Nuremberg Code:
http://helix.nih.gov:8001/ohsr/nuremburg.php3

Office of Human Subjects Research:
http://ohsr.od.nih.gov/

The World Medical Association Declaration of Helsinki (2000 Update):
http://www.wma.net/e/approvedhelsinki.html

US Code of Federal Regulations:
http://www4.law.cornell.edu/cfr/index.htm

US Code of Federal Regulations, Title 21: Food And Drugs:
http://www4.law.cornell.edu/cfr/21cfr.htm#start